AF515477

Textbook of

Lasers in Dermatology

Textbook of
Lasers in Dermatology

Editors

Koushik Lahiri MBBS DVD(CAL) FIAD FFAADV MRCPS(Glasgow) FRCP(Edin)
Senior Consultant Dermatologist
Apollo Gleneagles Hospitals and WIZDERM
Editor, Indian Journal of Dermatology
Director, International Society of Dermatology
Immediate Past President, Association of Cutaneous Surgeons (I)
Kolkata, West Bengal, India

Abhishek De MD FAGE
Associate Professor
Calcutta National Medical College
Deputy Editor, Indian Journal of Dermatology
Convenor of ACADEMY, Association of Cutaneous Surgeons (I)
Member, SIG Lasers and Aesthetics, IADVL
Kolkata, West Bengal, India

Aarti Sarda MD FAGE
Senior Resident
Department of Dermatology
KPC Medical College
Kolkata, West Bengal, India

Forewords

Thomas Ruzicka

Jorge Ocampo-Candiani

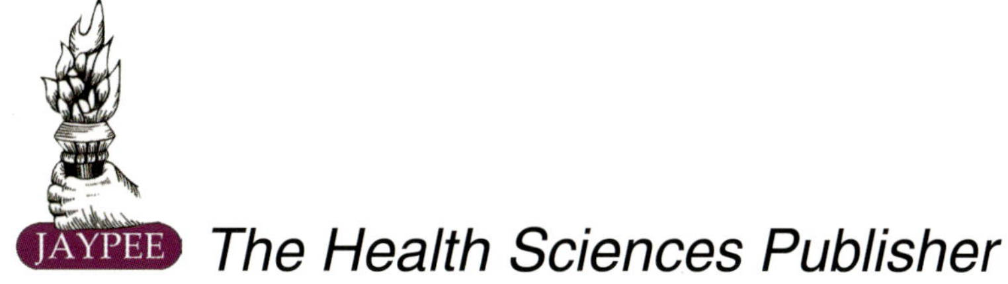

New Delhi | London | Philadelphia | Panama

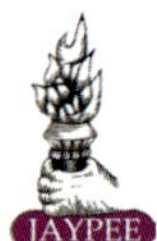

Jaypee Brothers Medical Publishers (P) Ltd

Headquarters
Jaypee Brothers Medical Publishers (P) Ltd
4838/24, Ansari Road, Daryaganj
New Delhi 110 002, India
Phone: +91-11-43574357
Fax: +91-11-43574314
Email: jaypee@jaypeebrothers.com

Overseas Offices

J.P. Medical Ltd
83 Victoria Street, London
SW1H 0HW (UK)
Phone: +44-2031708910
Fax: +02-03-0086180
Email: info@jpmedpub.com

Jaypee-Highlights Medical Publishers Inc
City of Knowledge, Bld. 235, 2nd Floor, Clayton
Panama City, Panama
Phone: +1 507-301-0496
Fax: +1 507-301-0499
Email: cservice@jphmedical.com

Jaypee Medical Inc
325 Chestnut Street
Suite 412, Philadelphia, PA 19106, USA
Phone: +1 267-519-9789
Email: support@jpmedus.com

Jaypee Brothers Medical Publishers (P) Ltd
17/1-B Babar Road, Block-B, Shaymali
Mohammadpur, Dhaka-1207
Bangladesh
Mobile: +08801912003485
Email: jaypeedhaka@gmail.com

Jaypee Brothers Medical Publishers (P) Ltd
Bhotahity, Kathmandu
Nepal
Phone: +977-9741283608
Email: kathmandu@jaypeebrothers.com

Website: www.jaypeebrothers.com
Website: www.jaypeedigital.com

Inquiries for bulk sales may be solicited at: jaypee@jaypeebrothers.com

Textbook of Lasers in Dermatology

First Edition: **2016**

ISBN: 978-93-85999-62-8

Printed at Replika Press Pvt. Ltd.

Dedicated to

My parents, partner, progenies, and patients

Koushik Lahiri

My parents and my wife

Abhishek De

My parents and my husband

Aarti Sarda

Contributors

EDITORS

Koushik Lahiri MBBS DVD(CAL) FIAD FFAADV MRCPS(Glasgow) FRCP(Edin)
Senior Consultant Dermatologist
Apollo Gleneagles Hospitals and WIZDERM
Editor, Indian Journal of Dermatology
Director, International Society of Dermatology
Immediate Past President, Association of Cutaneous Surgeons (I)
Kolkata, West Bengal, India

Abhishek De MD FAGE
Associate Professor
Calcutta National Medical College
Deputy Editor, Indian Journal of Dermatology
Convenor of ACADEMY, Association of Cutaneous Surgeons (I)
Member, SIG Lasers and Aesthetics, IADVL
Kolkata, West Bengal, India

Aarti Sarda MD FAGE
Senior Resident
Department of Dermatology
KPC Medical College
Kolkata, West Bengal, India

CONTRIBUTING AUTHORS

Madhuri H Agarwal MD
Consultant Dermatologist
Department of Dermatology
Yavana Aesthetics Clinic
Mumbai, Maharashtra, India

Ishad Aggarwal MBBS MD
Senior Resident
Department of Dermatology
Institute of Post-Graduate Medical
Education and Research
Kolkata, West Bengal, India

Emily M Altman MD
Fellow
Department of Dermatology
Summit Medical Group
Berkeley Heights, New Jersey, USA

Asad Ansari MBBS DDVL
Senior Resident
Department of Dermatology
Calcutta National Medical College
Kolkata, West Bengal, India

Shehnaz Z Arsiwala MD DDV
Honorary Dermatologist
Department of Dermatology
Prince Aly Khan Hospital,
Saifee Hospital, Renewderm Skin Hair
Laser and Aesthetics Centre
Mumbai, Maharashtra, India

Sanjeev J Aurangabadkar MBBS MD
Consultant Dermatologist
Skin and Laser Clinic
Hyderabad, Telangana, India

Projna Biswas MBBS MD
RMO
Department of Dermatology
Calcutta National Medical College and Hospital
Kolkata, West Bengal, India

Gillian R Britto MBBS MD
Consultant Dermatologist
Department of Dermatology and Aesthetic Medicine
MS Skin Center
Bengaluru, Karnataka, India

Chandrashekar BS MD DNB
Medical Director
Department of Dermatology
Cutis Academy of Cutaneous Sciences
Bengaluru, Karnataka, India

Manas Chatterjee MD DNB
Senior Adviser, Professor and Head
Department of Dermatology
INHS Asvini Hospital
Mumbai, Maharashtra, India

Banani Choudhury MD DNB
Consultant Dermatologist
Skin Secrets
Mumbai, Maharashtra, India

Rajetha Damisetty MD
Consultant dermatologist
Department of Dermatology
Mohana Skin and Hair Clinic
Hyderabad, Telangana, India

Anupam Das MD
Senior Resident
Department of Dermatology
KPC Medical College and Hospital
Kolkata, West Bengal, India

Nilay K Das MD
Associate Professor
Department of Dermatology
Medical College
Kolkata, West Bengal, India

Samujjala Deb MBBS MD
Fellow
Department of Dermatology
St. John's Medical College and Hospital
Bengaluru, Karnataka, India

Krupa Shankar DS MBBS DVD MD FRCP
Senior Consultant
Department of Dermatology
Mallige Medical Centre
Bengaluru, Karnataka, India

Abdullah Al Eisa MD
Consultant Dermatologist
National Center for Vitiligo and Psoriasis
Riyadh, Saudi Arabia

Anil Ganjoo MBBS MD
Senior Consultant
Department of Dermatology
Skinnovation Clinics
New Delhi, India

Deepti Ghia MD DNB FCPS DDV
Consultant Dermatologist
Mulekar Vitiligo Clinic
Mumbai, Maharashtra, India

Aparajita Ghosh MD
Assistant Professor
Department of Dermatology
KPC Medical College and Hospital
Kolkata, West Bengal, India

Chee-Leok Goh MBBS MRCP MMed FRCPE Hon FACD
Sr Consultant Dermatologist and Clinical Professor
Department of Dermatology
National Skin Centre
Singapore

Sunaina Hameed MD
Medical Director and Consultant Dermatologist
Skin Health Advanced Dermatology Center
Bengaluru, Karnataka, India

Stephanie G Ho BSc MBChB MRCP FAMS
Consultant Dermatologist
Stephanie Ho Dermatology
Singapore

Manmit K Hora MBBS
Junior Resident
Department of Dermatology
Institute of Post-Graduate Medical Education and Research and Seth Sukhlal Karnani Memorial Hospital
Kolkata, West Bengal, India

Ahmed Al Issa MD
Consultant Dermatologist
National Center for Vitiligo and Psoriasis
Riyadh, Saudi Arabia

Malavika Kohli MD
Medical Director
Department of Dermatology
Skin Secrets
Mumbai, Maharashtra, India

Muthuvel Kumaresan MD
Professor, Department of Dermatology
PSG Institute of Medical Sciences and Research
Coimbatore, Tamil Nadu, India

Imran Majid MBBS MD
Associate Professor
Department of Dermatology and STD
Government Medical College
Srinagar, Jammu and Kashmir, India

Vandana Mehta MD DNB
Consultant Dermatologist
Dr Hassan Al Abdulla Medical Centre
Doha, Qatar

Samipa S Mukherjee MBBS DDV DDVL FRGUHS
Pediatric Dermatologist and Dermatotrichologist
Department of Dermatology
Cutis Academy of Cutaneous Sciences
Bengaluru, Karnataka, India

Sanjeev V Mulekar MD
Consultant Dermatologist
National Center for Vitiligo and Psoriasis
Riyadh, Saudi Arabia

Venkataram Mysore MD DNB Dip RCPath FRCP FISHRS
President, IADVL
Director, Venkat Charmalaya -Centre for Advanced Dermatology
Bengaluru, Karnataka, India

Sudhir Nayak UK MD DDVL
Assistant Professor
Department of Dermatology
Venereology and Leprosy
Kasturba Medical College
Manipal, Karnataka, India

Shekhar Neema MD
Graded Specialist
Department of Dermatology
Command Hospital
Kolkata, West Bengal, India

Sathish B Pai MD DVD
Professor and Head
Department of Dermatology, Venereology and Leprosy
Kasturba Medical College
Manipal, Karnataka, India

Saumya Panda MD
Professor, Department of Dermatology
KPC Medical College and Hospital
Kolkata, West Bengal, India

Marisa Pongprutthipan MD
Clinical Instructor
Department of Medicine
Division of Dermatology
Chulalongkorn University
King Chulalongkorn Memorial Hospital
Bangkok, Thailand

Tolongkhomba Potsangbam MBBS MD
Consultant Dermatologist
Department of Dermatology
Shija Hospitals and Research Institute
Imphal, Manipur, India

Chakravarthi M Ravindran MD DVL
Consultant Dermatologist and Managing Director
Department of Dermatology
Mayil Skin Clinic
Mayil Laser Skin Clinic
Mayil Unit of Hair Restoration
Mayil Laser Dental Clinic
Erode, Tamil Nadu, India

Mukta Sachdev MBBS MD
Senior Consultant Dermatologist
Department of Dermatology and Aesthetic Medicine
MS Skin Center
Bengaluru, Karnataka, India

Amal H Al Salmi MD
Senior Specialist
Department of Dermatology
Al Buraimi Hospital
Al Buraimi, Oman

Archana Samynathan MBBS MD FRGUHS
Associate Consultant
Department of Dermatology
MS Skin Clinic
Bengaluru, Karnataka, India

Rashmi Sarkar MD MNAMS
Professor
Department of Dermatology
Maulana Azad Medical College
New Delhi, India

Warren B Seiler III MD Dip ABLS
Medical Director
Seiler Skin Cosmetic Laser and Aesthetics Center
Birmingham, Alabama, USA

Nidhi Sharma MBBS MD
Junior Resident
Department of Dermatology
Institute of Post-Graduate Medical Education and Research
Kolkata, West Bengal, India

Amrita Sil MD
Assistant Professor
Department of Pharmacology
Institute of Post-Graduate Medical Education and Research
Kolkata, West Bengal, India

Sirisha Singh MBBS MD
Consultant
Department of Dermatology
The Skin Centre
New Delhi, India

Chakravarthi R Srinivas MD
Professor and Head
Department of Dermatology
PSG Institute of Medical Sciences and Research
Coimbatore, Tamil Nadu, India

Ankur Talwar MD
Assistant professor
Department of Dermatology
Hind Institute of Medical Sciences
Safedabad, Lucknow, India

Kshama Talwar MD
Senior Resident
Department of Dermatology
Hind Institute of Medical Sciences
Safedabad, Lucknow, India

Atul Taneja MD
Senior Consultant Dermatologist
Department of Dermatology
Apollo Gleneagles Hospitals
Kolkata, West Bengal, India

Anurag Tiwari DVD DNB MNAMS
Consultant
Centre for Skin Diseases and Laser Treatment
Bhopal, Madhya Pradesh, India

Biju Vasudevan MD FRGUHS
Associate Professor
Department of Dermatology
INHS Asvini
Mumbai, Maharashtra, India

Aniketh Venkataram MS (MCh)
Department of Plastic Surgery
St Johns Medical College
Bengaluru, Karnataka, India

Jayashree Venkataram FRCOG
Surgeon and Director
Venkat Charmalaya -Centre for Advanced Dermatology
Bengaluru, Karnataka, India

Dhepe Niteen Vishwanath MD FAAD ASDS ASLMS EADV ISHRS IADVL ACSI
Medical Director
Department of Dermatology
Skin City PG Institute of Dermatology
Pune, Maharashtra, India

Bhawna Wadhwa MD
Junior Specialist, Department of Dermatology, Lok Nayak Hospital
New Delhi, India

Yousuf M Al Washahi MD
Senior Specialist
Department of Dermatology
Shinas Polyclinic
Shinas, Oman

Vijay P Zawar MD DNB DVD FAAD
Consultant Dermatologist
Department of Dermatology
Skin Diseases Center
Nashik, Maharashtra, India

Foreword

There have been significant advances in the development and use of lasers in dermatology in the past two decades. Medical science continues to progress at breakneck speed. Many entities which were not amenable to treatment a few decades back, can now be treated by lasers.

The advent and advances of lasers in dermatology has truly ushered in a sea change in our thought process as regards to the management of several entities is concerned.

There are various manuals of lasers, but true comprehensive textbooks on this topic are still not very common, especially from this part of the world. This title will surely plug that gap and certainly looks to be an exciting addition to the bookshelves of the dermatology departments anywhere in the world.

Another vital angle why this book is significant is its focus on the darker skin. Most publications on lasers deal with fairer skin and naturally, the parameters are 'biased' on that. Not many books have been written on lasers in dark skin.

This book is prepared by the pioneers in the field and will give the readers an insight about the parameters to be used in darker skin type to avoid complications. I find the chapters with a global flavor, with particular emphasis to darker skin.

This is a must read book for every dermatologist who wants to have a clear understanding of lasers, since it is an exhaustive and comprehensive book covering all the topics related to lasers in dermatology.

I congratulate the editors for their praiseworthy attempt and wish this book a grand success.

Thomas Ruzicka
Head, Department of Dermatology and Allergy
Ludwig Maximilian University of Munich
Munich, Germany

Foreword

"I suspect that no community will become humane and caring by restricting what its members can say."

Derek Bok

The publication of new works about aspects of dermatology will always be welcome. Especially, if they contribute significant information to particular communities and to the ways our colleagues have devised to cope with their contingencies and with the needs of the population. Generally, in dermatology, and especially in dermatologic surgery, the regional human variations are a fundamental factor in order to adapt the different procedures to their patients. We have seen texts appear which illustrate this aspect, in different geographical zones of the world.

This is perceived in the present work. Our colleagues from India present an excellent volume about laser applications on their population. Through this extensive and complete work, they enlighten us about the treatments on patients with particular characteristics of the skin that enhances our knowledge about these forms of treatment and, as a means to recognize our colleagues' work, it moves us to consider the need to disseminate texts that speak to us about the ways to solve regional problems.

The book has the intention of sharing with the Indian dermatologists, and with the entire world, a text which gathers the knowledge acquired and improved through time, and the successful ways of solving special situations. The book has thirty eight chapters, with more than three hundred pages, that cover all aspects of laser treatment, starting with the basic aspects, and continuing with the different kinds of lasers and how they are adapted to dark skins. It is written by about sixty authors, all of them great experts in the laser world in a light and entertaining fashion, demonstrating the authors' experiences with different aspects of this branch of dermatology. It provides us with a thorough review of this form of therapeutics. With very good and explicit illustrations, diagrams, and appropriate tables, they offer an extremely useful volume that will surely become a reference text. The high quality and academic authority of the authors are unquestionable, facts that backup their work. We are sure that their publication will be a fundamental contribution to the specialty not only in India, but in all the different regions of the planet, where the treatment of these types of skin is a real challenge.

As a first edition, the editorial work has been formidable. The task performed by Koushik Lahiri, Abhishek De, and Aarti Sarda has been exceptional and deserves broad recognition. The world of dermatology certainly appreciates relying on enterprising persons with an academic spirit, who demonstrate results of excellent team work and convening power. We can only wish their efforts continue and they keep working and contributing.

The production of knowledge is relentless. That is how it should be, and what is now accepted, most certainly will change in the future. At this moment, this book is at the frontline of knowledge about laser procedures. It is natural that it will need to be updated in the future. We wish that the authors and the editors keep up their spirit of academic advancement, so they continue with their work, and when that happens, they will let us present it.

This book is of immense value. Perhaps the greatest value being that it has given the Indian doctors, that are clearly telling us that they have been dedicated to care for their patients and to help them, a voice, and as the great educator from Harvard reminds us, doing this surely has made them more humane.

Jorge Ocampo-Candiani

Professor and Chairman, Department of Dermatology
University of Nuevo Leon, Monterrey, Mexico
President, Ibero-latinamerican College of Dermatology
Former President, International Society for Dermatologic Surgery
Former International Board Observer, American Academy of Dermatology
Mexico

Preface

In the pursuit of getting the best possible treatment options for our patients, and with the dawn of new millennium, when the three of us started our journey in the world of laser surgery, little idea did we have, what we considered to be just an extension of our routine dermatology practice, would slowly become a passion in our life. Training in lasers was difficult those days, and all three of us had to travel to different parts of the world to get ourselves trained in lasers. Roughly about 5 years back, when we started working together under one roof, we began tinkering with an idea to contribute more meaningfully to the world of lasers. We conducted various workshops, training programs for postgraduates and junior colleagues, to share what we have learnt over the years. However, even then, we could perceive,that much is left to be done beyond these sporadic efforts. Though a few good books on lasers are available, majority of them focus on Caucasian skin types. With lasers being used successfully for so many indications in dermatology, a comprehensive textbook was the need of the hour.

It was a coincidence and may be destiny that one of us was approached by the biggest publication house of the country to publish this title. The very next weekend, we were sitting together to chalk out the road map for the textbook of lasers, focusing on Indian skin types.

We decided to keep the book exhaustive, with chapters contributed by the very best of laser surgeons of India. After months of effort, today, as we write the preface for the book, we are very proud to present to you the work of the very bests of Indian Laser Surgeons, each one of them contributing in their respective field of expertize. The dreams of getting all of them together, kept us awake for long hours, but working late was never been so rewarding. Each of these authors has contrasting styles of expression, but we believe, we could manage to string their pearls of wisdom into a beautiful assembly. We also looked beyond boundaries to rope in some of the best international authors to make this book truly comprehensive.

The three of us had distinctive styles, but it suited the project best. To be precise, Dr Koushik Lahiri has been the brain of the concept; Dr Abhishek De has been the heart of the project, and Dr Aarti Sarda, the energetic spirit of the book.

The final result is a never before compilation on the subject, which we believe, suits your taste and requirement, just perfect.

This is our sincere and humble effort to bridge the gap in the learning of lasers in dermatology, and should be of great value to all dermatologists, postgraduates, plastic surgeons, and practitioners who are, or intend to be in laser practice. We know the road ahead is still long, but the beginning was necessary. We sincerely look forward to your feedback.

Koushik Lahiri

Abhishek De

Aarti Sarda

Acknowledgments

We were a little apprehensive when we first agreed to take the project.

It was surprising that, in spite of lasers now being widely practised in nearly all parts of India, no compendium of this magnitude was ever conceived from this part of the globe. Notwithstanding, the existence of astonishingly rich experience and expertize in using lasers in Indian skin types.

Our trepidation and edginess turned into pleasure and enthusiasm when all of the esteemed contributors, whom we approached, responded in a very positive way. They are virtually the topmost key opinion leaders in the field of lasers.

No words are enough for all the contributors of this book. In spite of their very busy schedule, they have done a stupendous job in writing so meticulously. The entire credit of the book goes to our brilliant contributors only.

We must thank M/s Jaypee Brothers Medical Publishers (P) Ltd, New Delhi, India, one of the most reputed and also one of the largest publishing houses in the world, for giving us the opportunity.

Shri Jitendar P Vij (Group Chairman) took personal care of this project, we owe a lot to him. Dr Neeraj Choudhary (Senior Acquisition Editor-Corporate), and his team were there with us at every step of the project with their untiring zeal to excel. We also thank Dr Swati Mishra and Gladden Savieo (Copy editors), Megha Kalra (Reader), Neha Bhatia (Development editor) and Manoj Kumar (DTP operator) from his team.

The icing on the cake was the forewords by Professor Thomas Ruzicka from Germany and Professor Jorge Ocampo-Candiani from Mexico which definitely add value and recognition to our humble effort.

Contents

CHAPTER 1

Advent and Evolution of Lasers in Dermatology

Anurag Tiwari

INTRODUCTION

Lasers are a relatively young technology which started as an analytical tool for physicists to look into the molecular structure but became one of the most sought after inventions. They were thought to be useful as weapons by some but failed. In medicine, lasers have been well accepted by doctors and patients for almost all the specialties.

HOW IT STARTED

In 1916, Einstein discussed the possibility of stimulating radiant energy based on Bohr's theory that atoms emitted energy in quanta when transitioning from excited states back to resting states.[1] Stimulated emission received little attention from experimentalists during the 1920s and 1930s when atomic and molecular spectroscopy were of central interest to many physicists.[2] Fabrikant defended his doctoral thesis *The emission mechanism of a gas discharge*, at the Lebedev Physical Institute in Moscow. It discussed experimental evidence for the existence of negative absorption (what was later called stimulated emission) and suggested experiments on light amplification.[3]

In early 1950s, physicists and electrical engineers began to collaborate with the research on monochromatic radiation of constant amplitude at very small wavelengths studying the microwave and radio frequency spectra of molecules. In this context, in 1953 and 1954, several physicists independently suggested the use of stimulated emission for microwave amplification, creating the acronym maser to stand for "microwave amplification by stimulated emission of radiation".[4]

Townes, Basov, and Prokhorov received the Nobel Prize in Physics in 1964 for their "fundamental work in the field of quantum electronics which has led to the construction of oscillators and amplifiers based on the maser–laser principle."[5] In 1958, Townes and his brother-in-law Schawlow, professor at Stanford University, showed that masers could theoretically be made to operate in the optical and infrared regions.[6] The same year, Makov et al. at the University of Michigan developed and built a solid state maser.[7] They used crystalline corundum (ruby) in a large magnetic field and a strategy similar to that known as optical pumping, suggested by Bloembergen at Harvard University in 1956.[8]

Maiman, in 1960, presented the first functional optical ruby maser excited by a xenon flash lamp to produce a bright pulse of 693.7 nm, deep red light of about a 1 ms duration, and a power output of about a billion watt per pulse.[9]

Maiman's invention rapidly led to the development of multiple other optical masers, now called laser (light amplification by stimulated emission of radiation). In 1961, McClung and Hellwarth introduced the quality-switching (Q-switching) technique to shorten the pulse length to nanoseconds with the use of an electro-optical shutter that permitted the storage and subsequent release of a peak power up to gigawatts of energy.[10,11]

Treatment of skin diseases with light has long been known. Lupus vulgaris with the Finsen lamp in 1899, wound healing and rickets with artificial UV light sources after 1901, and psoriasis with the combination of light and tar in 1925.

Goldman, in 1961, founded the first biomedical laser laboratory at the University of Cincinnati.[12] In 1963, Goldman and his coworkers published the first study on the effects of lasers on skin describing the selective destruction of pigmented structures of the skin including hair follicles with the beam of the ruby laser. They noted highly selective injury of pigmented structures (black hair) and no evident change in the white underlying skin.[13,14] He expected the laser to bring substantial benefits to the treatment of skin cancer; because of the accessibility and color, laser surgery can be used extensively in the field of skin cancer.

In 1973, Goldman published promising effects on angiomas with the continuous-wave neodymium doped yttrium-aluminium-garnet (Nd:YAG) laser. His book *Biomedical Aspects of the Laser*, published in 1967, is a comprehensive overview over the possibilities, problems, and ideas of the use of the laser in medicine at that time, also emphasizing the need for protection from laser energy. In addition, he discussed ideas of using the laser as a diagnostic tool (transillumination) to detect foreign bodies, hard tumors, or bone defects, and recommended the use of laser in dentistry.

Photoexcision (the optical scalpel) was possible with continuous wave lasers all invented. First the carbon dioxide (CO_2) laser, followed by the Nd:YAG laser and then the argon laser. The argon laser showed superior absorption by hemoglobin and was used for treating port wine stains and telangiectasia of the face and early rhinophyma.[15]

The early continuous wave lasers emitted an uninterrupted beam of light that was effective in destroying the desired target, but also damaged the healthy surrounding tissue. The result of this collateral damage was unacceptably high rates of scarring and pigmentary changes. The first attempt to minimize this nonspecific tissue injury involved making the continuous wave lasers discontinuous or quasi continuous by using a mechanical shutter to interrupt the beam of light.

In the treatment of vascular lesions, the development of the tunable yellow light dye laser with the absorption peak closer to oxyhemoglobin than the early argon lasers reduced the risk of side effects. In 1996, the erbium doped yttrium-aluminium-garnet laser with a very short wavelength of 2,940 nm allowed more superficial vaporization of tissue and was used together with CO_2 lasers for skin resurfacing. Very recently, the new technical concept of fractional photothermolysis was introduced. It received Food and Drug Administration (FDA) approval in 2004 for skin resurfacing and in 2005, for the treatment of melisma.[16]

Goldman wrote in 1967 "There is every indication that Q-switched lasers will remain an important tool in the physicists' laboratories."[17]

In 1980s, the pulsed ruby laser was commercialized in Japan for the treatment of tattoos and pigmented lesions, while being abandoned in Europe and the United States where tattoo removal was performed by CO_2 laser vaporization.[18] With the flashlamp-pumped pulsed dye laser in the early 1980s, Anderson and Parrish from Harvard Medical School in Boston developed the theory of selective photothermolysis that revolutionized the practice of cutaneous laser surgery.[19]

The authors recognized that the collateral thermal damage in the surrounding tissue of the target chromophore resulted from prolonged exposure to the laser's energy. By the appropriate manipulation of wavelength and pulse duration, and in dependence upon the chromophore's relaxation time, therapeutic destruction could be maximized while minimizing thermal damage to the surrounding tissue.[20] More than 3 decades later, a nearly identical ruby laser to the one used by Goldman in 1963 became the first device approved by the FDA in 1989 for permanent removal of pigmented hair, and the Q-switched Nd:YAG received FDA approval as a treatment modality for tattoos in 1991.[16,21]

CONCLUSION

The history is never complete; it is written with every passing moment. Lasers have become an integral part of any dermatology setup. The author is thankful all the physicists and physicians who founded and followed up on this technology.

REFERENCES

1. Einstein A. Zur Quantentheorie derStrahlung. Physikalische Gesellschaft Zürich. 1916;18:47–62. (The same paper was published on 15 March 1917, Physikalische Zeitschrift. 1917;18:121-8).
2. Townes CH. Production of coherent radiation by atoms and molecules: Nobel Lecture [Online]. 1964. Available from: http://nobelprize.org/nobel_prizes/physics/laureates/1964/townes-lecture.pdf [Accessed 30 October 2010].
3. Lukishova SG, Valentin A Fabrikant. Negative absorption, his 1951 patent application for amplification of electromagnetic radiation (ultraviolet,

visible, infrared and radio spectral regions) and his experiments. J Eur Optical Soc. 2010;5:10045s.
4. Townes CH. Early history of quantum electronics. J Modern Optics. 2005;52:1637-45.
5. Edlén B. (1964). Nobel prize award ceremony speech. [Online] Available from: http://nobelprize.org/nobel_prizes/physics/laureates/1964/press.html. [Accessed 30 Oct 2010].
6. Schawlow AL, Townes CH. Infrared and optical masers. Phys Rev. 1958;112:1940-9.
7. Makov G, Kikuchi C, Lambe J, Terhune RW. Maser action in ruby. Phys Rev. 1958;109:1399-1400.
8. Bloembergen N. Proposal for a new type solid state maser. Phys Rev. 1956;104:324-7.
9. Maiman TH. Stimulated optical radiation in ruby. Nature. 1960;187:493.
10. Hellwarth RW. Theory of the pulsation of fluorescent light from ruby. Phys Rev Lett. 1961;6:9-11.
11. Hellwarth RW, McClung FJ. Giant pulsations from ruby. Appl Phys. 1962;33:838-41 and Bull Am Phys Soc. 1962;6:414.
12. Coras B, Landthaler M, Leon Goldman. In: Loeser C, Plewig G, editors. Pantheon der Dermatologie–Herausragende historische Persönlich-keiten. Heidelberg: Springer; 2008. pp 357-61.
13. Goldman L, Blaney DJ, Kindel DJ Jr, Franke EK. Effect of the laser beam on the skin. Preliminary report. J Invest Dermatol. 1963;40:121-2.
14. Goldman L, Blaney DJ, Kindel DJ Jr, Richfield D, Franke EK. Pathology of the effect of the laser beam on the skin. Nature. 1963;197:912-4.
15. Goldman L. Historical perspective: personal reflections. In: Arndt KA, Noe JM, Rosen S. Cutaneous Laser Therapy: Principles and Methods. New York: Wiley; 1983. p. 7.
16. Houk LD, Humphreys T. Masers to magic bullets: an updated history of lasers in dermatology. Clin Dermatol. 2007:25;434-42.
17. Goldmann L. Biomedical Aspects of the Laser: The Introduction of Laser Applications into Biology and Medicine. Berlin: Springer; 1967.
18. Bailin PL, Ratz JL, Levine HL. Removal of tattoos by CO_2 laser. J Dermatol Surg Oncol. 1980;6:997-1001.
19. Anderson RR, Parrish JA. Selective photothermolysis: precise micro-surgery by selective absorption of pulsed radiation. Science. 1983:220:524-7.
20. Parrish JA, Anderson RR, Harrist T, Paul B, Murphy GF. Selective thermal effects with pulsed irradiation from lasers: from organ to organelle. J Invest Dermatol. 1983;80(suppl):75s-80s.
21. Anderson RR. Dermatologic history of the ruby laser: the long story of short pulses. Arch Dermatol. 2003;139:70-4.

CHAPTER 2

Physics of Light and Laser-tissue Interactions

Shekhar Neema, Manas Chatterjee

INTRODUCTION

Laser is one of the most significant discoveries in contemporary medicine. It has wide variety of uses in different branches of medicine and its scope is increasing in day-to-day practice. Laser is an acronym for Light Amplification by Stimulated Emission of Radiation. Laser differs from light as laser is collimated, coherent, and monochromatic.

HISTORY

In 1917, Einstein published *The Quantum Theory of Radiation* in which he conceptualized the theoretical basis to build a laser.[1] In 1960, the first laser, ruby laser was built by Maiman. In 1961, Goldman opened a laboratory to study the ruby laser, its safety, and medical uses of lasers. He realized the immense potential of lasers in treating human diseases and due to his pioneering work in lasers in respect of human diseases, he is known as father of laser medicine and surgery.[2,3] Discovery of ruby laser was followed by rapid development in the field of laser with development of the first gas laser, helium-neon laser in 1961,[4] neodymium-doped yttrium aluminium garnet (Nd:YAG) laser[5] and argon laser in 1962. In 1964, Patel invented the carbon dioxide (CO_2) laser and since then the field of laser is rapidly increasing with both development of new lasers as well as newer indications for laser treatment.[6]

BASIC LASER PHYSICS

What is Light?

Light is a radiant energy which exists in both particulate as well as wave forms. Light is composed of small packets of energy known as photons. The distance between two consecutive troughs or crests of waveform of light is known as wavelength (Fig. 1); light is arranged in electromagnetic spectrum depending upon the wavelength. Number of wave crests or trough, crossing a given point in a second determines the frequency of light.

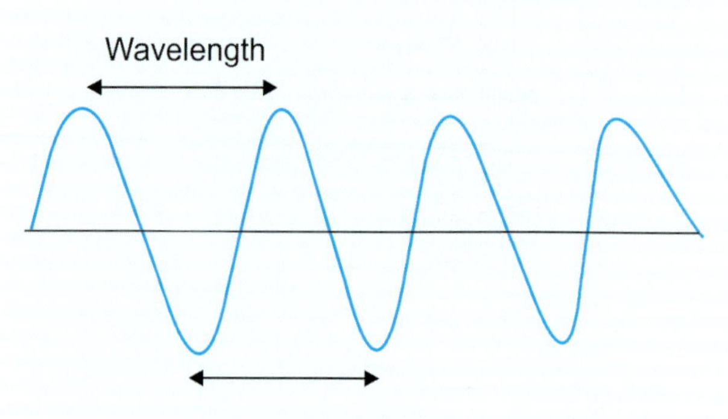

FIG. 1: Light in waveform

Understandably, wavelength and frequency are inversely related, i.e., light with shorter wavelength have higher frequency and vice versa. It can also be understood by the following formula:

$E = h\nu$

$E = hc/\lambda$

Where E, energy; h, Planck's constant; ν, frequency; c, velocity of light; λ, wavelength.

How is Laser Created?

It is important to understand the structure of atom to understand as to how laser is created. Atom consists of central nucleus surrounded by electrons which occupy the orbits around the nucleus. Nucleus contains protons which are positively charged particles and neutrons which are electrically neutral. Electrons are negatively charged particles. This electrical neutrality gives the atom a stable configuration. This is an oversimplified model of the atom as atom consists of numerous other particles which is beyond the scope of this book; nonetheless it is good for basic understanding (Fig. 2).

When an atom absorbs a photon of light, outer electron(s) move to higher energy orbit making the atom unstable. Atom releases a photon of light when electron returns to lower energy orbit and the atom once again achieves a stable configuration (Fig. 3). This release of light occurs in random fashion and results in incoherent light, as seen in the phenomenon of fluorescence. For amplification of light to occur, more atoms are required in unstable than resting configuration. This state is called as population inversion and is a prerequisite for creation of laser.

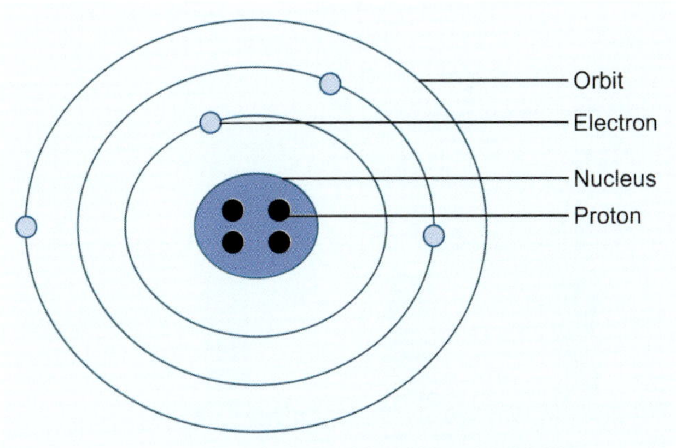

FIG. 2: Structure of an atom

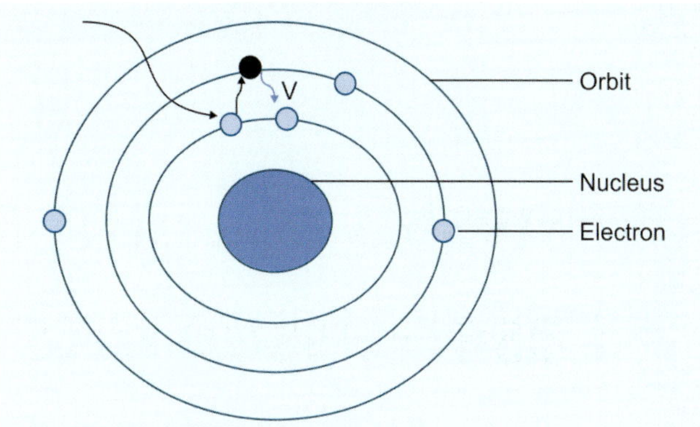

FIG. 3: Electron in excited state after absorbing energy and return to orbit by release of photon

What are the Basic Elements of Laser?

Laser consists of four basic elements:

1. Laser medium: wavelength of laser depends on the laser medium. Laser medium can be broadly divided into solid, liquid or gas. Type of laser is defined by its medium, for example carbon dioxide laser, argon laser, dye laser, and so on (Table 1)
2. Optical cavity: it surrounds the laser medium which is resonant and amplifies the light
3. Power supply: it excites the atom and creates population inversion
4. Delivery system: it can be articulating arm or fiber optic to deliver the laser precisely.

CHARACTERISTICS OF LASER

What are the characteristics of laser which differentiate it from normal light? Laser has three unique or special characteristics:

1. Collimation: all the waves are parallel to each other; convergence or divergence is minimum

TABLE 1: Types of laser based on optical medium

Name	Type	Wavelength (in nm)
Argon	Gas	488, 514
Copper vapor	Gas	511, 578
Carbon dioxide	Gas	10,600
Pulsed dye	Liquid	585
Ruby	Solid	694
Alexandrite	Solid	755
Diode	Solid	810
Nd:YAG	Solid	1,064

Nd:YAG, neodymium doped yttrium-aluminium-garnet.

Box 1: Laser terminology

- Power: rate of energy emitted from laser, expressed in watts
- Energy: product of power (watts) and pulse duration (time), expressed in Joule (watt-second)
- Irradiance: laser power per unit surface area (watt/cm^2), also known as power density

2. Coherence: all the waves are in phase with one another in both time and space. Temporal coherence means that frequency, wavelength, and speed of travel of all waves is same, while spatial coherence means that crest and trough of all waves coincide
3. Monochromaticity: all the waves are of same wavelength.

LASER-TISSUE INTERACTIONS

It is important to know laser-tissue interactions to understand the clinical effects of laser. Laser-tissue interactions lead to following phenomena:

- Reflection: reflection depends on the property of tissue and vary based on pigment present in the tissue; it also depends on the wavelength of the laser
- Transmission: rays which emerge distally from the tissue is termed as transmitted rays
- Scattering: scattering is change in the direction of light on interaction with tissue
- Absorption: absorption of laser energy by tissue leads to conversion of laser energy to heat energy.

As one can understand, absorption and scattering (change in the direction of light) lead to clinical effects produced in tissue.

Theory of Selective Photothermolysis

Theory of selective photothermolysis was proposed by Anderson and Parish in 1983.[7] This theory revolutionized the use of laser for dermatological diseases. It explains laser induced damage to selected types of tissue and minimal damage to adjacent tissue. This theory was proposed to explain the treatment of port wine stain by pulse dye laser. According to this theory, to cause only selective damage to target tissue, laser should fulfill the following criteria:

- It should emit a wavelength which is highly absorbed by targeted structure. This target is known as chromophore for particular laser. Example, pulse dye laser emitting 585 nm and oxyhemoglobin has peak absorption at 577 nm and is its target chromophore
- It should produce sufficient energy to inflict damage to target tissue
- Time of exposure should be short enough (pulse duration), so that damage is limited to target tissue and heat diffusion to surrounding structures is minimum.

Extended Theory of Selective Photothermolysis

When the target tissue does not absorb the laser very strongly, but surrounding tissue absorbs it strongly (chromophore), the theory of selective photothermolysis becomes inapplicable. According to theory of extended selective photothermolysis, target tissue can be damaged selectively by diffusion of heat from highly absorbing structure.

Thermal damage time is the time which is taken by a target to reach damage temperature by diffusion of heat from chromophore. This theory is utilized in treatment of unwanted hair, where chromophore is melanin but the target tissue is hair bulb.

Commonly used Lasers and Mechanism of Laser Delivery

Lasers can also be classified as ablative and nonablative. Ablative lasers are those lasers which remove the epidermis like CO_2 laser, while nonablative lasers do not remove the epidermis and act on deeper tissue.

There are various ways in which laser can be delivered to tissues. These different ways can be used to suit different clinical indications (Figs 4 to 6).

Continuous Wave

Laser is delivered continuously as long as switch is pressed.

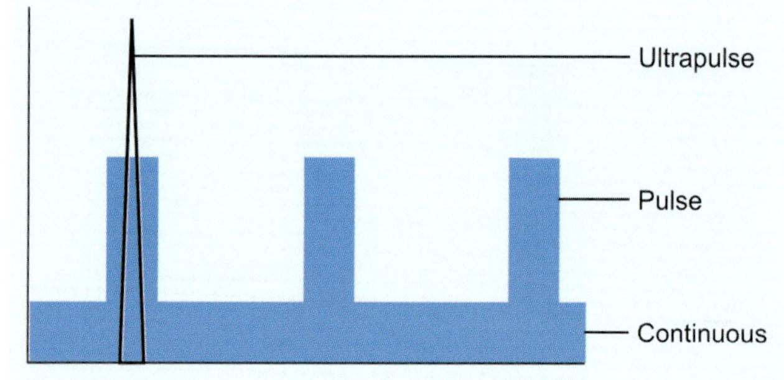

FIG. 4: Methods by which laser energy can be delivered to tissues

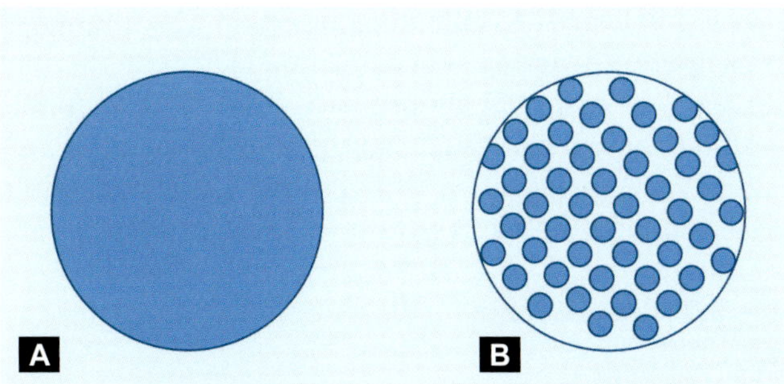

FIG. 5: Schematic representation of **A,** conventional mode of delivery of laser energy and **B,** fractional mode, with intervening untreated area

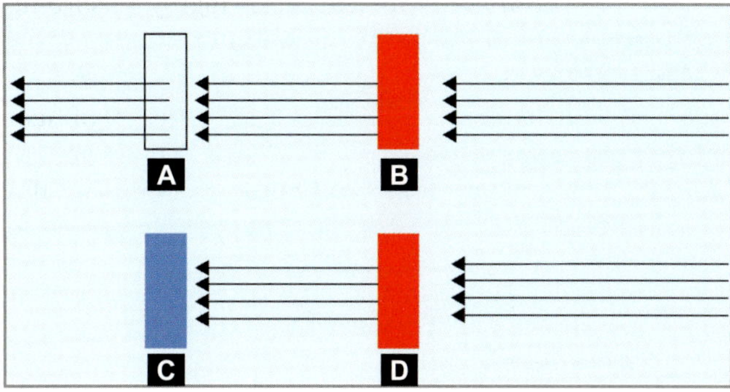

FIG. 6: Q-switching: system contains pockelcells (**A, C**) and polariser. On application of voltage, pockel cells become opaque; (**C**), thus allowing buildup of energy within the optical cavity. Energy is released when voltage is turned off, in short powerful pulse

Pulse Mode

Laser is delivered in pulses; pulse duration (interval between two pulses) can be changed depending on the requirement. If the pulse duration is less than thermal relaxation time (TRT) of the target tissue, damage to surrounding tissue is minimal.

Ultrapulse Mode

When pulse is so brief that it lasts only for microsecond(s), that mode of delivery is called ultrapulse. Ultrapulse delivers very high amount of energy for very short time, thus minimizing collateral damage.

Fractional

It is a novel way of delivery where only part of the target area is treated leaving behind untreated area in middle of treated area. This results in faster healing and less downtime.

Q-switching

Q or quality switching is a method of delivery of laser, where short pulses (5–20 ns) of high intensity (5–10 MW) are created. This system has polarizer and pockel cells within the optical cavity. Pockel cell is an optically transparent crystal which rotates the plane of polarization of light. On application of voltage, pockel cell becomes opaque, thus allowing buildup of energy in the optical cavity. Energy is released in short powerful pulse when voltage is turned off.

TYPES OF LASERS

Ablative Lasers

Carbon Dioxide Laser

This laser has wavelength of 10,600 nm and chromophore is water. The TRT of epidermis is approximately 1 ms; if laser-tissue interaction occurs for this time period or less, tissue will be vaporized with minimal residual thermal damage of 50–100 μm.[8,9] When CO_2 laser interacts with tissue, it leads to formation of three zones. First zone is zone of ablation where intracellular water gets vaporized. Second zone is of irreversible thermal damage, and the last zone is of reversible thermal damage in which collagen shrinkage occurs and leads to visible tightening of the tissues.

Erbium Doped Yttrium-Aluminium-Garnet Laser

Erbium yttrium aluminium garnet (Er:YAG) has wavelength of 2,940 mm and is highly absorbed by water. It is absorbed ten times more strongly by water than 10,600 nm CO_2 laser and hence, results in less collateral damage. One pass with erbium doped yttrium-aluminium-garnet laser ablates approximately 10–30 μm and zone of thermal damage of only 15–30 μm.

Pigment Removing Laser

Pigment removing lasers are those lasers which specifically remove the pigment with minimal damage to epidermis. Pigment should strongly absorb the corresponding wavelength of the laser without causing collateral damage. Q-switching is used in pigment lasers;

it generates nanosecond pulse which matches closely with TRT of melanosome or tattoo pigment. Photoacoustic effect created by short powerful pulses damages the melanosome or tattoo pigment which is subsequently removed by macrophages. Most common pigment removing system in use are Q-switched neodymium doped yttrium-aluminium-garnet (Nd:YAG) laser, Q-switched ruby laser, and Q-switched alexandrite laser.

Vascular Laser

Vessels can be destroyed selectively by attacking something which is unique to a vessel. Vessel contains blood and blood has hemoglobin. Oxyhemoglobin has three major absorption peaks namely 418, 542, and 577 nm. When hemoglobin absorbs laser energy, it transfers the energy and leads to destruction of endothelium. There are various host factors which decides laser wavelength and its parameters like fluence and pulse duration for management of certain lesions. These are depth, size, flow, and type of targeted vessel. Deeper vessels require larger spot size for better penetration and larger size of vessel require longer pulse duration which results in even diffusion of heat from hemoglobin to endothelium. Most commonly used vascular lasers are pulse dye laser (585 nm) and long pulse Nd:YAG laser (1,064 nm). Intense pulsed light with specific filters also work for these indications but is not the scope of this chapter.

Hair Removal Lasers

Hair bulb and shaft of pigmented hair contain melanin. This melanin can be used as target to destroy the unwanted hair. When melanin absorbs laser energy, it transfers the heat to the hair bulb thus damaging the stem cells present in bulb. The problem with this mechanism of hair damage is that epidermis also contains melanin and can also absorb the light leading to pigmentary alteration in dark skin. Longer wavelength penetrates deeper and are less absorbed by epidermal melanin, hence, longer wavelength lasers are safer in dark skin. In addition, there are epidermal cooling mechanisms to prevent thermal damage to epidermal melanin. By understanding this mechanism, one can understand that fair skin with dark hair have best response to hair removal lasers, while darker skin has higher risk of surface pigmentary changes and blonde or light hair is not amenable to hair removal laser as it does not contain the chromophore melanin.

CONCLUSION

Laser is a great tool in the hand of the dermatologist for management of myriads of diseases which are not amenable to treatment by other conventional methods. Understanding laser physics is an important step to utilize lasers to maximum potential and also prevent avoidable adverse effects.

REFERENCES

1. Einstein A. Zur Quanten Theory der Strahlung. Physical Zeitschr. 1917;18:121-8.
2. Goldman L. The CO_2 laser in dermatology: the perspective of Leon Goldman, M.D. "Father of laser surgery". Xanar Surgical Monograph. 1988.
3. Goldman L, Blaney D, Kindel DJ Jr, Franke EK. Effect of laser beam on the skin. J Invest Dermatol. 1963;40:121-2.
4. Javan A, Bennett W, Herriot D. Population inversion and continuous optical maser oscillator in a gas discharge containing a He–Ne mixture. Phys Rev. 1961;6:106-10.
5. Johnson L. Optical maser characteristics of rare-earth ions in crystals. J Appl Physiol. 1961;34:897-90.
6. Patel CKN, McFarlane R, Faust W. Selective excitation through vibrational energy transfer and optical maser action in N2–CO2. Phys Rev. 1964;136:617-9.
7. Anderson RR, Parrish JA. Selective photothermolysis: Precise micro-surgery by selective absorption of pulsed radiation. Science. 1983;220: 524-7.
8. Drake LA, Dinehart SM, Farmer ER, Goltz RW, Graham GF, Hordinsky MK, et al. Guidelines of care for photoaging/photodamage. American Academy of Dermatology. J Am Acad Dermatol. 1996;35(3 Pt 1):462-4.
9. Fitzpatrick RE, Tope WD, Goldman MP, Satur NM. Pulsed carbon dioxide laser, trichloracetic acid, Baker-Gordon phenol, and dermabrasion: a comparative clinical and histological study of cutaneous resurfacing in a porcine model. Arch Dermatol. 1996;132(4):469-71.

CHAPTER 3

Setting up a Laser Practice

Sathish B Pai, Sudhir Nayak UK

INTRODUCTION

Laser technology has revolutionized treatment procedures in dermatology and lasers are almost an integral part of a dermatologist clinic. It is very vital that the laser set-up is given due attention. This article gives a basic idea in setting up of a laser unit. The need of each dermatologist tends to vary and same needs to be followed. Make sure local, state, and national permits and regulations are followed. All safety, fire, building, and sanitation regulations should be met before starting a laser clinic.[1] The setting up of laser clinic involves not just buying a laser system. Various factors play an integral part in the proper and successful running of a laser like location of clinic, decor, front desk, auxiliary support staff, safety measures, etc.

PURCHASE OF A LASER MACHINE

This is perhaps the most important part in setting up a laser clinic. The main indication for which you need a laser decides the type of laser machine which needs to be purchased. The most common laser usually purchased initially are the hair removal laser and then, the fractional ablative laser.[2] Discuss with colleagues using a laser which you are planning to buy, and the merits and demerits of the laser machine. Assess the different types of laser machines available before buying one. It is prudent to decide whether you want to purchase a single machine or a platform device. While cost is the most important consideration in purchasing a laser, there are numerous other factors that need to be considered while purchasing a laser machine. These include the warranty, the make, availability of service center nearby, and availability of spare parts.[2] Signing of a contract with the manufacturer or dealer covering warranty, annual service, prompt inspection in case of machine breakdown etc. will be a good idea.

Always remember that a good laser machine is always better than a cheap imitator. You want your laser procedure to be a walking advertisement for your practice. Any complication or an unsatisfactory result is bad publicity for you.

LOCATION OF CLINIC

Laser clinic should be located at popular and easily accessible areas of the city or town. While changing of location may not be realistic for an already existing dermatological practice, dermatologists venturing into a new clinic may benefit from having a clinic here. Make sure adequate parking facilities exist or valet parking can be arranged.

LASER ROOM

The construction of a laser room should predate the purchase of a laser machine. The laser room should enforce confidentiality, safety, and convenience. The ideal dimension of the laser room should be 3.65 × 3.65 m (12 × 12 feet)[2]. The laser room needs to accommodate one procedure chair, one doctor chair, cooling device, treatment trolley, emergency trolley or tray, hand wash area, at least one laser machine, one cabinet, one doctor, and one assistant. In teaching institutes, the dimensions of the room needs to be increased accordingly. The door of the laser room should be wide and opaque to prevent transmission of laser rays. The door should be fitted with lock from inside to ensure privacy of patients. Avoid windows in laser room and if present should be opaque, especially, if facing outside or to the corridors. The floor of the laser room should be easily cleanable with mop. Reflective surfaces should be avoided in the laser room.[1] The lighting in the room should be bright and uniform. The cabinet in the laser room can be divided into compartments to store eye protection goggles, prescription pads, topical medications, preparatory material like disposable razors, surgical masks, gloves, marking pens, and other stationaries like post-treatment instructions. It is preferable to keep waste bins in a closed area. Separate waste bins for sharps, plastics, general, biological, and plastic wastes are required. It is also desirable to have a small table with lockable compartment for keeping patients belongings and valuables like jewelry. This is to ensure that patients do not complain of missing things. Providing a table for keeping things shows that the doctor is concerned about the storage of patient's belongings. If possible, a space for small refrigerator to store cooling gels and ice packs is desirable. Mirrors used for grooming of a patient postlaser should be kept in cabinets or drawers as they are reflective.

If you are constructing a laser clinic, make sure you have space for another machine in future.

TRAINING

Learning the basics of laser physics plays a vital role in the usage of a laser. Get yourself adequately trained in the laser you are planning to purchase. Read the instruction manual supplied with the laser machine before starting practising laser.

ELECTRICAL REQUIREMENTS

The electrical supply and portals are very important. Make sure there is adequate number of electrical sockets in the room. It is necessary to discuss with your clinic constructor at the initial stages itself where you want your electrical points, especially, for laser setup. The sockets needs to be located neither too high nor too low on the ground. Labeling of the uninterrupted power supply (UPS) sockets is a must. Electrical panels are best fitted in all walls of the laser room as sometimes you may decide to shift the machine to a different place in the same room. It is necessary to avoid wires running across the floor. Grounding or earthing of the socket board is to be done. It is vital to have a UPS for the laser machine. The ideal UPS requirements are minimum of 3 kVA with 16 batteries of 60 A each.[1,2] Check the requirements of your machine before plugging it to the socket. Discuss with the laser manufacturer and your electrician about the needs of the laser machine in advance.

External cooling systems like Zimmer are required as per the machine which you have purchased. If you have only a hair removal laser with an inbuilt cooling system, then, it may not be necessary. Lasers which do not have an inbuilt cooling system will require adequate cooling devices.

AIR CONDITIONING

Invest in a good air conditioning system. After having invested in a good laser, you do not want your laser to malfunction due to inadequate cooling of the room. Make sure the room is kept at an ambient temperature as instructed in the laser manual. Most lasers require about 18–22°C of ambient temperature.[2,3] Avoid keeping the laser room door open when not in use. Air conditioning the laser room usually ensures that it is dust free, which is needed for every laser machine.

TREATMENT CHAIR

Make sure the treatment or laser chair is comfortable. The chair should be minimum of 6 feet long and 22–24 inch wide.[3] Wider the chair, better would be the comfort of the patient. The increasing trend of obesity in India necessitates the purchase of wider chairs. The surface of the chair should be easily washable. It is advisable to lie down on the chair and see whether the chair is comfortable or not. Do not purchase a chair looking at the brochure.

WAITING AREA

Decorum of your laser clinic is necessity. Make sure it is appealing to the eye. Jarring colors are best avoided. The waiting area in the laser clinic should be well-ventilated and illuminated. Furniture should be comfortable. Magazines, papers, and patient information leaflets should be kept. Television for entertaining patients or for demonstration of common procedures may be kept. Ensure cleanliness of the waiting area as well as laser room. It is worthwhile to make sure that a separate area for keeping wet umbrellas and rain-coats is there in the waiting area and that patients do not carry these to the laser room.

PREPARATORY ROOM

Separate preparatory room, especially for hair removal lasers are desirable as you do not want your laser room being wasted for preparation. Interconnectivity between laser room and preparatory room as well of these rooms to the corridor will be useful in patient management.

STORAGE ROOM

A separate storage room to hold consumables, like towels, sheets, stationary etc., is a requisite. Disinfectants and other chemicals should be separately stored. The storage room should be as far as away from the laser room(s). In places where large storage rooms cannot be constructed in view of cost, then overhead cabinets or compartments may be constructed in rooms to store daily consumables.

RECORD KEEPING

Documentation is very vital in laser procedures. Records of the procedure and the consent forms needed to be stored safely. So, make sure you have adequate storage space for files you plan to maintain, if you are the one who prefers hard copies. Alphabetical storage of files is to be done for easy retrieval of files. For practices where multiple dermatologists work, storing files as per doctor will be useful. For those who are computer savvy, good backup of your files is necessary.

CONSENT FORM

Prepare a well-written consent form, preferably in English, Hindi, and the regional language(s) of the state or city. A standard dermatological consent form may be modified and adequate copies may be stored. If photography being taken and same is planned for publication or presentations, separate consent is required.

INSURANCE

Insurance for lasers from fire, breakdown, theft, etc., needs to be taken especially when laser devices are handled by multiple personnel. Try getting an extended warranty for your machine and spare parts. Clarify with your laser manufacturer beforehand what all are covered in both the warranty and extended warranty. If you are planning to shift laser machine in between different clinics, separate insurance clause may be needed.

EYE SAFETY MEASURES

Make sure you purchase adequate number of appropriate eye protecting glasses for the laser being purchased. The laser manufacturer is likely to give additional sets of glasses at the time of purchase as a complimentary one rather than later, when you will have to pay extra for that. This is very essential in institutes and medical colleges where teaching is conducted. Opaque eye protective wear are a must for patients and are usually provided along with the laser machine. In practices with more than one laser machine, storage of physician eye protective goggles needs to be separately stored and ensure that appropriate eye wear used for each laser. Any cracked or discolored goggles needs to be replaced as per laser machine guidelines.[4]

SMOKE EVACUATOR

For lasers generating smoke, it is desirable to have a smoke evacuator to filter irritants and viral particles.[5,6] Smoke evacuator may be purchased as per the recommendations of the laser manufacturer.

FIRE SAFETY MEASURES

Fire extinguishers should be placed at easily located areas and your staff should be adequately trained in using fire extinguishers. Fluorocarbon fire extinguishers are preferred over carbon dioxide fire extinguishers as they are unlikely to damage laser components.[6] Periodic checking of the fire extinguisher should be done.

SAFETY OF LASER MACHINE

Make sure one or two personnel are entrusted with the handling and daily maintenance of your laser machine. Instruct all your staff not to take water (cleaning and drinking purposes) near the laser machine.

SAFETY BOARDS

The required safety boards need to be installed on the laser room door. Light on top of the door, as in operation theatres, indicating that a procedure is going on, is desirable.

EMERGENCY TROLLEY

An emergency tray or trolley with necessary resuscitation medication and instruments should be kept handy.

PEST PROTECTION

Make sure the laser room is free from cockroaches and rodents which will damage the laser machine. Avoid cluttering in the laser room as this attracts rodents and other pests.

RECEPTIONIST

A good receptionist fluent in English and in the local language is needed. It is very important that there is no miscommunication between your laser patient or client and your clinic, especially with regard to timings of the laser sittings.

STANDARD OPERATING PROCEDURE

Standard operating procedure (SOP) may be developed when technicians are entrusted with using a laser machine. It is imperative that technical staff is well-versed in the SOP and periodic assessment of the technical staff in SOP and practice is done by the dermatologist.

PHOTOGRAPHY

As with all aesthetic procedures, good photography is needed for laser procedures. Invest in a good camera, preferably single-lens reflex (SLR). Have a separate photography room (if space permits), lest it interferes with your procedure or your consultation. Photography should be done in standardized condition with respect to illumination, background, position, distance etc.[1] It is preferable to have the same person take photograph for all the visits of the patient. It is necessary to have a plain background for photography. Storage and retrieval of pictures should be safe, confidential, and easily retrievable. Photographs before each setting are needed. Make sure you take pictures after marking area to be lased, especially in hair removal laser. Patients often tend to increase the borders of the laser area.

REST ROOMS FOR PATIENTS

Clean toilets for the patients are necessary. Some of your patients may be coming from far and some sittings of laser may go for few hours. Absence of toilet should not be a factor which a patient forgoes undergoing laser at your clinic.

AUXILIARY STAFF

The auxiliary staff should be preferably fluent in English, Hindi, and the regional language(s). It is best that all laser procedures are done by adequately trained dermatologist. In instances where technical staff is employed in performing laser procedures, it is the onus of the dermatologist to ensure that the technical staff is adequately trained and procedures are supervised. Regular evaluation of the procedures being performed by the technical staff should be done.

LINEN

Clean laundered linen like toilet sheets is an important requisite. Replacement of dirty and shabby is prudent. Contracts with local cleaners for laundering and ironing of towels may be done.

WASTE DISPOSAL MANAGEMENT

Appropriate waste disposal measures should be ensured. Separate bins for segregation of waste generated. Contracts with local waste disposal agencies need to be done.

CONCLUSION

While purchase of a laser machine maybe of prime importance, it is necessary to pay almost equal attention to other aspects in setting a laser unit. This chapter aims to suggest the basic requirements for setting up a laser unit. Modifications as per the needs of a dermatologist needs to be done. Safety, confidentiality, record keeping, convenience, and efficacy are some of the essential requirements of a laser unit and due attention to these is needed while establishing a laser unit.

REFERENCES

1. Aurangabadkar SJ, Mysore V, Ahmed ES. Buying a laser-tips and pearls. J Cutan Aesthet Surg. 2014;7:124-30.
2. Dhepe N. Minimum standard guidelines of care on requirements for setting up a laser room. Indian J Dermatol Venereol Leprol. 2009;75:101-10.
3. Dheepe NV. Setting up a Laser theatre. In: Venkataram M (Ed). ACS (I) textbook on cutaneous and aesthetic surgery. New Delhi: Jaypee Brothers Medical Publishers Pvt Ltd; 2012. pp. 763-70.
4. Association of surgical technologists. AST Standards of Practice for Laser Safety. [Online]. Available from: http://www.ast.org/uploadedFiles/Main_Site/Content/About_Us/Standard%20Laser%20Safety.pdf [Accessed March 2016].
5. Centers for disease control and prevention. The National Institute for Occupational Safety and Health (NIOSH). [Online]. Available from: http://www.cdc.gov/niosh/docs/hazardcontrol/hc11.html [Accessed March 2016].
6. Oberoi C, Parasramani SG. Laser basics. In: Sacchidanand S, Oberoi C, Inamadar A (Eds). IADVL textbook of Dermatology, 4th edition. Mumbai: Bhalani Publishing House; 2015. pp. 2535-50.

CHAPTER 4

Ethical Issues in Laser Practice

Nilay K Das, Amrita Sil

INTRODUCTION

Aesthetics and cosmetic medicine is one of the fastest growing fractions of medicine. Laser in dermatology are widely used for a plethora of indications, be it hair reduction, fade or remove vascular and pigmented birthmarks, tattoos, telangiectasia, and many acquired pigmentary disorders, without a visible scar or change in texture.[1] Conditions such as wrinkles, sun damaged skin, unsightly veins, acne scars may be treated with the laser. Laser can be used as a cutting instrument. Cosmetic concerns, which could not be addressed before the advent of lasers, are now within the reach of mankind. Thus, laser caters a target population for whom the zeal of beautification can make them vulnerable. Thus, it is a doctor's moral responsibility to make sure that patients are not exploited.

Recent advancements and modifications in laser technology have greatly expanded the laser surgeon's armamentarium and resulted in better results. However, with great power comes great responsibility. On one hand, laser is a powerful tool for the right patient treated by the right physician for the right indication, and on the other hand, the technology can be misused and unethically turned into a profit-only-machine regardless of its actual requirement or indication. This makes the patient more vulnerable and the physicians ethically responsible for their patients who come to undergo a laser procedure.

Ethics are the moral values of human behavior and the principles which govern these values. The principles of ethics rest on the four pillars of autonomy, beneficence, nonmaleficence, and justice.[2]

AUTONOMY

Autonomy is the respect for the patient's "right to self-governance, choice for care, and the right to accept or refuse treatment".[3,4]

The principle of autonomy states that the patient has the right to make his or her own choice as to what procedure he or she aspires to have. Thus, the patient's right to an informed consent must be respected. The patient must be given the right information as what to expect, the risks involved, and the alternative options available.

Patients have unrealistic expectations encouraged by media advertisements. Some may even turn to cosmetic therapy to tide emotional and personal crisis. In these cases, the physician is ethically bound to understand the patient's mind set, make him aware of the pros and cons of the procedure, and refuting the laser treatment if the procedure is contraindicated.

Informed Consent

The informed consent is a process by which the physician sensitizes the patient about the nature of the procedure to be done on him. The informed consent document has two parts: first, the "subject information sheet" and the "informed consent form". Prior to a laser procedure, the physician should obtain written informed consent from his patient.

The components of the subject information sheet are as follows:

- Purpose and background of need of laser therapy: to provide information about the procedure, the laser instrument to be used, and the indications that can be dealt with in the clinical setup
- Risks and complication: risks of infection, scarring, color changes, burns, delayed healing, unsatisfactory result, etc. should be properly mentioned
- Alternative treatment(s): alternative forms of treatment include procedures other than the proposed laser procedure. This may include chemical peels, dermabrasion, radiofrequency ablation, and surgical excision. Also, shaving, plucking, depilatory creams, waxing, and electrolysis are alternative treatment of laser hair removal. Benefits and risks of the alternative methods compared to laser procedure should be mentioned
- Cost: laser surgery requires payment at the time of service which is before the full degree of improvement may be determined. Most uses of laser are considered cosmetic and they are generally not reimbursable. Additional costs may occur if complications arise
- Consent for photographs: consent should be taken for photographs to be taken during course of treatment. If the clinic wants to utilize the "before-after" photographs of the patient for advertisements or presentation in journals or conferences, that too should be consented beforehand
- Confidentiality: all aesthetic procedures including laser treatment should be done maintaining the confidentiality of the patient.

The information provided in the subject information sheet is explained to the patient in vernacular, queries and doubts handled and the patient signs on the informed consent form to complete the process. One copy of the informed consent document is retained by the physician and another copy is handed to the patient.

Informed Assent

Informed consent process in a child less than 18 years entails not only the patients' "assent" but also the parental consent. Also, the physician should always remember that the child is in a growing phase and drastic laser surgery should be refrained from.

BENEFICENCE

The principle of beneficence requires the practitioner to act in the patient's "best interest". It is important for the practitioner to assess the risks versus the benefits of the procedure and maximize benefits, minimize harms. The motivation of the patient for having the procedure and how it will affect quality of life should be gauged by the physician. The physician should be specialized in the procedure and should be able to handle risks and side effects that might occur.

NONMALEFICENCE

The principle of nonmaleficence requires the practitioner to "do no harm" to the patient. The practitioner should be unwilling to perform a procedure on a patient who has impractical expectations. Discussion of the possible side effects and complications of the procedure, the postprocedure treatments and the follow-up procedures that may be required is a must. At this point, the practitioner may suggest alternative procedures and treatments that may be more beneficial for the patient or refer the patient to another medical professional that specializes in other treatments that would yield the desired result.

JUSTICE

This principle seeks "fair treatment". Exploitation of the patient economically should be refrained. Fair practice regarding the correct choice of laser, number of sessions required are to be decided according to the pathology of concern. The practitioner should be respectful to the patients' wishes, understand the depth of the problem, and educate the patient about the expectation from the procedure.

ETHICAL ISSUES IN LASER PRACTICE

Ethical conflicts arise when the physician struggles with beneficence versus economic interest. Few interesting situations have been described below.

Not the Correct Indication

Let us consider an example where a patient with Fitzpatrick skin type VI wishes intense pulsed light hair reduction. Such an indication should not be entertained as the risk of postinflammatory pigmentation is high. Even if the patient insists, the physician remains ethically bound to refuse the treatment even if it means a loss of revenue to him.

Not the Right Machine

The right type of laser for the correct indication can work wonders. No such laser is "jack of all trades" which will work for all indications. It seems logical and ethical to use laser fittingly instead of carrying out all procedures with the single laser that one owns, e.g., flashlamp pumped pulsed dye Laser (PDL) of wavelength 577 nm coincides to one of the absorption peak of oxyhemoglobin and is the laser of choice for vascular lesion.[5] Variable pulse width frequency doubled neodymium doped: yttrium-aluminium-garnet (Nd:YAG) laser (532 nm) may be used but effectiveness is not as good as PDL. Thus, someone not having PDL in his clinic can compromise with the ethics if he counsels for Nd:YAG in vascular lesions (the reason being his/her clinic is equipped with frequency doubled Nd:YAG). Referring the patient to the setup which owns the particular laser which can address the problem seems an ethical approach to the situation or else informed consent may be obtained with proper explanation that both of the lasers work in vascular lesions, but PDL is better than frequency doubled Nd:YAG (532 nm). If the patient is willing, then a doctor is ethically correct even in doing a vascular lesion with Nd:YAG. At times, a doctor can also explain his action by published reports wherein the use of Nd:YAG is justified.

Not the Right Person

The issue of training in laser and the persons qualified in it are a serious problem. Weekend crash courses are way too less to understand and work with the machine. Even hands-on training held by manufacturing companies might not involve real patients but simulations. More so, proper assessments of the skin types regarding development of iatrogenic skin damage, dealing with complications postprocedure, and legal issues that may follow require experience.

If a doctor acquires laser equipment, his initial patients should not be the victim of his inexperience. In such situations, ethical practice can be done if the doctor performs the procedure along with an experienced laser surgeon who can monitor the procedure.

Unrealistic Expectations

It should be remembered that it is not the diseased skin that is primarily treated but the healthy skin is injured upon respecting the patients' wishes and concerns. The patient may be emotionally insecure, facing a career crisis, or suffer from body dysmorphic disorder. These individuals are subjects of unrealistic expectations fed by impractical "before-after" advertisements on the media and internet. They look at the laser procedure as an answer to repair a damaged marriage, acquiring a job, or for emotional security.

Assessing the individual remains utmost important during the first visit and taking time to counsel the patient regarding the expectation, risks, and feasibility of the laser procedure falls within the pillars of ethical practice.

Newly Developed Lasers

When a laser is marketed, there are often no dependable data available from studies, thus, the physician has to depend on the advertising claims of the manufacturer. This is a real serious issue because with laser, there are no randomized controlled trials and the system must change for laser companies to introduce a new laser after going through the same routine as for introduction of new drug by doing clinical trials.

Business Pressure of Cosmetic Clinics

The number of cosmetic clinics is on the rise and the business pressure imposed by the clinic owners on the doctor is enormous. The financial gain has the potential to undermine the ethics, just like in any other profession. Keeping a balance between business and ethics and to tackle the pressure is a challenge.

Unrealistic Claims

Unrealistic claims unsupported by evidence are a source of malpractice and unethical. Here too, the prioritizing business over ethics is the major driving force.

Record Keeping

The clinic should keep records of the various laser sessions of the patient and maintain confidentiality as a part of ethical practice. If any advertisement is to feature "before-after" photographs of an individual, prior written consent should be obtained.

CONCLUSION

Aesthetics and lasers are that branch of medicine where the outcome of the procedure is the happiness and contentment of the patient, which is subjective in nature. The transaction here is more akin to business. However, the physicians' better sense of judgment and responsibility should take over the financial pressures while treating his patient and this alone can lead to an ethical laser practice.

REFERENCES

1. Wheeland RG. Cosmetic use of lasers. Dermatol Clin. 1995;13(2):447-59.
2. Beauchamp TL, Childress JF. Principles of Biomedical Ethics, 5th edition. Oxford: Oxford University Press; 2001. pp. 454.
3. Chung KC, Pushman AG, Bellfi LT. A systematic review of ethical principles in the plastic surgery literature. Plast Reconstr Surg. 2009;124(5):1711-8.
4. Kennelly J. Medical ethics: four principles, two decisions, two roles and no reasons. J Prim Health Care. 2011;3(2):170-4.
5. Nouri K, Trent JT. Lasers. In: Nouri K, Leal-Khouri S (eds). Techniques in Dermatologic Surgery, 1st edition St Louis: Mosby; 2003. pp. 245-58.

CHAPTER 5

Pre- and Postoperative Care in Laser Surgery

Sirisha Singh

INTRODUCTION

Taking adequate precautions in the preoperative and postoperative period will:

- Minimize the side effects and complications associated with laser therapy
- Enhance the effectiveness of the treatment with the potential advantage of higher patient satisfaction.

In general, the higher the risk of complications, the more important it is to ensure a good skin care protocol before and after laser procedure. Therefore, the following situations merit more attention to pre- and postoperative care as they are more likely to result in complications:

- Ablative lasers like carbon dioxide lasers. The fractionated technologies are safer than the non-fractionated technologies
- People with darker skin tones, especially people with Fitzpatrick skin types III-VI. Studies on ablative fractionated lasers have found that the ideal candidates for laser interventions by fractional technologies are Fitzpatrick skin types I-III individuals and side effects develop more readily in individuals with darker skin type[1]
- People with keloidal tendency or a tendency to develop postinflammatory hyperpigmentation (PIH).

PREOPERATIVE CARE

Two to Four Weeks Before the Procedure

Sunscreens

Sun avoidance is mandatory in the preoperative period to minimize the risks of skin burns with lasers. The duration of use of sunscreen is very variable. In the preoperative period, it is important that the skin is not tanned as that increases the risks of laser burns. Most practicing laser physicians will counsel the patient on the use of sunscreen for at least 2–4 weeks before the laser procedure.

Priming of the Skin

The most common side effects seen in Indian skin is post-laser erythema and PIH. The incidence of PIH can be reduced by using tretinoin, hydroquinone, and desonide cream in the pre-and postoperative period.[2] There are no clear guidelines on the duration of priming required but 2–4 weeks may be ideal for ablative lasers in pigmented skin types.

Immediate Preoperative Care

This is the care to be undertaken just before and during the laser procedure to minimize complications while the patient is on the treatment table.

Numbing Gel

Use of a numbing gel like Emla or Prilox can reduce the pain and increase the tolerability of the laser procedure. However, care should be taken in some cases as some lasers like the diode laser and intense pulsed light systems (not truly a laser but a light based device) rely on feedback from the patient about the pain levels. In such systems, if the patient complains of pain, then the settings need to be revisited. It is strongly advised that the doctor read the instruction manual of the laser or light based device being used to avoid complications.

Cooling the Skin

Melanin in the skin is an important chromophore and tends to absorb light energy and hence, the risk of skin burns and pigmentation. Cooling of the skin using ice packs, cool gel packs, or zimmer coolers may reduce the epidermal skin temperature and reduce the risks of burns.

Application of Gels

Application of cool gels helps in moving the handpiece across the skin and helps the physician avoid excessive treatment overlap as the marking of the handpiece can be seen on the gel. This reduces the risk of bulk heating and complications.[3] Some lasers do not need the use of gels, the manual of the laser will state whether or not a gel is to be used and it is strongly recommended that the doctor reads the manual before using the laser device. With some lasers, especially the ablative lasers, one must ensure that the skin to be treated is not cleansed with spirit, the instruction manual will give this instruction and should be followed strictly.

Use of Compression

Compression of the skin while performing the laser helps to reduce purpura and hyperpigmentation.[3] Compression can be carried out using the handpiece. This is particularly true for diode lasers and Q-switched lasers. The laser manual will again state whether or not compression is to be used with a particular device.

POSTOPERATIVE CARE

Immediate Postoperative Care

This is the care to be undertaken soon after the laser procedure has been carried out.

Cooling the Skin

Soon after the laser procedure, the gel should be wiped off gently and the skin cooled using ice, gel pack, or other cooling devices. This cooling helps reduce the erythema and discomfort in the immediate postoperative period. It is suggested that aggressive cooling in the immediate post-treatment period may help reduce the incidence of PIH.[1]

Dressing

This depends upon the laser device used. Nonablative laser devices need application of barrier repair cream such as one containing ceramides. A mild steroid cream may also be used to minimize the postlaser erythema. With ablative lasers an antibiotic cream or a dressing may be applied to keep the wound moist. Studies suggest that the use of a skin barrier repair cream such as one containing ceramides and free fatty acids reduces fluid oozing during the first two postoperative days and allows quick restoration of the skin barrier hence reducing the incidence of wound infections.[4]

Antibiotics

The risk of postlaser infection is quite low. A study involving the use of ablative fractional lasers in a military setup showed that the incidence of infections was less than 1%.[5]

Postoperative Care (2–4 weeks)

The care to be undertaken from the day after the procedure till complete reepithelialization which can take 2–4 weeks depending upon the type of laser, the energy, and the density used.

Sunscreens

They need to be used to minimize the risk of complications like PIH. In the postoperative period, sunscreen needs to be used until the postlaser erythema settles down.[6]

Moisturizers

Ablative lasers cause epidermal denudation. The skin then heals in the post-treatment period by reepithelialization from cutaneous appendages. Maintaining a moist wound is the key prevent Escher development and promote reepithelialization and healing.[7] A barrier repair cream, such as one containing ceramides, may be used in the postoperative period to keep the wound moist. The barrier repair cream may be used 2–3 times a day until complete reepithelialization is seen.[4]

Other Cosmeceuticals

Creams containing steroids, retinol, retinaldehyde, vitamin C, and vitamin K and skin lightening creams containing hydroquinone, kojic acid, and other such ingredients have been used in the postlaser period to minimize the risk of PIH. One or more such cosmeceutical may be used depending upon the individual's skin type, the area treated, and the risk of PIH. The physician may use their discretion based on individual requirement and risk assessment.

CONCLUSION

Pre- and postoperative care is very important when dealing with lasers to minimize risk and maximize efficacy. Attention to pre- and postoperative care also allows us to use optimal settings on the lasers. The care needs to be customized according to the skin type and also the type of laser procedure undertaken. The highest risk is development of PIH in the Indian skin types. Therefore, utmost care must be taken while using ablative lasers on photoexposed skin.

REFERENCES

1. Hwang YJ, Lee YN, Lee YW, Choe YB, Ahn KJ. Treatment of acne scars and wrinkles in asian patients using carbon-dioxide fractional laser resurfacing: its effects on skin biophysical profiles. Ann Dermatol. 2013;25(4):445-53.
2. Alexiades-Armenakas MR, Dover JS, Arndt KA. The spectrum of laser skin resurfacing: nonablative, fractional, and ablative laser resurfacing. J Am Acad Dermatol. 2008;58(5):719-37.
3. Weinstein C, Ramirez O, Pozner J. Postoperative care following carbon dioxide laser resurfacing. Avoiding pitfalls. Dermatol Surg. 1998;24(1):51-6.
4. Ho C, Nguyen Q, Lowe NJ, Griffin ME, Lask G. Laser resurfacing in pigmented skin. Dermatol Surg. 1995;21(12):1035-7.
5. Kono T, Groff WF, Chan HH, Sakurai H, Nozaki M. Comparison study of a Q-switched alexandrite laser delivered with versus without compression in the treatment of dermal pigmented lesions. J Cosmet Laser Ther. 2007;9(4):206-9.
6. Mortensen JT, Bjerring P, Cramers M. Locobase repair cream following CO2 laser resurfacing reduces interstitial fluid oozing. J Cosmet Laser Ther. 2001;3(3):155-8.
7. Anderson RR, Donelan MB, Hivnor C, Greeson E, Ross EV, Shumaker PR, et al. Laser treatment of traumatic scars with an emphasis on ablative fractional laser resurfacing: consensus report. JAMA Dermatol. 2014;150(2):187-93.

CHAPTER 6

Anesthesia in Laser Practice

Sunaina Hameed, Warren B Seiler III

INTRODUCTION

Anesthesia in its many forms is critical to patient comfort and overall treatment experience and satisfaction. Proper and safe anesthesia also promotes the treating physician/surgeon's procedure efficacy. This efficacy comes in being able to perform a proper strength procedure if the patient is adequately anesthetized. This chapter will describe the basic as well as the more advanced applications and techniques of anesthesia used in today's laser and light/energy-based procedures. This will include both outpatient and inpatient procedures. Pictures and videos have been included to demonstrate advanced applications and techniques.

DEFINITION

The literal meaning of anesthesia is "lack of sensation". While local anesthetics (LAs) block pain sensation to the area localized to application or infiltration, general anesthetic drugs lead to loss of pain, touch, vibration, and temperature sensations along with a reversible loss of consciousness.

MECHANISM OF LOCAL ANESTHETIC ACTION

Local anesthetic drugs diffuse across the neural membrane and bind to the intracellular receptors. They work by blocking nerve depolarization while interfering with the influx of Na^+ ions. This inhibits nerve impulse conduction as the action potential of the nerve fails to reach threshold levels. Small fibers are blocked first. Therefore, autonomic fibers are blocked first, followed by sensory fibers conducting temperature and pain, and finally those transmitting touch, pressure, and vibration. Recovery of function occurs in the reverse order.[1] However, the myelinated A fibers which carry the pain sensation are more sensitive to the actions of LAs. Hence, patients can continue to appreciate sensation of pressure and vibration while being insensitive to pain.

CLASSIFICATION OF LOCAL ANESTHETIC AGENTS

The molecular structure of LAs consists of three components: an aromatic ring, an intermediate chain and an amine group (Fig. 1). The aromatic ring is lipophilic and the lipophilicity is directly proportional to the potency of the anesthetic. The intermediate chain connects the aromatic and amine components and determines the classification of the drug as ester or amide:

- Esters include procaine (available in 0.5, 1, and 2%) and tetracaine (available in 0.1 and 0.25%)
- Amides include lidocaine (0.5, 1, and 2%), mepivicaine (1 and 2%), bupivicaine (0.25, 0.5, and 0.75%) and etidocaine (0.5 and 1%). One can remember these as amides because each has an extra "i" in the name like the "i" in "amide" as opposed to the word "ester" not containing an "i" in the word

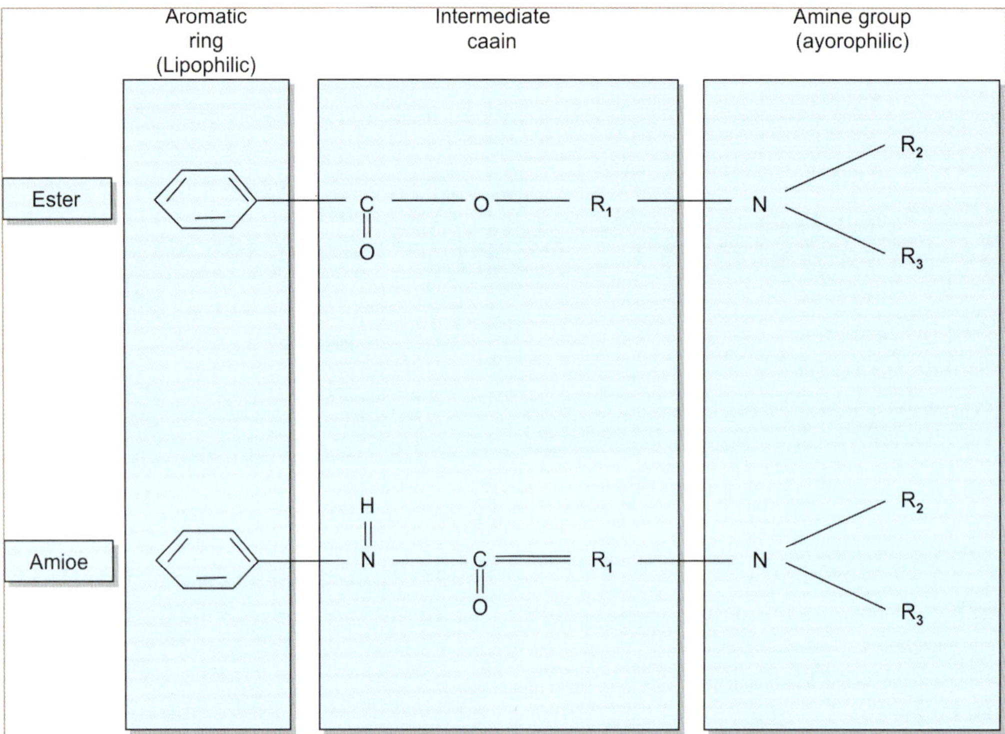

FIG. 1: Basic structure of local anesthetic drugs

- Esters are rapidly hydrolyzed by plasma cholinesterases and excreted in the urine. They form para-aminobenzoic acid, which is allergenic
- Amides are metabolized by microsomal enzymes in the liver, and are less allergenic
- Lidocaine and procaine are rapid-acting and have a short duration of anesthesia. Tetracaine is slow-acting but has a longer duration of anesthesia. Tetracaine has been associated with potential toxicity and can cause a local erythema reaction when used topically in numbing creams/gels.

PATIENT EVALUATION

- History of allergy to lidocaine or any other LA
- Pregnancy [eutectic mixture of local anesthetics (EMLA) and lidocaine is category B]
- Medical history—rule out hypertension, epilepsy, hepatic illness, methemoglobinemia, paroxysmal supraventricular tachycardia (PSVT), glucose-6-phosphate dehydrogenase (G6PD) deficiency, etc.
- Drug history including substance abuse
- Intradermal testing for infiltrative anesthesia, which must be specifically mentioned in the informed consent form.

COMBINING EPINEPHRINE WITH ANESTHETIC DRUG

All LA agents increase vasodilation, resulting in enhanced drug elimination, leading to shorter duration of action. Hence, combining vasoconstrictors like epinephrine leads to decreased absorption, decreased systemic toxicity, longer duration of action, and reduced bleeding at the operative site. Epinephrine is usually incorporated in an extremely diluted form (1:100,000) which maintains drug efficacy while eliminating the risk of tissue necrosis.

Absolute Contraindications

Uncontrolled hypertension, hyperthyroidism, ischemic heart disease, PSVT, Raynaud's disease, and other peripheral vascular disease and pheochromocytoma.

Relative Contraindications

Mental illnesses (adrenaline can precipitate acute psychosis), pregnancy (induces preterm labor), use of β-blocking drugs, sites like digits, lips, nose and penis (areas with endarterial supply), and skin grafting procedures (vasoconstriction leads to ischemia, and delayed rebound bleeding uplifts the graft).[1]

TECHNIQUES TO ADMINISTER ANESTHESIA IN LASER PROCEDURES

These are broadly categorized as topical anesthesia, injectable anesthesia, and supervised anesthesia

Topical Anesthesia (Noninvasive Anesthesia)

Topical anesthesia is the surface application of a LA to the skin or mucous membrane by means of a cream or refrigerant sprays.

Indications

It allows laser ablation of small benign growths and superficial laser surgeries (resurfacing, rejuvenation, pigmentary lasers, pulsed dye laser), and allows painless insertion of the needle.

Depending on the agent used, the product is left in place for 30–60 minutes or longer depending on desired depth of effect (determined by depth of potential laser treatment). Occlusion using plastic wraps or Tegaderm dressing enhances cutaneous drug absorption. However, one must be knowledgeable of maximum allowable body surface area (BSA) to be covered so as to avoid toxicity and systemic absorption. Occlusion versus open application should include the consideration of this maximum applicable BSA. Complete removal of residual cream with cosmetic toner is important before laser procedures, especially with alcohol containing topical anesthetics because of their incendiary and combustible potential.[2] Liposomal encapsulation is another technology that facilitates percutaneous drug delivery. This also protects the drug from metabolic degradation, allowing prolonged duration of action.[3]

Topical creams are available as:

- Eutectic mixture of local anesthetics (EMLA): eutectic mixtures allow individual anesthetic compounds, which are normally in the solid state at room temperature, to be combined as liquids.[3] It facilitates application to the skin and allows higher concentrations of anesthetics to be used safely

  Eutectic mixture of local anesthetics cream is a 5% mixture of 25 mg/mL lidocaine and 25 mg/mL prilocaine in an oil-in-water emulsion cream.

  At sites with thin or absent stratum corneum (the eyelids, penis, mucosae), EMLA is more readily absorbed and anesthesia is achieved in a short duration of time. At other sites, analgesia is achieved to a depth of 3 mm after 60 minutes of application and a maximum dermal depth of 5 mm is reached after 120 minutes of application.[3]

  After application to skin, EMLA produces a biphasic response with initial vasoconstriction and blanching that peaks after 90 minutes of application and a rebound vasodilatation after 2–3 hours. It is recommended to advise the patient of this effect (and its visual consequences)
- Lidocaine: brand names include Ela-Max (4–5% lidocaine in liposomal delivery system) and Topicaine (4% lidocaine)
- Tetracaine: brand names include Tetracaine gel and Amethocaine (both contain 4% tetracaine)
- Betacaine: this ointment contains lidocaine, prilocaine, dibucaine, and a vasoconstrictor (phenylephrine), compounded into a petrolatum base.[4] The exact concentration of its ingredients are a trade secret and it is not advocated for use in children. It is not approved by Food and Drug Administration
- S-Caine peel and S- Caine patch: the peel is novel eutectic mixture of 7% lidocaine and 7% tetracaine in a cream base. After application, the cream dries in 30 minutes to form a flexible film that fixes the anesthetic into position. Distribution was finally terminated because of an inability to obtain consistent product viscosity.[3] The S-Caine patch contains a 1:1 eutectic mixture of lidocaine and tetracaine base with a disposable, oxygen-activated heating element. When the patch is applied to the skin, it increases local skin temperature by 5°C. The mean depth of analgesia has been measured to at least 6.8 mm.[5]

Advantages

It provides a safe and effective means of anesthesia in needle-phobic patients or those with multiple lesions (like double-pointed needles), where infiltration anesthesia of individual lesions is not practical.

Disadvantages

Erythema, blanching, and edema are the most commonly observed local reactions. The milk:plasma ratio of lidocaine is 1:4, so caution must be exercised in nursing mothers.[3] Prilocaine can cause contact urticaria and allergic contact dermatitis.[6] Vascular lesions must be marked before application of EMLA as the cream produces local blanching. Other disadvantages include postinflammatory hyperpigmentation and short duration of action. Accidental eye exposure can result in severe corneal irritation.

Eutectic mixture of local anesthetics may have to be supplemented with oral analgesics, oral diazepam, nerve blocks, or intravenous sedation to maximize patient comfort during full face carbon dioxide laser resurfacing and other more aggressive treatments.

Special Delivery Techniques for Topical Anesthesia

These include iontophoresis (small low voltage and continuous constant current) and use of fractional ablative lasers like erbium doped:yttrium-aluminium-garnet to enhance penetration and absorption of lidocaine by disrupting the stratum corneum.[7] Needleless Dermojet®, electroporation (short duration high voltage current), and sonoporation (low frequency ultrasound) have also been tried. All of these techniques must be incorporated only after evaluation of their potential side effects and resulting change in laser application, efficacy, and safety. Simple strategies like tape stripping and degreasing with acetone can also enhance percutaneous drug absorption.

Complications and Adverse Events

Prolonged application, use of inappropriately high concentrations, use on damaged or inflamed skin, and application to and/or occlusion of large surface areas (2,000 cm^2 or more) increases the risk of cardiotoxicity (bradycardia and hypotension) and central nervous system (CNS) toxicity[3] (Table 1). The CNS is generally more susceptible to pharmacological actions of LAs.

Methemoglobinemia from prilocaine is another dreaded complication. Prilocaine can oxidize the iron in red blood cells from the ferrous to the ferric state, impairing oxygen transportation by hemoglobin. Patient presents with cyanosis when blood levels reach 15–30%. When the levels reach 30–50%, it results in dyspnea, tachycardia, and headache, and levels greater than 50% are associated with lethargy and coma.[3]

Avoid topical anesthetics on eroded skin, in neonates, and those with hepatic failure. It is also not recommended to dispense any of the topical numbing agents to the patient to take home and apply before coming in for a treatment. Topical anesthetic should always be administered by a trained practitioner in a medical/surgical setting.

TABLE 1: Signs and symptoms of lidocaine toxicity[3]

Blood lidocaine levels, (µg/mL)	Signs and symptoms
1–5	Tinnitus, lightheadedness, circumoral numbness, diplopia, metallic taste in mouth
5–8	Nystagmus, slurred speech, localized muscle twitching, fine tremors
8–12	Focal seizure activity, which may progress to tonic-clonic seizures
20–25	Respiratory depression which can lead to coma

Injected Anesthesia

Advantages

- Ease of administration
- Rapid onset of action
- Stronger and more profound effect for deeper laser treatments
- Longer duration of anesthesia.

Disadvantages

- One of the major disadvantages is patient anxiety due to use of needles, especially among needle-phobic patients
- When large volumes of anesthetic are needed, it can cause tissue distortion, which is desirable in some cases (full face laser resurfacing) and undesirable in other cases
- Nerve blocks require considerable practice and experience to avoid neurapraxia. Neurapraxia is nerve injury leading to temporary loss of motor and sensory function due to blockages of nerve conduction, generally lasting an average of 6–8 weeks before complete recovery. Although rare, permanent loss of function is possible
- Other complications include bruising, vasovagal syncope, and CNS complications related to lidocaine toxicity from drug overdose.

Infiltrative Anesthesia

Lidocaine with or without epinephrine is the most commonly used drug in this technique. Sodium bicarbonate (lidocaine:bicarbonate ratio is 10:1) may be added to reduce the acidity of the lidocaine and, therefore, make for a more comfortable injection for the patient. Local anesthesia is injected intradermally and/or subcutaneously. Intradermal injections are more painful but have a rapid onset of action in comparison to subcutaneous infiltration. Gentle massage postinjection will hasten the onset of action. Always aspirate prior to injecting to confirm that the needle tip has not entered a vessel. Use epinephrine unless contraindicated and warn the patient of potential visual blanching of the skin for several hours after injection. Lidocaine and its metabolites are excreted through the kidneys.

Indications

Laser ablation, vaporization or excision of benign skin tumors, large warts, various keratosis and precancerous lesions, small basal cell carcinomas, xanthelasmas, rhinophyma, neurofibromas, and large acrochordons.[8]

Complications with Infiltrative Anesthesia

With lidocaine

Systemic complications are similar to complications with topical lidocaine (previously mentioned).

Local reactions include pain, bruising, infection and abscess, contact dermatitis, and paresthesia.

With epinephrine

Systemic complications include palpitations, hypertension, chest pain, angina, arrhythmias, excitation, tremors, anxiety, and headaches.

Local reactions include pain, tissue necrosis (from severe and prolonged vasoconstriction), delayed/rebound bleeding, delayed wound healing, and rejection of grafts.

Techniques used with Infiltrative Anesthesia

There are a few variations and extensions in injection techniques using infiltrative anesthesia, based on indications and site of treatment. These include:

Field block

This is a technique where the entire operative field is anesthetized by injecting circumferentially around the site to be treated so that no nerve impulse can escape the surgical field.[1] The injection is given both intradermally and subcutaneously. Anesthesia can be achieved with smaller amount of drug but onset of action is delayed. It can be used for laser excision of larger tumors or laser-assisted narrow-hole extrusion of cysts. This technique is of particular advantage when a large area needs to be anesthetized, as it limits the amount of LA needed.

Digital nerve block

this is the commonly performed nerve block used in any laser surgeries involving the digits (laser ablation of multiple verrucae, laser treatment of onychomycosis, and laser removal of pyogenic granuloma on the digit). The anesthetic is injected around the two dorsal and two ventral branches of the nerves innervating each digit. It is usually recommended to exclude the incorporation of adrenaline in these injections.

The fingers are supplied by the radial and ulnar nerve on dorsal surface, and median and ulnar nerve on palmar surface.

The toes are supplied by peroneal nerve on dorsal surface and tibial nerve on plantar surface.

There are two techniques of achieving a digital block—ring block technique and metacarpal or metatarsal head technique. Ring block is more commonly used in day-to-day practice.

1. Ring block: 0.5–1 mL of LA (without epinephrine) is injected using a 26 G 0.5 inch needle at the dorsolateral margin of the desired digit at the level of webspace. The needle is advanced further across the dorsal aspect of the digit and LA is injected in superficial (subcutaneous) and then deep plane (periosteum). Aspiration to avoid vessel insertion is recommended. It is then withdrawn up to the insertion point and rerouted along the palmar surface in a similar manner and after depositing 0.5–1 mL, the needle is completely removed. The hand is turned over and needle inserted at the palmar medial surface at level of webspace of the same digit. It is pushed across laterally and solution injected, withdrawn to insertion point, and redirected medially to complete the block.[1] Another technique is the serial puncture use of four injections straight into the skin down to the periosteum with small but sufficient bolus injections (after aspiration). This generally allows enough anesthetic to be introduced without too many injection points or needle movement for infiltration and thus making the experience more tolerable for the patient. Occasionally, in the apprehensive patient, topical anesthetic may be applied first to decrease the pain of needle insertion.

2. Metacarpal or metatarsal head techniques: Here, the nerves are anesthetized before they enter the digit. The needle is introduced in the space between the heads of metacarpals/metatarsals, proximal to the webspace and perpendicular to skin. It is advanced in a similar direction towards the palmar/plantar aspect of hand/foot, till it reaches the subcutaneous level.[1]

Local anesthetic is used without epinephrine as the digits are supplied by terminal arteries. The volume injected to produce block should not exceed 8 mL as larger volume can produce mechanical compression on the vessels leading to ischemia and digital necrosis.

Disadvantages of digital nerve block techniques

Ring block carries more risk of nerve damage and paresthesia. The metacarpal/metatarsal head technique is more painful and has a slower onset of action. These techniques require some amount of practice and experience, without which anesthesia may fail or be incomplete.

There is a higher risk of vascular injury and vascular compression as each nerve is generally accompanied by a vessel. This can result in hematoma, ischemia and systemic toxicity.

Temporary paralysis, needle breakage, and periostitis (from periosteal injury) are other rarer complications.

Peripheral nerve block

A nerve block involves placing LA at and around the main trunk of a peripheral nerve, to block nerve impulses along the nerve trunk rather than at the level of terminal nerve endings.

Indications

Full face anesthesia for carbon dioxide laser ablative resurfacing, laser surgeries on the penis (penile block), e.g., ablation of pearly penile papules, ankle block (laser ablation of multiple mosaic warts), etc.

Large areas can be anesthetized using a small amount of LA without any distortion of the surgical site and the surgeon can enjoy a longer duration of anesthetic action.

A set of the seven blocks can anesthetize the entire face.[9]

Infraorbital nerve

The infraorbital foramen is located on a line dropped from the medial limbus of the iris. If the patient stares straight ahead, the infraorbital foramen is located 4–7 mm below the orbital rim on that line. The alveolar branch of the infraorbital nerve supplies sensation to the anterior gingival and maxillary teeth. This nerve, usually visible by tilting up the mucosa superior to the canine teeth (pulling up the lip) can be blocked using the perpendicular transcutaneous route or an intraoral technique. With your left index finger on the infraorbital rim, ask the patient to look straight ahead. Holding the syringe like a pen, advance the needle in a perpendicular direction to bone toward the designated point about 4–7 mm down from the rim (Fig. 2). It is advisable to use a 28 G 1.5 inch needle and inject 1–2 mL of LA.

Depending on the physician's comfort, the transcutaneous (intraoral) route may be used and can be equally effective when performed correctly. This route may also avoid the superficial swelling, blanching and/or bleeding sometimes accompanied by the transcutaneous route. To perform this anesthesia, elevate the lip and insert a 1 inch 30 G needle in the vestibular sulcus between the canine and the first premolar tooth, and direct superiorly toward the infraorbital foramen (Fig. 3). Usually, a small bleb of anesthetic is injected immediately upon mucosal

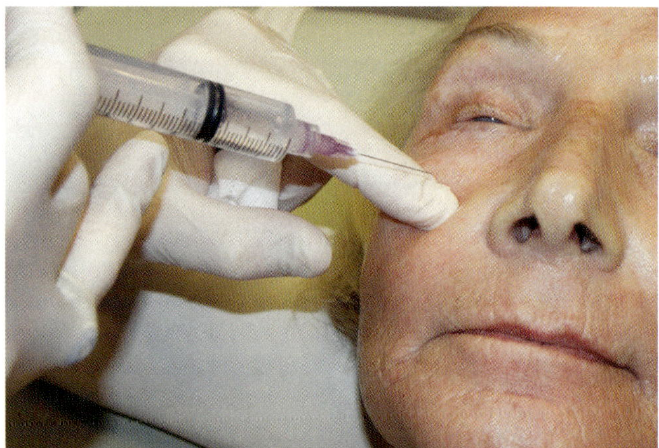

FIG. 2: Position for percutaneous infraorbital nerve block

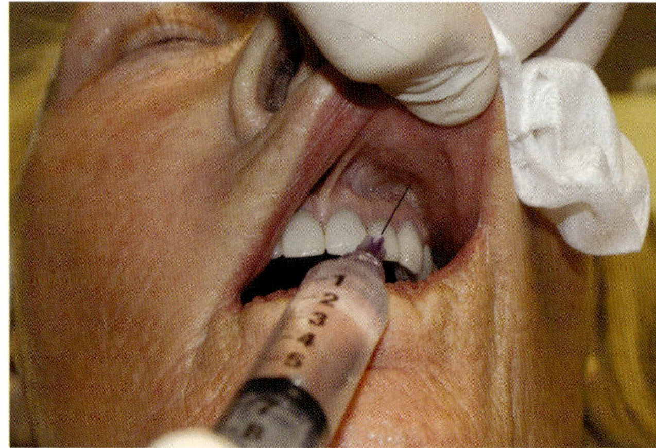

FIG. 3: Intraoral alveolar to infraorbital nerve block for upper lip, anteromedial cheek and lower eyelid

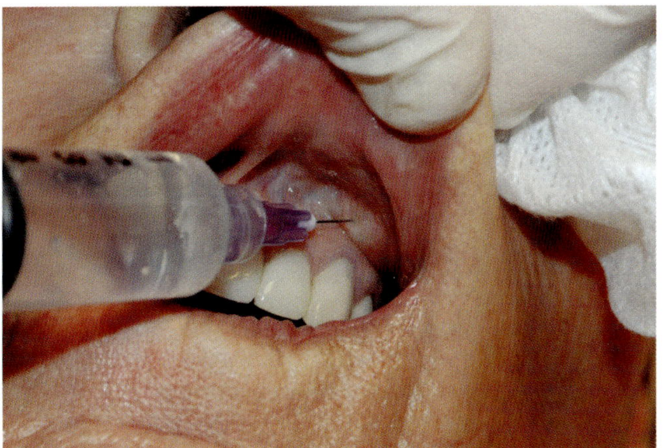

FIG. 4: Intraoral approach to infraorbital nerve block and extended "field" block for upper and lateral cheek

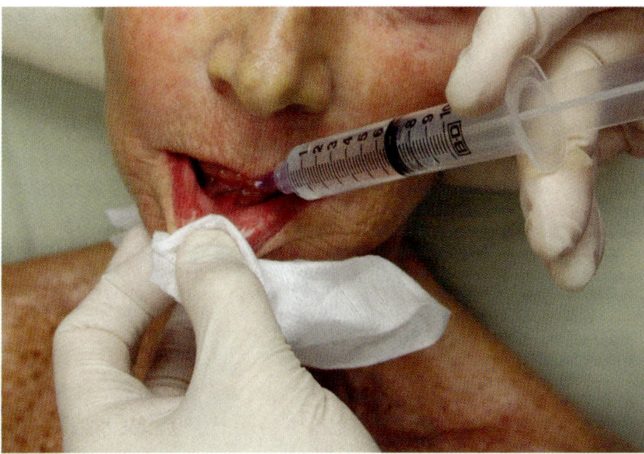

FIG. 5: Intraoral mental nerve block for chin and lower jaw

puncture to anesthetize the alveolar branch. Then, use the nondominant hand to palpate the infraorbital rim to avoid injecting superior to the orbit.[10] Inject 2–4 mL of anesthetic and feel the bolus below the infraorbital nerve to confirm the correct placement. Proper technique includes aiming the needle towards the infraorbital rim once in the mucosa (tilting the hand up so as to infiltrate deeper as opposed to staying more superficial by "riding" teeth and gums instead of tilting the syringe up and needle down). If the transoral approach does not provide complete anesthesia then one may add more anesthetic from the transcutaneous approach directly towards the infraorbital foramen. Additional "field block" can be added through the transoral approach by infiltrating and injecting in a fanning direction laterally towards the cheek and ear (Fig. 4).

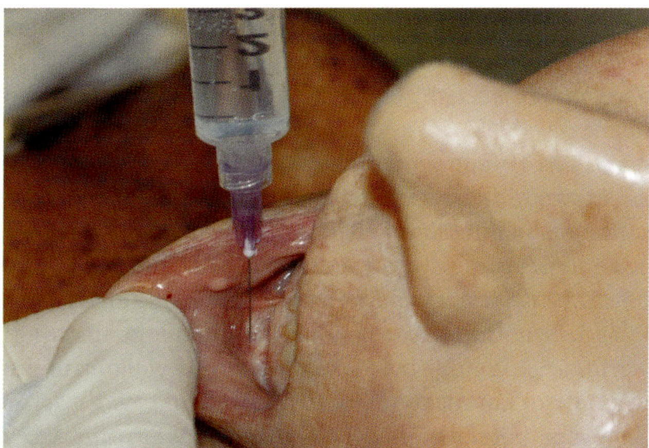

FIG. 6: Intraoral mental nerve block and extended chin/lateral jaw "field" block

Areas of anesthesia: nose, cheek, lip, and lower eyelid.

Mental nerve

The mental nerve usually exits from a foramen below the apex of the second bicuspid. The variability of this foramen is 6–10 mm anterior or 6–10 mm posterior to this point. One can usually palpate the mandibular flare or bony prominence of the lower jaw where the foramen should be located. After exiting from the foramen, it divides into two to three branches. These branches provide sensation to the lip and the skin of the chin. The mental nerve can be submucosally blocked at the mental foramen or a few centimeters after it leaves the foramen. To block it at the foramen, locate the second lower bicuspid. Use the thumb of one hand to pull out the lower lip, lateral to the lower canine tooth. The nerve is visible submucosally about 85% of the time.[9] Place the needle tip vertically down in the buccal sulcus, near the base of the second premolar tooth, and inject 2–4 mL[10] (Figs 5 and 6). Even if the foramen is not directly injected, bolus anesthesia in the area is usually sufficient for effect.

Alternatively, the mental nerve can also be blocked using a transcutaneous approach, although this is not recommended due to patient discomfort.

Area of anesthesia: this injection only anesthetizes the lower lip down to the chin.

Supraorbital, supratrochlear, and infratrochlear nerves

The supraorbital notch, rarely the foramen, is easily palpable at the supraorbital rim just above the medial limbus. The supraorbital nerve arising from it supplies the forehead. The supratrochlear nerve supplies sensation to the midforehead. It can be found under the medial centimeter of the eyebrow. The infratrochlear nerve is a branch of the nasociliary that runs along the medial orbital wall and leaves the orbit below the trochlea to supply the skin in the medial eyelids, the side of the nose above the medial canthus, the conjunctiva and lacrimal apparatus.[11]

The block is performed by injecting along the supraorbital rim from lateral to medial. Stretch the eyebrow laterally and pierce the lateral part of the middle-third of the eyebrow. Aim the needle at the supraorbital notch (which is palpable) (Fig. 7). After injecting 1–2 cc prior to the notch under the muscle, the needle moves medially about 10 mm along the rim and another 1 cc is deposited at the supratrochlear notch (which is not palpable) (Fig. 8). An additional 1 cc is deposited as the needle advances toward and touches the nasal bones.[9] Alternatively, separate injections may be used for each nerve.

Areas of anesthesia: forehead, the upper eyelid, and a few millimeter of the frontoparietal scalp.

Zygomaticotemporal nerve

This nerve is a terminal branch of the zygomatic nerve. It emerges through a foramen which is posterior to the zygoma on the lateral orbital rim, around 1 cm below the level of the lateral canthus.[9] From behind the patient, a27 G 1.5 inch needle must be inserted behind the concave portion of the lateral orbital rim (Fig. 9). This is about 10–12 mm behind and just below the zygomaticofrontal suture (which is palpable).[11]

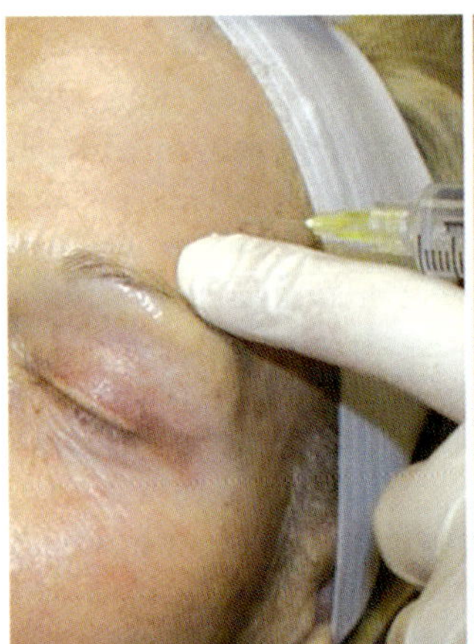
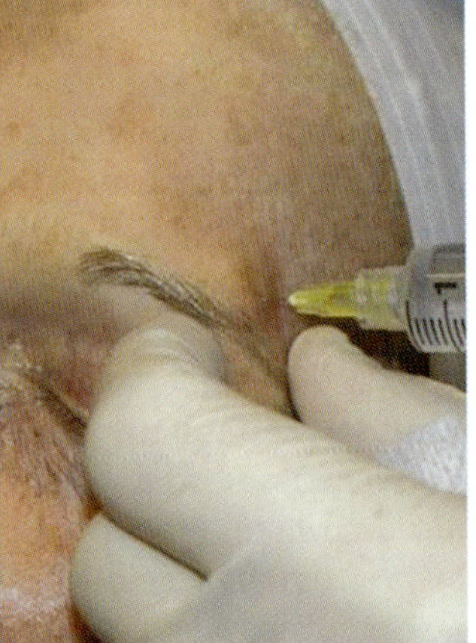

FIG. 7: Supraorbital nerve block for brow, eyelid and lower forehead anesthesia

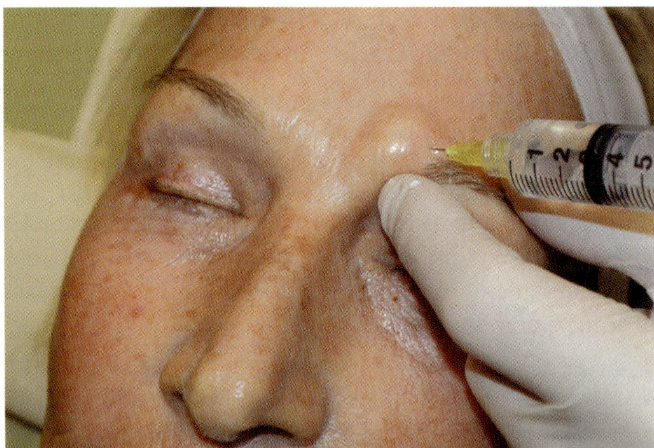

FIG. 8: : Supratrochlear nerve block for medial brow, medial upper eyelid and lower medial forehead anesthesia

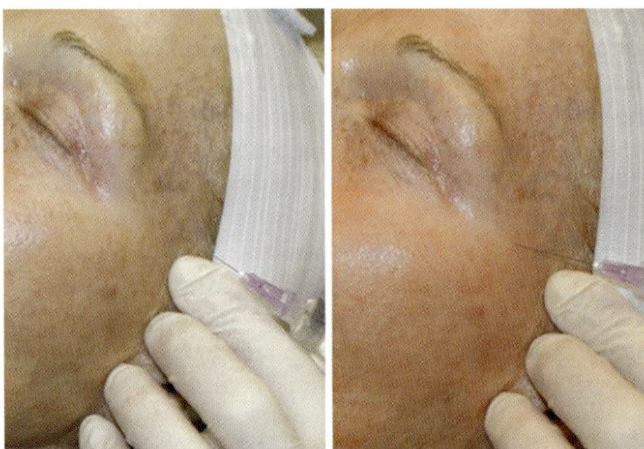

FIG. 9: Position for zygomatic nerve block and lateral temple "field" block

Area of anesthesia: this nerve provides sensory innervation to a fan-shaped area posterior to the lateral orbital rim extending into the hair.

Zygomaticofacial nerve

This nerve exits through a foramen in the inferior lateral portion of the lateral orbital rim at the zygoma. By palpating the portion and injecting just lateral to the palpating finger with 1–2 mL of LA, this nerve is successfully blocked (Fig. 9).

Area of anesthesia: The zygomaticofacial block is always done right after the zygomaticotemporal block.[9] The anesthesia is achieved in a triangular area on the cheek prominence.

Disadvantages: Requires greater level of skill and experience, difficult to perform, and higher risk of more serious complications like nerve injury, neurapraxia and blood vessel cannulation/damage.

Tumescent anesthesia

Tumescent anesthesia is a specialized form of injected anesthesia that involves the infiltration of large volumes of dilute anesthetic solutions with lidocaine into the subcutaneous fat compartment over a large area, resulting in the bulging of targeted areas.[12] Using this technique, larger volumes of lidocaine, even up to 45–55 mg/kg weight can be administered safely.[13] This is due to the poor vasculature of subcutaneous tissue and addition of epinephrine to the solution. The large volume of tumescent solution compresses blood vessels, leading to further limitation of systemic absorption. Hence the rate of absorption of lidocaine is slow, leading to slower peak values and therefore less chance of toxicity.[13]

Composition of solution

- Normal saline 1,000 cc
- Lidocaine (2%) 50 cc
- Epinephrine (1:1000) 1 cc
- Sodium bicarbonate (8.4%) 10 cc.

Effective concentration of lidocaine is 0.1%, which is safe up to 55 mg/kg as per the American Academy of Dermatology guidelines of care for liposuction.

Indications

Tumescent anesthesia of face for ablative resurfacing, laser correction of rhinophyma, laser-assisted endovenous ablation of varicose veins, and laser-assisted or power-assisted liposuction. In laser resurfacing, nerve blocks are often combined with a "horseshoe" shaped tumescent block on each side of the face, beginning at the temporal hair line and extending sequentially to the preauricular area, jaw, and chin.[13]

Advantages

- Injection is nearly painless, as it is placed in the lax tissue of the subcutaneous compartment
- Ballooning up and stretching of the skin, provides a cushioning effect to deeper structures, so less chance of damage
- Hemostasis due to compression of subcutaneous vasculature by large volume of anesthetic solution
- Hydrodissection of the subcutaneous layer, which provides a safer plane for tissue dissection
- Smaller amount of LA needed, hence lower risk of systemic toxicity
- Prolonged duration of action as a result of reservoir effect of LA
- Adrenaline in the solution increases the duration of action, while sodium bicarbonate helps to adjust the pH of the solution to a level close to that of tissue fluid (reducing tissue irritation and pain)
- Elimination of general anesthesia, hence lower cost of surgery and better safety
- No need for infusion pumps
- Postanesthesia recovery is immediate and anesthetic effect lasts for several hours postoperatively.

Disadvantages

Delayed onset of action (10–15 minutes), and a time consuming process (which increases procedure time) requiring multiple needle pricks.[12] One must also be careful not to increase the water content in the dermis by infiltrating too superficially. This would change the skin's physiology by increasing the water content and, therefore, the reaction to ablative (water-targeting) lasers.

Regional anesthesia

This includes instillation of LA in a region of the body,[1] e.g., spinal anesthesia, epidural analgesia, penile block, axillary block, cervical plexus block, etc. This can be used for laser ablation of large condyloma acuminata and pearly penile papules. Onset of action is in 5–20 minutes and the anesthesia lasts from 150–240 minutes.

Conscious Sedation (Supervised Anesthesia)

Many patients fear undergoing procedures with only local anesthesia due to perceived pain and conscious awareness during surgery. Conscious sedation allows the optimization of patient comfort and physician efficacy. Conscious sedation is defined as a medically controlled state of depressed consciousness that: (i) allows protective reflexes to be maintained; (ii) retains the patient's ability to maintain a patent airway continuously; and (iii) permits appropriate responses by the patient to physical stimulation or verbal command.[14] Recovery from conscious sedation is rapid (3–7 minutes after discontinuation of anesthetic) with minimal confusion.[14]

The Ramsey Sedation Scale is used to determine the level of sedation. Level 2–3 is appropriate for an office procedure, as the patient is cooperative and able to respond to commands. Level 5–6 constitute the onset of general anesthesia.[12]

The office should be equipped with the following (some countries require facility certification and practitioner certification and registration for anesthesia permission):

- Portable oxygen tanks
- Suction sources
- Emergency cardiac medications (atropine, epinephrine, dopamine, diazepam, naloxone, hydrocortisone, succinylcholine, aminophylline)
- Nasal oxygen cannulas
- Ambubag
- Oral and nasal airways
- Endotracheal tubes
- Laryngoscope
- Continuous pulse oximeter
- Electrocardiogram
- Sphygmomanometer
- Temperature monitor
- Intravenous access.

The facility must also have hospital transport mechanisms in place with written protocols and algorithms for all staff and procedures (general and emergency).[12] Extreme caution must be used with the use of oxygen during laser procedures to avoid the danger of ignition.

Drugs Used in Conscious Sedation

Midazolam

It is used at a dose of 0.05–0.075 µg/kg. It has a rapid onset of action is an anxiolytic and induces sedation and amnesia. It may cause vomiting and respiratory arrest at high dosage, which can be reversed with intravenous Flumazenil.

Fentanyl

It is used at a dose of 1–2 µg/kg. It is hundred times more potent than morphine and is highly lipophilic. Peak analgesic effect is reached in 2–3 minutes of intravenous injection. It can cause "tight chest syndrome" and bradycardia at high doses which can be reversed with naloxone.[15]

Propofol

It is used at a dose of 25–50 µg/kg/min. Propofol is a sedative hypnotic with a half-life of 2–8 minutes. It offers the benefit of a clear head postoperatively. Adverse effects include painful injection, apnea and hypoxemia. It does not contain preservatives and has soybean oil, egg lecithin, and glycerol, so strict asepsis must be maintained.

Methohexital

It was used prior to propofol but is less analgesic and causes nausea more often.

Ketamine

It is a good agent when used in small doses (<1 mg/kg) in combination with diazepam and/or propofol. Adverse effects include dysphoria and hallucinations.

Diazepam and Meperidine

They are older agents, generally used in conjunction with each other and more commonly used for less/lighter sedation.

Oral Sedation

There are many forms of mild-to-moderate oral sedation. In this segment, the basic guidelines will be provided but details of dosing and such are beyond the scope of this chapter. The following are recommendations:

- Oral sedation typically comes through anxiolytics such as benzodiazepines, analgesics such as hydrocodone/oxycodone or demerol, and antinausea through phenergan or zofran
- Individual prescriptions to each unique patient should be given and have the patient fill them and bring the medicines with them to the treatment. This allows one to be FDA/DEA compliant and keeps the practitioner from the legal risk and requirements of dispensing medication
- You may recommend having them take small doses before arriving to the treatment as they will need a driver to take them to and fro from the treatment
- Additional doses can then be given in the office/clinic under supervision (usually while topical numbing agents are setting in)
- Certain medications like Fentanyl, Halcion, and Phenergan can be compounded in low doses into an oral lollipop or lozenge, given under direct supervision
- Although monitoring the patient is usually not necessary, it is sometimes recommended to use a pulse oximeter and/or cardiac monitor depending on the level of expected sedation
- The supervising practitioner should be knowledgeable of the medications, uses, complications and what do to in the case of over-sedation (including having

Naloxone and Flumazenil available) and access to emergency medical help

- A thorough preoperative evaluation should be obtained before prescribing and/or administering these medications (such as anesthesia/medical/cardiac/renal/hepatic history, availability of a ride to and from the treatment, etc.)
- Although there are risks with these medications, their use can greatly ease the patient's pain and anxiety and therefore allow for a more thorough, safe and effective treatment and better overall patient experience.

Finally, the most invasive and risky form of anesthesia is "general anesthesia with endotracheal intubation". It allows for quickly administered airway control and allows the administration of adequate narcotic without concern for respiratory depression.[15] Disadvantages include increased number of equipment and trained personnel, increased level of care and facilities required, and increased cost of treatment. The patient is also at risk of malignant hypertension from inhaled halogenated anesthetics.[14]

USE OF ANESTHESIA FOR LASER PROCEDURES IN CHILDREN

Indications

Laser ablation of verruca, molluscum, laser treatment of vascular lesions and nevi, and "prenumbing" prior to lidocaine injection.

The use of EMLA in neonates, infants, and children has been associated with complications like allergic contact dermatitis, eye irritation, purpura, petechia, and methemoglobinemia (especially in those with G6PD deficiency with use of topical Prilocaine). In view of these risks and its uncertain efficacy, EMLA is best avoided in children less than 3 months of age (Table 2).

The usual lidocaine concentration used in pediatric patients is a 1% solution (10 mg/mL). The maximum pediatric dose of lidocaine without epinephrine is 5 mg/kg (0.5 mL of 1% lidocaine/kg). The maximum recommended dose of 1% lidocaine with epinephrine is 7 mg/kg (0.7 mL of 1% lidocaine/kg).[16]

Acetaminophen and codeine has been used for perioperative analgesia.[16] For conscious sedation, Midazolam is used as the retrograde amnesia it induces is particularly useful in children who may need repeated sessions of laser treatments. Ketamine may cause nightmares and hallucinations in children and this must be taken into consideration when choosing a sedative.[16]

TABLE 2: Dosage of eutectic mixture of local anesthetics in pediatric patients[12]

Age and weight	Maximum total dose and time	Maximum application area (in cm^2)
1–3 months or less than 5 kg	1 g (1 h)	10
4–12 months and more than 5 kg	2 g (1 h)	20
1–6 years and more than 10 kg	10 g (1 h)	100
7–12 years and more than 20 kg	20 g (1 h)	200

In conclusion, disposition, maturity, gender, and stage of development often dictate the type of anesthesia that is indicated for various cutaneous laser surgeries performed on children.[16]

NONPHARMACOLOGICAL ANESTHESIA

Talkesthesia and Hypnosis

Holding the patient's hand with or without gentle stroking, keeping the patient engaged in conversion as a diversionary tactic, soothing verbal and tactile reinforcement from doctor, and (in some cases) a loved one can increase the patient's pain tolerance.

Vibration Anesthesia

A vibratory massager is used for 2–3 seconds prior to injection or laser firing and continued throughout the procedure. The mechanism can be explained by "gate theory of pain control", according to which, simultaneous and continuous vibratory stimulation excites large A fibers, which activates inhibitory interneurons at the gate and mitigates the perception of pain in the brain.

Cooling Techniques

Spray (cryoanesthesia) and contact cooling are the two most popular methods used in photoepilation, laser skin rejuvenation, and treatment of vascular lesions. The cooling process should ideally be nonstationary and dynamic in character.[17] Further details on precooling, parallel cooling, and postcooling will be covered in subsequent chapters. One must consider the possibility of "overcooling" the target with these methods, so efficacy could be affected.

GUIDELINES TO AVOID COMPLICATIONS

Hypersensitivity reactions can be potentially lethal although true allergic reactions to LA are rare and vasovagal syncopal attacks are often mistakenly considered as hypersensitivity reactions.[13]

Sensitivity to LA can be either type I (anaphylaxis) or type IV (delayed hypersensitivity).

Skin testing with topical anesthetic cream using a patch test is not recommended as routine in all cases. However, it can be performed by applying a 1–2 mm thick layer of EMLA over 1 cm^2 area for 30 minutes and checking for itching or rash.[13]

Intradermal testing on the other hand is mandatory in all first-time cases. This is performed by injecting 0.1 mL of lidocaine on flexural forearm about 1–2 inches below the antecubital fossa. Appearance of itching, erythema, or urticaria indicates a positive test for hypersensitivity.[13]

In case of hypersensitivity to amide group of LA, an ester group LA can be used and vice versa. In case of hypersensitivity to both ester and amide, the physician may consider cryospray, ethyl chloride spray, diphenhydramine, benzyl alcohol, or intravenous sedation according to the circumstances.

Sensitivity to these drugs and to epinephrine may be known to the patient. The practitioner should obtain a full anesthetic history. Often, the patient will know of his/her sensitivity from past experience, commonly with a dental procedure.

Optimizing Patient Comfort and Pain Minimization during Infiltrative Anesthesia

Pain experienced during the administration of LA is due to the needle puncture of the skin, tissue irritation from the solution, and tissue distension from infiltration.

Techniques for Minimization of Needle Prick Pain

Explanation of procedure—talkesthesia—using EMLA for prenumbing, precooling with ice, using local vibratory stimuli or stress balls, use of oral analgesic or anxiolytic, use of smaller gauge needle, using longer needle or field block technique to anesthetize larger area, slow introduction of needle, and reinserting the needle in an area already anesthetized.[18]

Techniques for Minimizing Pain due to Tissue Irritation

Lidocaine solution is acidic in nature and stings during infiltration. The solution can be buffered through several means to increase the pH. This includes mixing lidocaine with epinephrine with plain lidocaine or adding sodium bicarbonate in a 1:10 dilution (one part sodium bicarbonate to ten parts lidocaine with epinephrine) to increase the pH to near tissue fluid levels.[19]

Techniques for Minimizing Pain Due to Tissue Distension

Slow injection of LA, injecting only the required amount, injecting into subcutaneous tissue, use of field block and anterograde injection technique.[20]

MANAGEMENT OF COMPLICATIONS

Central nervous system complications can be managed with 5–10 mg slow intravenous diazepam, maintaining airway and ventilatory support, and transferring the patient to emergency room or intensive care unit in case of seizures.

Cardiovascular system (CVS) complications require oxygen mask, cardiopulmonary resuscitation, vasopressors, and intravenous fluids. On the other hand, CVS complications due to epinephrine (palpitations and hypertension) require vasodilators like hydralazine and sublingual nifedipine.

In case of anaphylaxis and angiodema, administer antihistamines, subcutaneous adrenaline, oxygen, and steroids.

Vasovagal and psychogenic syncope are the most common complications. These can be managed by placing the patient in Trendelenburg position, loosening buttons/ties/belts, cold compresses to forehead and neck, fanning the patient, sipping a cool beverage, splashing water droplets on the face, sucking on hard candy, and/or making the patient sniff an ammonia ampoule.

CONCLUSION

Different forms of anesthesia can be safely and effectively used to allow a comfortable experience for the patient. One must understand the information, physiology, pharmacology, techniques, and safety measures explained in this chapter. The practitioner should also comply with medical laws regarding the different levels of anesthesia. Finally, as proper anesthesia can make a significant difference in the patient's experience and in procedure efficacy and result. Hence one should train to be adept and comfortable with various anesthesia techniques.

REFERENCES

1. Atal-Shah R. Anaesthesia in dermatosurgery. In: Savant SS, editor. Textbook of dermatosurgery and cosmetology. 2nd edition. Mumbai: ASCAD; 2005. pp. 53-64.
2. Railan D, Alster TS. Use of topical lidocaine for cosmetic dermatologic procedures. J Drugs Dermatol. 2007;6(11):1104-8.
3. Sobanko JF, Miller CJ, Alster TS. Topical anesthetics for dermatologic procedures: a review. Dermatol Surg. 2012;38(5):709-21.
4. Friedman PM, Mafong E, Friedman ES, Geronemus RG, et al. Topical anesthetic update: EMLA and beyond. Dermatol Surg. 2001;27(12):1019-26.
5. Shomaker TS, Zhang J, Love G, Basta S, Ashburn MA. Evaluating skin anesthesia after administration of a local anesthetic system consisting of an S-Caine patch and a controlled head-aided drug delivery (CHADD) patch in volunteers. Clin J Pain. 2000;16(3):200-4.
6. van den Hove J, Decroix J, Tennstedt D, Lachapelle JM. Allergic contact dermatitis from prilocaine, one of the local anesthetics in EMLA cream. Contact Dermatitis. 1994;30(4):239
7. Yun PL, Tachihara R, Anderson RR. Efficacy of erbium:yttrium-aluminum-garnet laser-assisted delivery of topical anesthetic. J Am Acad Dermatol. 2002;47(4):542-7.
8. Krupashankar DS. Standard guidelines of care: CO2 laser for removal of benign skin lesions and resurfacing. Indian J Dermatol Venereol Leprol. 2008;74 Suppl:S61-7.
9. Zide BM, Swift R. How to block and tackle the face. Plast Reconstr Surg. 1998;101:840-51.
10. Sachdev M, Hameed S. Applied surgical anatomy in relation to facial rejuvenation. In: Mysore V, editor. ACSI Textbook of Cutaneous & Aesthetic Surgery. 1st ed. New Delhi: Jaypee Brothers Medical Publishers (P) Ltd.; 2012. pp. 10-32.
11. Niamtu J, Carruthers J. Pain control in cosmetic facial surgery. In: Carruthers J, Carruthers A, editors. Soft tissue augmentation, 1st edition. New Delhi: Jaypee Brothers Medical Publishers (P) Ltd.; 2006. pp. 11-8.
12. Gaitan S, Markus R. Anesthesia methods in laser resurfacing. Semin Plast Surg. 2012;26(3):117-24.
13. Mysore V, Nischal KC. Guidelines for administration of local anesthesia for dermatosurgery and cosmetic dermatology procedures. Ind J Dermatol Venereol Leprol. 2009;75(Suppl 2):S68-75.
14. Hanke CW. The tumescent facial block: tumescent local anesthesia and nerve block anesthesia for full-face laser resurfacing. Dermatol Surg. 2001;27(12):1003-5.
15. Abeles G, Warmuth IP, Sequeira M, Swensen RD, Bisaccia E, Scarborough DA. The use of conscious sedation for outpatient dermatologic surgical procedures. Dermatol Surg. 2000;26(2):121-6.
16. Fitzpatrick RE, Williams B, Goldman MP. Preoperative anesthesia and postoperative considerations in laser resurfacing. Semin Cutan Med Surg. 1996;15(3):170-6.
17. Chen BK, Eichenfield LF. Pediatric anesthesia in dermatologic surgery: when hand-holding is not enough. Dermatol Surg. 2001;27(12):1010-8.
18. Zenzie HH, Altshuler GB, Smirnov MZ, Anderson RR. Evaluation of cooling methods for laser dermatology. Lasers Surg Med. 2000;26(2):130-44.
19. Arndt KA, Burton C, Noe JM. Minimizing the pain of local anesthesia. Plast Reconstr Surg. 1993;72(5):676-9.
20. Skidmore RA, Patterson JD, Tomsick RS. Local anesthetics. Dermatol Surg. 1996;22(6):511-22.

CHAPTER 7

Cooling Devices in Laser Practice

Amal H Al Salmi, Yousuf M Al Washahi

INTRODUCTION

Since the start of cutaneous laser surgery, many side effects including pain, blistering, scarring, and dyspigmentation started to appear on the treated sites. These side effects result from the thermal damage caused by the nonspecific absorption of direct or scattered light in 500–1,200 nm wavelengths by either melanin or hemoglobin.

Darker skinned patients pose more challenges because of their increased epidermal melanin which competes as significant chromophore for laser energy, leading to increased rate of these unintended side effects. Furthermore, this increased absorption by epidermal melanin results in reduction in the laser energy reaching the intended targets and hence reducing laser efficacy.

With the introduction of the cooling methods and devices in 1990s, those side effects along with the pain were all reduced, causing reduction in the need for topical or injectable anesthetics and even analgesia.[1] In addition, darker skin types started to benefit from light and laser therapy with minimal number of patient visits due to the use of higher energy fluencies, which were not possible previously.[1]

This chapter will cover the different types of cooling devices used in cutaneous laser surgery, and will discuss some practical implementation of their use.

TYPES OF COOLING DEVICES IN LASER PRACTICE

Different cooling devices have been described in the literatures which are based on two main methods of cooling—contact cooling and noncontact cooling (Table 1).

TABLE 1: Types of cooling methods in laser practice

Type of cooling	Advantages	Disadvantages
Contact cooling		
Ice or cold gels (passive)	Simple, bulk cooling	Limited protection, messy
Metal tips, e.g., copper, sapphire windows (active)	Efficient cooling, skin compression (deep targets)	Frequent cleaning
Noncontact cooling		
Cryogen spray (evaporative)	Efficient precooling	Cryogen cost, risk of frostbite
Cold air (convective)	Inexpensive, fast, not disturbing laser beam	Poor thermal conductor

These devices can be used to cool the epidermis before, during, and after laser exposure (precooling, parallel cooling, and postcooling).[2]

In contact cooling, tissue cooling is achieved by conduction of heat from the skin to the cooling device or substance placed directly onto the skin. This method is further divided to passive contact cooling and active contact cooling.[2] Ice and chilled transparent gels are considered one of the simplest methods of passive contact cooling which causes an average temperature increase of the cooling agent after contact with skin, thereby limiting its epidermal protection.[2] However, ice and chilled gels can be easily used to cool large areas of skin (bulk cooling); although, it is messy in clinical practice. While in active contact cooling, more integrated cooling devices are developed by different laser manufacturers and include chilled metal tips and transparent glass or sapphire windows. Heat is actively removed from these device through chilled liquid or gas circulating in closed loop; therefore, keeping the average temperature of the cooling device constant at (3–4°C).[3] In addition to being more efficient in heat extraction, active contact cooling offers manually controlled skin compression, diminishing the blood flow in superficial blood vessels; therefore, decreasing the oxyhemoglobin which is an active chromophore. Also skin compression brings deeper targets like the hair follicles closer to the skin surface thus, maximizing the absorption of the laser energy, so less fluence can be used to heat these targets.[4] However, these devices require frequent cleaning after every 5–10 pulses to remove debris and disinfection of the tip between patients is mandatory to prevent skin infections.

In noncontact cooling, heat is actively removed from tissues through either evaporative cooling using cryogen spray or convective cooling by cold air.[3] These devices can be used to access difficult areas like mucous membranes, ears and skin folds since tissue cooling is not dependent on the surface topography and no substance to be applied directly onto the skin.

In the first method, a cryogen, usually the nontoxic 1,1,1,2-tetrafluoroethane also known as R-134a (boiling point: -26.2°C) is delivered in programmed pulses of not more than (10–100 ms) duration with same time delay between the cryogen pulse and the laser pulse.[3] This type is considered the most efficient precooling method.[1] Furthermore, it has a proven benefit in port wine stains treatment allowing higher fluencies use and better results,[5] but the disposable cryogen cost and the very high global warming potential (GWP: 1,300) are disadvantageous.[3,6]

In trials to find another cryogen rather than the R-134a, a study done in 2007 showed that liquid carbon dioxide (GWP: 1) used in skin cooling is as effective as R-134a and more environmentally accepted, but its higher amount of consumption needed to reach the desired cooling effect might be problematic.[6]

The newest generation of noncontact cooling devices uses convective cooling by delivering continuous flow of chilled air at -30°C at adjustable flow rates and without interfering with the laser beam. This method was first evaluated in laser therapy by Raulin et al. in 2000 and found to be safe and inexpensive.[7] Studies done on the use of cold air during treatment of facial telangiectasia and port wine stains with pulse dye laser demonstrated significant reduction in pain, improved patient satisfaction, and minimized adverse effects.[8,9] However, air is considered poor thermal conductor and slightly inferior to sapphire contact cooling when used on darkly pigmented subjects during 810 nm diode laser application.[10]

PRACTICAL IMPLEMENTATIONS

Cooling devices are now used with almost all laser applications to protect the epidermis except for ablative skin resurfacing which targets epidermal water. However, some dermatologist may still use postcooling with ice packs in ablative lasers to reduce the erythema, edema, and discomfort caused by the thermal injury to the epidermis. For Q-switched laser, precooling is more suitable because of the very short pulse duration (nanoseconds). In contrast, lasers with long pulse durations (>100 ms), parallel cooling using contact cooling devices provides best epidermal protection.[2]

Nevertheless, aggressive tissue cooling is not without any risk especially in pigmented skin. Datrice et al.[11] found that longer durations of cryogen spurts and multiple cryogen spurt patterns can cause side effects like acute erythema, urticaria (lasting 1–24 h) and even hyperpigmentation in skin types III–VI which was self-limited over 8 weeks time in his study. Arcuate shaped hyperpigmentation has been also reported with cryogen skin cooling.[12] Furthermore, increased incidence of postinflammatory hyperpigmentation has been demonstrated with continuous cold air cooling.[13]

CONCLUSION

Cooling devices/methods are now available in most laser systems and aims to protect the epidermis, reduce pain, and improves laser efficacy. These can be divided into contact cooling and noncontact cooling methods. Cooling may also be divided into three phases in relation to the timing of laser irradiation, namely, precooling, parallel cooling, and postcooling.

REFERENCES

1. Lowe NJ. Minimally invasive treatments and procedures for ageing skin. In: Burns T, Breathnach S, Cox N, Griffiths C, editors. Rook's textbook of dermatology (vol. 4), 8th ed. Oxford, Wiley Blackwell; 2010. pp. 80.10-1.
2. Zenzie HH, Altshuler GB, Smirnov MZ, Anderson RR. Evaluation of cooling methods for laser dermatology. Lasers Surg Med. 2000;26(2): 130-44.
3. Vallee JA, Kelly KM, Rohrer TE, Arndt KA, Dover JS. Lasers in the treatment of vascular lesions. In: Kaminer MS, Arndt KA, Drover JS, Rohrer TE, Zachary CB, editors. Atlas of cosmetic surgery. 2nd ed. Irvine: Elsevier Saunders; 2009. pp. 138-9.
4. Klavuhn KG. Epidermal protection: a comparative analysis of sapphire contact and cryogen spray cooling. Laser Hair Removal Technical Note. CA: Coherent Medical; 2000.
5. Chang CJ, Nelson JS. Cryogen spray cooling and higher fluence pulsed dye laser treatment improve port-wine stain clearance while minimizing epidermal damage. Dermatol Surg. 1999;25(10):767-72.
6. Jia W, Svaasand LO, Nguyen TB, Nelson JS. Dynamic skin cooling with an environmentally compatible alternative cryogen during laser surgery. Lasers Surg Med. 2007;39(10):776-81.
7. Raulin C, Greve B, Hammes S. Cold air in laser therapy: first experiences with a new cooling system. Lasers Surg Med. 2000;27(5):404-10.
8. Hammes S, RaulinC. Evaluation of different temperatures in cold air cooling with pulsed-dye laser treatment of facial telangiectasia. Laser Surg Med. 2005;36(2):136-40.
9. Hammes S, Roos S, Raulin C, Ockenfels HM, Greve B. Does dye laser treatment with higher fluences in combination with cold air cooling improve the results of port-wine stains? J Eur Acad Dermatol Venereol. 2007;21(9):1229-33.
10. Chang CW, Reinisch L, Biesman BS. Analysis of epidermal protection using cold air versus chilled sapphire window with water or gel during 810 nm diode laser application. Lasers Surg Med. 2003;32(2):129-36.
11. Datrice N, Ramirez-San-Juan J, Zhang R, Meshkinpour A, Aguilar G, Nelson JS, et al. Cutaneous effects of cryogen spray cooling on in vivo human skin. Dermatol Surg. 2006;32(8):1007-12.
12. Lee SJ, Park SG, Kang JM, Kim YK, Kim HD. Cryogen-induced arcuate shaped hyperpigmentation by dynamic cooling device. J Eur Acad Dermatol Venereol. 2008;22(7):883-4.
13. Manuskiatti W, Eimpunth S, Wanitphakdeedecha R. Effect of cold air cooling on the incidence of postinflammatory hyperpigmentation after Q-switched Nd:YAG laser treatment of acquired bilateral nevus of Ota like macules. Arch Dermatol. 2007;143(9):1139-43.

CHAPTER 8

Ablative Carbon Dioxide Lasers in Dermatology Practice

Krupa Shankar DS, Chakravarthi M Ravindran

INTRODUCTION

Over the past decade, advances in laser technology have allowed dermatologists to improve the appearance of scars and wrinkles and to remove benign skin growths using both ablative and nonablative lasers. Carbon dioxide (CO_2) laser treatment ensures minimal discomfort and rapid recovery, enabling a quick return to daily routine. The CO_2 laser is the gold standard in ablative lasers. Detailed knowledge of the machines is essential.[1]

HISTORY

After the invention of CO_2 laser by Kumar Patel in 1960, it soon became popular and its applications became wider and wider in the various fields. Carbon dioxide laser was first tested in the human skin by an American dermatologist Leon Goldman.[2]

Initially used for resurfacing, gradually its indications in dermatology became wider. Over the past decade, advances in laser technology have allowed dermatologists to improve the appearance of scars and wrinkles and to remove benign skin growths using CO_2 laser.

COMPONENTS OF CARBON DIOXIDE LASER

- Energy source: Electricity
- Optical cavity (Fig. 1)
    - Active medium
    - Optical resonator: totally reflective (M1) and partially transmissive mirrors (M2)
- Delivery system (Fig. 2)
    - Articulated arm
    - Hallow tube
    - Mirror joint
    - Lens
    - Handpiece.

PRINCIPLES

The optical cavity contains active medium which contains a mixture of CO_2, nitrogen and helium gases. It also

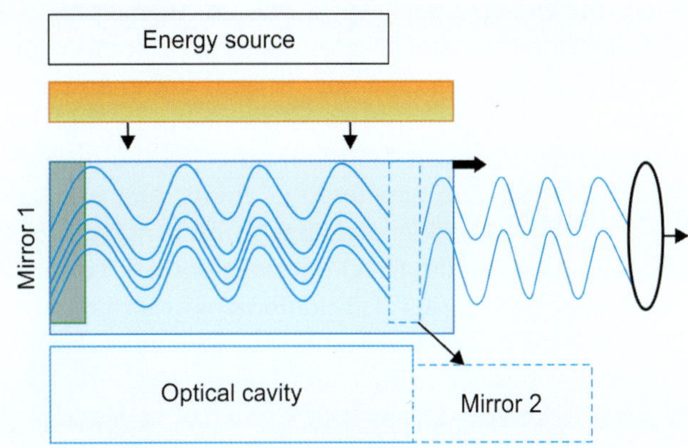

FIG. 1: Illustration of generation of laser

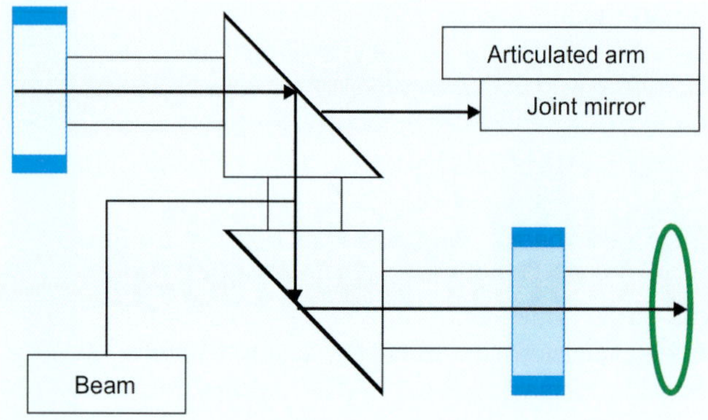

FIG. 2: Schematic illustration of laser articulated arm

TABLE 1: Energy calculations

Power	Irradiance (w/cm^2)	Fluence
0.5	6369.43	5.14
1.0	12738.85	11.46
2.0	25477.7	22.93
3.0	38216.56	34.39
4.2	53503.18	48.15
6	76433.12	68.79
6.3	80254.78	72.23
9	114547.54	103.09

consists of two parallel mirrors placed either side of the active medium. One is totally reflective and other is partially transmissive.

When the external electric source enters the optic cavity, the active medium CO_2 molecules are pumped to the high energy vibrational state. They release infrared photon to the wavelength of 10,600 nm and subsequently decay back to the ground state.

The reflective mirror helps the photons to reenters the active medium to stimulate the release of more photons to maintain the steady supply of photons. To maintain this population inversion, continuous is provided, which continuously pumps atom to excited state.

The mirrors collimate photons perpendicular to the mirrors. The light that escapes the partially transmissive mirror will be converged to one beam using convex lens. These beams are reflected to the target, using mirrors in the articulated arm.

Energy Calculations (Table 1)

- Irradiance: the rate at which photons are poured into skin
- Fluence: the total amount of photons poured into unit volume of tissue in unit time.

Calculations

- Power = joules/second or watts
- Spot size = πr^2
- R = radius = diameter/2 cm
- Irradiance = power/spot size
- Fluence = irradiance × time in second.

If

- Diameter = 0.1 mm = 0.01 cm
- Time = 0.9 m s = 0.0009 s
- Radius = 0.005 cm
- Radius 2 = 0.000025 cm
- Spot size = πr^2 = 0.00007857.

Modes of Carbon Dioxide Laser (Fig. 3)

There are two modes in CO_2 lasers—continuous and pulsed. When there is continues emission of laser waves as long as foot pedal is pressed is called continuous mode, the pulsed emission is achieved by timed electronic

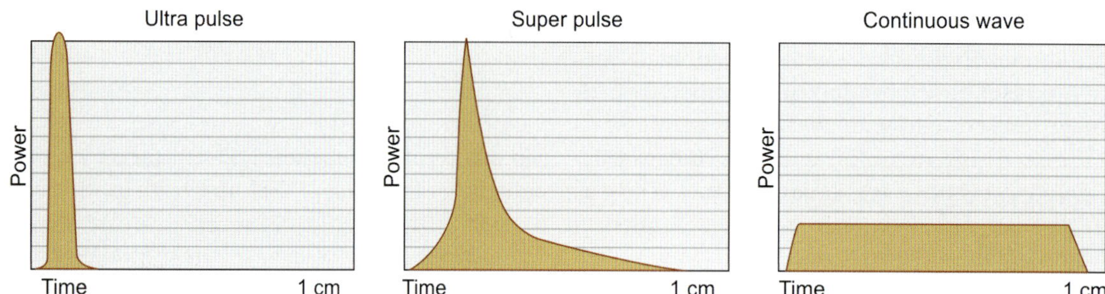

FIG. 3: Illustrated modes of carbon dioxide laser

control connected to the shutter positioned at the beam path. This timing can be controlled by the control panel.

Tissue-laser Interaction

Absorption

When the laser energy is absorbed by the chromophore water, four basic effects can occur, namely, photothermal, photochemical, photomechanical, and photoacoustic.

Photothermal Reaction

Photothermal reaction occurs at the surface of the skin. The laser energy vaporizes the water and causes thermal damage to the skin. The skin exposed to laser is called the vaporization plane.

The high and rapid heat from the laser results in vaporization of cellular water and complete destruction of cellular protein and also the cell itself.

The thermal coagulation causes cell necrosis, hemostasis, tissue welding, and ceiling of nerve endings.

Indications[2]

Nonesthetic indications actinic and seborrheic keratosis,[3-7] deep penetrating nevus (DPN) variety of warts like verruca vulgaris,[8] verruca plana, plantar wart;[9] and subungual and periungual wart;[10] moles; skin tags; epidermal and dermal nevi;[11-16] xanthelasma;[17] dermatofibroma;[18] rhinophyma;[19-23] severe cutaneous photodamage (observed in Favre-Racouchot syndrome); sebaceous hyperplasia; syringomas;[3,24,25] actinic cheilitis;[26-29] angiofibroma;[30-32] scar treatment;[33-35] keloid;[36-39] skin cancer;[40-43] neurofibroma;[44-46] diffuse actinic keratoses; granuloma pyogenicum;[47] and pearly penile papules.[48]

Materials Needed

For surgery

Carbon dioxide laser, povidone iodine solution, normal saline, syringe and needle (size according to requirement), lignocaine with or without adrenaline, sterile gauze, artery forceps (both curved and straight), toothed forceps, suture materials, antibiotic cream or ointment, and dressing materials.

For safety

Wavelength rated spectacles for surgeon and assistants, eye shield for patients, oxygen cylinder, ambu bag, and emergency drug tray.

Ocular protection

Ocular injuries are more serious hazard with CO_2 laser for surgeon, assistant and patient. Carbon dioxide laser which emits 10,600 nm will get absorbed by tissue water will particularly affect the cornea and can cause opacity of the cornea, but the degree of burn will depend upon duration of exposure.

For all these complications, patient should be protected by opaque eyewear, if the treatment area is close to the eyes like eyelids, opaque intraocular eyeshield can be used. For surgeon and assistant, wavelength rated spectacles should be used, for CO_2 laser clear polycarbonate fiber spectacle with high thermal capacity will block the beam.

Protection from Plume

Carbon dioxide laser vaporizes the tissue from the surgical area. The plume contains not only the water vapor but also the tissue particles in aerosol state. Several studies have been reported the presence of viral deoxyribonucleic acid in laser plume.[49] Especially the human papilloma virus is highly infective, several reports of laryngeal papilloma has been reported.[50,51] Surgical mask will protect these infections. The some evacuator will remove the viral particle along with the smoke.

Mechanical Hazard

It is essential to know the emergency cut off switch before using the laser, laser can be emitted even without pressing the foot pad. In that case point the laser beam away from the patient and assistant and press the emergency button to cut the supply.

Preoperative Investigations

Complete blood picture, random blood sugar, bleeding time, clotting time, viral marker, prothrombin time, and activated prothrombin time, only if indicated, and histopathology (in suspected cutaneous malignancy).

Preoperative Preparation

Written Informed Consent

To be taken after explaining the disease and the need for procedure, possible postoperative appearance, complications and need for postoperative care.[49]

Control of Systemic Diseases

Diabetes mellitus and hypertension optimization.

Positioning of Patient

- Face, chest, upper limb, abdomen, genitalia, and ventral aspect of lower limb: supine position
- Sides of face, neck, and body: lateral position
- Nape of the neck, back, gluteal region, and dorsal aspect of lower limb: prone position
- Palms: supine position with palms above the head
- Soles: prone position with extended ankles.

Part Preparation

- Shave the area minimum 2 cm radius from the lesion
- Painting with povidone iodine or ioprep (spirit should not be used because it is inflammable).

Anesthesia

Depending upon the site and type of lesions, one of the following types of anesthesia can be given:

- Topical anesthesia: eutectic mixture of local anesthesics (eutectic mixture of local anesthetics) cream is used. Apply 2 mg/cm^2 topically under occlusion for 60 minutes. The occlusion should be removed just before the procedure
- Local infiltration: lignocaine 2% with or without adrenaline 1:100,000 is used. Dosage of lignocaine plain is 3 mg/kg and lignocaine with adrenaline is 7 mg/kg. Lignocaine with adrenaline should be avoided at areas with end arteries like fingers, toes, earlobes, nose and penis. Local anesthesia (LA) is injected as follows:
    - Using 30 G needle with bevel pointing upward LA is injected immediately below the planned area of laser. Pinching the lesion before injection will reduce the pain
    - In case of palms and soles, insert the needle with 45 angulations to the skin surface
    - Inject the anesthesia while withdrawing and slowly to minimize the pain
    - Insert the needle at a distance from the lesion such that the tip of the needle is below the lesion after it is pushed in to its full length, failing which anesthesia will be deposited distal to the lesion
    - Anesthesia must be infiltrated slowly and not pushed in briskly to avoid pain
    - For the injection near the eyes always be parallel to the surface to avoid injury to eyes

Ring Block

Ring block is employed to anesthetize fingers, toes, and penis. The needle is inserted at the base of the fingers and toes on either side or a ring of anesthesia is deposited around the digit. The LA is injected while withdrawing. A distal digital nerve block on either side of lateral nail folds can supplement a ring block for nail surgeries. In case of penile region, LA is given at the base of the shaft.

Field Block

Local anesthesia is infiltrated circumferentially around the site blocking the nerve impulse from leaving the area. The actual surgical site is not injected. They are particularly useful when a large area needs to be anesthetized.

General Instructions for the Operation of Laser

- Hold the handpiece like holding a pen
- Hold the handpiece perpendicular to the lesion and press the foot pedal to fire the laser. Vaporize the lesion in coiled, whorled, centrifugal, vertical, or horizontal fashion. Vaporize the flat lesions from the top
- Pedunculated lesions can be excised by lasing from the base of the lesion. Hold the lesion with toothed forceps on the top, pull it to the side on the top of the wet gauze (to prevent charring of the normal skin). Always use wet gauze as dry gauze can catch fire
- Wipe the vaporized lesions with wet gauze. Always make sure to dry the area or wipe the water with dry gauze. Look for the raw areas. Coagulate the bleeding spots if any by defocusing the laser beam.

Practical Tips on use of Carbon Dioxide Laser

- Always use handpiece pointer on skin to cut
- Remember lens focuses beam and renders it collimated
- Moving hand piece away (defocusing) leads to logarithmic fall in irradiance; use this to coagulate
- Super-pulse CO_2 laser reduces dwell time, maximizes power
- Use continuous wave in highly vascular lesions and areas, debulking, and where esthetics is not an issue, e.g., foot
- Undertreat, eschew therapeutic greed
- Laser settings in texts are often for collimated hand pieces, read carefully before applying. One-third to one-fourth the irradiance suggested in the texts seems to deliver the results
- The newer CO_2 lasers with advanced output control software, when used in the super-pulsed mode for carrying out free hand procedures, are versatile devices with numerous therapeutic options.

Bleeding Control

- Small ooze from venules can be controlled by lasing at defocused mode and pressure for 5 minutes will be sufficient
- For arterial bleeding, sutures may be needed, use 3-0 absorbable can be used
- At the end arteries like finger and toes, tourniquet can be used
- Pressure dressing with elastic adhesive bleeding should be done.

Postoperative Care and Follow-up

- For superficial lesions like seborrheic, keratosis, DPNs topical antibiotic cream, bland face wash, and sunscreen will be sufficient and postoperative follow-up is 7th day, and 1 month
- Superficial lesions in cover area can be treated only with topical antibiotics
- For deeper facial lesions like moles, hydrocolloid dressing is important and follow-up is 7 days, 1 month, 3 months, and 1 year
- Allow the scabs to fall on own. Avoid picking
- Emphasize on sunscreen application three times a day from day one for the lesions on the face and neck
- Treat for postinflammatory hyperpigmentation if any with Kligman's formula
- Allow occlusive pressure dressing to remain in place for 3–7 days and not to wet the area
- Look for healthy granulation tissue after removal of the occlusive dressing
- Avoid contact with dust. Use handyplast if needed for a couple of days for protection.

Hydrocolloid Dressing Instruction

- Remove the dressing before bath
- Wipe the pus-like material with wet cotton
- Wash the area with soap and water when you take bath
- Press the area dry after bath
- Paint the area and skin around it with Betadine solution. Wait for 3 minutes for the Betadine to dry
- Apply the dressing, so that the sticky side of the dressing which adheres to the paper sticks to the wound
- Please remember that when you change the dressing you will find a yellowish brown material which may look and smell like pus, but this is not pus, it is the material in the dressing which melts when it comes into contact with the wound.

Complications[52]

Minor complications

It is frequent, are usually of minimal consequence. Postinflammatory hyperpigmentation, milia formation, perioral dermatitis, acne and/or rosacea exacerbation and contact dermatitis, hyperpigmentation or erythema. However, this is temporary, lasting for only about 6 weeks and gradually improves.

Major complications

Viral, bacterial, and candidial infection delayed hypo-pigmentation, persistent erythema, and prolonged healing. The most severe complications are—hypertrophic scarring, disseminated infection, and ectropion.

Nail deformity can happen if the treatment area is at nail matrix, in care of wart over the nail matrix.

CONCLUSION

In conclusion, the CO_2 laser is a versatile device that treats a large number of benign lesions and needs to be a part of every dermatology practice.

It would be useful to have a pre op check list on hand that addresses eye protection , lung protection, theatre safety. A fluence chart to follow guidelines, a pre op look at lab test results and a post op instructions sheet prepared in advance before the surgery in order to avoid oversight.

The post op instructions should mention dates of follow up and detailed written instructions on management or change of dressings. I should also indicate address of emergency medical care facility, urgent phone call number and email id of the treating physician.

REFERENCES

1. Krupa Shankar D, Chakravarthi M, Shilpakar R. Carbon dioxide laser guidelines. J Cutan Aesthet Surg. 2009;2:72-80.
2. Goldman L, Blaney DJ, Kindel DJ, Franke EK. Effect of the laser beam on the skin. J Invest Dermatol. 1963;40:121-2.
3. Trimas SJ, Ellis DA, Metz RD. The carbon dioxide laser. An alternative for the treatment of actinically damaged skin. Dermatol Surg. 1997;23(10):885-9.
4. Phahonthep R, Sindhuphak W, Sriprajittichai P. Lidocaine iontophoresis versus EMLA cream for CO_2 laser treatment in seborrheic keratosis. J Med Assoc Thai. 2004;87(Suppl 2):S15-8.
5. Fulton JE, Rahimi AD, Helton P, Dahlberg K, Kelly AG. Disappointing results following resurfacing of facial skin with CO_2 lasers for prophylaxis of keratoses and cancers. Dermatol Surg. 1999;25(9):729-32.
6. Fitzpatrick RE, Goldman MP, Ruiz-Esparza J. Clinical advantage of the CO_2 laser superpulsed mode. Treatment of verruca vulgaris, seborrheic keratoses, lentigines, and actinic cheilitis. J Dermatol Surg Oncol. 1994;20(7):449-56.
7. Quaedvlieg PJ, Ostertag JU, Krekels GA, Neumann HA. Delayed wound healing after three different treatments for widespread actinic keratosis on the atrophic bald scalp. Dermatol Surg. 2003;29(10):1052-6.
8. Tukac S. The CO2 laser and verruca vulgaris. Med Pregl. 2000;53(7-8):389-93.
9. Landsman MJ, Mancuso JE, Abramow SP. Carbon dioxide laser treatment of pedal verrucae. Clin Podiatr Med Surg. 1992;9(3):659-69.
10. Lim JT, Goh CL. Carbon dioxide laser treatment of periungual and sub-ungual viral warts. Australas J Dermatol. 1992;33(2):87-91.
11. Hohenleutner U, Wlotzke U, Konz B, Landthaler M. Carbon dioxide laser therapy of a widespread epidermal nevus. Lasers Surg Med. 1995; 16(3):288-91.
12. Khoo L. Carbon dioxide laser treatment of benign skin lesions. National Skin Centre Experience. 2001;12:2.
13. Verma KK, Ovung EM. Epidermal and sebaceous nevi treated with cabon dioxide laser. Indian J Dermatol Venereol Leprol. 2002;68(1):23-4.
14. Ratz JL, Bailin PL, Wheeland RG. Carbon dioxide laser treatment of epidermal nevi. J Dermatol Surg Oncol. 1986;12:567-70.
15. Boyce S, Alster TS. CO_2 laser treatment of epidermal nevi: Long-term success. Dermatol Surg. 2002;28(7):611-4.
16. Hohenleutner U, Landthaler M. Laser therapy of verrucous epidermal naevi. Clin Exp Dermatol. 1993;18(2):124-7.
17. Alster TS, West TB. Ultrapulse CO2 laser ablation of xanthelasma. J Am Acad Dermatol. 1996;34:848-9.
18. Krupa Shankar DS, Kushalappa AA, Suma KS, Pai SA. Multiple dermatofibromas on face treated with carbon dioxide laser. Indian J Dermatol Venereol Leprol. 2007;73(3):194-5.
19. Simo R, Sharma VL. The use of the CO_2 laser in rhinophyma surgery: personal technique and experience, complications and long-term results. Facial Plast Surg. 1998;14(4):287-95.
20. Goon PK, Dalal M, Peart FC. The gold standard for decortication of rhinophyma: combined erbium-YAG/CO_2 laser. Aesthetic Plast Surg. 2004;28(6):456-60.
21. Bohigian RK, Sharpshay SM, Hybels RL. Management of rhinophyma with carbon dioxide laser: Lahey Clinic experience. Lasers Surg Med. 1988;8(4):397-401.
22. Sharpshay SM, Strong MS, Anatasi GW, Vaughan CW. Removal of rhinophyma with the carbon dioxide laser: a preliminary report. Arch Otolaryngol. 1980;106(5):257-9.
23. Greenbaum SS, Krull EA, Watrick K. Comparison of CO_2 laser and electrosurgery in the treatment of rhinophyma. J Am Acad Dermatol. 1988;18:363-8.
24. Wang JI, Roenigk HH. Treatment of multiple facial syringomas with the carbon dioxide (CO_2) laser. Dermatol Surg. 1999;25(2):136-9.
25. Wheeland RG, Bailin PL, Reynolds OD, Ratz JL. Carbon dioxide (CO2) laser vaporization of multiple facial syringomas. J Dermatol Surg Oncol. 1986;12(3):225-8.
26. Duane C, Whitaker MD. Microscopically proven cure of actinic cheilitis by CO_2 laser. Lasers Surg Med. 2005;7:520-3.
27. Laws RA, Wilde JL, Grabski WJ. Comparison of electrodessication with CO_2 laser for the treatment of actinic cheilitis. Dermatol Surg. 2000;26:349-53.
28. Alamillos-Granados FJ, Naval-Gias L, Dean-Ferrer A, Alonso del Hoyo JR. Carbon dioxide laser vermilionectomy for actinic cheilitis. J Oral Maxillofac Surg. 1993;51(2):118-21.
29. Zelickson BD, Roenigk RK. Actinic cheilitis: treatment with the carbon dioxide laser. Cancer. 1990;65(6):1307-11.
30. Belmar P, Boixeda P, Baniandrés O, Fernández-Lorente M, Arrazola JM. Long-term follow up of angiofibromas treated with CO2 laser in 23 patients with tuberous sclerosis. Actas Dermosifiliogr. 2005;96(8):498-503.
31. Papadavid E, Markey A, Bellaney G, Walker NP. Carbon dioxide and pulsed dye laser treatment of angiofibromas in 29 patients with tuberous sclerosis. Br J Dermatol. 2002;147(2):337-42.
32. Verma KK, Ovung EM, Sirka CS. Extensive facial angiofibromas in tuberous sclerosis treated with carbon dioxide laserbrasion. Indian J Dermatol Venereol Leprol. 2001;67(6):326-8.
33. Lupton JR, Alster TS. Laser scar revision. Dermatol Clin. 2002;20(1):55-65.
34. Ostertag JU, Theunissen CC, Neumann HA. Hypertrophic scars after therapy with CO2 laser for treatment of multiple cutaneous neurofibromas. Dermatol Surg. 2002;28(3):296-8.
35. Kang DH, Park SH, Koo SH. Laser resurfacing of smallpox scars. Plast Reconst Surg. 2005;116(1):259-65.
36. Nowak KC, McCormack M, Koch RJ. The effect of superpulsed carbon dioxide laser energy on keloid and normal dermal fibroblast secretion of growth factors: A serum-free study. Plast Reconstr Surg. 2000;105(6):2039-48.
37. Apfelberg DB, Maser MR, Lash H, White D, Weston J. Preliminary results of argon and carbon dioxide laser treatment of keloid scars. Lasers Surg Med. 1984;4(3):283-90.
38. Cheng ET, Pollard JD, Koch RJ. Effect of blended CO2 and erbium: YAG laser irradiation on normal and keloid fibroblasts: A serum-free study. J Clin Laser Med Surg. 2003;21(6):337-43.
39. Krupa Shankar DS, Gupta V. Management of ear rim keloid with carbon dioxide laser. Indian J Dermatol Venereol Leprol. 2007;73:445.
40. Kim ES, Kim KJ, Chang SE, Lee MW, Choi JH, Moon KC, et al. Metaplastic ossification in a cutaneous pyogenic granuloma: A case report. J Dermatol. 2004;31:326-9.

41. Vaïsse V, Clerici T, Fusade T. Bowen disease treated with scanned pulsed high energy CO2 laser. Follow-up of 6 cases. Ann Dermatol Venereol. 2001;128(11):1220-4.
42. Nouri K, Chang A, Trent JT, Jiménez GP. Ultrapulse CO2 used for the successful treatment of basal cell carcinomas found in patients with basal cell nevus syndrome. Dermatol Surg. 2002;28(3):287-90.
43. Humphreys TR, Malhotra R, Scharf MJ, Marcus SM, Starkus L, Calegari K. Treatment of superficial basal cell carcinoma and squamous cell carcinoma in situ with a high-energy pulsed carbon dioxide laser. Arch Dermatol. 1998;134(10):1247-52.
44. Lapid-Gortzak R, Lapid O, Monos T, Lifshitz T. CO2-laser in the removal of a plexiform neurofibroma from the eyelid. Ophthalmic Surg Lasers. 2000;31(5):432-4.
45. Becker DW. Use of the carbon dioxide laser in treating multiple cutaneous neurofibromas. Ann Plast Surg. 1991;26(6):582-6.
46. Roenigk RK, Ratz JL. CO_2 laser treatment of cutaneous neurofibromas. J Dermatol Surg Oncol. 1987;13:187-90.
47. Raulin C, Petzoldt D, Werner S. Granuloma pyogenicum—removal with the CO_2 laser. Hautarzt. 1997;48:402-5.
48. Magid M, Garden JM. Pearly penile papules: treatment with the carbon dioxide laser. J Dermatol Surg Oncol. 1989;15:552-4.
49. Rosio TJ. Basic laser physics. In: Roenigk RK, Ratz JL, Roenigk HH (eds). Roenigk's dermatologic surgery. 3rd ed. New York: Informa Healthcare; 2007. pp. 607-24.
50. Wisniewski PM, Warhol MJ, Rando RF, Sedlacek TV, Kemp FE, Fisher JC. Studies on transmission of viral disease via CO2 laser plume and ejecta. J Reprod Med. 1990;35(12):1117-23.
51. Kunachak S, Sithisarn P, Kulapaditharom B. Are laryngeal papilloma virus infected cells viable in the plume derived from a continuous mode carbon dioxide laser, and are the infectious? A preliminary report on one laser mode. J Laryngol Otol. 1996:110(11):1031-3.
52. Naouri M, Delage M, Khallouf R, Georgesco G, Atlan M. CO_2 fractional resurfacing: side effects and immediate complications. Ann Dermatol Venereol. 2011;138(1):7-10.

CHAPTER 9

Treatment of Benign Tumors of Skin with Carbon Dioxide Laser

Krupa Shankar DS, Chakravarthi M Ravindran

INTRODUCTION

Benign tumors of the skin are the most common among all neoplasms. It causes cosmetic disfigurement and anxiety to the patient. Lasers became an effective alternate for the treatment of benign tumors of the skin.[1] Three types of lasers are used to treat cutaneous neoplasms—carbon dioxide (CO_2) lasers,[2] argon lasers, and neodymiumdoped yttrium-aluminium-garnet lasers.[3] Each of these can shrink or destroy tumor. Among these lasers, CO_2 laser gained advantages over other two and became versatile tool to treat variety of skin tumors.

TUMORS OF SKIN

To know the level of the tumor in the integument is important before treating it. The tumors of skin are basically classified into many types. They are macular, papular, nodular, pigmented, vascular, subepidermal, and rare tumors.

Macular or Slightly Papular

- Actinic keratosis[4,5]
- Seborrheic keratosis[6,7]
- Nevus sebaceous[8]
- Bowen's disease
- Sebaceous hyperplasia
- Dermatofibroma.

Papular

- Acrochordon
- Keratoacanthoma
- Cutaneous horn
- Keloid
- Nevus both junctional and intradermal
- Dermatofibroma.

Pigmented

- Dermatosis papulosa nigra (DPN)
- Dermatofibroma
- Warts.

Subepidermal

- Neurofibroma
- Lipoma
- Schwannoma
- Dermoid cyst
- Sebaceous cyst.

Vascular

- Cherry angioma
- Pyogenic granuloma.

Uncommon Tumors

- Trichilemmoma
- Trichoepithelioma
- Pilomatrixoma
- Angiofibroma
- Pearly penile papule.

CONTRAINDICATIONS

Systemic Disorder

- Uncontrolled diabetes
- Hypertension
- Cardiovascular disorders
- Bleeding dyscrasia
- Collagen vascular disease.

Other Contraindications

Any infection at the site has to be treated, history of keloid formation, isotretinoin use in past 6 months, current ultraviolet radiation and radiation treatment at the site, on anticoagulants, chemical peel, and dermabrasion.

Preoperative Investigations

Complete blood picture, random blood sugar, bleeding time, clotting time, viral marker, prothrombin time, and activated prothrombin time only if indicated and histopathology (in suspected cutaneous malignancy).

Preoperative Preparation

Written Informed Consent

To be taken after explaining the disease and the need for procedure, possible postoperative appearance, complications, and need for postoperative care.

Control of Systemic Diseases

Diabetes mellitus and hypertension optimization.

Positioning of Patient

- Face, chest, upper limb, abdomen, genitalia, and ventral aspect of lower limb: supine position
- Sides of face, neck, and body: lateral position
- Nape of the neck, back, gluteal region, and dorsal aspect of lower limb: prone position
- Palms: supine position with palms above the head
- Soles: prone position with extended ankles.

Part Preparation

- Shave the area minimum 2 cm radius from the lesion.
- Painting with povidone iodine or ioprep (spirit should not be used because it is inflammable).

Anesthesia

Depending upon the site and type of lesions, one of the following types of anesthesia can be given:

- Topical anesthesia
- Local infiltration
- Ring block
- Field block.

ACTINIC AND SEBORRHEIC KERATOSIS

- Anesthesia: topical anesthesia
- Laser settings: 4–7 watts, super-, or ultrapulsed mode
- Procedure: vaporize from above and wipe it with wet gauze till the pinpoint bleeding is seen. Ablation should be done not more than epidermis.

DERMATOSIS PAPULOSA NIGRA

- Anesthesia: topical anesthesia
- Laser settings: 1–5 watts, super- or ultrapulsed repeat mode of 0.1 second on and 0.1 second off
- Procedure: Vaporize superficially and wipe with wet gauze till it disappears.

WARTS

Verruca Vulgaris and Plana

- Anesthesia: topical for verruca plana and local infiltration or topical for verruca vulgaris

- Laser settings: 8–9 watts, continuous mode and continuous wave for verruca vulgaris, 4–5 superpulsed for the flat warts
- Procedure: vaporize from above, with 2 mm margin to prevent recurrence.

Plantar Wart

- Anesthesia: Local infiltration
- Laser settings: 10–12 watts, continuous mode and continuous wave
- Procedure: first vaporize the margin of the wart with 3 mm away from the lesion, and then vaporize from above. Wipe the area with wet gauze; wart may separate from the base, if not repeat until it happens. After separating the wart fire the base unto 1 mm depth and arrest the bleeding by defocusing.

Periungual and Subungual Wart

- Anesthesia: digital block
- Laser settings: 4.5–7.5 watts, continuous mode and continuous wave
- Procedure: avulse the nail to find the exact area of involvement. Then vaporize 2 mm away from the lesion and vaporize from the above, wipe it with wet gauze till you find the clear area.

Skin Tags, Filiform Wart, and Cutaneous Horn

- Anesthesia: topical/local infiltration
- Laser settings: 4.2–5 watts, continuous mode
- Procedure: avulse as described for pedunculated lesion and vaporize the base.

NEVI

Melanocytic nevi, verrucous epidermal nevi and other dermal and epidermal nevi.

- Anesthesia: local infiltration
- Laser settings: 4.5–7.5 watts, ultrapulsed mode
- Procedure: vaporize from above and wipe with wet gauze, repeat the procedure till the pigments disappear, apply hydrocolloid dressing to avoid scar.

SYRINGOMA, XANTHOMA, ANGIOFIBROMA, AND SENILE COMEDONE

- Anesthesia: topical anesthesia
- Laser settings: with 4.5–6.5 watts
- Procedure: mark each lesion with thin surgical pen. Vaporize from above till the clear surface is seen. In case of senile comedone, comedone extraction should precede the laser.

PYOGENIC GRANULOMA

- Anesthesia: local infiltration
- Laser settings: 9–10 watts, continuous mode
- Procedure: vaporize in defocusing mode, to avoid torrential bleeding. Vaporize till the arrest of bleeding.

KERATOACANTHOMA

- Anesthesia: local infiltration
- Laser settings: 4.5–6 watts
- Procedure: vaporize from the top till the base is clear.

MUCOCELE AND PEARLY PENILE PAPULE

- Anesthesia: local infiltration
- Laser settings: 2–3.5 watts, ultrapulsed mode using fixed pulses of 0.1–0.5 second
- Procedure: vaporize from the top till the base is clear.

EARLOBE KELOID

- Anesthesia: local infiltration
- Laser settings: 9–15 watts, continuous mode and continuous wave
- Procedure: ablate from the base and inject triamcinolone into the lesion.

SEBACEOUS CYST

- Anesthesia: local infiltration
- Laser settings: 4.5–6 watts, continuous mode and continuous wave
- Procedure: narrow hole made using the laser followed by squeezing out the sebaceous material and excision of wall through the narrow hole.

Bleeding Control

- Small ooze from venules can be controlled by lasing at defocused mode and pressure for 5 minutes will be sufficient
- For arterial bleeding sutures may be needed, 3-0 absorbable can be used
- At the end arteries like finger and toes tourniquet can be used

- Pressure dressing with elastic adhesive bleeding should be done.

Postoperative Care and Follow-up

- For the superficial lesions like seborrheic keratosis, DPNs; topical antibiotic cream, bland face wash, and sunscreen will be sufficient and postoperative follow-up is 7th day, and 1 month
- Superficial lesions in cover area can be treated only with topical antibiotics
- For deeper facial lesions like moles, hydrocolloid dressing is important and follow-up is 7th days, 1 month, 3 months, and 1 year
- Allow the scabs to fall on own. Avoid picking
- Emphasize on sunscreen application three times a day from day one for the lesions on the face and neck
- Treatment for postinflammatory hyperpigmentation if any is with Kligman's formula
- Allow occlusive pressure dressing to remain in place for 3–7 days and not to wet the area
- Look for healthy granulation tissue after removal of the occlusive dressing
- Avoid contact with dust. Use hansaplast if needed for a couple of days for protection.

COMPLICATIONS

Minor Complications

- Postinflammatory hyperpigmentation
- Milia formation
- Perioral dermatitis
- Acne and/or rosacea exacerbation
- Contact dermatitis.

Hyperpigmentation or erythema over the treated area is common in colored skin and causes anxiety to patients. However, this is temporary, lasting for only about 6 weeks and gradually improves.

More serious complications include localized viral, bacterial and candidal infection, delayed hypopigmentation, persistent erythema, and prolonged healing. The most severe complications are hypertrophic scarring, disseminated infection, and ectropion. Early detection of complications and rapid institution of appropriate therapy are extremely important. Delay in treatment can have severe deleterious consequences including permanent scarring and dyspigmentation.

Nail deformity can happen if the treatment area is at nail matrix; in care of wart over the nail matrix explain the patient about the risk of nail deformity.

CONCLUSION

Carbon dioxide laser has several advantages over the other modalities of treating tumors of skin. It produces cosmetically acceptable results and recovery down time is short. Though, the oldest laser in the field of dermatology, it is still the gold standard for the ablative lasers.

REFERENCES

1. Khoo L. Carbon dioxide laser treatment of benign skin lesions. National Skin Centre Experience. 2001;12:2.
2. Krupa Shankar D, Chakravarthi M, Shilpakar R. Carbon dioxide laser guidelines. J Cutan Aesthet Surg. 2009;2(2):72-80.
3. Cohen JL. Minimizing skin cancer surgical scars using ablative fractional Er:YAG laser treatment. J Drugs Dermatol. 2013;12(10):1171-3.
4. Trimas SJ, Ellis DA, Metz RD. The carbon dioxide laser: An alternative for the treatment of actinically damaged skin. Dermatol Surg. 1997;23(10):885-9.
5. Quaedvlieg PJ, Ostertag JU, Krekels GA, Neumann HA. Delayed wound healing after three different treatments for widespread actinic keratosis on the atrophic bald scalp. Dermatol Surg 2003;29(10):1052-6.
6. Phahonthep R, Sindhuphak W, Sriprajittichai P. Lidocaine iontophoresis versus EMLA cream for CO_2 laser treatment in seborrheic keratosis. J Med Assoc Thai. 2004;87(suppl 2):S15-8.
7. Fitzpatrick RE, Goldman MP, Ruiz-Esparza J. Clinical advantage of the CO_2 laser superpulsed mode. Treatment of verruca vulgaris, seborrheic keratoses, lentigines and actinic cheilitis. J Dermatol Surg Oncol. 1994;20(7):449-56.
8. Verma KK, Ovung EM. Epidermal and sebaceous nevi treated with carbon dioxide laser. Indian J Dermatol Venereol Leprol. 2002;68(1):23-4.

CHAPTER 10

Laser- and Light-assisted Hair Reduction: Principles and Options

Deepti Ghia, Ahmed Al Issa, Abdullah Al Eisa, Sanjeev V Mulekar

INTRODUCTION

Unwanted body hair removal is a worldwide requirement. Using lasers or other light-based technologies is highly sought after service especially as it is nearly permanent and convenient.

The laser and light device companies are permitted to claim permanent hair reduction, but not permanent hair removal by the Food and Drug Association, United States.

Permanent hair reduction is defined as the long-term, stable reduction in the number of hair regrowing after a treatment regime, which may include several sessions, but does not necessarily imply that all hair within the treatment area are eliminated.[1]

NEED FOR LASER HAIR REDUCTION

Excess hair growth needs to be differentiated from unwanted hair. Excess hair growth may present as hypertrichosis or hirsutism. Hypertrichosis means excess hair growth at any body site more than usual norms, whereas hirsutism manifests as excess hair growth in women at androgen-dependent sites. However, cosmetic reason of having a hair free appearance in people with normal hair pattern (unwanted hair) is the most common indication for hair removal treatments.[2] With few exceptions, such as pseudofolliculitis barbae, acne keloidalis, pilonidal sinus, and hidradenitis suppurativa, hair removal is almost solely driven by personal preferences rather than being a medical requirement.[1]

BASIC HAIR BIOLOGY

There are three main types of hair: 1) lanugo, 2) vellus, and 3) terminal. Lanugo hairs cover the fetus and are shed within the neonatal period. Vellus hair are usually nonpigmented, having a diameter ranging from 30 to 50 µm. Terminal hair shafts range from 150 to 300 µm in diameter. Individual follicle is capable of change from vellus to terminal or vice versa.

The hair follicle is a hormonally active structure, anatomically divided into infundibulum (i.e., hair follicle orifice to opening of the sebaceous gland), isthmus (opening of sebaceous gland to insertion of erector pili muscle) and inferior segment (insertion of erector pili to the base of the hair follicle). The dermal papilla provides the neurovascular support to the follicle (Fig. 1).

Hair follicle is controlled by a programed cycle. The hair cycle consists of anagen, catagen, and telogen phases. Anagen is characterized by a period of active growth. Catagen is a transition period in which the lower part of the hair follicle undergoes apoptosis. Telogen is a resting period that ensures regrowth to occur when anagen resumes. The hair regrowth is dependent on stem cells within the hair bulb matrix and follicular bulge area.

The amount and type of pigment in the hair shaft determines the hair color. Melanocytes produce two types of melanin, eumelanin, a brown black pigment and pheomelanin, a red pigment. Melanocytes are located in the upper portion of the hair bulb and outer root sheath of infundibulum.[3]

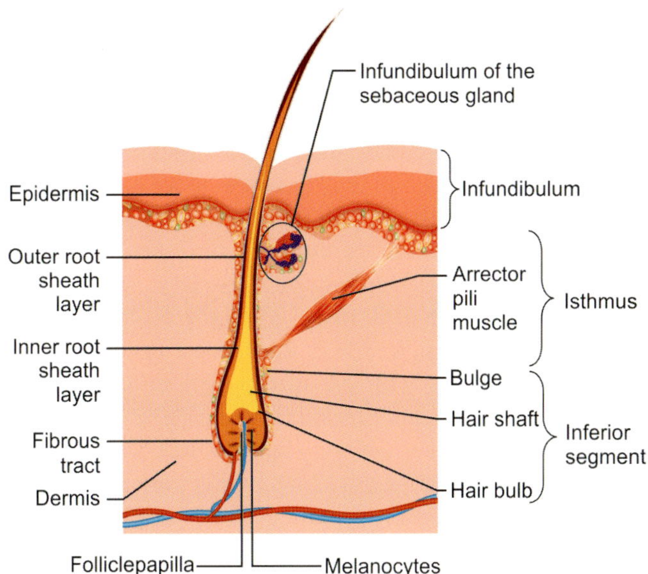

FIG. 1: Anatomical structure of hair follicle

PRINCIPLE

The melanin in the hair shaft is the targeted chromophore. Melanin absorbs light in the wavelength of the red and the infrared part of electromagnetic spectrum.[2] This light energy absorbed transforms to heat energy in the tissue and causes damage to the hair. The bulge area and the dermal papilla have the stem cells which need to be destroyed by heat diffusion for permanent hair reduction.

Theory of Selective Photothermolysis

The word photothermolysis comes from three Greek root words-"photo" meaning light, "thermo" meaning heat, and "lysis" meaning destruction.

This theory proposes targeting a structure or tissue using a specific wavelength of light with the intention of absorbing light into that target area alone. The energy directed into the target area produces sufficient heat to damage the target, while allowing the surrounding area to remain relatively untouched.

Since the desired target is away from the chromophore and the heat energy needs to diffuse from melanin to stem cells, the pulse duration must be longer than the thermal relaxation time of melanin for heat to diffuse. This is the extended theory of selective photothermolysis.

Absence of melanin in gray hair, light colored hair, white hair, and vellus hair makes photothermolysis difficult, hence, these cannot be targeted easily with laser.[4]

Cooling

Laser light passes through the epidermis and is then absorbed by target hair follicles in the dermis. Hence, the laser fluence at the skin surface must be high enough so that sufficient photons are delivered to the depth of the follicle. Simultaneously, the epidermis must be cooled to avoid thermal damage. A variety of techniques for skin cooling have been devised to lower the epidermal temperature through direct contact (aqueous gel or chilled transparent optical handpiece tips) or through the delivery of cold air or cryogen sprays to the skin surface.

TREATMENT PARAMETERS

The main parameters to consider when using lasers and light for hair removal are wavelength, fluence, spot size, and pulse duration. The wavelength is usually fixed for each device type, whereas the operator selects the remaining parameters.

Wavelength

Melanin within the hair shaft is the chromophore for laser hair removal. Although melanin absorbs all wavelengths throughout the ultraviolet, visible, and near-infrared (NIR) regions, only the longer wavelength photons (i.e., red to NIR) are capable of penetrating the skin to the level of the growing hair follicle.[1]

The wavelength is constant for each device. A shorter wavelength is safe for lighter skin types and a longer wavelength is better for darker or tanned skin types.

Hence, the ruby and the alexandrite laser are suitable for Fitzpatrick skin type II–IV, diode laser is suitable for Fitzpatrick skin types II–V, and the long-pulsed neodymium doped yttrium-aluminum-garnet (Nd:YAG) laser is suitable for skin types III–VI (Fig. 2).

Spot Size

The spot size is the diameter of the laser beam or the linear dimensions of the skin contact probe. According to the phenomenon of lateral scattering of light, once it penetrates the skin, the spot size affects the effective depth of light penetration. If all other parameters are held constant, a larger spot size will result in an overall greater depth of effect, which is desirable for targeting hair follicles (Fig. 3). For dermal targets, larger spot size is better. This phenomenon is valid for a spot size of up to 10 mm.

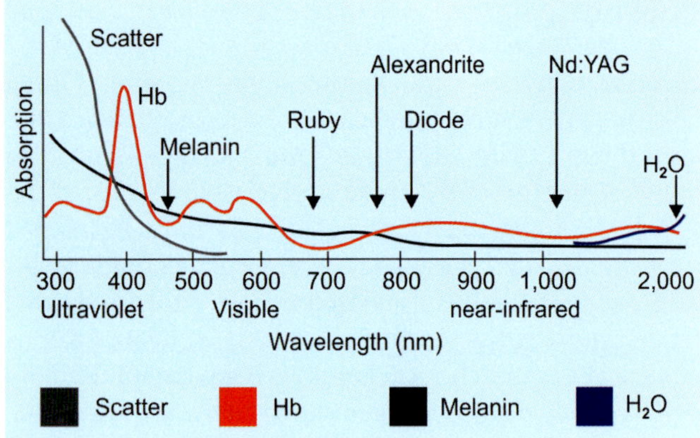

Hb, hemoglobin; Nd:YAG, neodymium doped yttrium-aluminium-garnet.

FIG. 2: Absorption of light by different chromophores versus wavelength of different lasers used for hair removal

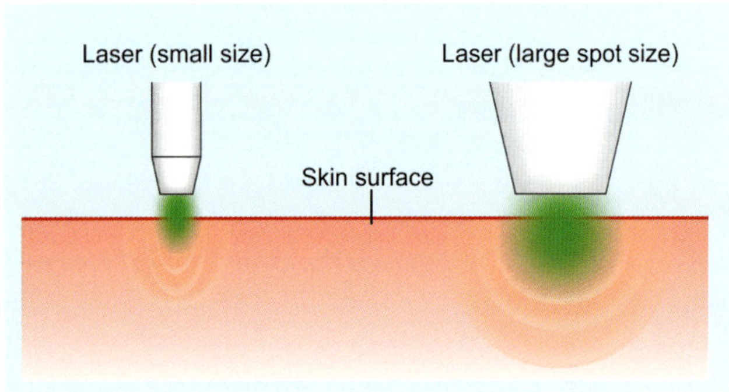

FIG. 3: Effect of spot size on scattering

Pulse Duration

Pulse duration refers to the subsecond duration of each light exposure, and is inversely proportional to the peak power density of the laser or light pulses.

According to the theory of selective photothermolysis, thermal effects within tissue can be confined to a specific structure through heating that structure faster than it cools. The rate at which any tissue component cools is largely dependent on the square of its physical diameter and is usually specified by its thermal relaxation time, which in turn is the time it takes for the target to dissipate half of its heat to the surrounding tissue.

To achieve selective photothermolysis, the optimal pulse duration is roughly equal to or shorter than the thermal relaxation time. Hair-bearing skin contains melanin as a chromophore both within the hair shaft and the interfollicular surface epidermis. During laser hair removal, epidermal melanin represents an unintended bystander target. Clinical effects on the epidermis can be minimized through selecting pulse durations that are longer than epidermal melanin thermal relaxation time, but do not exceed the follicular thermal relaxation time. Thermokinetic selectivity states that smaller structures (e.g., epidermal melanin) will lose heat more quickly than larger structures (e.g., dermal hair follicles).

Longer pulse durations allow for more gentle heating of the epidermis by slowing the deposition of the light energy into the skin; the more gradually the pigmented epidermis absorbs light, the slower its conversion to heat, making cooling more efficient and limiting any deleterious thermal effects on the interfollicular epidermis. Usually, the pulse durations in laser and light devices have a range from 1 to 600 ms; pulse durations longer than 100 ms are preferred in darker skin types.

Fluence

The amount of energy delivered to a unit area in a single pulse is defined as fluence. Higher fluencies deliver more photons to the hair follicle, and therefore, higher energy results in more hair reduction. However, the risk of side effects increase with a higher fluence. From a practical point of view, the fluence should be gradually titrated upward until the clinical threshold of immediate perifollicular erythema and edema is reached; this determines the appropriate optimal fluence setting.[4] The fluence should be gradually increased until this is observed.

Frequency and Number of Treatments

Multiple laser treatments are necessary to achieve long-term reduction of hair, typically in the range of 5–7 sessions spaced approximately 4–8 weeks apart. With each session, an estimated 15–30% of hairs are removed.[4] Treated hairs usually shed 2 weeks after the laser treatment. Treated sites will manifest a decrease in the total hair density and miniaturization of hair.

DEVICES AVAILABLE FOR LASER HAIR REMOVAL (TABLE 1)

Long-pulsed ruby lasers were the first lasers used for hair removal. Ruby lasers are indicated in Fitzpatrick skin types I, II, and III with dark hair. Due to their relative inefficiency and high cost, ruby lasers are no longer commercially available in North America.

TABLE 1: Devices available for photoepilation[1]

Wavelength	Pulse duration (ms)	Fluence (J/cm^2)	Spot size (mm)
Nd:YAG	1,064	0.1–10,000 up to 900	1.5–30 × 30
Diode	800–810	5–500 up to 100	5–22 × 35
IPL	400–1,400	0.3–500 up to 500	Up to 50 × 25
Alexandrite	755	0.1–300 up to 600	1.5–18

IPL, intense pulsed light; Nd:YAG, neodymium doped yttrium-aluminum-garnet.

Neodymium doped Yttrium-Aluminium-Garnet

The long-pulsed Nd:YAG laser is best indicated for patients with Fitzpatrick skin phototype VI. The Nd:YAG laser system operates at a longer wavelength (1,064 nm) than the alexandrite laser, allowing deeper penetration into the dermis. The Nd:YAG laser is less absorbed by epidermal melanin, and therefore, is possibly more suitable for darker skin types because of lesser side effects in these patients.

Alexandrite Laser

The long-pulsed alexandrite (755 nm) laser has been shown to be effective for hair removal. Patients with Fitzpatrick skin phototypes I–IV can be treated with long-pulsed alexandrite lasers.

Diode Laser

The long-pulsed diode laser has been used for laser hair removal, and is recommended for patients with Fitzpatrick skin phototypes I–V. Multiple arrays of semiconductor diodes provide a laser light of 800–810 nm. Diode lasers are generally considered reliable devices.

Nonlaser Devices

Intense pulsed light (IPL) devices emit polychromatic noncoherent light with wavelengths ranging from 400 to 1,400 nm. With these light sources, different filters are used to target different chromophores.

The light delivery systems for IPLs consist of broad rectangular crystal probes that are held in contact with the skin. Good alignment of each adjacent rectangular exposure pulse and maintenance of skin contact over the entire crystal surface are important for uniform treatment.

Radiofrequency Combined with Intense Pulsed Light

Dual energy technology is based on the delivery of synchronous pulses of bipolar radiofrequency current and pulsed visible light within the same pulse to reduce the light intensity and side effects.

EFFICACY OF LIGHT-BASED HAIR REMOVAL

Multiple studies have shown efficacy of different lasers in reducing unwanted hair. In long-term clinical trials, photoepilation devices have been shown to reduce hair counts by approximately 50% after a series of multiple treatments.[5]

Efficacy of different lasers have been compared through the analysis of randomized controlled studies. In a study by Toosi et al.,[6] efficacy of diode was comparable to the alexandrite laser and the IPL at 6 months of treatments, where 3–6 sessions were given to each patient. The side effects of diode were more than that of the alexandrite laser and the IPL. Studies by Smith et al.[7] in 2006 and Hamzavi et al.[8] in 2007 have demonstrated that efficacy of hair removal laser combined with eflornithine application is more efficacious than laser alone. Davoudi et al.[9] in 2008 compared Nd:YAG laser versus alexandrite laser versus a combination of Nd:YAG and alexandrite laser for 18 months with four treatment sessions. There was no significant difference in the hair reduction in all the groups. Braun et al.[10] in 2009 compared high fluence low frequency diode with a low fluence and high frequency diode. The results in both groups were comparable, but lesser pain was seen in the lower fluence group. Pai et al.[11] in 2011 compared low fluence high repetition rate versus high fluence low repetition for 810 diode laser. There was a comparable reduction in the hair thickness in both the groups, however, pain was lesser in low fluence high repetition rates.

A study by Mustafa et al.[12] in 2014 showed that for darker skin types, the diode laser is safer than alexandrite laser.

PRELASER WORKUP

- Identify the cause of hirsutism or hypertrichosis
- Note the previous methods of hair removal
- Give oral acyclovir prophylaxis to patients with history of herpes labialis and herpes genitalis

- Rule out relative contraindications, like isotretinoin therapy in last 6 months, photosensitizing dermatoses and drugs, pregnancy, gold therapy, or history of keloids
- Obtain informed consent including potential complications, expected results about hair reduction from the patient
- Instruct patients to avoid plucking, waxing, or electrolysis 2 weeks before treatment. If necessary, shaving or trimming may be permitted.

ANESTHESIA AND PAIN CONTROL

Topical lidocaine and prilocaine combinations are appropriate anesthetic agents. They can be applied 1 hour prior to the laser session covered by occlusive dressing or moistened gauze. Sometimes, the topical anesthetic creams can cause sensitization and inflammatory side effects.[13] Pneumatic skin flattening (PSF) technology can reduce pain by invoking the "gate theory" of pain transmission.

LASER SAFETY

- Eye protection is essential for laser- or light-based hair removal
- Enamel of teeth should be protected by gauze when working around lips
- Optimal cooling reduces risk of pigmentary changes and postlaser burns.

POSTLASER CARE

- Apply ice and a topical corticosteroid to shorten duration of perifollicular erythema and edema
- A shedding growth may be seen after the session which usually falls off after 2 weeks
- Apply sunscreen and avoid excessive sun exposure to prevent postinflammatory dyspigmentation
- Avoid swimming and parlour activities till the erythema settles.

COMPLICATIONS

Paradoxical Hypertrichosis

It is defined as an increase in the density of hair or coarseness at laser site or surrounding areas occurring in the absence of any other cause of hypertrichosis. The incidence can range from 0.01 to 10%.[14] The cause of this is poorly understood. A proposed theory states that the subtherapeutic thermal injury may stimulate the vellus hairs and also lead to synchronization of the hair cycle causing this growth. Individuals with darker skin type and black hair are more prone to it. Treatment with suboptimal fluencies, superficial depth of treatment, and hormonal imbalances can cause paradoxical hair growth. This condition is treated with laser therapy at moderate to high fluence.[15]

Urticaria

This can occur within 72 hours postlaser photoepilation due to delayed hypersensitivity reaction to ruptured hair follicles[16] which can be managed with antihistamine drugs.

Discoloration

There can be hyper- or hypopigmentation after a laser session due to inflammatory effect of the laser which usually gets better with time.

Scarring

Sometimes, scarring can occur due to higher laser fluence or by inexperienced operators. These scars need to be moisturized frequently which may heal subsequently.

CONCLUSION

Laser- and light-based hair removal techniques have become one of the most commonly performed procedures on the skin. No single device is better than the other, and individual customization may be required for optimal treatment outcomes.

REFERENCES

1. Zandi S, Lui H. Long-term removal of unwanted hair using light. Dermatol Clin. 2013;31(1):179-91.
2. Haedersdal M, Wulf HC. Evidence-based review of hair removal using lasers and light sources. J Eur Acad Dermatol Venereol. 2006;20(1):9-20.
3. Zenzie HH, Altshuler GB, Smirnov MZ, Anderson RR. Evaluation of cooling methods for laser dermatology. Lasers Surg Med. 2000;26:130-44.
4. Ibrahimi OA, Avram MM, Hanke CW, Kilmer SL, Anderson RR. Laser hair removal. Dermatol Ther. 2011;24:94-107.
5. Haedersdal M, Beerwerth F, Nash JF. Laser and intense pulsed light hair removal technologies: from professional to home use. Br J Dermatol. 2011;165 Suppl 3:31-6.
6. Toosi P, Sadighha A, Sharifian A, Razavi GM. A comparison study of the efficacy and side effects of different light sources in hair removal. Lasers Med Sci. 2006;21:1-4.

7. Smith SR, Piacquadio DJ, Beger B, Littler C. Eflornithine cream combined with laser therapy in the management of unwanted facial hair growth in women: a randomized trial. Dermatol Surg. 2006;32:1237-43.
8. Hamzavi I, Tan E, Shapiro J, Lui H. A randomized bilateral vehicle-controlled study of eflornithine cream combined with laser treatment versus laser treatment alone for facial hirsutism in women. J Am Acad Dermatol. 2007;57:54-9.
9. Davoudi SM, Behnia F, Gorouhi F, Keshavarz S, Nassiri Kashani M, Rashighi Firoozabadi M, et al. Comparison of long-pulsed alexandrite and Nd:YAG lasers, individually and in combination, for leg hair reduction: an assessor-blinded, randomized trial with 18 months of follow-up. Arch Dermatol. 2008;144:1323-7.
10. Braun M. Permanent laser hair removal with low fluence high repetition rate versus high fluence low repetition rate 810 nm diode laser–a split leg comparison study. J Drugs Dermatol. 2009;8:s14-7.
11. Pai GS, Bhat PS, Mallya H, Gold M. Safety and efficacy of low-fluence, high-repetition rate versus high-fluence, low-repetition rate 810-nm diode laser for permanent hair removal–a split-face comparison study. J Cosmet Laser Ther. 2011;13:134-7.
12. Mustafa FH, Jaafar MS, Ismail AH, Mutter KN. Comparison of alexandrite and diode lasers for hair removal in dark and medium skin: which is better? J Lasers Med Sci. 2014;5(4):188-93.
13. Hahn IH, Hoffman RS, Nelson LS. EMLA-induced methemoglobinemia and systemic topical anesthetic toxicity. J Emerg Med. 2004;26:85-8.
14. Moreno-Arias G, Castelo-Branco C, Ferrando J. Paradoxical effect after IPL photoepilation. Dermatol Surg. 2002;28:1013-6.
15. Alster TS, Khoury RR. Treatment of laser complications. Facial Plast Surg. 2009;25:316-23.
16. Bernstein EF. Severe urticaria after laser treatment for hair reduction. Dermatol Surg. 2010;36:147-51.

CHAPTER 11

Intense Pulsed Light Therapy

Mukta Sachdev, Archana Samynathan

INTRODUCTION

Laser and nonlaser light therapies gained tremendous reception in the field of dermatology owing to their noninvasive character, convenient skilled execution with relatively lesser time for the procedure with low downtime. The science of laser made its way in 1983 after the original publication of "selective photothermolysis" theory by Anderson and Parrish. The various conditions in which laser and other light therapies are indicated were close to not being treatable before the advent of this technology. Laser and other light energy sources like radiofrequency, intense pulsed light (IPL), long pulsed laser are fast gaining momentum in the treatment of vascular lesions, pigmentary lesions, and hair reduction.

Intense pulsed light was for the first time used in 1995 to treat telangiectasias. The fundamental principle of selective photothermolysis is packets of light called photons of a particular wavelength are absorbed by certain chromophores (oxyhemoglobin, deoxyhemoglobin, melanin, water in the skin) and the light energy is then converted to heat energy which is made use for cellular destruction. Intense pulsed light is derived from xenon flash lamps that produce high output bursts of lights with a broad wavelength spectrum ranging between 400 and 1,200 nm. Filters are used to derive variable wavelength, thus enabling the light source to target multiple chromophores, therefore, addressing vascular lesions, pigmentary lesions, hair reduction, and photorejuvenation. Shorter wavelengths have lesser energy and attack more superficial chromophores, longer wavelengths, on the other hand, contain more energy and penetrate deeper into the skin. Cooling is used to protect the skin in contact with the device.

INDICATIONS OF INTENSE PULSED LIGHT[1]

- Aesthetic
  - Hair reduction
    - Hirsutism
    - Hypertrichosis
    - Pseudofolliculitis barbae
  - Photo rejuvenation.
  - Fine lines
  - Wrinkles
  - Skin texture
  - Enlarged pores
- Therapeutic
  - Photo damage (dyspigmentation and vascular changes)[2,3]
  - Pigmented lesions
    - Birthmarks
    - Lentigines
    - Freckles
    - Postinflammatory hyperpigmentation (PIH)
    - Epidermal melasma
    - Poikiloderma of civatte

- Vascular lesions
  - Thread veins
  - Rosacea and vascular dyschromia
  - Telangiectasias
  - Cherry hemangioma
  - Spider angioma
  - Diffuse redness (vascular dyschromia)
- Acne vulgaris
- Sebaceous gland hyperplasia
- Actinic keratosis[2,3]
- Bowen's disease (squamous cell carcinoma)
- Basal cell carcinoma.

CONTRAINDICATIONS[1]

- Extensively tanned skin, owing to a higher risks of laser burn and PIH
- In case of hair removal, waxing, epilation, tweezing, and bleaching must be avoided 10–20 days prior depending on growth of hair
- Hypopigmentation (e.g., vitiligo, PIH, etc.)
- Active dermatitis or infection at the treatment site (eczema, herpes simples, etc.)
- Pregnancy and lactation until the periods return to normal. As the hormonal imbalances may interfere with the treatment sessions planned
- Endocrine disorders, such as polycystic ovarian syndrome, hypothyroidism, hyperthyroidism, etc., must be evaluated as the outcome of light therapy may be influenced by the course of these disorders
- Keloidal tendency of an individual
- Epileptic disorders as laser may initiate seizures
- Oral isotretinoin and other photosensitizing drugs intake 3–6 months prior to treatment
- Antidiabetic medications and blood thinner therapy
- Cancer and anticancer medications
- Presence of pacemaker or other metal implants in the tissues underlying the area to be treated.

HAIR REMOVAL[4-6]

Intense pulsed light in hair reduction made its first appearance in the year 1997. A study was conducted in 2006 which showed no significant statistical difference between lasers (alexandrite and diode) and IPL. The most significant results were observed in patients with fair skin and dark coarse hair, however, all skin types do respond to IPL hair removal, the darker skin types poses an inherent tendency to postprocedural dyspigmention, hyperpigmentation has been more commonly recorded. Lighter hair color and finer textures are relatively less responsive to this treatment and are opted to be treated with other technologies better suited for this phenotype. Broad spectrum light is applied to the area to be treated, which targets the melanin, more concentrated in the bulb which is eventually destroyed along with the hair producing papilla, and also the darker capillaries that feed the papilla. The photothermal energy attacks the follicle, papilla, and its blood supply to cause follicular miniaturization, delaying the growth cycle duration by complete disruption of the intracellular melanocytes and tissue coagulation.

Intense pulsed light targets active follicles in the anagen phase of the hair cycle. Not all follicles are active at a given point of time, thus, 8–10 sessions, 4–6 weeks apart are required for effective hair reduction. There is no strict protocol; the sessions are decided based on the expertize of the physician to aptly suit the skin and hair type of an individual patient. Perifollicular erythema is the desired end point. As the epidermal melanin is too capable of absorbing the light energy, appropriate energy levels must be chosen for effective outcome without causing damage to the surrounding skin tissue. Darker skin, darker coarser hair, and high density of hair will require lesser energy, while lighter skin, lighter finer hair may necessitate the use of high energy levels. Longer pulses are needed for thick coarse hair whereas shorter pulses are required for finer hair. Longer pulses also cause lesser collateral damage as the tiny melanin particles have time to lose the absorbed heat.

Wavelengths between 500 and 1,000 nm are exploited for the purpose of long-term hair reduction. The longer of these rays penetrate deeper to reach the deeper follicles, while the shorter of the wavelengths target the more superficial follicles and scatter more readily.

Long-term stable hair reduction is achieved after multiple sessions. The results may vary based upon the phenotype of the patient and the skill with which the procedure has been executed.

The area to be treated is shaved clean of any hair, cleansed, and must be free of any sunburn. A test patch is treated to ascertain parameters. Liberal use of clear refrigerated gels and ice packs reduce the pain and discomfort of patients. Postprocedure, a topical antibiotic may be used. A broad spectrum sunscreen is mandatory. The importance of keeping the skin hydrated and avoidance of other therapies in the same area treated, like chemical peeling, microdermabrasion, etc. must be stressed upon. Contact with chemicals, like perfumes, strong makeup, and bleaching must be avoided for a couple of days post-treatment.

PHOTOREJUVENATION AND ANTI-AGING[7.]

The term "photorejuvenation" was coined to describe the simultaneous improvements in brown spots, red spots, and fine wrinkles with IPL devices,

The wavelengths useful for this purpose span 400–1,200 nm in the visible and infrared range of the electromagnetic spectrum. Cutoff filters are used to specifically match the components of the skin. Simultaneous usage of different wavelengths can be used to target multiple facets of photoaging. In other words, the numerous components for photorejuvenaton can be targeted concurrently. Photoaged skin is a comprehensive description of skin characterized by mottled pigmentation, roughened skin texture, fine vessels (thread veins), enlarged pores, and skin laxity. Asian photoaged skin has more pigment dyschromia whereas Caucasian skin exhibits more telangiectatic component of photoaging.

The working principle relies on the fact that energy is built up in the sun damaged skin by electromagnetic rays' absorption of melanin in the pigmentation and hemoglobin in the vascular lesions to eliminate them to a significant extent. Photothermal damage to the blood vessels resulting in the release of inflammatory growth factors stimulates the formation of new collagen. The effect of which is shown as improvement of skin texture, translucence, pore size reduction, hydration, and elasticity of skin. Caucasian skin is the most challenging to treat owing to their prolonged sun.

The treatment is done in phases; the epidermal superficial pigmentation is targeted first followed by vascular lesions and finally, the collagen stimulation. Increased collagen production evens out fine lines and flattens wrinkles to present a younger appearance. Multiple sessions are required with an interval of 4–6 weeks in between each session. Subtle improvements are seen in patients, regarding which patients are sufficiently counseled. The patients approved as candidates for the treatment must be introduced to a regular skin care regime including a good moisturizer and a broad spectrum sunscreen; an antiaging cream may be used for a synergistic outcome which must be strictly used before and after procedure sessions. Laughter lines, frown lines, and nasolabial folds do not respond significantly owing to the underlying muscle patterns. They may be corrected with botulinum toxin, dermal fillers, or ablative laser techniques. The therapy may be combined with chemical peels and nonaggressive cosmetic procedures like microdermabrasion.

The area to be treated is cleansed. A test patch must be performed to optimize the energy levels for a patient; the whole face and neck are treated. Areas of bony prominence, around eyes and mouth, and problem areas are dealt with caution. Treatment gels and fluids are applied in sufficient amounts to ensure uniform penetrance of the light energy. Postprocedural skin care is made mandatory.

PIGMENTARY LESIONS[8,9]

The ideal wavelengths used are in the range of 530–1,200 nm. Melanin is the primary target for pigment specific lasers. The other less important target is hemoglobin. Short-pulsed lasers cause more effective membrane disruption of melanosomal membranes and structural disruption which is evidenced by electron microscopy. Shorter pulse durations measuring in 40–750 nanoseconds efficiently destroy melanosomes.

Most effectively treated are the lesions with epidermal pigmentation. The pigmented lesions are usually treated in stages. Intense pulsed light therapy can be combined with bleaching agents like hydroquinone, azelaic acid; topical tretinoin and glycolic acid more for their desquamating action and along with chemical peels. Pigmented lesions usually require about 4–6 sessions at monthly intervals. Each session may last 5–15 minutes depend upon the size of the lesion. They mostly require topical anesthesia applied 45 minutes to 1 hour prior to therapy. The laser beams are guided within the pigmented lesion. The beams cause superficial to deep epidermal injury. The primary chromatophore is melanin; hemoglobin in the feeding vessels is also targeted. The desired end point is the lesional and perilesional erythema along with immediate darkening of the lesion. The lesion further darkens progressively for about 24–48 hours following which scab formation and exfoliation may occur over the next 7–14 days. The lesions heal with a mild hypopigmentation which eventually pigment to become indistinguishable.

Postprocedure skin care including antibiotic cream, moisturizer, and sunscreen is applied based upon the lesion. The patients may feel a pricking or a mild discomfort. The procedure normally has a downtime. Adverse effects may range between postprocedural hypopigmentation, erythema, swelling, and bleeding lasting for a few to several hours. Scarring may occur very rarely.

The advent of broad spectrum noncoherent flashlamp source allowed the modulations of wavelengths so as to target multiple skin blemishes simultaneously unlike the laser which required a specific wavelength for a particular lesion.

Excellent response is observed in epidermal lesions including freckles, lentigines. The higher the contrast between the lesion and the surrounding normal skin, the faster is the response. Improvement of the pigmented lesions with lesser contrast takes about twice to thrice the time taken by individuals with lighter skin types with dark pigmented lesions.

Some of the pigmented lesions that can be treated with lasers and light technology are:

Epidermal Lesions

- Lentigines: lentigines are very responsive to IPL. Q-switch lasers have proven to be less effective than IPL in patients with PIH
- Café au lait macules: café au lait macules are more effectively treated by short-pulsed lasers. Clearance of lesions does occur followed by recurrence which is not uncommon
- Becker's nevus: recurrence is the rule with Becker's nevus.

Mixed Epidermal/Dermal and Dermal Lesions

- Nevus of Ota: IPL finds a supportive role in the management of pigmentory lesions with some success. IPL sources pose less of a PIH risk but require a greater number of treatment sessions
- Melasma: lasers and light therapy play a role in adjuvant treatment. Melasma responds poorly to IPL, the primary modality being the use of bleaching creams with a broad spectrum sunscreen in the day
- Postinflammatory hyperpigmentation: this resists laser and light therapy. The inability of the available light technologies to target the scattered melanosomes in the dermis unlike the intracellular melanosomes. With the advent of newer technologies equipped with ultrashort pulses in femto and picoseconds, such particles may become treatable
- Nevus spilus: the results of light technologies are variable. The treatment must be done cautiously as melanomas are known to arise in nevus spilus
- Melanocytic nevus: the use of lasers and IPL are a controversy in melanocytic nevi. Recurrence of the lesion after procedure must be biopsied and the histopathology must be determined.

Intense pulsed light in darker skin types requires a special mentioning as the constituent epidermal melanin which imparts the skin with color, competes with the lesional melanocytes. This is rationale why darker skin has more chances of PIH. It is here that the knowledge and skill of the physician help to set a dose. A test patch is performed to establish the dose and the fluence is progressively increased in the following sessions. Sufficient skin cooling during the procedure along with liberal use of broad spectrum sunscreen further minimize PIH.

Vascular Lesions[10]

Vessels are components of the papillary and reticular dermis. Apart from perfusion, all skin types have a vascular contribution to the skin color. Large vessels of diameter more than 1 mm do not respond to IPL. They are treated either with long-pulsed neodymium doped yttrium-aluminium-garnet or sclerotherapy. Very fine vessels lesser than 0.1 mm do not clear completely with ILP either necessitating the use of pulsed dye or potassium titanyl phosphate laser. Vessels with diameter in the range 0.1–0.5 mm respond effectively to IPL.

Multiple sessions may be required. Higher fluencies with multiple pulsing setting permit time for epidermal cooling amid the pulses and thus, minimizing the chances of burns and PIH. Results are achieved faster and superior in the lighter skin types (Fitzpatrick types I–III).

INTENSE PULSED LIGHT IN THE TREATMENT OF ACNE VULGARIS[11]

One of the major contributions to the pathogenesis of acne is *Propionibacterium acnes* overcolonization of the sebaceous glands. The bacterium manufactures the proinflammatory factors to cause inflammatory lesions. The bacteria also generate porphyrins in high concentrations. The basis of IPL in treating acne is due to the fact that porphyrins are light sensitive and comprise the property to absorb light and convey the light to the surrounding oxygen molecules converting them to free radicals and singlet oxygen particles which attack and destroy the bacterial cell components. The wavelength spectrum delivering beneficial response falls between 530 and 950 nm.

It is a process requiring multiple sessions. Typically, 5–6 sessions 10–15 days apart induce significant response. Longer wavelengths may be used to target the deeper seated bacteria. The therapy is used as an adjuvant along with other opted treatments.

Patient Prepping[1]

- Refrain from tanning as the epidermal melanin absorbs the IPL energy to result in an IPL burn. The risk of a burn increases with darker photo types

- A broad spectrum sunscreen must be prescribed several weeks prior
- A skin lightening cream may be used for several weeks to reduce the risk of IPL burn
- Activities like swimming, trekking, etc. are discouraged 4–6 weeks before a treatment session
- Topical anesthetic creams may be used as per indication and requirement
- The eyes of the patient as well as the persons performing and assisting the procedures require protection
- A clear gel is applied to the area to be treated to ensure maximal transmission of light
- The energy levels are individualized depending on the nature of the skin type undergoing treatment
- Light is delivered in specified pulses.

Morbidity Association of Intense Pulsed Light

Appropriate usage of IPL may not lead to severe adverse effects. Mild to moderate discomfort and redness are the most commonly encountered adverse effects.

Inappropriate use of IPL may possibly lead to the following:

- Immediate adverse effects:
  - Tingling
  - Burning
  - Discomfort
  - Pain
  - Scaling
  - Swelling
  - Bleeding
  - Blistering
  - Scab formation
- Delayed adverse effects:
  - Dyspigmentation
  - Prolonged itching or discomfort
  - Skip areas
  - Scarring (very rarely).

MANAGEMENT OF ADVERSE REACTIONS

Ice packs, applied to the treated areas postprocedure, cool the area, thus, reducing the tingling, discomfort, and pain to an extent. Pain can be controlled with an analgesic. In case of intense discomfort or pain, the energy levels may be decreased; further the session may be deferred for 24–48 hours and started with a lower energy test patch, before the entire session. Sterile gauze with normal saline can be used to clean the scaling and scab. Scabs should not be forcefully peeled as they form natural barriers from the external environment and also help in healing. Pressure bandages can be used in bleeding lesions. Antibiotic creams may be used in deep wound to prevent secondary infections.

Hyperpigmentation is treated with corticosteroids. Both hypo- and hyperpigmentation lesions involve the use of moisturizers and sun protection with the use of a good broad spectrum sunscreen.

CONCLUSION

Intense pulsed light technology made it possible for one device to be used for the treatment of umpteen varied indications including hair reduction, vascular lesions, pigmentary lesions, and photorejuvenation. The modality of therapy is relatively safe with not much of harsh idea effects limiting its usage.

REFERENCES

1. Khunger N, Sachdev M. Practical Manual of Cosmetic Dermatology and Surgery. Pune: Mehta Publishers; 2010; pp. 314-428.
2. Gilbert DJ. Treatment of actinic keratoses with sequential combination of 5-fluorouracil and photodynamic therapy. J Drugs Dermatol. 2005;4:161-3.
3. Dover JS, Bhatia AC, Stewart B, Arndt KA. Topical 5-aminolevulinic acid combined with intense pulsed light in the treatment of photoaging. Arch Dermatol. 2005;141:1247-52.
4. Haedersal N, Wulf HC. Evidence-based review of hair removal lasers and light resources. J Eur Acad Dermatol Venerol. 2006;20:9-20.
5. Fodor L, Menachem M, Ramon Y, Oren S, Yaron R, Liron E, et al. Hair removal using intense pulse light (EpiLight):patient satisfaction, our experience, and literature review. Ann Plast Surg. 2005;54:8-14.
6. Hee Lee J, Huh CH, Yoon HJ, Cho KH, Chung JH. Photo-epilation results of axillary hair in dark-skinned patients by intense pulsed light: comparison between different wavelengths and pulse width. Dermatol Surg. 2006;32:234-40.
7. Brazil J, Owens P. Long-term clinical results of IPL photorejuvenation. J Cosmet Laser Ther. 2003;5:168-74.
8. Bjerring P, Christiansen K. Intense pulsed light source for treatment of small melanocytic nevi and solar lentigines. J Cutan Laser Ther. 2000;2:177-81.
9. Chan H. The use of lasers and intense pulsed light sources for the treatment of acquired pigmentary lesions in Asians. J Cosmet Laser Ther. 2003;5:198-200.
10. Angermeier MC. Treatment of Asian vascular lesions with Intense pulsed light. J Cutan Laser Ther. 1999;1:95-100.
11. Papageorgiou P, Katsambas A, Chu AC. Phototherapy with blue (417 nm) and red (660 nm) light in the treatment of acne vulgaris. Br J Dermatol. 2000;142:973-8.

CHAPTER 12

Laser Hair Removal: Diode Laser

Mukta Sachdev, Gillian R Britto

INTRODUCTION

Laser hair removal is one of the fastest growing procedures in cosmetic dermatology.[1] The International Society of Aesthetic Plastic Surgeons estimated the total number of laser hair removal procedures done as of 2013 is 1,440,252. The desire to remove unwanted hair is a trend that continues to become more prevalent in our society.[1]

Excess hair growth ranges in severity and may present as hypertrichosis (excess hair growth in any body site) or hirsutism (abnormal hair growth in women in androgen dependent sites).[2] Many methods are available to remove unwanted hair, including bleaching, plucking, shaving, waxing, chemical depilators, and electrolysis.[3] However, these procedures can produce unwanted side effects such as irritation and cutaneous infection. Laser hair removal provides easy, painless, and long-term hair reduction. No wonder it has been appropriately called “the next big thing in cosmetic dermatology”.

HISTORY

Laser hair removal was an accidental discovery. Reduction in the number or density of hair, vaporization of the hair shaft and even bleaching of the hair root was observed when Q-switched ruby laser was being used to remove a tattoo. This observation was documented by Dover et al. in 1989 in guinea pigs. The first human trial was conducted on 13 patients by Grossman et al. using a 270 microseconds ruby laser. Follow-up of these patients showed a significant hair reduction in four patients.[4]

Q-switched neodymium doped yttrium-aluminium-garnet (Nd:YAG) laser was the next to undergo trial in 1995. But, there was only 25% reduction in hair density by a 3 months follow-up. The use of selective photothermolysis in laser hair removal was first demonstrated in 1996, by a 694 nm ruby laser. Soon a chain of clinics spawned, offering permanent hair removal. They were faced with a law suit in 1998 for using false claims of permanent hair removal and ultimately wound up. However, things changed for the better with the dawn of new devices such as long-pulsed alexandrite laser (755 nm) in 1997, pulsed diode laser (800 nm) in 1998, long-pulsed Nd:YAG in 1999 as well as intense pulsed light (IPL), and variants of the IPL which include optical synergy technology (electro-optical synergy.[4]

DIODE LASER

Diode laser is an electrically pumped semiconductor laser in which the active medium is formed by a PN junction of a semiconductor diode. The new diode lasers have an inbuilt cooling device. The nozzle of the device’s handpiece incorporates a sapphire chill window technology through which a coolant is in constant circulation; therefore, there is no need for other cooling methods.[5]

MECHANISM OF ACTION

Laser hair removal is based on the theory of selective photothermolysis, which states that utilizing an appropriate wavelength of light targeted at a specific chromophore which absorbed and transformed the energy into heat that is capable of damaging the surrounding tissues (Table 1). Melanin acts as the chromophore for targeting hair follicles; the lasers or light sources that are used for hair removal lie within the optical window of the electromagnetic spectrum where absorption by melanin and deep penetration into the dermis are combined (Fig. 1). Within the 600–1,100 nm region, deep and selective heating of the hair shaft, hair follicle epithelium, and hair matrix is possible, while selective cooling of the epidermis minimizes epidermal injury and damage to epidermal melanin.[1,2,6,7]

Appropriate selection of wavelength, pulse duration, fluence, and spot size are important in optimizing the hair removal while minimizing any potential side effects (Figs 2 and 3).[1]

Light can also destroy hair follicles by two more mechanisms such as 1) mechanical (via shock waves or violent cavitation) and 2) photochemical through generation of toxic mediators, like singlet oxygen or free radicals[6] (Table 1).

TABLE 1: Mechanisms of laser hair removal[1]

Mechanism	Effect
Mechanical	Shock waves or violent cavitation
Photochemical	Generation of toxic mediators such as singlet oxygen or free radicals
Selective photothermolysis	Melanin acts as the chromophore for the lasers or light sources

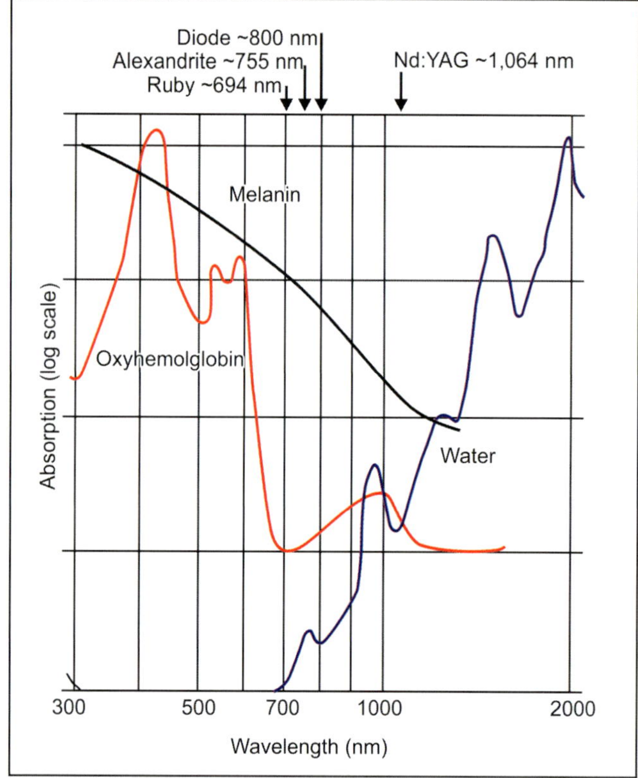

FIG. 1: Absorption spectrum for skin chromophores according to wavelength for different lasers[3]

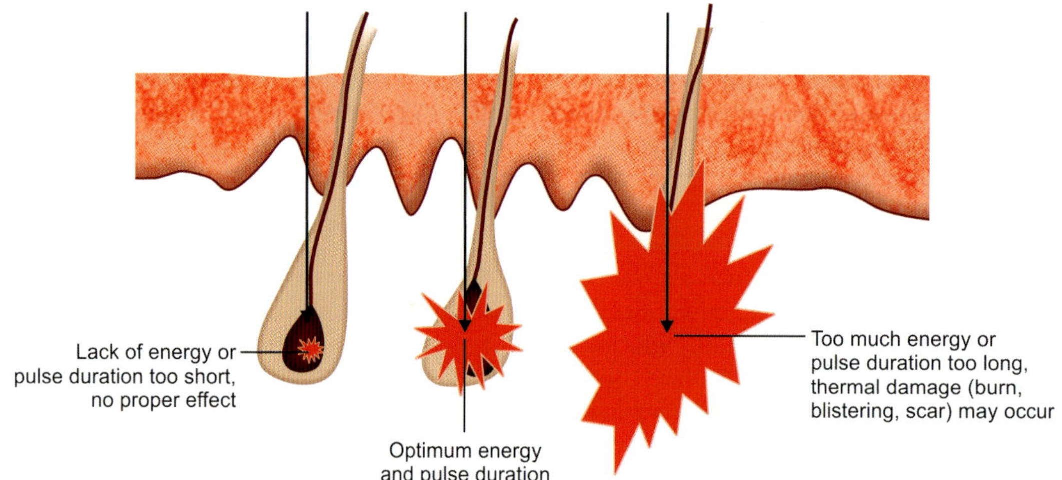

FIG. 2: Laser hair removal: optimal combination of pulse duration and energy[7]

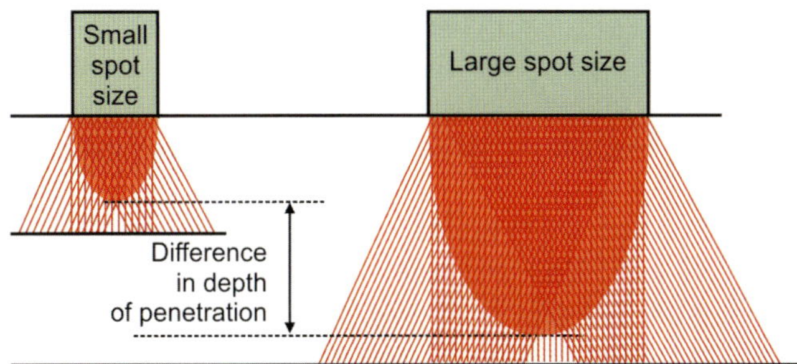

FIG. 3: Effect of dermal scatter on beam propagation[6]

DISCUSSION

Diode lasers are solid state laser devices that have been used successfully over the past several years. Because of their reliability and their ability to penetrate into the much deeper part of the skin, even darker skin individuals are successfully treated for the epilation of unwanted hair. Clinical studies using diode lasers have shown their effectiveness in permanent (long-term hair removal) and have had minimal adverse effects.[5] Long-pulsed diode lasers ranges from 800 to 810 nm. There are many companies which are manufacturing machines with different wavelength output such as 800, 808, and 810 nm. Among diode lasers, 810 nm seems a better wavelength as it penetrates deeper and scatters lesser than 800 nm. However, 800 nm wavelength proved to be a better treatment option than other lasers as it requires lesser sessions, is less painful and more effective.[8] According to a study by D Kopera, the mean hair plucking interval after use of a 800 nm diode laser was extended by 4.11 times giving a welcome increase in the quality of life and self-consciousness. Side effects were not noted, however, post-treatment folliculitis was seen in three cases.[7] Adrian et al. observed in their study that 800 nm diode laser was effective in hair removal in all African-American women who were presented with facial and neck hair. Men noted a significant reduction in pseudofolliculitis barbae after a single treatment and were pleased with the results regardless of overall hair reduction success.[9]

Diode laser systems for hair removal have traditionally used a long pulse width with high energy densities to treat hair, which can increase the risk of skin burns during the course of treatment. As well as, many patients have noted that there is pain associated with the treatment without adequate cooling. The reason for pain and discomfort following treatment is because the laser light energy is converted into heat which is then dissipated to the surrounding areas such as the sensory nerve endings supplying the hair follicle, therefore, causing pain and discomfort.[10]

These systems have also been shown to be associated with slow hair removal treatments when treating large surface areas.

Halachmi et al. evaluated the safety and efficacy of low fluence, large spot size treatments in laser hair removal and compared it to traditional diode high fluence treatments. The results demonstrated that both laser systems provided significant hair reduction with 3 months follow-up after five treatments. However, a mild difference was noted after the third treatment session with a slightly more rapid regrowth of hair in the low fluence, large spot size laser relative to the traditional diode laser. They concluded that the major benefit with a low fluence diode laser is the reduced risk of adverse events.[6]

Recently, aerodynamics has been incorporated into laser hair removal technology. The technology uses a vacuum suction to expand the skin to be treated which thereby increases the transparency of the skin and reduces the energy required during the treatment session. The vacuum generates negative pressure which draws the skin into the vacuum chamber. The feeling of pressure and touch sensations activate the respective receptors, thereby preventing the transmission of pain to the brain. Pain is also reduced because the density of the melanin is lesser in the expanded skin and therefore, the energy absorbed is also lesser.[11]

Using low fluences with repetitive millisecond pulses to achieve heat stacking in the hair bulb and bulge represents a paradigm shift in laser hair removal. A study done by Pai et al. which compared the efficacy, safety, and treatment speed of a low fluence, rapid pulse, and multiple passes 810 nm diode laser and a single, high fluence pass 810 nm diode concluded that both the laser treatments produced hair reduction in excess of 80% in 6 months following the first treatment. But, the treatment of low fluence and multiple passes showed a more significant reduction in hair thickness in subsequent sessions.[10]

HOME USE DEVICES

The 810 nm diode Tria laser is the current Food and Drug Administration approved hair removal home use device. Wheeland's study using the Tria diode laser produced an average hair reduction of 41% after three treatments at 6 months follow-up. Side effects noted were blisters (8%) in skin types V and 33% in skin type IV. Subjects with lighter skin types did not experience any blistering. Pain was more in the dark skinned individuals.[3]

COMPARING THE DIODE LASER WITH OTHER HAIR REMOVAL LASERS

Neodymium Doped Yttrium-aluminium-garnet Laser

Studies have shown that Nd:YAG lasers are safe and effective lasers for hair removal. They are best to be used in patients with darker skin types such as Fitzpatrick IV–VI. The study by Ruohong et al. showed that both Nd:YAG laser and diode laser are safe and effective lasers for hair removal, but the diode laser seemed to be more efficacious and less painful than the of Nd:YAG laser. The hair growth rate is about 270–400 μm/day and in this clinical trial, the regrowth rate slowed down after the use of the lasers, however, the hair diameter reduction was more apparent on the diode laser side compared to the Nd:YAG laser after the first session of treatment. Bouzari et al. retrospectively studied the efficacy of the two laser systems in 75 patients with Fitzpatrick skin type I–IV; hair reduction for the diode laser was 42.4% and Nd:YAG laser was 46.9%.[12]

Chan et al. also compared the efficacy of the two laser systems in 15 Chinese women with skin types IV and V and found that the regrowth rate from the diode and Nd:YAG laser was 23 and 19%, respectively.[12]

Treatments with Nd:YAG laser are known to be more painful than diode laser. Rogachefsky et al. considered pain from laser hair removal to be related to a variety of factors such as treatment sites, fluence, spot sizes, and longer wavelengths.[12]

Another study by Wanitphakdeedecha et al. done to observe the effect of low fluence, high repetition rate 810 nm diode versus a high fluence, low repetition rate 1,064 nm Nd:YAG for axillary hair removal showed that both laser systems are effective in reducing the axillary hair, with minimal down time and adverse effects. But, the high fluence, low repetition rate Nd:YAG laser is superior in hair reduction and provides higher patient satisfaction. However, the low fluence, high repetition rate diode laser is less painful.[13]

Alexandrite Laser (755 nm) and Diode Laser (810 nm)

It was Finkel in 1997 who first reported effective hair removal on the face, arms, legs, and bikini line using an alexandrite laser.

These lasers are more suited for lighter skin types such as Fitzpatrick I–III due to their shorter wavelength and paucity of competing with epidermal melanin and therefore, low risk of laser induced dyspigmentation or burns.

Both alexandrite and diode lasers produce good long-term hair reduction of about 84–85% after four repetitive treatments. Bouzari and colleagues did not find any significant difference in efficacy between the alexandrite and diode laser in treating patients with skin types I–V. Similar results were seen by Handrick et al. too.

Treating patients sequentially with diode laser followed by alexandrite laser did not produce greater mean hair reduction than an equivalent number of treatment sessions with alexandrite laser used alone.

Also, the alexandrite laser may be better suited for treating fine vellus hairs as it is capable of shorter pulse durations.[14-16]

Comparison with Many Lasers

Navid et al. reported that alexandrite and diode lasers have almost equal efficacy whereas Nd:YAG laser is the least efficacious, with a mean hair reduction of 42.4, 65.6, and 46.9% for Nd:YAG, alexandrite, and diode lasers, respectively. They also reported that neither laser systems had any advantage over any particular skin types. And the occurrence of side effects was not significantly different between the three lasers.[14-17]

Intense Pulsed Light Lasers

Intense pulsed light lasers also work on the principle of selective photothermolysis. It has the ability to emit a spectrum of wavelengths; therefore, a single light exposure can excite multiple chromophores in the skin at one time. Hence, only trained physicians should use these lasers. When using the device, an optical coupling gel application and direct skin contact with the handpiece is required which hinders the visualization of the immediate local reaction. In addition, the perifollicular erythema and edema seen with other lasers is infrequently encountered with the IPL which makes it difficult to administer the next pulse adjacent to the previous pulse.

No statistical significant difference in efficacy between IPL and diode laser was noted by Amin and colleagues. Another study compared split face treatments of a diode laser and IPL in 31 hirsute women and noted a

TABLE 2: Comparison of various types of hair removal lasers[3,11]

Features	Diode	Nd:YAG	Alexandrite	Ruby	Intense pulsed light
Wavelength	810 nm	1,064 nm	755 nm	694 nm	550–1,200 nm
Best outcome: skin type	Darker skin types: VI–VI	Darker skin types Fitzpatrick: VI–VI type (best for darker skin types)	Lighter skin types: I–III		Lighter skin types: I–III
Long-term efficacy in hair removal	22–59% hair reduction	46.9%	65–80.6%	40.1%	40%
Fluence (J/cm^2)	5–15	30–50	15–25	30–60	Depends on skin type
Pulse duration (ms)	5–30	20–30	5–20	270 µsec	Depends on skin type
Pain	Less painful	Painful	±	±	Painful
Side effects	Paradoxical hypertrichosis mild crusting, transient hypo- and hyperpigmentation Mild crusting transient hypo- and hyperpigmentation	Transient erythema and hyperpigmentation	Blistering with smaller incidence of folliculitis, transient hyperpigmented excoriation	Blistering and pigmentary changes	Perifollicular erythema, edema is difficult to observe. However, blistering and pigmentary changes are the common side effects noted

hair reduction of 40% with IPL and 34% with diode laser, however, this difference was not statistically significant. Pain was consistently greater with IPL than diode laser.[1,3,11]

Comparison of various types of hair removal lasers is provided in table 2.

HISTOPATHOLOGY (FIGS 4 TO 8)

Immediate Changes

Treated follicles display changes of keratinocyte swelling, scattered apoptotic and necrotic keratinocytes, and full thickness necrosis of the follicle depending on the amount of energy absorbed.

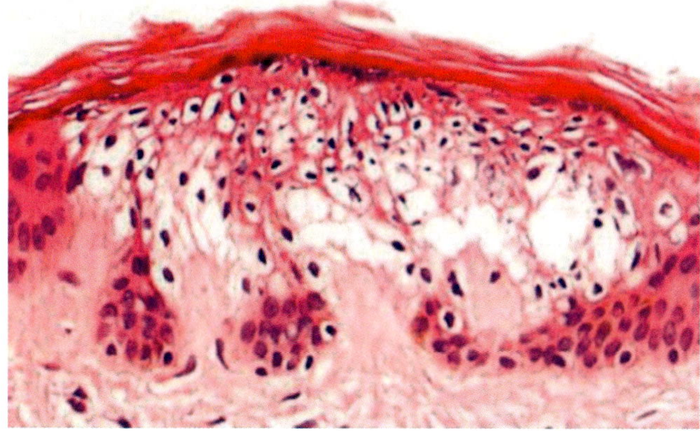

FIG. 4: Skin × 125 hematoxylin and eosin staining. Cytopathic and vacuole changes at the keratinocyte level are clearly seen[19]

Late Changes

Most follicles are in telogen phase 1 month after treatment, whereas fibrosis with a foreign body giant cell reaction replaces others.[5,18]

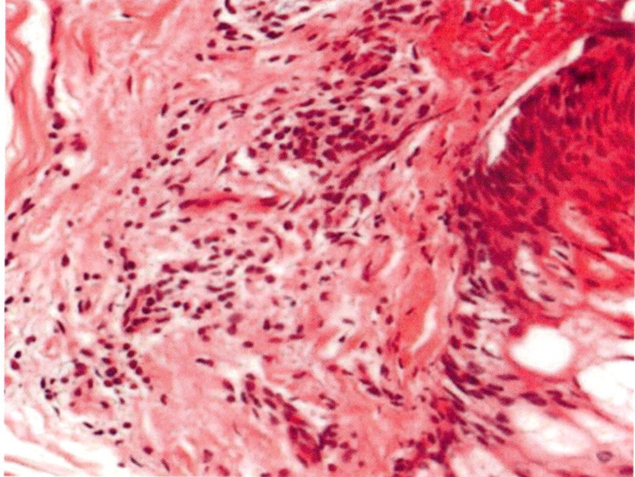

FIG. 5: Skin × 400 hematoxylin and eosin staining. Perifollicular edema and peribulb thermal damage, represented by darker staining, and polymorphic nuclear cell inflammatory infiltration are noticed respecting the integrity of the neighboring tissue[19]

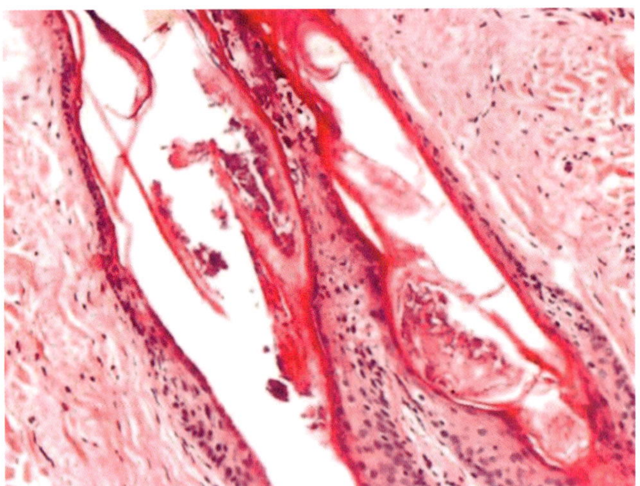

FIG. 6: Skin × 250 hematoxylin and eosin staining. Images of hemorrhaging are seen in between the collagen fibers at the stroma hair level[19]

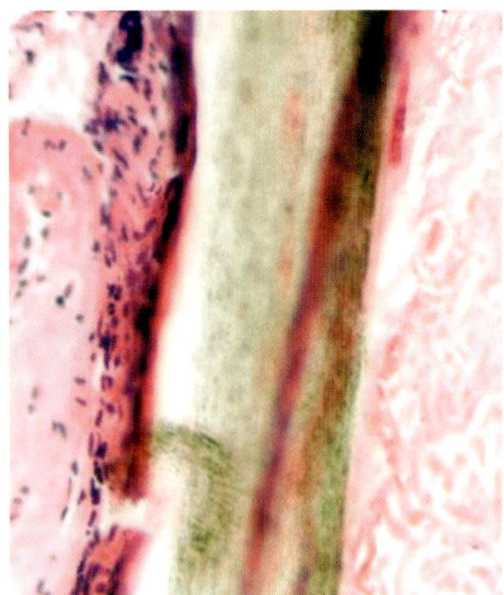

FIG. 8: Skin × 400 H&E. Presence of hair disruption with detachment from its shaft. Peri-isthmic fibrosis is observed together with inflammatory infiltration[19]

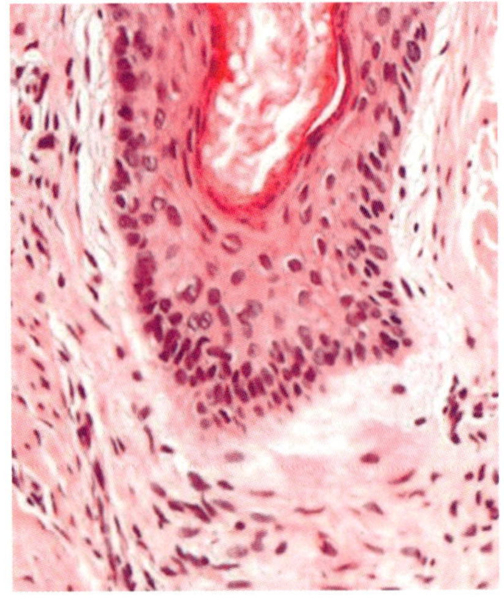

FIG. 7: Skin × 400 hematoxylin and eosin staining. Perifollicular edema is clearly noticed as a consequence of thermal effects[19]

CONCLUSION

The ruby laser (694 nm), alexandrite laser (755 nm), diode laser (810 nm), IPL source (550–1,200 nm), and the Nd:YAG laser (1,064 nm) work on the principle of selective photothermolysis. The chromophobe is the melanin in the hair follicles. Regardless of the type of laser being used, to achieve satisfactory results, multiple treatments are necessary. On an average, after repeated treatments, hair clearance of 30–50% is generally reported 6 months after the last treatment. Patients with dark skin (Fitzpatrick skin types VI, V) can be treated effectively with comparable morbidity to those with lighter skin. Although there is no obvious advantage of one laser system over the other in terms of treatment outcome (except the Nd:YAG laser which is found to be less efficacious, must more suited to patients with darker skin) laser parameters may be important when choosing the ideal laser for a patient.

REFERENCES

1. Casey AS, Goldberg D. Guidelines for Laser Hair Removal. J Cosmet Laser Ther. 2008;10:24-33.
2. Dierickx CC. Laser Hair Removal: Scientific Principles and Practical Aspects.
3. Gan SD, Graber EM. Laser Hair Removal: A Review. Dermatol Surg. 2013;39:823-38.
4. Omprakash HM. History and Physics of Lasers: Dermatologic Lasers and their Evolution. Textbook on Cutaneous and Aesthetic Surgery, 1st edition. New Delhi: Jaypee Brothers Medical Publishers (P) Ltd; 2012.
5. Ilknur T, Bicak MU, Eker P, Ellidokuz H, Ozkan S. Effects of the 810-nm diode laser on hair and on the biophysical properties of skin. J Cosmet Laser Ther. 2010;12(6):269-75.
6. Halachmi S, Lapidoth M. Low Fluence hair removal: A contralateral control non-inferiority study. J Cosmet Laser Ther. 2012;14:2-6.
7. Kopera D. Hair reduction: 48 months of experience with 800nm diode laser. J Cosmet Laser Ther. 2003;5:146-9.
8. Gupta G. Diode Laser: Permanent hair "reduction" not "removal". Int J Trichology. 2014;6(1):34.
9. Adrian RM, Shay KP. 800 nanometer diode laser hair removal in African American patients: a clinical and histologic study. J Cosmet Laser Ther. 2000;2:183-90.
10. Pai GS, Bhat PS, Mallya H, Gold M. Safety and efficacy of low-fluence, high-repetition rate versus high-fluence, low-repetition rate 810-nm diode

laser for permanent hair removal–A split-face comparison study. J Cosmet Laser Ther. 2011;13(4):134-7.
11. Ibrahimi OA, Avram MM, Hanke W, Kilmer SL, Anderson RR. Laser Hair Removal. Dermato Ther. 2011;24:94-107.
12. Li R, Zhou Z, Gold MH. An efficacy comparison of hair removal utilizing a diode laser and an ND: YAG laser system in Chinese women. J Cosmet Laser Ther. 2010;12:213-7.
13. Wanitphakdeedecha R, Thanomkitti K, Sethabutra P, Eimpunth S, Manuskiatty W. A split axilla comparison study of axillary hair removal with low fluence high repetition rate 810 nm diode laser vs. high fluence low repletion rate 1064 nm Nd:YAG laser. JEACV. 2012;26:1133-6.
14. Eremia S, Li C, Newman N. Laser hair removal with alexandrite versus diode laser using four treatment sessions: 1-year results. Dermatol Surg. 2001;27:927-30.
15. Rao J, Goldman Mitchel. Prospective, comparative evaluation of three laser systems used individually and in combination for axillary hair removal. Dermatol Surg. 2005;31:1671-7.
16. Bouzari N, Tabatabai H, Abbasi Z, Firooz A, Dowlati Y. Laser hair removal: comparison of long pulsed ND: YAG, long-pulsed alexandrite, and long-pulsed diode lasers. Dermatol Surg. 2004;30:498-502.
17. Khoury JG, Saluja R, Goldman MP. Comparative evaluation of long-pulse alexandrite and long-pulse ND:YAG laser systems used individually and in combination for axillary hair removal. Dermatol Surg. 2008;34:665-71.
18. Lepselter J, Elman M. Biological and clinical aspects in laser hair removal. J. Dermatolog. Treat. 2004;15:72-83.
19. Trelles MA, Urdiales F, Al-Zarouni M. Hair structures are effectively altered during 810 nm diode laser hair epilation at low fluences. J Dermatolog Treat. 2010;21(2):97–100.

CHAPTER 13

Laser Hair Reduction with Neodymium Doped Yttrium-aluminium-garnet Lasers

Anil Ganjoo

INTRODUCTION

Laser hair reduction (LHR) has come as welcome boon to all the patients of excessive hair growth. These patients used to be a harried lot running from pillar to post getting all sorts of modalities done to get rid of their unwanted hair. With the availability of lasers, we now have a much better option of reducing this unwanted hair.

Laser hair reduction has evolved from permanent hair removal to permanent hair reduction. We now know that wc cannot cradicate the hair completely and can only reduce the hair growth and delay the growth considerably.

Lot has been learnt and understood about this procedure since its approval by the FDA in 1996. We have now developed specific parameters to suit our kind of dark skins that are safe and provide better clinical outcomes. There has also been an explosive growth in the type of technologies available for LHR now.

The laser systems useful for LHR include the long-pulsed ruby, alexandrite, diode, neodymium doped yttrium-aluminium-garnet (Nd:YAG), intense pulsed light, electro-optical synergy (ELOS) and the micro-delivery systems.

All these have their advantages and disadvantages, with one being better than the other in a particular situation. For example, ruby laser at 694 nm has the maximum melanin absorption and therefore, is the most effective laser to reduce hair, but at such short wavelength, it is easily absorbed by the epidermal melanin and can be quite damaging to the epidermis, particularly in our kind of darker skins. So, this wavelength is never used in darker skins. On the other hand, the long-pulsed Nd:YAG laser at 1,064 nm can penetrate deep into the dermis and is less absorbed by the competing melanin in the epidermis making it the safest option for LHR in the skin of color.

Laser light can destroy hair follicles by selective photothermal damage (due to local heating), mechanical damage (due to generation of shock waves), or by photomechanical damage (due to generation of mediators like singlet oxygen and free radicals). Nd:YAG laser is capable of destroying the hair follicle both by photothermal damage using the endogenous chromophore, melanin as well as by photomechanical damage using exogenous chromophores, like carbon (Fig. 1).

Nd:YAG lasers were developed way back in 1964 and lot has been learnt about their efficacy and applications since then. They are one of the most versatile laser systems available for the treatment of various laser amenable conditions. Available as Nd:YAG 1,064 nm wavelength and the frequency doubled 532 nm wavelength where a potassium titanyl phosphate (KTP) crystal is used to halve the 1,064 nm wavelength. The applications of Nd:YAG lasers range from LHR to pigmented lesion and tattoo removal to vascular lesions.

Hair reduction with Nd:YAG lasers is done by both versions including the long-pulsed 1,064 nm and the Q-switched 1,064 nm using the external chromophore.

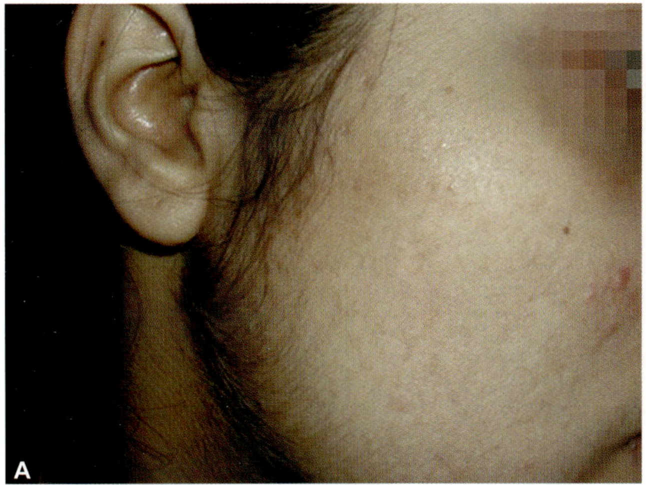

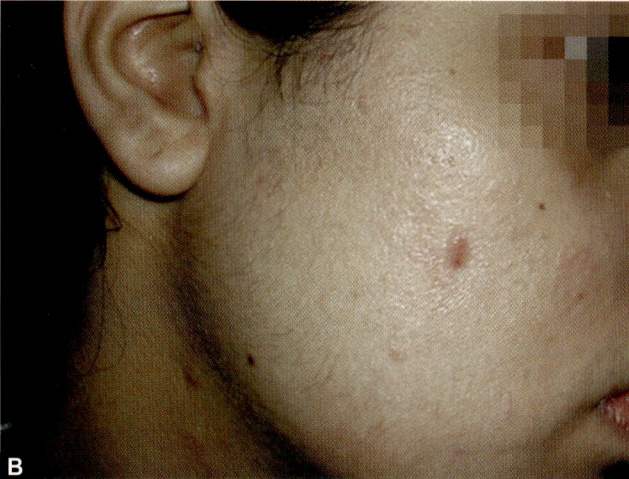

FIG 1: Hair reduction after six sessions of long-pulsed neodymium doped yttrium-aluminium-garnet at 6-week interval

LONG PULSED NEODYMIUM DOPED YTTRIUM-ALUMINIUM-GARNET LASERS[1-4]

Several long-pulsed Nd:YAG lasers (1,064 nm wavelength), which deliver pulses in the milliseconds domain, are now available for LHR treatment for all skin types. These lasers include Lyra or Gemini, CoolGlide, Ultrawave, Profile, VascuLight, SmartEpiII and Acclaim, Athos, Dualis, Varia, Mydon, and GentleYAG.

The long-pulsed Nd:YAG lasers have deeply penetrating 1,064 nm wavelength. The reduced melanin absorption at this wavelength necessitates the need for high fluences in order to adequately damage hair. However, the poor melanin absorption at this wavelength coupled with epidermal cooling makes the long-pulsed Nd:YAG a potentially safe laser treatment for darker skin types, up to VI. Overall a very effective technique for LHR (Figs 1A and B). The Nd:YAG laser is also often used for treatment of pseudofolliculitis barbae, a skin condition commonly seen in persons with darker skin types.

Q-SWITCHED NEODYMIUM DOPED YTTRIUM-ALUMINIUM-GARNET 1,064 NM[5-8]

A high-powered, 1,064 nm Q-switched Nd:YAG laser (MedLite IV; Hoya ConBio, Fremont, Calif) is also available for hair removal. It has very short pulse duration in the nanosecond range, a 4 mm spot, a repetition rate of 10 Hz, and a fluence of up to 8–10 J/cm^2.

An external chromophore, like carbon is applied to epilated skin and rubbed in for a long time to ensure that the external chromophore percolates down into the empty hair canal. The skin is then irradiated with Q-switched 1,064 nm to target the carbon and damage the hair follicle (Fig. 2).

The high repetition rate (10 Hz) delivers the laser pulses very rapidly; therefore, larger areas can be covered easily and operative time is significantly shortened. The longer wavelength (1,064 nm) makes it useful for darker skin types. Although, capable of inducing a growth delay, it appears to be ineffective for long-term hair removal.

TECHNIQUE

Preoperative Considerations

We need to take the following history before treatment:

- Presence of conditions that may cause hypertrichosis: these may include hormonal, familial, drug-related, or tumor-related conditions. If present, need to be addressed medically before LHR
- History of herpes simplex, especially perioral (for facial treatment)
- History of herpes genitalis (for pubic or inguinal treatment)
- History of keloids or hypertrophic scarring
- History of previous treatment modalities: methods, (e.g., shaving, waxing, tweezing, depilatory creams, electrolysis, lasers), frequency, last treatment session, and response all should be considered
- Present medications, e.g., isotretinoin (accutane) intake in the previous 6–12 months.

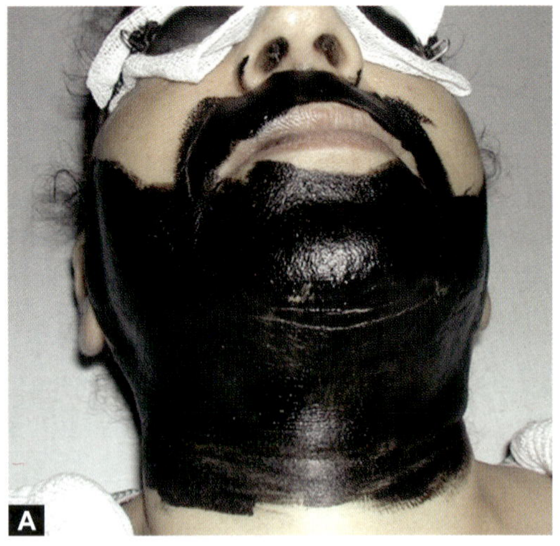

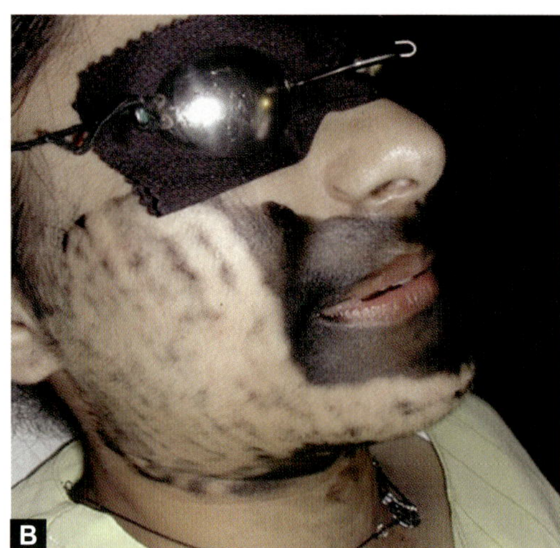

FIG. 2: Carbon used as an external chromophore with Q-switched neodymium doped yttrium-aluminium-garnet laser for light colored and thin hair

Preoperative Care 6 Weeks before Laser Treatment

- Sunscreen: a broad spectrum sunscreen is recommended, and sun avoidance must be practiced, if hair removal is planned in exposed sites
- Bleaching cream: a bleaching cream such as hydroquinone (Solaquin Forte) may be prescribed to patients with darker skin types or a recent suntan
- Plucking, waxing, or electrolysis: the patient should avoid these activities. Research has shown greater hair loss at shaved versus epilated sites, suggesting that light absorption by the pigmented hair shaft itself plays an important role
- Shaving and depilatory creams: these may be used up to the day before laser treatment. The patient is instructed to shave the area to be treated; however, the area must not be irritated. If the patient is uncomfortable with the idea of shaving the area, a depilatory cream can be used instead
- Antivirals: the patient should start prophylactic antiviral medications (e.g., acyclovir, valacyclovir, famciclovir) when indicated
- Antibiotics: the patient should start oral antibiotics when indicated (e.g., nasal, perianal skin infections).

Day of Treatment

- Cleansing and makeup: The area to be treated should be clean and free of makeup or powder
- Preprocedure anesthesia: If desired, a thick layer of a topical anesthetic cream (e.g., Emla, Ela-Max, topicaine) can be applied under occlusion (plastic wrap) for 30 minutes to 2 hours before the scheduled laser treatment.

Procedure

- Skin preparation: remove all anesthetic cream, makeup, or other skin creams or powders
- Apply anesthesia, if needed, as described above in the anesthesia section
- Visibility: a treatment grid can be applied in order to provide the operator with an outline of the area to be irradiated. A grid may be manually drawn using a white makeup pencil or a yellow fluorescent highlighter. Dark markers or ink should be avoided in delineating treatment grids since darker colors may interfere with the device optics. In the absence of a grid, careful attention must be given to prevent double laser pulsing and missing areas. Visibility can also be increased by a polarized headlamp with a magnifying loupe (Seymour light)
- Treatment fluence: the ideal treatment parameters must be individualized for each patient; test sites can be placed at inconspicuous regions of the area to be treated. The fluence is carefully increased while observing the skin for signs of acute epidermal injury, such as whitening, blistering, ablation, or the Nikolsky sign (forced epidermal separation). In general, the treatment fluence should be at 75% of the Nikolsky threshold fluence
- Technique: nonoverlapping or minimally overlapping laser pulses are delivered with a predetermined spot

size. The largest spot size and the highest tolerable fluence should be used in order to obtain the best results.

Postoperative Changes

The ideal immediate response of treated skin is vaporization of the hair shaft with no other apparent effect. After a few minutes, perifollicular edema and erythema should be evident. The intensity and duration of these tissue changes depend on the hair color and density. The fluence should be reduced if signs of epidermal damage develop. Perifollicular edema is the end point for effective LHR.

Postoperative Care

Ice packs reduce postoperative pain and minimize swelling. Analgesics are not usually required unless extensive areas are treated. Prophylactic courses of antibiotics or antivirals should be completed. Topical antibiotic ointment application twice daily is indicated if epidermal injury has occurred. Potent topical steroid creams, such as clobetasol or fluocinonide, may be prescribed for 1–2 days to reduce immediate swelling and erythema.

Avoid any trauma such as picking or scratching of the area. Avoid sun exposure. Use sunscreen with a sun protection factor of 30. Makeup may be applied on the next day unless blistering or crusting has developed. Shedding of hair casts (especially on the face) may be seen; the damaged hair follicle is often shed during the first week after treatment. Patients should be reassured that this is not a sign of hair regrowth.

INTERVAL BETWEEN SESSIONS

The repeat sessions can be done as soon as the growth reappears. This will depend on the hair growth cycle and varies from region to region. On an average, the growth cycle is 6–8 weeks, being slightly shorter on the face compared to the other body areas.

SIDE EFFECTS

Although most typical complications are minor and easily manageable, all patients should provide verbal and written consent prior to treatment and they should be informed of the possible risks, benefits, and alternatives.[9]

The most common risks with light- and laser based hair removal systems include intraoperative burns (Fig. 3), skin discoloration (hyper- or hypopigmentation) (Fig. 4), pain

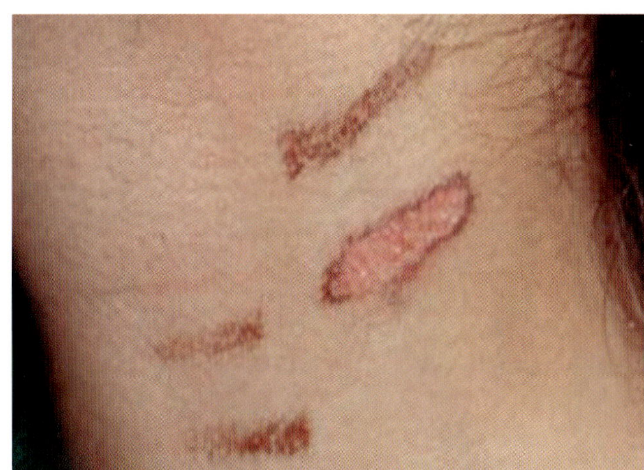

FIG. 3: Intraoperative burns due to use of high fluences. We need to use the appropriate fluences which may vary from patient to patient

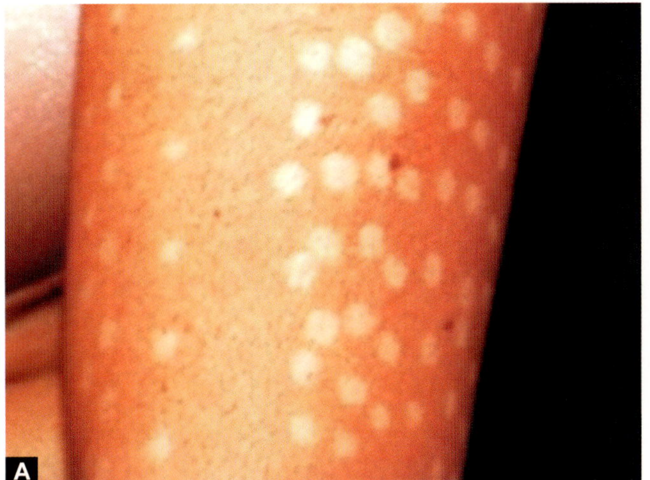

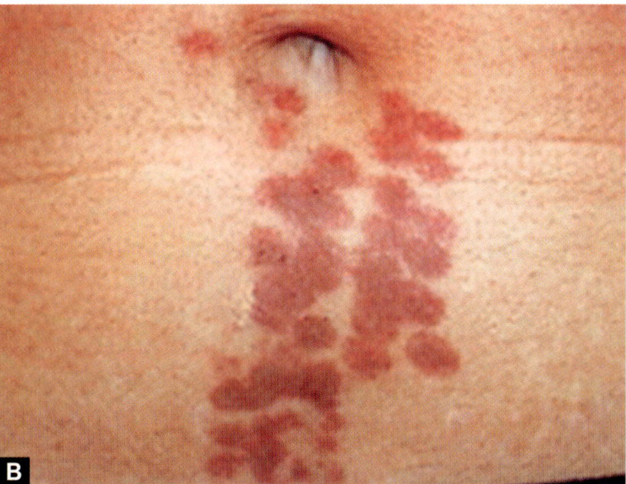

FIG. 4: Postinflammatory hypopigmentation (**A**) and hyperpigmentation (**B**) following laser burns. We need to reduce the fluence as soon as signs of epidermal injury like graying or blanching are evident.

or discomfort, itching, folliculitis, ingrown hairs, herpes virus reactivation, blistering, infection, temporary result, failure to achieve desired result, or worsening/increased symptoms (paradoxical hypertrichosis).[10]

Perifollicular erythema and edema are expected in all patients treated at the threshold fluence. The intensity and duration depend on hair color, hair density and fluence. The reaction may last from a few minutes to 1-3 days.[11]

Rare complications include permanent scars, permanent darkening or lightening of tattoo or permanent makeup pigments, eye injury, blindness, headache, persistent redness, and bruising.

CONCLUSION

Laser hair reduction has met the unmet need of treating excessive hair growth to a large extent. These patients are much more satisfied now than they used to be with the older physical modalities like shaving, waxing, threading, etc. Out of the various laser-assisted hair removal devices available Nd:YAG laser is one of the most effective and safe lasers. The long wavelength ensures that the epidermal scattering and absorption is minimal which makes it the safest out of all the LHR devices. The need is to:

- Select your patient properly
- Counsel your patient thoroughly
- Do an extensive workup
- Manage medically, if required
- Select the best wavelength, pulse width, and fluence suited for a particular patient before starting the procedure
- Get a satisfactory outcome.

REFERENCES

1. Alster TS, Bryan H, Williams CM. Long-pulsed Nd:YAG laser-assisted hair removal in pigmented skin: a clinical and histological evaluation. Arch Dermatol. 2001;137(7):885-9.
2. Kilmer SL, Chotzen V, Calkin J. Laser hair removal with the long-pulse 1064nm coolglide laser system. Lasers Surg Med. 2000;12:84.
3. Raff K, Landthaler M, Hohenleutner U. Optimizing treatment parameters for hair removal using long-pulsed Nd:YAG-lasers. Lasers Med Sci. 2004.18(4):219-22.
4. Tanzi EL, Alster TS. Long-pulsed 1064-nm Nd:YAG laser-assisted hair removal in all skin types. Dermatol Surg. 2004;30(1):13-7.
5. Goldberg D. Laser hair removal with a millisecond Q-switched Nd:YAG laser. Lasers Surg Med. 1999;11(suppl):88.
6. Goldberg DJ, Littler CM, Wheeland RG. Topical suspension-assisted Q-switched Nd:YAG laser hair removal. Dermatol Surg. 1997;23(9):741-5.
7. Kilmer SL, Chotzen VA. Q-switched Nd-YAG laser (1064 nm) hair removal without adjuvant topical preparation. Lasers Surg Med. 1997;9(suppl):145.
8. Nanni CA, Alster TS. Optimizing treatment parameters for hair removal using a topical carbon-based solution and 1064-nm Q-switched neodymium:YAG laser energy. Arch Dermatol. 1997;133(12):1546-9.
9. Vachiramon V, Brown T, McMichael AJ. Patient satisfaction and complications following laser hair removal in ethnic skin. J Drugs Dermatol. 2012;11(2):191-5.
10. Fontana CR, Bonini D, Bagnato VS. A 12-month follow-up of hypopigmentation after laser hair removal. J Cosmet Laser Ther. 2013;15(2):80-4.
11. Lapidoth M, Shafirstein G, Ben Amitai D, Hodak E, Waner M, David M. Reticulate erythema following diode laser-assisted hair removal: a new side effect of a common procedure. J Am Acad Dermatol. 2004;51(5):774-7.

CHAPTER 14

Evidence Based Approach in Hair Reduction

Biju Vasudevan, Samipa S Mukherjee, Chandrashekar BS

INTRODUCTION

Unwanted hair growth is a therapeutic challenge as the desire of the society for the same continues to become more prevalent. The use of photoepilation and lasers for effective removal of hair has revolutionized the therapy for hair removal, however, the quest for a safe, effective, long-lasting, cost effective means of permanent hair reduction still continues.

Excess hair growth covers a broad range of severity and may present as hypertrichosis or hirsutism.[1] Hypertrichosis means excess hair growth at any body site, whereas hirsutism presents as excess hair growth in women at androgen-dependent sites. However, hair removal treatments are performed in a large number of patients with normal hair pattern predominantly for cosmetic reasons. There are many methods that temporarily treat unwanted hair, including bleaching, plucking, shaving, waxing, and chemical depilatories which are tedious, need to be repeated and painful.[2,3]

The Food and Drug Administration has defined permanent hair removal as the long-term stable reduction in the number of hairs regrowing after a treatment regime, which may include several sessions. The number of regrowing hairs must be stable over time greater than the duration of the complete growth cycle of hair follicles, which varies from 4 to 12 months according to body location. Permanent hair reduction does not necessarily imply the elimination of all hairs in the treatment area,[4] although till date no method of permanent hair removal is available. Lasing has become one of the most effective ways of permanent hair reduction since it leads to significant reduction of hair follicles at any given time of treatment and improves the cosmetic appearance in a patient.

LASERS FOR HAIR REDUCTION

The various lasers in use for laser hair removal have been listed in table 1.

Understanding the Hair Cycle and Its Importance in Laser Hair Removal

The human hair follicle grows in three successive phases: active growth (anagen), regression (catagen), and resting (telogen). During anagen, mitotic activity occurs in the hair matrix and hair is generated by

TABLE 1: Types of lasers used for laser hair removal

Type of laser	Wavelength
Ruby	694 nm
Alexandrite	755 nm
Diode	800–810 nm
Neodymium doped yttrium-aluminium-garnet	1,064 nm
Intense pulsed light	590–1,200 nm

TABLE 2: Variation in the percentage of hairs in anagen phase in various parts of the body

Area	Percentage of hairs in anagen
Scalp	85%
Face	56–76%
Limbs	42–51%

these proliferating cells.[5] The mechanism of laser hair removal works on the hypothesis that growth delay and permanent hair loss may be caused by telogen induction and miniaturization of terminal hairs follicle.[6] There is a variation in the percentage of hair in anagen phase in various parts of the body as given in table 2.[7]

Mechanism of Laser Hair Removal

Destruction of the hair follicle using light can occur by the three mechanisms; thermal using heat energy, mechanical through the generation of shock waves, and photochemical through the generation of reactive oxygen species.[8] Laser hair removal is thought to work through selective damage to the hair follicles and this mechanism is based on the principles of selective photothermolysis with melanin as the chromophore.[9] The selection of laser for hair removal depends on the thickness of hair, phase of the hair cycle, site, and density whereas appropriate selection of the laser parameters are useful for minimizing side effects and increasing effectiveness.

Prior to treatment, the possibility of adverse effects must be discussed with patients. Adverse events include but are not limited to: hyperpigmentation, hypopigmentation, erythema, edema, scarring, pain, and blistering.[10]

Ideal Time Interval

The ideal time interval between each session (Table 3) is based on the fact that anagen hair bulbs contain the highest concentration of melanin and in humans, the melanin within the pigmented hair shaft serves as the dominant chromophore.[1] Hair follicles contain a greater density of melanocytes and larger melanosomes when compared with the epidermis.[11] Another proposed mechanism of laser hair removal is through the destruction of follicular stem cells that regenerate the epidermis and its adnexal structures; there is experimental evidence to suggest that selective destruction of follicular stem cells will prevent hair regrowth.[12] However, immunohistochemistry done before and after lasing a patient did not show any change in the staining pattern, thereby questioning the second postulate of the mechanism of hair removal and also reaffirming the safety of lasers as the stem cells were not affected.

TABLE 3: Ideal interval between treatment sessions for laser hair removal[13]

Median hair-free interval was 8 weeks after four consecutive laser treatments	Chana et al.
45 days	Bouzari et al.
4 weeks	Gorguet et al.
4–6 weeks	Eremia et al.
4–8 weeks	Drosner and Adatto
6–8 weeks	Anecdotal evidence

Factors influencing laser hair removal include:

- Wavelength (nm): concentration on follicle
- Pulse duration: influence on thickness of hair
- Fluence: effectiveness of permanent hair removal
- Cooling temperature: stability of treatment.

Optimal Wavelengths for Laser Hair Removal

The optimal wavelengths for laser hair removal are given in table 4.

Lasers for Hair Removal and their Evidences

The available lasers and light sources operate in the red or near-infrared wavelength regions: ruby laser (694 nm), alexandrite laser (755 nm), diode laser (800–810 nm), neodymium doped yttrium-aluminium-garnet (Nd:YAG) laser (1,064 nm), and noncoherent intense pulsed light (IPL) (590–1,200 nm).

Ruby Laser

Randomized controlled trial (RCT) and controlled trials (CT) have shown better short-term reduction in hair growth as compared to epilation, electrolysis, shaving,

TABLE 4: Optimal wavelengths for laser hair removal

Hair color	Fitzpatrick skin type	Wavelength (nm)
Brown	I, II	694,755,800
Brown, black	III, IV, V	8,001,064
Red, grey	I, II	694, 755
Blond, white	I, II	694

and waxing. No long-term hair reduction was obtained 12 months after three ruby laser treatments, whereas Dierickx et al. found obvious hair loss in four of seven individuals 1 and 2 years after one ruby laser treatment.[6,14] Side effects have been reported with low incidences in one RCT and one CT, hypopigmentation being the most frequently reported adverse reaction in pigmented skin and less epidermal damage being found for 20 versus 1 ms pulse duration in skin of dark complexion.[15,16]

Alexandrite Laser

Randomized controlled trial and CT were evaluated to evaluate the efficacy of hair removal. In comparison with shaving, the short-term hair removal efficacy was transiently superior after one alexandrite laser treatment 3 months postoperatively, whereas complete regrowth was seen 6 months postoperatively.[17] A large study (n = 144 Asian patients) evaluated the hair removal efficacy after repetitive treatments up to 9 months postoperatively and found a significantly improved short-term and long-term clearing after two and three treatments (overall 55% hair reduction) versus a single treatment (overall 32% hair reduction) with the alexandrite laser.[18] In one of the studies, slightly more pain, blistering, and hyperpigmentation were seen after diode laser than after alexandrite laser, whereas no scarring or atrophy occurred at all.[19]

Diode Laser

The hair removal efficacy after diode laser treatment was evaluated in three RCTs and four CTs. Two repetitive treatments with the diode laser (34–53% hair reduction) were superior to a single treatment (28–33% hair reduction) at an average follow-up time of 20 months.[20] Two studies compared the diode laser with the alexandrite laser and similar treatment outcomes were seen.[19,21] One study compared the diode laser with the Nd:YAG laser and similar almost complete hair regrowth was seen for both lasers 9 months postoperatively.[22]

Neodymium doped yttrium-aluminium-garnet Laser

The hair removal efficacy after Nd:YAG laser treatment was evaluated in two RCTs and four CTs. The long-pulsed Nd:YAG laser was superior to shaving in both short-term and long-term studies and the short-pulsed Q-switched Nd:YAG laser was transiently superior to wax epilation 3 months postoperatively, whereas full regrowth was seen 6 months postoperatively. Repetitive treatments improved the long-term treatment outcome with 40% of patients obtaining greater than 50% hair reduction 12–16 months after five treatments versus 100% of patients obtaining less than 25% of hair reduction after one treatment.[23] The short-term hair removal efficacy was limited and similar for long-pulsed Nd:YAG laser and IPL treatment as well as for Q-switched Nd:YAG laser and alexandrite laser.[24,25]

Intense Pulsed Light

One each of RCT and CT were available for evaluation. One treatment with long-pulsed Nd:YAG laser and IPL resulted in similar limited hair removal efficacy 6 weeks postoperatively, whereas IPL treatment more often resulted in postinflammatory pigmentation as compared with the Nd:YAG laser.[24] Adverse effects in the form of pain, discomfort, crusting, and time until skin normalizes were more as compared to Nd:YAG and ruby lasers.

Comparison of the Laser Modalities

Five different lasers and light sources were evaluated and the best available evidence was found for the alexandrite (three RCTs, eight CTs) and the diode (three RCTs, four CTs) lasers, followed by the ruby (two RCTs, six CTs) and Nd:YAG (two RCTs, four CTs) lasers, whereas limited evidence was available for IPL photoepilation (one RCT, one CT) by Haedersdal and Wulf.[1] They also concluded that substantial evidence exists for a partial short-term hair removal efficacy up to 6 months after treatment with ruby laser, alexandrite laser, diode laser, Nd:YAG laser, and IPL. As noted in the various studies, the efficacy improved with repeated sessions. The long-term efficacy was found better with diode and alexandrite lasers based on the studies. The best long-term hair reduction was reported for the alexandrite and diode lasers after four repetitive axillary treatments with 84–85% hair reduction 12 months postoperatively (maximum tolerated fluences).[21] Permanent hair removal still remains elusive as the maximum follow-up time in the studies have been up to 2 years post-therapy. Haedersdal and Wulf suggested that patients are preoperatively informed that:[1]

- Epilation with lasers and light sources induces a partial short-term hair reduction up to 6 months postoperatively
- The efficacy is improved when repeated treatments are given

- The efficacy is superior to conventional treatments (shaving, wax epilation, electrolysis)
- Evidence exists for a partial long-term hair removal efficacy beyond 6 months postoperatively after repetitive treatments with alexandrite and diode lasers and probably after treatment with ruby and Nd:YAG lasers, whereas evidence is lacking for long-term hair removal after IPL treatment
- Today there is no evidence for a complete and persistent hair removal efficacy after laser and photoepilation.

Ideal Number of Sessions for Hair Removal

There is no firm recommendation on the number of sessions required till date and studies in this field are lacking. It is possible that the number of sessions depend on various parameters like thickness of the hair, density, site, growth characteristics, and the type of lasers used.

The alexandrite and diode lasers produce good long-term hair reduction (84–85%) 12 months postoperatively after four repetitive axillary treatments.[21] The success rates with alexandrite laser as noted were: 25% for patients receiving four or fewer treatments, 76% for five treatments, 58% for six treatments, and 15% for seven treatments. The lower rate of success in the six and seven treatments groups is attributed to a higher incidence of side effects such as hyper- and hypopigmentation, blister, and folliculitis.[26]

Toosi et al. found similar results in that the efficacy of diode laser hair removal (n576) on facial and neck hair was significantly related to the number of treatment sessions as an increased number of sessions improved the results; the number of treatments ranged from three to seven with a mean of 4.29.[27]

Regardless of skin type or targeted body region, patients who underwent three treatment sessions with the long-pulsed ruby laser demonstrated an average 35% regrowth in terminal hair count 6 months after initial therapy compared with baseline pretreatment values.[28]

Repetitive treatments have been shown to be more effective than single session with Nd:YAG as well. More than 50% hair reduction was obtained in 44.9% of the areas 1 month after a single treatment and with two treatments this percentage increased to 71.5%.[29]

Although there have been studies showing that there has not been significant improvement post the first session, most studies suggest otherwise. In the guidelines set forth by the European Society for Laser Dermatology, Drosner and Adatto recommend three to eight treatments to achieve satisfactory results.[30]

Recommendations for Shaving, Plucking, and Waxing before Lasing

Sunscreen and/or sun avoidance is universally recommended prior to laser hair removal because melanin is the principle chromophore for laser hair removal. As melanin is the target chromophore in laser hair removal, it is imperative that the hair needs to be trimmed to a short length in order to avoid absorption of the laser beam by the superficial hair.

Wax epilation converts normally telogen hairs into anagen and therefore increases the susceptibility of these hairs to thermal damage. During anagen, keratinocytes are dividing rapidly to create the hair shaft and rapidly dividing tissues are more susceptible to extreme heat and the oxidative products created during laser treatment.[31] In the guidelines set forth by the European Society for Laser Dermatology, Drosner and Adatto recommend avoiding any pretreatment plucking, waxing, or electrolysis because the light needs the melanin in the hair shaft as a chromophore in order to produce successful photoepilation. They also state that cutting, shaving, or using a depilatory cream are all acceptable prior to treatment.[30]

Recommendations for Sun Exposure before and after the Procedure

Persistent erythema and pigmentary disturbances are the most frequently encountered complications more commonly seen in patients with a pigmented skin. Sun avoidance would prevent further stimulation of the melanocytes,[32] thereby reducing the risk of postinflammatory pigmentary changes. Casey and Goldberg routinely recommend that our patients avoid sun exposure for 6 weeks before and after laser treatment as we have found that additional inflammation to the area tends to lead to irritation and rarely, hyperpigmentation. They have found that sun avoidance is a relatively easy recommendation for patients to adhere to and they recommend minimal sun exposure to all patients in order to reduce the short, and long-term complications of ultraviolet light exposure.[13]

The Laser Paradox

There have been several reports of hair growth induced by laser treatment. Bouzari et al. noted the conversion of vellus hairs to terminal hairs following laser treatment.[33] In their study, they note that 27, 12, and 3% of patients receiving treatment with the Nd:YAG, alexandrite, and diode lasers, respectively experienced terminalization; overall, 10% of patients experienced this side effect in their study. The authors hypothesized that the produced heat is less than the temperature necessary for thermolysis and that the heat shock may induce follicular stem cell differentiation and growth via increased heat shock proteins and other growth factors.[34] Moreno-Arias et al. describe a "paradoxical effect" following IPL treatment of facial hirsutism in 10.2% of patients undergoing IPL photoepilation. They define the paradoxical effect as the growth of fine dark hair in an untreated area in close proximity to the treated area which resulted due to the stimulation of the dormant follicles.[35]

Optimizing Laser Outcomes in a Darker Skin

- Grey hairs: electrolysis
- Light/blond hairs: more sittings, higher power, low pulse width
- Appropriate laser safety precautions must be followed
- Explain postoperative sequelae.

Discussion Points

- Risks and benefits before the treatment
- Long-term results
- Treatment alternatives and cost
- Treatment failure and recurrence of hair growth.

POINTS TO REMEMBER

- Darker skinned individuals have an increased risk of side effects
- Type VI skin absorbs 40% more energy when compared to type I
- To achieve maximum benefit, an appropriate wavelength, pulse duration, and fluence must be tailored to each individual
- Choose minimum fluence producing desired tissue effect
- Lower fluence in highly dense areas
- Some dark skin patients may have lighter skin but their ethnic background and genetic darker skin decent must be kept in mind
- Cooling allows higher fluences to be used for more permanent hair removal
- Cooling is important but avoid cold injuries
- A laser test spot should be considered for any patient in whom there is a concern about the potential for side effects like dark skin
- Wait for 48 hours to decide about optimum parameters as there may be delayed reaction to exposure
- Avoid jawline vellus hairs as chances of paradoxical hair stimulation risk is more
- Darker skin may require more number of sessions more than 10, sometimes
- Discuss potential risk of scarring/hypo-/hyper-pigmentation.
- Insist on 1 mm hair before procedure/trim hairs to 1 mm length—helps in area demarcation and ensures intact roots
- Wait for 6 weeks after waxing/plucking
- Avoid direct sun exposure for at least 2 weeks
- Receive specialized training for darker skin types.

CONCLUSION

Laser hair removal is a promising way to tackle unwanted and cosmetically unacceptable hair growth. In spite of the wide variety of lasers in the dermatologist's armamentarium, the search for the ideal laser still continues. Laser hair removal continues to be a safe and effective modality. There are limited studies to date regarding recommendations before, during, and after treatment guidelines. Thorough knowledge regarding the hair cycle, cell dynamics, and laser physics forms the base towards optimum use of the laser machine.

REFERENCES

1. Haedersdal M, Wulf HC. Evidence-based review of hair removal using lasers and light sources. J Eur Acad Dermatol Venereol. 2006;20(1):9-20.
2. Lanigan SW. Management of unwanted hair in females. Clin Exp Dermatol. 2001;26(8):644-7.
3. Shapiro J, Lui H. Treatments for unwanted facial hair. Skin Therapy Lett. 2006;10(10):1-4.
4. Food US, Drug Administration, CDRH Consumer Information. Laser facts. Hair removal. Updated 5/17/2002. [online] Website available from http://www.fda.gov/cdrh/consumer/laserfacts.html [Accessed February, 2016].
5. Philpott MP, Green MR, Kealey T. Human hair growth in vitro. J Cell Sci. 1990;97:463-71.
6. Dierickx CC, Grossman MC, Farinelli WA, Anderson RR. Permanent hair removal by normal-mode ruby laser. Arch Dermatol. 1998;134(7):837-42.
7. Chana JS, Grobbelaar AO. The long-term results of ruby laser depilation in a consecutive series of 346 patients. Plast Reconstr Surg. 2002;110(1):254-60.
8. Dierickx C. Laser-assisted hair removal: state of the art. Dermatol Ther. 2000;13:80-9.
9. Grossman MC, Dierickx C, Farinelli W, Flotte T, Anderson RR. Damage to hair follicles by normal-mode ruby laser pulses. J Am Acad Dermatol. 1996;35(6):889-94.
10. Lim SP, Lanigan SW. A review of the adverse effects of laser hair removal. Lasers Med Sci. 2006;21(3):121-5.

11. Kolinko VG, Littler CM, Cole A. Influence of the anagen:telogen ratio on Q-switched Nd:YAG laser hair removal efficacy. Lasers Surg Med. 2000;26(1):33-40.
12. Ito M, Liu Y, Yang Z, Nguyen J, Liang F, Morris RJ, et al. Stem cells in the hair follicle bulge contribute to wound repair but not to homeostasis of the epidermis. Nat Med. 2005;11(12):1351-4.
13. Casey AS, Goldberg D. Guidelines for laser hair removal. J Cosmet Laser Ther. 2008;10(1):24-33.
14. Polderman MC, Pavel S, le Cessie S, Grevelink JM, van Leeuwen RL. Efficacy, tolerability, and safety of a long-pulsed ruby laser system in the removal of unwanted hair. Dermatol Surg. 2000;26(3):240-3.
15. Haedersdal M, Egekvist H, Efsen J, Bjerring P. Skin pigmentation and texture changes after hair removal with the normal-mode ruby laser. Acta Derm Venereol. 1999;79(6):465-8.
16. Elman M, Klein A, Slatkine M. Dark skin tissue reaction in laser assisted hair removal with a long-pulse ruby laser. J Cutan Laser Ther. 2000;2(1): 17-20.
17. Nanni CA, Alster TS. Long-pulsed alexandrite laser-assisted hair removal at 5, 10, and 20 millisecond pulse durations. Lasers Surg Med. 1999;24(5):332-37.
18. Hussain M, Polnikorn N, Goldberg DJ. Laser-assisted hair removal in Asian skin: efficacy, complications, and the effect of single versus multiple treatments. Dermatol Surg. 2003;29(3):249-54.
19. Handrick C, Alster TS. Comparison of long-pulsed diode and long-pulsed alexandrite lasers for hair removal: a long-term clinical and histologic study. Dermatol Surg. 2001; 27(7):622-6.
20. Lou WW, Quintana AT, Geronemus RG, Grossman MC. Prospective study of hair reduction by diode laser (800 nm) with long-term follow-up. Dermatol Surg. 2000;26(5):428-32.
21. Eremia S, Li C, Newman N. Laser hair removal with alexandrite versus diode laser using four treatment sessions: 1-year results. Dermatol Surg. 2001;27(11):925-9.
22. Chan HH, Ying SY, Ho WS, Wong DS, Lam LK. An in vivo study comparing the efficacy and complications of diode laser and long-pulsed Nd:YAG laser in hair removal in Chinese patients. Dermatol Surg. 2001; 21(11): 950-4.
23. Lorenz S, Brunnberg S, Landthaler M, Hohenleutner U. Hair removal with the long pulsed Nd:YAG laser: a prospective study with one year follow-up. Lasers Surg Med. 2002;30(2):127-34.
24. Goh CL. Comparative study on a single treatment response to long pulse Nd:YAG lasers and intense pulse light therapy for hair removal on skin type IV to VI—is longer wavelengths lasers preferred over shorter wavelengths lights for assisted hair removal? J Dermatolog Treat. 2003;14:243-7
25. Rogers CJ, Glaser DA, Siegfried EC, Walsh PM. Hair removal using topical suspension-assisted Q-switched Nd:YAG and long-pulsed alexandrite lasers: a comparative study. Dermatol Surg. 1999;25(11):844-50.
26. Bouzari N, Nouri K, Tabatabai H, Abbasi Z, Firooz A, Dowlati Y. The role of number of treatments in laser-assisted hair removal using a 755-nm alexandrite laser. J Drugs Dermatol. 2005;4(5):573-8.
27. Toosi P, Sadighha A, Sharifian A, Razavi GM. A comparison of the efficacy and side effects of different sources in hair removal. Lasers Med Sci. 2006;21(1):1-4.
28. Williams R, Havoonjian H, Isagholian K, Menaker G, Moy R. A clinical study of hair removal using the long-pulsed ruby laser. Dermatol Surg. 1998;24(8):837-42.
29. Lorenz S, Brunnberg S, Landthaler M, Hohenleutner U. Hair removal with the long pulsed Nd:YAG laser: A prospective study with one year follow-up. Lasers Surg Med. 2002;30(2):127-34.
30. Drosner M, Adatto M, European Society for Laser Dermatology. Photo-epilation: guidelines for care from the European Society for Laser Dermatology (ESLD). J Cosmet Laser Ther. 2005;7(1):33-8.
31. Lehrer MS, Crawford GH, Gelfand JM, Leyden JJ, Vittorio CC. Effect of wax epilation before hair removal with a long-pulsed alexandrite laser: a pilot study. Dermatol Surg. 2003;29(2):118-22.
32. Pathak MA, Stratton K. Free radicals in human skin before and after exposure to light. Arch Biochem Biophys. 1968;132(3):468-76.
33. Bouzari N, Firooz AR. Lasers may induce terminal hair growth. Dermatol Surg. 2006;32(3):460.
34. Bouzari N, Tabatabai H, Abbasi Z, Firooz A, Dowlati Y. Laser hair removal: comparison of long-pulsed Nd:YAG, long pulsed alexandrite, and long-pulsed diode lasers. Dermatol Surg. 2004;498-502.
35. Moreno-Arias GA, Castelo-Branco C, Ferrando J. Side-effects after IPL photodepilation. Dermatol Surg. 2002;28(12):1131-4.

CHAPTER 15

Lasers and Light for Pigmented Lesion: Opportunities and Limitations

Sanjeev J Aurangabadkar

INTRODUCTION

Laser technology has made rapid strides over the past decade, considerably enhancing our ability to treat pigmented lesions and tattoos with great deal of efficacy and safety. With the wide availability and accessibility to laser technology, significant experience and data has been collecting with regards to treatment of darker skin types particularly in Southeast Asia. New developments in the field of laser physics, refinement, and modification of techniques have opened new vistas for targeting pigment in the skin. Though laser treatment of pigmented lesions is generally gratifying, challenges do exist such as unpredictable and variable response, prolonged treatment duration, difficulty in treating colored skin, and inability to clear certain pigments in tattoos. Though these limitations are real, a better understanding of laser-tissue interaction at the subcellular level, new innovations, and improvisation of techniques have opened up opportunities in laser treatment of pigmented lesions and tattoos.

The Q-switched lasers have been at the forefront of laser technology when it comes to treating these conditions. Their ability to deliver very high energy in ultrashort pulses (typically nanoseconds) has allowed the dermatosurgeon to specifically target melanosomes and ink particles in epidermis and dermis. Other lasers and light devises such as millisecond infrared lasers and intense pulsed light (IPL) systems have also been used effectively in certain indications. The commercial availability of picoseconds lasers and the concept of combining lasers have given additional impetus to the management of pigmentary disorders.

LASER-TISSUE INTERACTION: CURRENT CONCEPTS

Laser therapy of pigmented lesions is based on the principle of selective photothermolysis that was pioneered by Anderson and Parrish.[1]

In addition to its selectivity, the Q-switched lasers also produce an additional photoacoustic effect that results in the generation of shock waves following laser irradiation of tissue.[2] The instantaneous selective heating of the chromophore (the structures absorbing the laser irradiation-melanosomes and ink particles in this case) and rapid progression of these shock waves leads to explosion and fragmentation of the pigment granules which are then cleared by the macrophages and lymphatics to regional lymph nodes and/or eliminated trans-epidermally.[3]

Irradiation of the skin with Q-switched laser pulse leading to rapid thermal expansion and production of shock waves produces a brisk whitening of the lesion due to intracellular steam formation and vacuolization.[4] An audible popping sound can be heard during treatment due to shock wave generation in the treated tissue. The whitening is followed by erythema and edema which are transient. During this period of whitening, the cells become opaque to further Q-switched pulses due to scattering of laser light, thus closing the optical window to further immediate lasing. The clinical significance of this will be dealt with further in the chapter.

The concept of subcellular selective photothermolysis has recently been proposed where low fluence Q-switched laser pulses are used in order to damage only the micro-organelles, such as melanosomes, in the keratinocytes and melanocytes without killing or rupturing the cells they are contained in.[5] This technique of laser toning has been widely used in Southeast Asia for the treatment of melasma. Low fluence Q-switched pulses induce selective photothermolysis of stage IV melanosomes and produce "dendrectomy" (reduced number of dendrites of melanocytes in the epidermis compared to pretreatment after laser toning).

INDICATIONS

Indications of lesions are given in table 1.

Lasers used for Pigmented Lesions and Tattoos

Ultrashort Pulse Lasers

The pulse duration (PD) is in nanoseconds and picoseconds—Q-switched neodymium doped:yttrium-aluminium-garnet (Nd:YAG) laser (1,064 nm and 532 nm), Q-switched alexandrite laser (755 nm), Q-switched ruby (694 nm).

Picosecond Lasers

Pulse duration in picoseconds (PS)—PS alexandrite (755 nm)

Long-pulsed Lasers

Pulse duration in milliseconds (ms)—Long-pulse alexandrite (755 nm), long-pulse diode (810 nm). These lasers act by causing intracellular protein coagulation followed by denaturation and cellular apoptosis.

TABLE 1: Types of lesions and their response to laser treatments

Lesions	Types	Response to laser
Epidermal lesions	• Lentigines • Freckles • Café au lait macules • Nevus spilus • Pigmented seborrheic Keratosis	Respond well to lasers, recurrence a problem
Dermal lesions	• Nevus of Ota • Nevus of Ito • Blue nevus • Hori's nevus • Drug induced pigmentation	Respond well to laser therapy
Mixed epidermal and dermal lesions	• Melasma • Postinflammatory hyperpigmentation • Becker's nevus • Junctional and compound nevi	Controversial and unpredictable outcomes
Tattoos	• Decorative, traumatic, cosmetic, medical, fire work, gunpowder tattoos • Professional or amateur	Respond well to laser therapy
Others	• Laser toning-low fluence mode/fractional mode—for rejuvenation, melasma	Newer concepts—need further evaluation

Ablative Lasers

Carbon dioxide laser (10,600 nm), erbium doped yttrium-aluminium-garnet laser (Er:YAG) (2,940 nm) due to their high absorption in tissue water can also be used to ablate epidermal pigment. Fractional ablative lasers can also be used for certain lesions either alone or in combination with Q-switched lasers.

Intense Pulsed Light

High intensity polychromatic noncoherent light sources that use cutoff filters to deliver multiple wavelengths. They are generally used for epidermal lesions only.

Patient Selection

Proper patient selection is the key to achieving optimal results in pigmented lesions and tattoos. General medical history, health problems if any, and current medication, history of allergies, past procedures performed, bleeding tendency, and wound healing should be recorded. Assessment of patients' skin type is important as the choice of wavelength and parameters used will depend on it. It is important to avoid a tanned patient while treating pigmented lesions and it is best to wait until tan clears before taking up the patient for laser therapy. Priming of the patient with sunscreens and skin lightening agents helps minimize tan. There has been controversy regarding use of laser therapy in patients on oral isotretinoin and the general recommendation is that it is best to avoid a patient on oral retinoids. Patients may be taken up after 6 months following discontinuation. In the authors experience (and based on a just concluded large multicenter study in India), it seems relatively safe to perform laser therapy in such patients. It is best exercise caution and performs test spots before taking up such patients for pigmented lesion laser treatments. Establishing a proper diagnosis in pigmented lesions is essential and if in doubt, a skin biopsy must be performed in order to rule out any malignancy. Laser therapy is best avoided in pregnancy due to lack of data regarding its safety.

Preoperative Preparation and Priming

It is paramount to ensure that the patient is not tanned, particularly in darker individuals (skin types IV, V) as the epidermal pigment induced by ultraviolet exposure may interfere with laser treatment and increase the risk of dyschromias. Patient should be encouraged to use regular sunscreens, sun protecting clothing before, during, and after treatment sessions. Use of skin lightening agents such as hydroquinone (HQ) and non-HQ products such as kojic acid, licorice extract, etc. may help reduce tan before treatment initiation.

It is recommended to perform test spots to determine the treatment parameters for a given individual and lesion. Evaluate the response to the test spots 4–6 weeks following that to access response to therapy. This helps fine tune the future sessions and predict results.

TREATMENT PROTOCOL

Counseling: pretreatment counseling with explanation of the procedure, expected outcomes, adverse effect profile, and realistic expectation by the patient all go a long way in ensuring compliance and cooperation.

Consent and photographs: taking a written informed consent is necessary and photo documentation with high quality pre- and post-treatment photographs should be done in every case as this will be useful in the objective evaluation and for medicolegal purposes.

Wavelength selection: the frequency doubled 532 nm Q-switched Nd:YAG wavelength is used for epidermal lesions and red tattoo ink removal. This wavelength has very high melanin absorption, has shallow depth of penetration, and should be used carefully in darker skin types as the risk of hyper- and hypopigmentation is higher. Always start with lower fluences and perform test spots.

Q-switched Nd:YAG 1,064 nm wavelength is used for dermal lesions, green ink, blue-black ink tattoos, and laser toning as it has deeper penetration. It is poorly absorbed by epidermal melanin and is relatively safer to use. Fluence depends on indication. Test spots recommended but not mandatory while using this wavelength.

Spot Size

Choosing the correct spot size is critical for getting the desired outcomes. Spot sizes of Q-switched lasers range from 2 to 10 mm. Large spot sizes allow deeper penetration. For epidermal lesions always use spot to match the size of lesion. For dermal lesions it is advisable to use the largest spot that elicits immediate brisk whitening of the irradiated area.

Pulse duration: typically, Q-switched laser pulses are in the nanosecond domain. These ultrashort pulses generate very high peak power and selectively target the melanosomes and ink particles. Typically, the PD is 3–10 nanoseconds for Q-switched lasers. Shorter the PD, higher the peak power. High fluences or standard fluences are used for dermal melanosis, tattoo removal, etc. Low fluence is used for laser toning in melasma. A top-hat beam profile is preferable over a Gaussian beam profile as it allows uniform distribution of the laser energy over a given area without producing hot-spots (areas of uneven high energy within a spot). Pulse width should be shorter than the thermal relaxation time (TRT) of its chromophores in order to only affect its chromophore without unnecessary thermal damage to nearby tissues. For example, the TRT of tattoo particles has been calculated as approximately 0.1–10 nanosecond. But current evidence shows this to be even lower with values approaching 10–100 picosecond. Hence, the newer generation picoseconds lasers may be more effective in laser tattoo removal. Similarly the TRT for melanosomes ranging in size from 0.5–1 μm in diameter is approximately 0.25–1 millisecond.

Anesthesia: Q-switched laser treatment generally does not require anesthesia, but if the area being treated is large, topical anesthesia in the form of eutectic mixture of local anesthetics can be used 45 minutes to 1 hour under occlusion prior to laser therapy.

Eye protection: Q-switched laser pulses can be extremely harmful to the eye as it may cause retinal damage and vision loss. It is mandatory to use laser protecting eye glasses/goggles by the operator and those present in the room during laser exposure. Optically coated laser eye glasses provided by the manufacturer with an optical density of at least four must be worn at all times. Protective eye shields in the form of an anodized external metal eye cup must be worn by the patients. While treating the eyelids, metal corneal eye shields or disposable laser specific corneal eye shields must be inserted after applying topical anesthesia in order to protect the globe.

Epidermal lesions: the wavelength used is 532 nm Q-switched Nd:YAG in lighter skin individuals whereas the 1,064 nm can be used for patients with darker skin tones. On an average, one to three sessions are enough for epidermal lesions. Good clearing in most patients even with one session. Chance of recurrence high with epidermal lesions, such as lentigines, freckles, etc., should be explained to the patient during counseling. Patients can be retreated safely if lesions recur.

Dermal lesions: the wavelength of choice here is the 1,064 nm Q-switched Nd:YAG due to its deeper penetration and excellent safety profile in treating skin types III-VI. An average of six to eight sessions is required for dermal lesions and tattoos (range 2–20). The interval is usually 6–8 weeks or longer between each session. Amateur tattoos require fewer sessions than professional tattoos. Serial photographs must be taken to access improvement. The dermal melanoses have a low chance of recurrence generally but it is prudent to have a long-term follow-up to look for recurrences with pigmented lesions or complications (Fig. 1).

Fluence: start with lowest fluence which elicits brisk whitening. If the response to lasing is suboptimal, then the fluence can be increased. If there is too much epidermal debris/tissue splatter or purpura then the fluence needs to be lowered.

Treatment endpoint: Q-switched laser irradiation at standard fluences produce a brisk whitening of the area treated. Whereas the endpoint while treating with low-fluence (e.g., as in laser toning mode) is erythema without whitening. The treatment endpoint with IPL is mild erythema. If too much whitening or tissue splatter is noted then the fluence needs to be reduced (Fig. 2).

Repetition rate: the number of shots delivered in a second is the repetition rate. Most Q-switched lasers have a frequency of 1–10 Hz. For better control, it is advisable to use a frequency of 2–5 Hz. For covering a larger area of in laser toning, 10 Hz can be used as it allows faster treatment times.

Laser procedure: the area to be treated is cleansed, surface anesthesia if applied is removed, and the patient

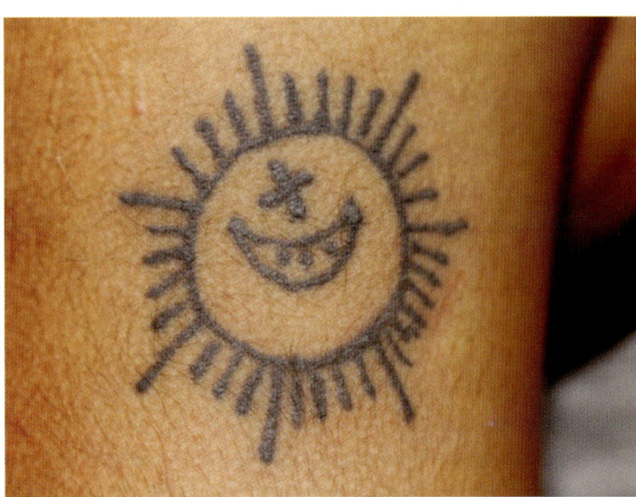

FIG. 1: Amateur tattoo on the right arm of a male patient

is placed in a comfortable position under adequate illumination and treatment initiated. Use of magnifying lamps and loupes are helpful while treating small lesions and fine tattoos. After choosing the parameters for a given patient/lesion, the handpiece is held perpendicular to the skin and the treated with minimal overlap (about 10% overlap is acceptable). Avoid too much overlap and stacking as this may lead to collateral thermal damage, blistering, and scarring. A popping sound may be heard during lasing which is due to the photoacoustic phenomenon explained above. Cooling the area under treatment with continuous air cooling or ice pack application may provide additional comfort to the patient.

Postoperative instructions and care: immediately after procedure, the whitening of the treated area clears and mild erythema and edema may follow (Figs 3 and 4). This usually clears in a few hours. The patient may experience a burning sensation and postoperative ice pack application is helpful to alleviate burning and pain. Patient is asked to apply broad spectrum sunscreen of at least sun protection factor 30 and above every 3–4 hours daily between treatment sessions. Topical emollient generally suffices for a few days following treatment but topical steroid and antibiotic combination may be used topically for 3–5 days postoperative if the area appears abraded or shows signs of excessive inflammation. Treatment interval varies with the indication.

Tattoo Removal

Laser therapy remains the gold standard for tattoo removal and Q-switched lasers remain the mainstay of therapy. The choice of laser depends on the skin type, tattoo ink, and type of the tattoo to be treated. The characteristics of the laser, i.e., spot size, pulse width, and fluence are key to successful treatments. Type of the ink used (organic or inorganic, heavy metals, etc.), amount of ink placed, and the depth of ink placement also affect the outcomes. Until now, multiple sessions spaced over a period of time have been the protocol for tattoo removal. The limitations

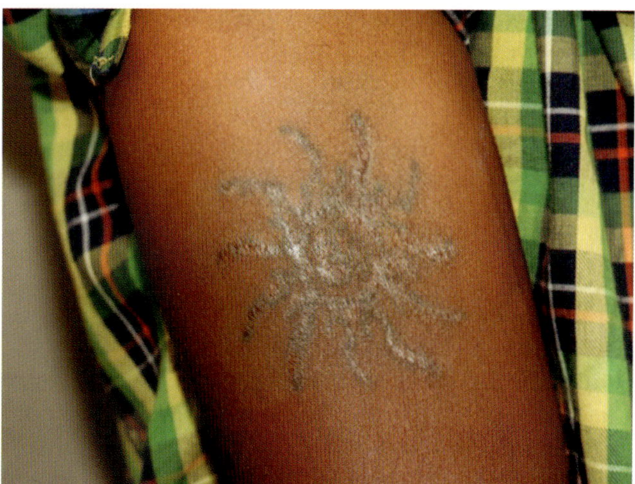

FIG. 3: Amateur tattoo on left right arm of a male with skin type V

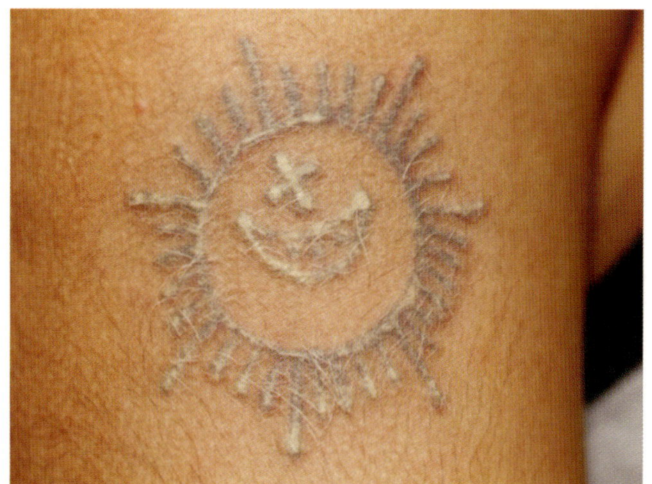

FIG. 2: Immediate whitening following Q-switched neodymium doped:yttrium-aluminium-garnet laser treatment; this is the endpoint to look for

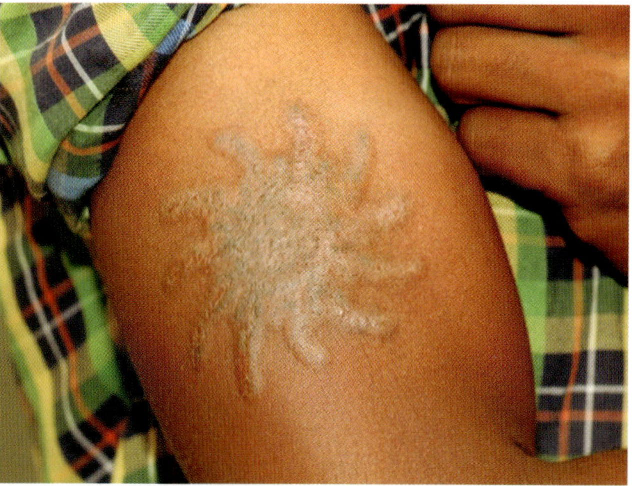

FIG. 4: Post-Q-switched neodymium:yttrium-aluminiumgarnet treatment erythema and edema following laser irradiation

included incomplete clearance, long total treatment duration, and ineffective removal of some colors. Other problems faced in laser tattoo removal include allergic reactions to certain ink, darkening of cosmetic tattoos, tattoo resistance, etc.

The types of tattoos commonly found are:

- Amateur (decorative)
- Professional (decorative)
- Cosmetic
- Traumatic
- Medical
- Gun powder and firearm tattoos.

Amateur tattoos: they are made of carbon-based ink. They tend to be less dense than professional tattoos. These types of tattoos respond readily to Q-switched laser treatment. Wavelength of 1,064 nm is the preferred wavelength as it targets black ink in the dermis. Generally, less number of sessions is needed for removal as compared to professional tattoos (Figs 5–8).

Professional tattoos: they are more complex and can be multicolored. Inks used include organic (azo dyes) or inorganic compounds (cadmium, mercury, cobalt, copper, cinnabar, ferric oxide, TiO_2, carbon ink, etc.). Professional tattoos are more dense and intricate than amateur tattoos. These generally need multiple treatments and yet may not clear fully.

Wavelengths used for tattoo removal:

- Q-switched Nd:YAG 1064 nmn—blue black tattoos
- Q-switched Nd:YAG 532 nm—red tattoo ink
- Q-switched 755 nm alex—purple and teal colors
- Q-switched ruby 694 nm—green color
- Picosecond 755 nm alex—blue and green color tattoos.

FIG. 5: Amateur tattoo on chin and cheek

Estimation of number of sessions needed for tattoo removal: as a general rule, amateur tattoos clear more rapidly than professional tattoos. The older the tattoos, the better the response to laser therapy as macrophages are already present and are trying to phagocytose the pigment. Older tattoos have blurred, indistinct margins.

The Kirby-Desai Scale used to estimate the approximate number of sessions needed for a given tattoo based on the following factors:[6]

- Fitzpatrick skin type
- Location
- Color

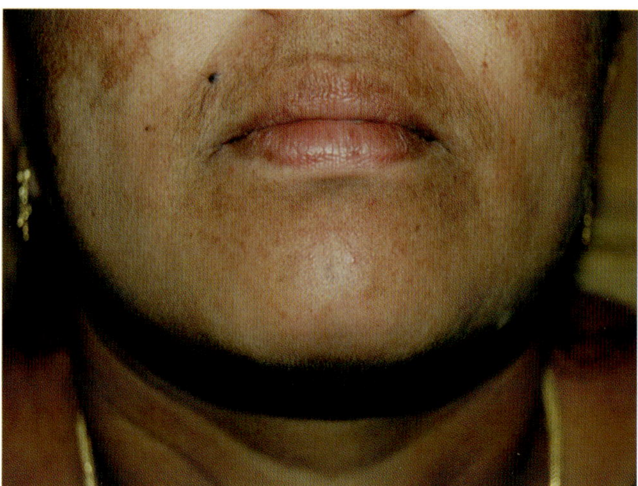

FIG. 6: Complete clearance after a single Q switched neodymium doped:yttrium-aluminiumgarnet laser session

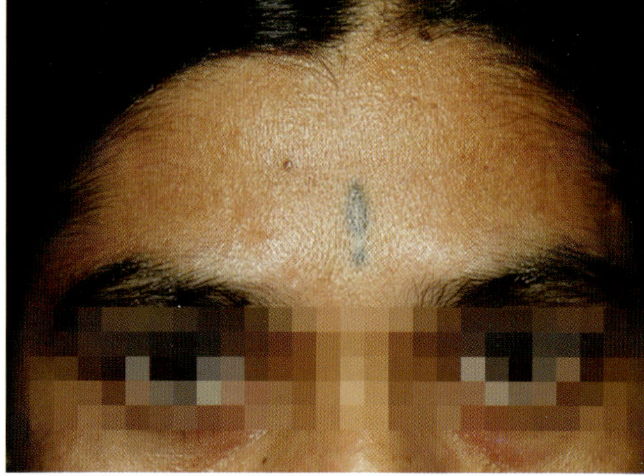

FIG. 7: Amateur bindi tattoo in skin type V female

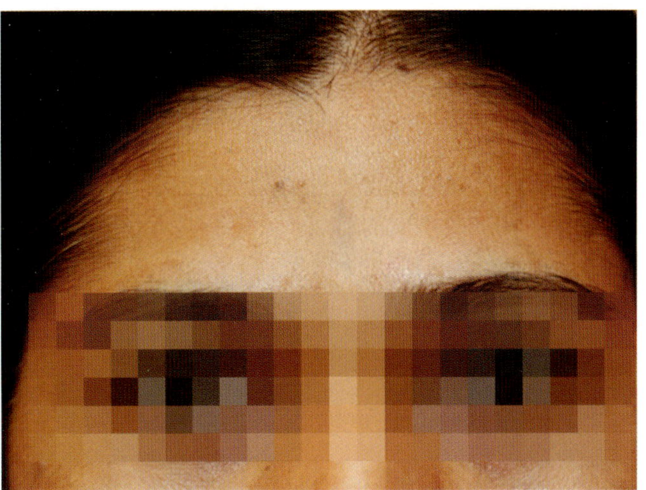

FIG. 8: Near complete clearing after 4 Q-switched neodymium doped:yttrium-aluminium-garnet sessions

- Amount of ink used
- Scarring and tissue damage
- Ink layering.

Each of these six factors are given numerical score and the total of these will give an estimate of the approximate number of sessions required for tattoo removal.

Newer techniques for laser tattoo removal: the limitations of conventional protocol of tattoo removal led to the development of newer techniques.[7] These limitations include a long total duration of treatment (interval of 6–8 weeks between treatments), ink retention despite multiple sessions (which could be due to wrong or ineffective wavelength choice for multicolored tattoos, poor technique, insufficient interval between sessions, etc.), ghosting (shadow or outline of the residual tattoo), and complications such as hyper- and hypopigmentation, blistering, and scarring.

The newer protocols attempt to overcome these short comings by modifying the technique or combining multiple lasers to achieve optimal results and minimize adverse effects.

The newer techniques for laser tattoo removal are:

- R20 technique
- R0 technique
- Combining fractional lasers with Q-switched lasers.

R20 method: tattoo removal in a single laser session, based on method of repeated exposure.[8,9,10] Four treatment passes are done with an interval of 20 minutes between passes. Immediate whitening is seen on the first pass with

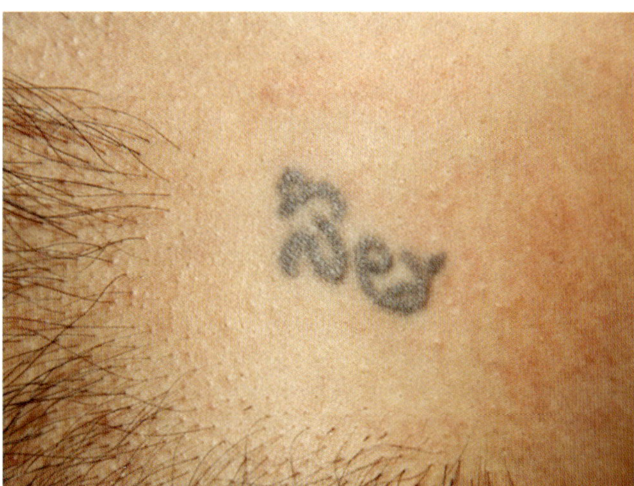

FIG. 9: Amateur tattoo on left chest of a male

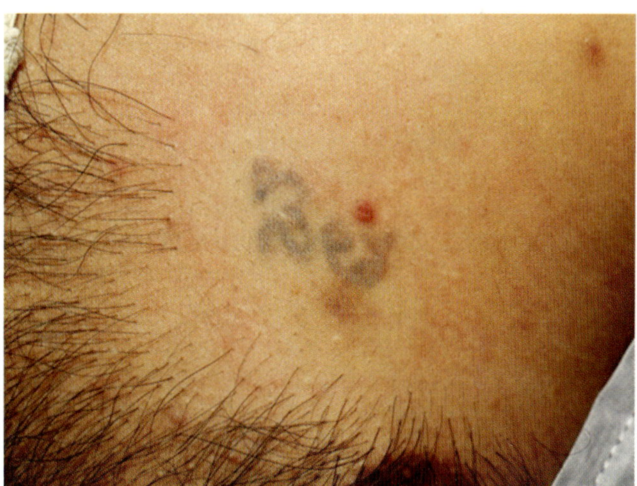

FIG. 10: Amateur tattoo after R20 session

little or no whitening on subsequent passes. Kossida et al. in a study found that treatment with the R20 method was much more effective than conventional single-pass laser treatment (Q-switched alex 755 nm laser was used in the study) (Figs 9 and 10).[8]

R0 method: repeated exposure on same day with no waiting period by applying perfluorodecalin (a per fluorocarbon compound), immediately after lasing.[11] This compound dissolves the gas bubbles formed upon initial laser exposure thus opening the optical window by reducing scatter. This allows an immediate next pass to be performed without the waiting time of 20 minutes as in the R20 technique.

Combining lasers: monotherapy with Q-switched laser (QSL) is often effective for tattoo removal but combining QSL with an alcoholic fatty liver or nonalcoholic fatty liver may yield faster clearing, minimize number of sessions and reduce side effects. Combination can be in any order; fatty liver followed by QSL helps reduces blister formation.

A study by Weiss and Geronimus found that after multiple sessions of QSL followed immediately by either nonablative fractional resurfacing (NAFR) or ablative fractional resurfacing (AFR) increases tattoo clearance, eliminates blistering, shortens recovery and diminishes treatment induced hypopigmentation. They noted the addition of AFR to QSL enhances the rate of pigment clearance. Addition of NAFR to QSL may decrease the degree of treatment-induced hypopigmentation.[12]

Marini et al. proposed a combination of fractional Er:YAG laser skin conditioning followed by Q-switched Nd:YAG laser for laser tattoo removal. In their two-steptechnique, they used a fractional Er:YAG laser to drill microholes into the skin which was followed by QSL treatment. According to the authors, this fractional Er:YAG laser conditioning protects the skin from damages at higher fluences by allowing the escape of gases through these microholes and thus relieving the internal pressure generated by QSL treatment. This also aided in repeating the next pass after 20 minutes. They concluded that this procedure led to a 30% reduction in the number of sessions.[13]

Bencini et al. studied the variables influencing the outcomes in QSL tattoo removal. The authors assessed the prognostic factors affecting the outcomes in a large cohort of patients and found that smoking, the presence of colors other than black and red, a tattoo larger than 30 cm^2, a tattoo located on the feet or legs or older than 36 months, high color density, treatment intervals of 8 weeks or less, and development of a darkening phenomenon were associated with a reduced clinical response to treatment.[14]

Au et al. analyzed the incidence of bulla formation after tattoo treatment using the combination of the picoseconds alexandrite laser and a fractionated carbon dioxide (CO_2) laser ablation. In their study, 32% of patients treated with the picoseconds laser alone experienced blistering, whereas none of the patients treated with the combination developed blistering. The study showed a statistically significant decrease in bulla formation associated with tattoo treatment when fractionated CO_2 ablation was added to the picosecond alexandrite laser.[15]

Picosecond lasers:Alexandrite 550 picoseconds and 755 picoseconds lasers are available now and picosecond Nd:YAG laser is also under development and trails. There is a possibility to have both nanosecond and picoseconds pulse width in same system in future. Picosecond lasers useful for blue and green colors which were difficult to remove earlier.

Brauer et al. reported successful and rapid removal of blue and green pigment with a novel picosecond alexandrite laser. They found more than two-thirds of the tattoos treated achieved near 100% clearance.[16]

Ross et al. compared the response of tattoos to a nanosecond and a picoseconds Q-switched Nd:YAG lasers. This group compared two Nd:YAG lasers for effectiveness at removing black tattoo pigment, one a 10 nanosecond PD laser and the other a 35 picosecond PD laser. Sixteen tattoos were treated at 4-week intervals for four treatments. In 12 of the 16 tattoos, the picosecond laser yielded greater removal of tattoo pigment.[17]

Treatment of Epidermal Pigmented Lesions

Epidermal lesions respond readily to Q-switched lasers with few exceptions. Since the melanin pigment is superficial, shorter wavelength that are highly absorbed by the chromophore and which penetrate to a lesser depth are generally chosen. Q-switched Nd:YAG 532 nm, Q-switched ruby 694 nm, Q-switched 755 nm alexandrite, and Q-switched Nd:YAG 1,064 nm are the wavelength often used. In darker individuals, it is safer to use Q-switched Nd:YAG at 1,064 nm as it offers greater safety. Intense pulsed light with a 530–900 nm filter can also be used for epidermal pigmented lesions. Typically, epidermal lesions require one to three sessions for complete removal. Exceptions to this include café au lait macules (CALMs), nevus spilus, etc., which show variable response to Q-switched lasers and the number of sessions are more difficult to predict.

Café au Lait Macules

These are very light to dark brown patches which occur as isolated lesions or associated with genodermatoses, e.g., neurofibromatosis. They contain giant melanosomes in epidermis. The lesions are thin and superficial that are difficult to treat. Multiple sessions are generally needed with Q-switched lasers and recurrence rate of up to 50% at the end of one year are common (Box 1).

Shimbashi et al. in a study observed that multiple treatments over months to years are required with Q-switched ruby laser and recurrences occur in 50% patients up to 1 year following clearance.[18] This could be

Box 1: Treatment protocol for Café au lait macules

- Avoid tanned patients
- Perform test spots
- Best option—532 nm Q-switched Nd:YAG laser (light skin patients)
- Risk of PIH and hypopigmentation higher in darker patients
- Recurrence, residual hyperpigmentation, incomplete pigment removal common

Nd:YAG, neodymium doped:yttrium-aluminium-garnet, PIH, postinflammatory hyperpigmentation

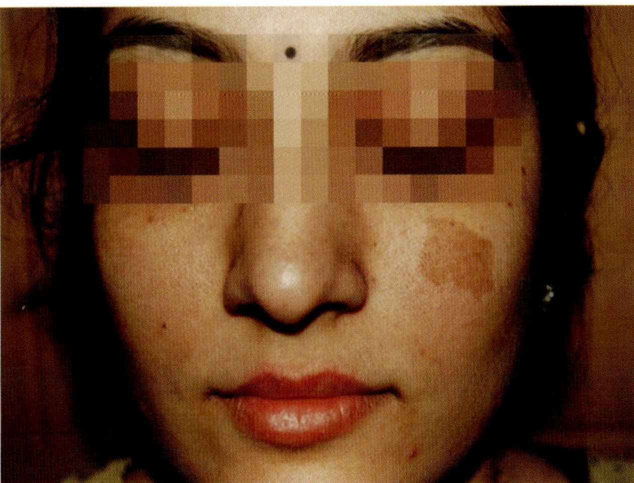

FIG. 11: Café au lait macule on left cheek

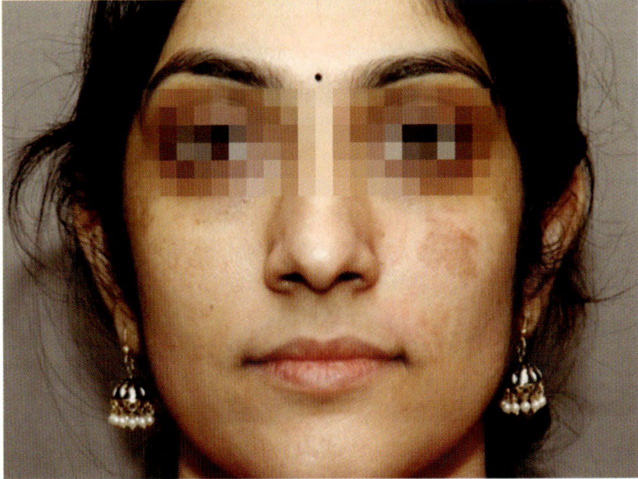

FIG 12: Café au lait macule after 5 Q-switched neodymium doped:yttrium-aluminium-garnet laser sessions showing partial clearing

due to dermal induction of epidermal hyperpigmentation in CALMs (Figs 11 and 12).

Due to the unpredictable response to QSL, ablative lasers have been tried in the treatment of CALM. Alora et al. successfully treated a "QSL-resistant" CALM with an Er:YAG ablative laser.[19]

Freckles, Lentigenes, and Solar Lentigo

These superficial epidermal pigmented macules respond readily to laser therapy (Figs 13 and 14).[20] Pigment specific lasers such as QSL, long-pulsed mid infrared lasers such as alexandrite, diode as well as nonselective lasers such as ablative CO_2 and Er:YAG lasers can be used. Intense pulsed light with a 530–570 nm filter can also be used. Most lesions respond one to two sessions but recurrences are high and continued sun protection and

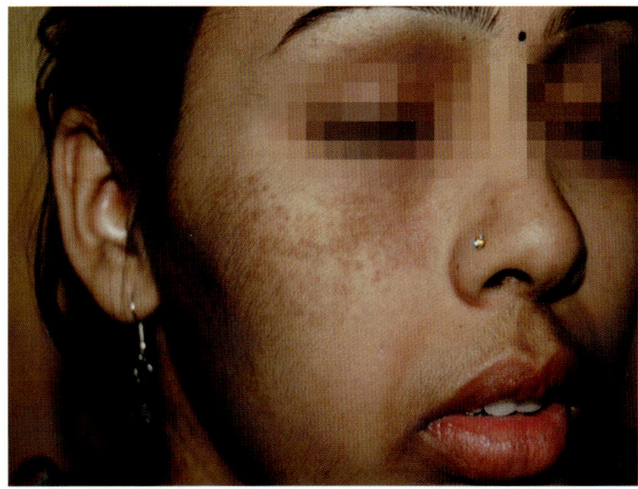

FIG. 13: Zosteriform lentiginosis on right cheek of a female

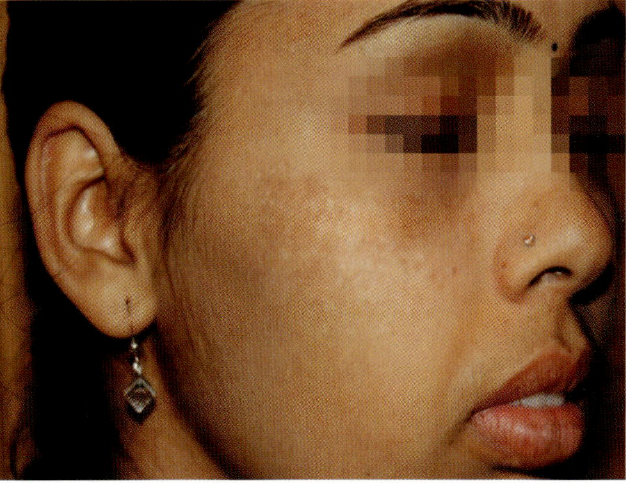

FIG. 14: Zosteriform lentiginosis after 5 Q-switched neodymium doped:yttrium-aluminium-garnet (Nd:YAG) 532 nm laser sessions

repeat treatments may be necessary. Studies have shown the QSL to be more effective than other modalities such as liquid nitrogen, trichloroacetic acid peels or glycolic acid peels.[21-27]

In the author's experience, a QSL at 1,064 nm is the ideal tool for treating lentigines and freckles in dark skin. The 532 nm wavelength is seldom needed and with appropriate spot size and fluence (spot size should either match or be within the size of the lesion), the 1,064 nm QSL can effectively treat most lesions in a short time. Mucosal lentigines can also be safely treated with the 1,064 nm QSL. Most lesions clear in two to three sessions at 1 month interval.

Nevus Spilus

This epidermal melanosis has two components. A background CALM and scattered darker junctional or compound melanocytic nevi within it. The lighter background lesion does not respond as well as the junctional component and either 532 or 1,064 nm Q-switched Nd:YAG laser can be used with preference towards 1,064 nm in darker patients. Multiple reports suggest that QSL and IPL are effective in treating nevus spilus.[28,29]

Dermal Lesions

Nevus of Ota: also known as oculodermal nevus. It is a rare pigmented dermal nevus often seen at birth or early in life involving the ophthalmic and/or maxillary division of the trigeminal nerve seen clinically as bluish, grey macular pigmentation on skin and the sclera of the eye. The lesion is often unilateral but bilateral involvement may also be seen. Mucosal pigmentation on the hard palate, pigmentation on the ears, and tympanic membrane may also occur.

The nevus responds well to 1,064 nm Q-switched Nd:YAG laser. Multiple sessions spaced at 2–3 months intervals yield excellent results with significant clearing. As the lesion is dermal in location, the use of a large spot size and longer wavelength is recommended. Recurrences are very rare after Q-switched Nd:YAG treatment.[30,31]

Periocular area can be treated by inserting a laser protecting ocular eye shields to protect the globe from inadvertent laser irradiation.

It has been observed that the number of treatments required varies significantly according to the lesional color and site: grey lesions and those on the forehead/temple are most resistant.

In dark skin types, the use of lower fluences are recommended and test spots are useful in deciding the parameters in a given case and to minimize the risk of hyper- and hypopigmentation (Figs 15 and 16). But the results are generally very satisfactory even in skin types IV-VI.[30,31]

Newer concepts such as the use of low fluence 1,064 nm Q-switched Nd:YAG laser treatment performed once in 2 weeks has also been tried with reasonable success. Combination of fractional lasers with QSL has also been explored for treating nevus of Ota.[32-35]

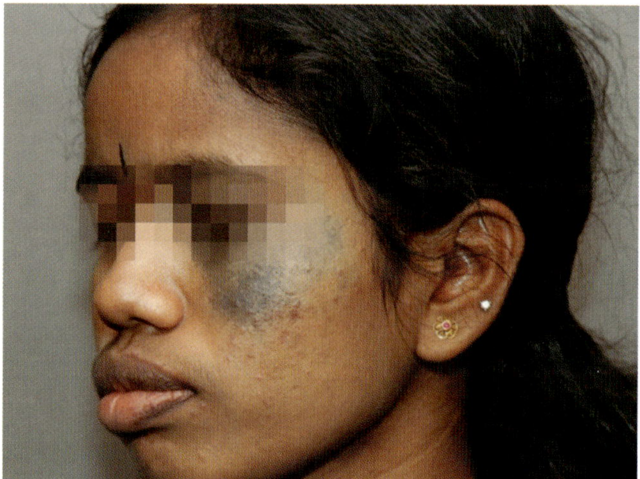

FIG. 15: Nevus of Ota on left cheek and periorbital area before treatment

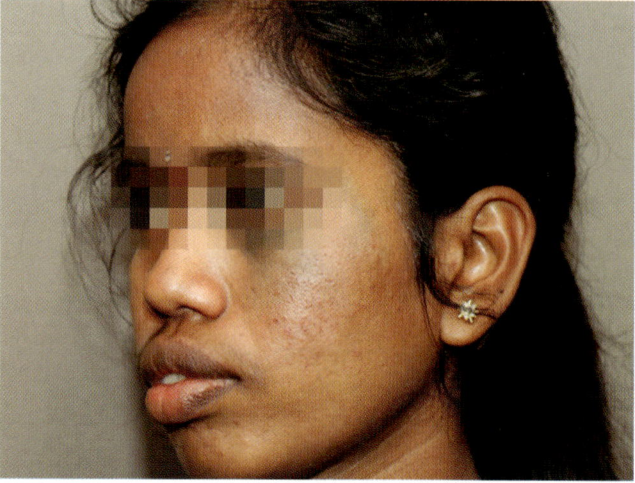

FIG. 16: Nevus of Ota after 6 Q-switched neodymium doped: yttrium-aluminium-garnet laser sessions with 3 month interval between sessions

Hori's Nevus

Acquired bilateral nevus of Ota-like macules (ABNOM) or Hori's macules can mimic nevus of Ota but they differ in their late age of onset, lack of mucosal involvement, and are bilateral in distribution. They respond well to QSL but multiple sessions are generally necessary. The recommended interval between sessions is 4–6 weeks between sessions.[36-38]

In the authors experience, Hori's nevi tend to be more stubborn than nevus of Ota and a combination of fractional Er:YAG or fractional CO_2 with Q-switched Nd:YAG laser may yield better results.

Blue Nevus

The deep dermal location of these nevi allows them to be conveniently treated with 1,064 nm Q-switched Nd:YAG. They respond readily to Q-switched Nd:YAG treatment unless the lesion is extending into the subcutaneous tissue.[39] The blue coloration is due to the Tyndall effect.

Acquired Dermal Melanosis

This is an increasingly recognized entity comprising of varied inflammatory dermatoses that lead to pigment incontinence and dermal melanosis. Entities such as lichen planus pigmentosus (LPP), fixed drug eruptions (FDE), and ABNOM, are some examples that are included in this group (Figs 17–20).

Since the abnormal pigment is located in the dermis, the longer wavelength QSL, such as 1,064 nm Q-switched Nd:YAG, can potentially target these lesions aiding in clearing of pigment.

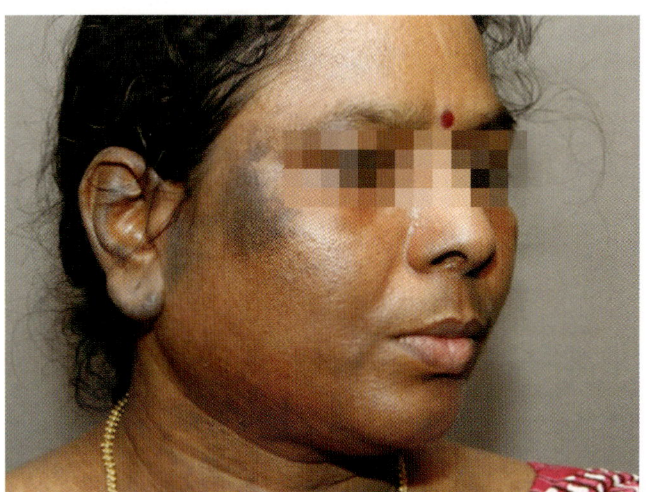

FIG. 17: Lichen planus pigmentosus before laser

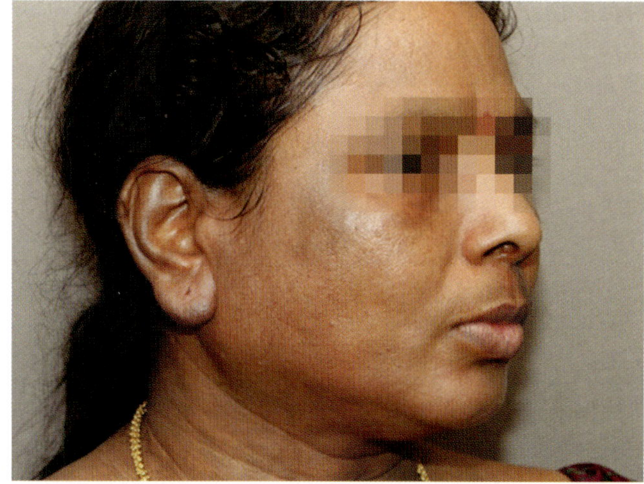

FIG. 18: Lichen planus pigmentosus after 5 Q-switched neodymium doped: yttrium-aluminium-garnet laser treatment sessions

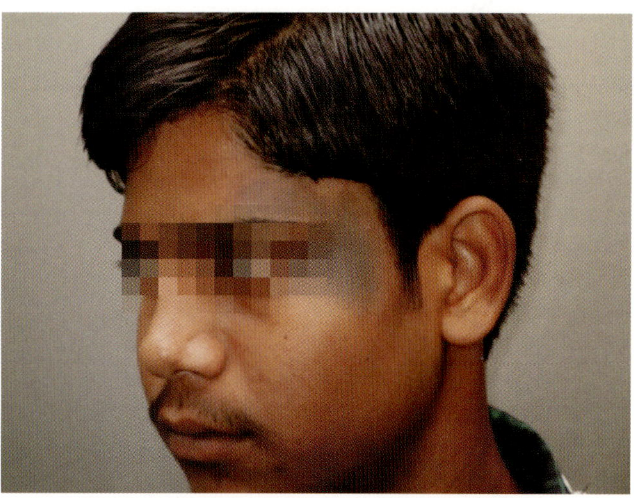

FIG. 19: Lichen planus pigmentosus before treatment

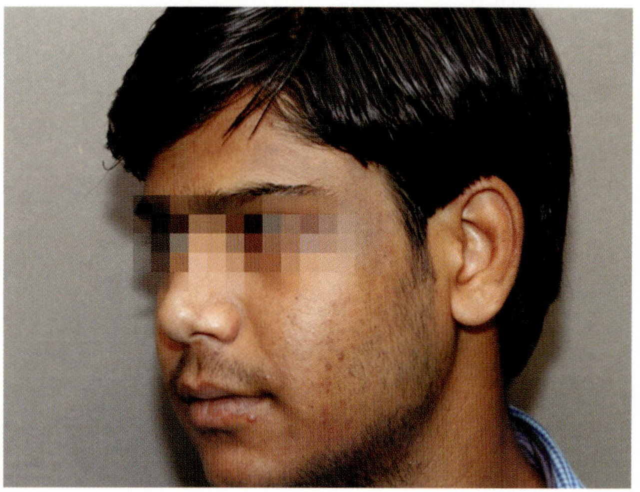

FIG. 20: Lichen planus pigmentosus after 5 Q-switched neodymium doped:yttrium-aluminiumg-arnet laser sessions

In the author's experience, these lesions respond favorably to 1,064 nm Q-switched Nd:YAG, requiring on an average five to six laser sessions spaced 4–8 weeks apart. Conditions such as LPP and FDE need to be managed medically and stabilized prior to initiating laser therapy.

MIXED EPIDERMAL AND DERMAL PIGMENTED LESIONS

Melasma

Melasma is best managed medically. Fixed triple combination creams and sunscreens remain the mainstay of therapy followed by maintenance with HQ and non-HQ skin lightening agents. Peels have successfully been used as well as an adjunct to medical management. A variety of lasers and light devices have been used with varying degrees of success in melasma. Q-switched lasers, fractional lasers, ablative lasers, IPLs, copper bromide laser, thulium laser, and combinations have all been used but response can be unpredictable and the pigment frequently recurs. Lasers can be used in selected patients with resistant melasma after thorough counseling and after conducting test treatments if necessary (Fig. 21).

A number of studies have reported the use of low-fluence Q-switched Nd:YAG laser treatment (laser toning) at weekly intervals for eight to ten sessions with some success.[40-44] Though effective, the risk of mottled hypopigmentation following multiple Q-switched Nd:YAG laser sessions at frequent intervals has been reported in literature. Hence, caution needs to be exercised while performing this procedure and the risks need to be explained to patients. In the author's experience, modified laser toning with treatments performed once in 2 weeks instead of weekly treatments for six to eight sessions is better as it decreases the risk of hypopigmentation (Fig. 22).

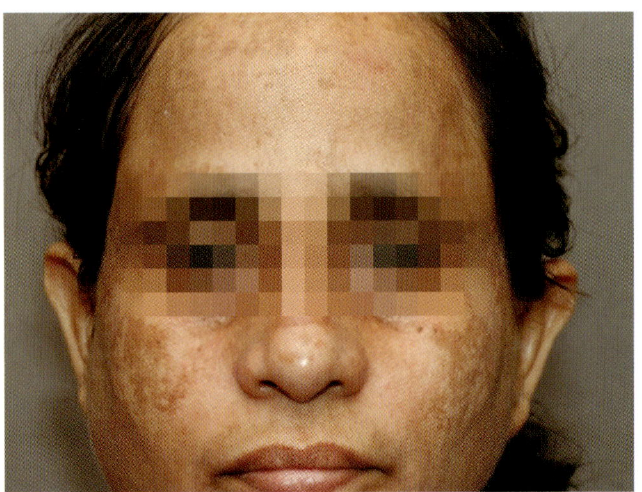

FIG. 21: Melasma before Q-switched neodymium doped:yttrium-aluminum-garnet laser

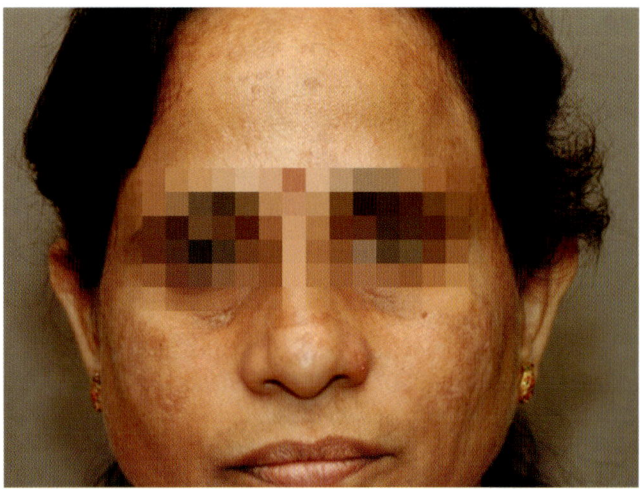

FIG. 22: Melasma after eight Q-switched neodymium:yttrium-aluminium-garnet low-fluence laser treatments, performed once in every 2 weeks

Becker's Nevus

Becker's nevus is a pigmented, hairy nevus that appears at adolescence or young adulthood. It is a hamartoma and does not respond well to laser treatment. Intense puled light, long-pulsed lasers, ablative lasers such as Er:YAG laser, and QSLs, have all been used either alone or in combination but the results are unpredictable with either incomplete clearance or recurrence.[45,46] Test spots with individual or combination of lasers is recommended to determine which laser or combination works best in a given case.

Postinflammatory Hyperpigmentation

Postinflammatory hyperpigmentation can be managed conservatively with sunscreens, skin lightening agents (HQ and non-HQ) and peels. Lasers have a limited role in its management as the response is either ineffective suboptimal, or unpredictable. Q-switched Nd:YAG laser can be used but with caution and after performing test spots.[47] In the author's experience, use of low-fluence 532 nm QS Nd:YAG in combination with 1,064 nm may improve PIH after three to five sessions at monthly intervals.

Nevocellular Nevi

Laser treatment of nevocellular nevi is controversial and a subject of ongoing debate. Nevocellular nevi may be congenital or acquired and acquired nevi can be junctional, compound or dermal in type. Congenital melanocytic nevi are usually varied in size (some small and others very large) and are generally dark and bulky lesions with a deep dermal component.

Any QSL can be used to treat junctional nevi, with the Q-switched Nd:YAG being the treatment of choice in dark skin. The 532 nm wavelength and 1,064 nm wavelength of Q-switched Nd:YAG laser can both be used (with preference for 1,064 nm in darker skin). The long-pulsed millisecond lasers with PD up to 3 millisecond can also be used for nevi. On an average, one to three treatment sessions are generally necessary. The response is usually variable, with risk of partial clearing, lightening, and recurrence. Compound and dermal nevi are best addressed by radiofrequency surgery or surgical excision.

Congenital melanocytic nevi often need a combination approach involving serial excision, grafting, and/or lasers. A combination of QSL, followed by longer-pulsed lasers has been reported to be effective with most lesions needing three to five sessions. Again, laser treatment is plagued by unpredictable response and partial clearing.

Due to the risk of potential malignant transformation in some of these laser irradiated nevi and the possibility of persistence of amelanotic nests of nevus cells in some of these lesions, it is suggested that a biopsy be performed if felt necessary prior to laser treatment of suspicious lesions and a long-term follow-up is recommended to watch for any morphological change in these lesions.[48-54]

Classification of pigmented lesions according to response to laser therapy:

- Excellent: 532/IPL—ephelids, lentigines, labial melanosis, and seborrheic melanosis
- Very good: 1,064 nm—nevus of Ota, Hori's nevus, junctional nevus, black tattoos, and acquired dermal melanosis
- Variable: CALMs, nevus spilus, mongolian spots, and segmental lentigines
- Poor: melasma, Becker's melanosis.

COMPLICATIONS

As with any laser procedure, complications can and sometimes do occur with pigment lasers. Most are transient and clear in due course with minimal sequel. Most complications are due to improper patient selection (such as tanned skin) and poor priming. Poor technique or wrong choice of parameters such as excessive stacking/overlapping, and excessive fluence are another reason why complications occur. Proper postoperative instructions need to be given and followed by the patient and noncompliance could increase risk of complications.

The complications following QSL treatment are listed below:

- Immediate erythema, edema, mild burning, and pain occasionally purpura, blistering (Figs 23–26)
- Postinflammatory hyperpigmentation (Fig. 27)
- Postinflammatory hypopigmentation (Fig. 28)
- Textural changes and scarring

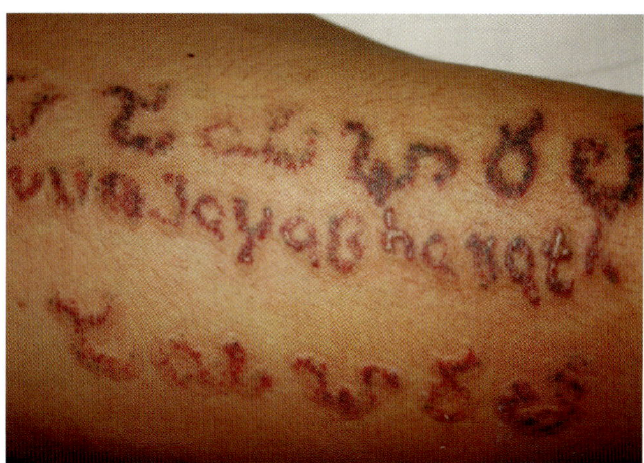

FIG. 23: Erythema and edema immediately after Q-switched neodymium doped: yttrium-aluminium-garnet treatment of amateur tattoo on the arm

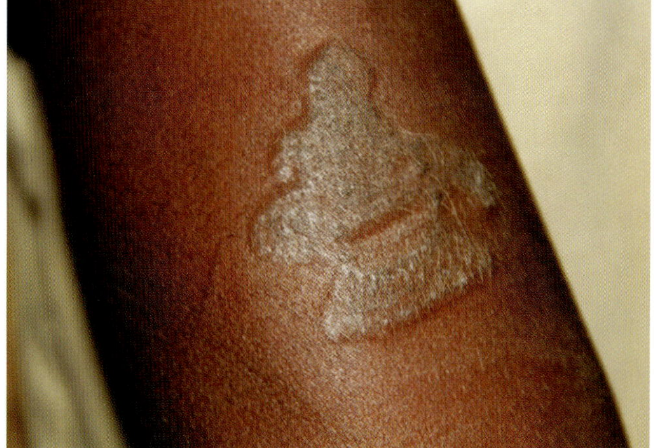

FIG. 24: Blistering immediately after Q-switched neodymium doped:yttrium-aluminium-garnet treatment (need citation)

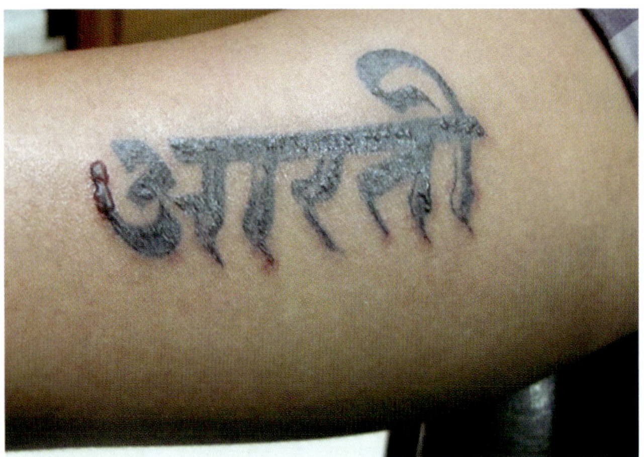

FIG. 25: Hypopigmentation following Q-switched neodymium doped:yttrium-aluminium-garnet tattoo removal (need citation)

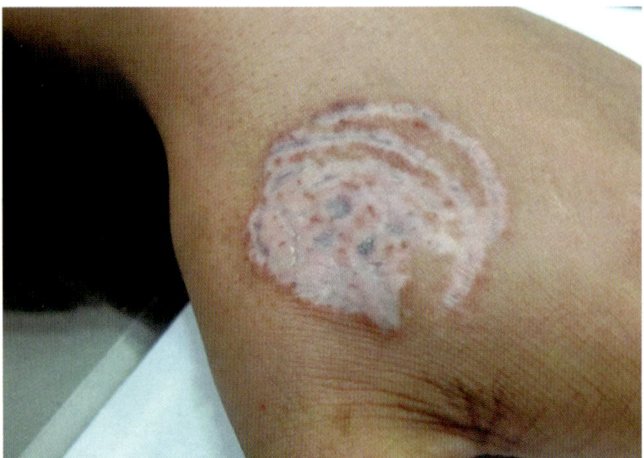

FIG. 26: Hypertrophic scar following Q-switched neodymium doped:yttrium-aluminium-garnet laser tattoo removal (need citation)

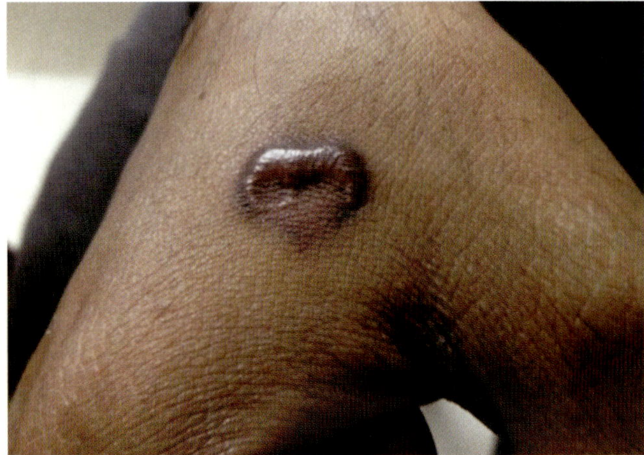

FIG. 27: Hypopigmentation on right cheek following Q-switched neodymium doped:yttrium-aluminium-garnet laser treatment of nevus of Ota

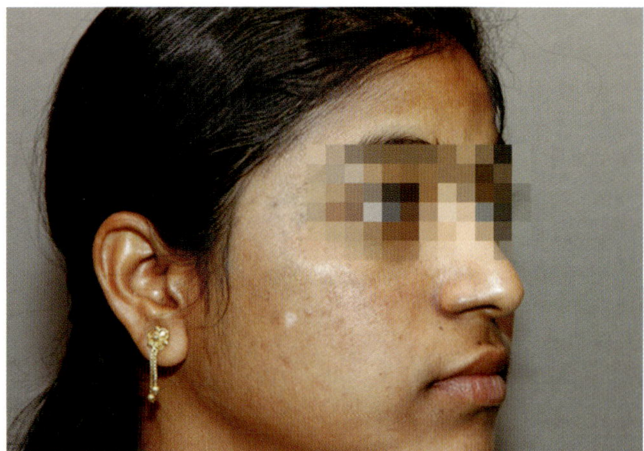

FIG. 28: Postinflammatory hypopigmentation after multiple Q-switched neodymium doped:yttrium-aluminium-garnet 1,064 nm laser treatments

- Allergic reactions to tattoo pigment
- Red tattoo ink (cinnabar/Hg) common cause of allergic reaction and granulomatous inflammation
- Laser treatment of red ink dispersion of antigen resulting in urticaria and systemic allergic reactions
- Darkening of skin-colored cosmetic tattoos
- Tattoo darkening: laser pulse can reduce rust-colored ferric oxide to jet-black ferrous oxide.

CONCLUSION

Q-switched Nd:YAG laser is the gold standard for pigment and tattoo removal in dark skin. Due care needs to be taken with regards to technique and patient selection to avoid complications. Proper sun protection and priming goes a long way in minimizing complications and achieve satisfactory outcomes. Newer techniques and advancement in laser technology have aided in improving efficacy and minimizing adverse effects.

REFERENCES

1. Anderson RR, Parrish JA. Selective photothermolysis: precise microsurgery by selective absorption of pulsed radiation. Science. 1983;220(4596):524-7.
2. Polla LL, Margolis RJ, Dover JS, Whitaker D, Murphy GF, Jacques SL, et al. Melanosomes are a primary target of Q-switched ruby laser irradiation in guinea pig skin. J Invest Dermatol. 1987;89(3):281-6.
3. Murphy GF, Shepard RS, Paul BS, Menkes A, Anderson RR, Parrish JA. Organelle-specific injury to melanin-containing cells in human skin by pulsed laser irradiation. Lab Invest. 1983;49(6):680-5.
4. Dover JS, Margolis RJ, Polla LL, Watanabe S, Hruza GJ, Parrish JA, et al. Pigmented guinea pig skin irradiated with Q-switched ruby laser pulses. Morphologic and histologic findings. Arch Dermatol. 1989;125(1):43-9.

5. Mun JY, Jeong SY, Kim JH, Han SS, Kim IH. A low fluence Q-switched Nd:YAG laser modifies the 3D structure of melanocyte and ultrastructure of melanosome by subcellular-selective photothermolysis. J Electron Microsc (Tokyo). 2011;60(1):11-8.
6. Kirby W, Desai A, Desai T, Kartono F, Geeta P. The Kirby-Desai Scale: A Proposed Scale to Assess Tattoo-removal Treatments. J Clin Aesthet Dermatol. 2009;2(3):32-7.
7. Luebberding S, Alexiades-Armenakas M. New tattoo approaches in dermatology. Dermatol Clin. 2014;32(1):91-6.
8. Kossida T, Rigopoulos D, Katsambas A, Anderson RR. Optimal tattoo removal in a single laser session based on the method of repeated exposures. J Am Acad Dermatol. 2012;66(2):271-7.
9. Bunert N, Homey B, Gerber PA. Successful treatment of a professional tattoo with the R20 method. Hautarzt. 2014;65(10):853-5.
10. Zawar V, Sarda A, De A. Bindi tattoo on forehead: success with modified R-20 technique using low fluence q-switched nd yag laser: a case report. J Cutan Aesthet Surg. 2014;7(1):54-5.
11. Reddy KK, Brauer JA, Anolik R, Bernstein L, Brightman L, Hale E, et al. Topical perfluorodecalin resolves immediate whitening reactions and allows rapid effective multiple pass treatment of tattoos. Lasers Surg Med. 2013;45(2):76-80.
12. Weiss ET, Geronemus RG. Combining fractional resurfacing with Q-S ruby laser for tattoos. Dermatol Surg. 2010;36:1-3.
13. Marini L, Kozarev J, Grad L, Jezersek M, Cencic B. Fractional Er:YAG skin conditioning for enhanced efficacy for Nd:YAG Q switched laser tattoo removal. J Laser Health Acad. 2012;1:35-40.
14. Bencini PL, Cazzaniga S, Tourlaki A, Galimberti MG, Naldi L. Removal of tattoos by q-switched laser: variables influencing outcome and sequelae in a large cohort of treated patients. Arch Dermatol. 2012;148(12):1364-9.
15. Au S, Liolios AM, Goldman MP. Analysis of incidence of bulla formation after tattoo treatment using the combination of the picosecond Alexandrite laser and fractionated CO2 ablation. Dermatol Surg. 2015;41(2):242-5.
16. Brauer JA, Reddy KK, Anolik R, Weiss ET, Karen JK, Hale EK, et al. Successful and rapid treatment of blue and green tattoo pigment with a novel picosecond laser. Arch Dermatol. 2012;148(7):820-3.
17. Ross V, Naseef G, Lin G, Kelly M, Michaud N, Flotte TJ, et al. Comparison of responses of tattoos to picosecond and nanosecond Q-switched neodymium: YAG lasers. Arch Dermatol. 1998;134(2):167-71.
18. Shimbashi T, Kamide R, Hashimoto T. Long-term follow-up in treatment of solar lentigo and café au lait macules with Q-switched ruby laser. Aesthetic Plast Surg. 1997,21(6):445-8.
19. Alora MB, Arndt KA. Treatment of a café-au-lait macule with the erbium:YAG laser. J Am Acad Dermatol. 2001;45(4):566-8.
20. Kilmer SL, Wheeland RG, Goldberg DJ, Anderson RR. Treatment of epidermal pigmented lesions with the frequency-doubled Q-switched Nd:YAG laser. A controlled, single-impact, dose-response, multi-center trial. Arch Dermatol. 1994;130(12):1515-9.
21. Jang KA, Chung EC, Choi JH, Sung KJ, Moon KC, Koh JK. Successful removal of freckles in Asian skin with a Q-switched alexandrite laser. Dermatol Surg. 2000;26(3):231-4.
22. Wang CC, Sue YM, Yang CH, Chen CK. A comparison of Q-switched alexandrite laser and IPL for the treatment of freckles and lentigines in Asian persons: a randomized, physician-blinded, split-face comparative trial. J Am Acad Dermatol. 2006;54(5):804-10.
23. Jiang SB, Levine V, Ashinoff R. The treatment of solar lentigines with the Diode (Diolite 532 nm) and the Q-switched ruby laser: a comparative study. Laser Surg Med Suppl. 2000;12-55.
24. Todd MM, Rallis TM, Gerwels JW, Hata TR. A comparison of 3 lasers and liquid nitrogen in the treatment of solar lentigines: a randomized, controlled comparative trial. Arch Dermatol. 2000;136(7):841-6.
25. Li YT, Yang KC. Comparison of frequency-doubled Q-switched Nd:YAG laser and 35% trichloroacetic acid for the treatment of face lentigines. Dermatol Surg. 1999;25(3):202-4.
26. Bjerring P, Christiansen K. Intense pulsed light source for treatment of small melanocytic nevi and solar lentigines. J Cutan Laser Ther. 2000;2(4):177-81.
27. Kono T, Manstein D, Chan HH, Nozaki M, Anderson RR. Q-switched ruby versus long-pulsed dye laser delivered with compression for treatment of facial lentigines in Asians. Lasers Surg Med. 2006;38(2):94-7.
28. Gold MH, Foster TD, Bell MW. Nevus spilus successfully treated with an intensed pulsed light source. Dermatol Surg. 1999;25(3):254-5.
29. Moreno-Arias GA, Bulla F, Vilata-Corell JJ, Camps-Fresneda A. Treatment of widespread segmental nevus spilus by Q-switched alexandrite laser (755 nm, 100 nsec). Dermatol Surg. 2001;27(9):841-3.
30. Felton SJ, Al-Niaimi F, Ferguson JE, Madan V. Our perspective of the treatment of naevus of Ota with 1,064-, 755- and 532-nm wavelength lasers. Lasers Med Sci. 2014;29(5):1745-9.
31. Aurangabadkar S. QYAG5 Q-switched Nd:YAG laser treatment of Nevus of Ota: An Indian study of 50 Patients. J Cutan Aesthet Surg. 2008;1(2):80-4.
32. Moody MN, Landau JM, Vergilis-Kalner IJ, Goldberg LH, Marquez D, Friedman PM. 1,064-nm Q-switched neodymium-doped yttrium aluminum garnet laser and 1,550-nm fractionated erbium-doped fiber laser for the treatment of nevus of Ota in Fitzpatrick skin type IV. Dermatol Surg. 2011;37(8):1163-7.
33. Landau JM, Vergilis-Kalner I, Goldberg LH, Geronemus RG, Friedman PM. Treatment of Nevus of Ota in Fitzpatrick skin type VI with the 1064-nm QS Nd:YAG laser. Lasers Surg Med. 2011;43(2):65-7.
34. Choi CW, Kim HJ, Lee HJ, Kim YH, Kim WS. Treatment of nevus of Ota using low fluence Q-switched Nd:YAG laser. Int J Dermatol. 2014;53(7):861-5.
35. Turnbull JR, Assaf Ch, Zouboulis C, Tebbe B. Bilateral nevus of Ota: a rare manifestation in a Caucasian. J Eur Acad Dermatol Venereol. 2004;18(3):353-5.
36. Kunachak S, Leelaudomlipi P. Q-switched Nd:YAG laser treatment for acquired bilateral nevus of Ota-like maculae a long-term follow-up. Laser Surg Med. 2000;26(4):376-9.
37. Polnikorn N, Tanrattanakorn S, Goldberg DJ. Treatment of Hori's nevus with the Q-switched Nd:YAG laser. Dermatol Surg. 2000;26(5):477-80.
38. Lee B, Kim YC, Kang WH, Lee ES. Comparison of characteristics of acquired bilateral nevus of Ota-like macules and nevus of Ota according to therapeutic outcome. J Korean Med Sci. 2004;19(4):554-9.
39. Milgraum SS, Cohen ME, Auletta MJ. Treatment of blue nevi with the Q-switched ruby laser. J Am Acad Dermatol. 1995;32:307-10.
40. Angsuwarangsee S, Polnikorn N. Combined ultrapulse CO2 laser and Q-switched alexandrite laser compared with Q-switched alexandrite laser alone for refractory melasma: split-face design. Dermatol Surg. 2003;29(1):59-64.
41. Nouri K, Bowes L, Chartier T, Romagosa R, Spencer J. Combination treatment of melasma with pulsed CO2 laser followed by Q-switched alexandrite laser: a pilot study. Dermatol Surg. 1999;25(6):494-7.
42. Wang CC, Hui CY, Sue YM, Wong WR, Hong HS. Intense pulsed light for the treatment of refractory melasma in Asian persons. Dermatol Surg. 2004;30(9):1196-200.
43. Manaloto RM, Alster T. Erbium:YAG laser resurfacing for refractory melasma. Dermatol Surg. 1999;25(2):121-3.

44. Rokhsar CK, Fitzpatrick RE. The treatment of melasma with fractional photothermolysis: a pilot study. Dermatol Surg. 2005;31(12):1645-50.
45. Nanni CA, Alster TS. Treatment of a Becker's nevus using a 694-nm long-pulsed ruby laser. Dermatol Surg. 1998;24(9):1032-4.
46. Trelles MA, Allones I, Moreno-Arias GA, Vélez M. Becker's nevus: a comparative study between erbium:YAG and Q-switched neodymium:YAG; clinical and histopathological findings. Br J Dermatol. 2005;152(2):308-13.
47. Taylor CR, Anderson RR. Ineffective treatment of refractory melasma and postinflammatory hyperpigmentation by Q-switched ruby laser. J Dermatol Surg Oncol. 1994;20(9):592-7.
48. Goldberg DJ, Stampien T. Q-switched ruby laser treatment of congenital nevi. Arch Dermatol. 1995;131(5):621-3.
49. Grevelink JM, van Leeuwen RL, Anderson RR, Byers HR. Clinical and histological responses of congenital melanocytic nevi after single treatment with Q-switched lasers. Arch Dermatol. 1997;133(3):349-53.
50. Rosenbach A, Williams CM, Alster TS. Comparison of the Q-switched alexandrite (755 nm) and Q-switched Nd:YAG (1064 nm) lasers in the treatment of benign melanocytic nevi. Dermatol Surg. 1997;23(4):239-44.
51. Waldorf HA, Kauvar AN, Geronemus RG. Treatment of small and medium congenital nevi with Q-switched ruby laser. Arch Dermatol. 1996;132(3):301-4.
52. Ueda S, Imayama S. Normal-mode ruby laser for treating congenital nevi. Arch Dermatol. 1997;133(3):355-9.
53. Kono T, Erçöçen AR, Chan HH, Kikuchi Y, Nozaki M. Effectiveness of normal-mode ruby laser and the combined (normal-mode plus q-switched) ruby laser in the treatment of congenital melanocytic nevi: a comparative study. Ann Plast Surg. 2002;49(5):476-85.
54. Kono T, Erçöçen AR, Nozaki M. Treatment of congenital melanocytic nevi using the combined (normal-mode plus Q-switched) ruby laser in Asians: clinical response in relation to histological type. Ann Plast Surg. 2005;54(5):494-501.

CHAPTER 16

Evidence Based Approach for Hyperpigmentary Diseases by Laser

Aparajita Ghosh, Saumya Panda

INTRODUCTION

Therapeutic options, other than chemical agents, have been proposed for hyperpigmentation since long, such as cryotherapy with liquid nitrogen, laser surgery, superficial dermabrasion, etc.[1,2] Since the first demonstration,[3] treatments of pigmented lesions with numerous lasers like argon, Carbon dioxide (CO_2), neodymium doped yttrium-aluminium-garnet (Nd:YAG), Q-switched ruby, alexandrite, erbium doped yttrium-aluminium-garnet (Er:YAG) laser, etc. have been reported.[4] The theory of a selective photothermolysis suggests that laser therapy would allow discriminating destruction of pigment without injuring the surrounding tissue.[5] Selective melanin photothermolysis can be obtained with any laser light having a wavelength in the absorption spectrum of melanin and sufficient energy levels to target melanosomes.[6] Laser induces extreme heating of melanosomes with subsequent thermal expansion, local vaporization and generation of acoustic waves that damage the nucleus, and, eventually, destroy the pigment-laden cells. The released melanin is then removed through transepidermal elimination or phagocytosis by dermal macrophages. To be effective and specific, wavelengths that avoid absorption by other skin chromophores and penetrate to the desired depth have to be used.[7]

This review has searched extensively the English language literature in the PubMed for studies on the use of laser in all congenital and acquired disorders presenting with hyperpigmentation, namely melasma, lentigines, ephelides, postinflammatory hyperpigmentation (PIH), melanocytic nevus and its many variants, e.g., nevus of Ota, Hori's nevus, etc. As the number of randomized controlled trials (RCTs) is not very large, uncontrolled trials and even retrospective studies were also taken into account in this review.

USE OF LASERS IN MELASMA

Melasma is the most common facial pigmentation disorder and a notoriously recidivist condition. Despite significant advances in medical therapy consisting of hydroquinone (HQ) and non-HQ products including botanicals, therapy of melasma remains a challenge. The challenges in treatment are contributed largely by as-yet-unanswered queries about its causation and pathophysiology. Over the last decade, however, a lot of new findings have provided sufficient insight regarding the pathogenesis of this ubiquitous, yet enigmatic, condition that necessarily demand a thorough revision of our basic concepts about the disease and the principles of its management. Use of lasers in the treatment of melasma has been addressed in case reports and few recent trials, but there is no consensus in the literature regarding the safety, efficacy, or durability of laser-based treatments. Furthermore, given the potential risks of laser intervention in hyperpigmented skin, the relative risks and benefit of laser must be compared to more conservative and traditional treatment approaches.[8]

The original concept of subdividing melasma into epidermal, dermal, and mixed type, floated 35 years ago by Sanchez et al.,[9] has been rendered redundant with recent *in vivo* reflectance confocal microscopic findings that demonstrated heterogeneous distribution of melanin between different regions of the melasma lesion and within a particular region of a melasma lesion. These findings have given rise to a host of concepts that may be summarized as:

- There is probably no true dermal melasma; rather all melasma are in essence mixed
- True primary histologic target in melasma is the epidermal melanin in lesional skin.[10]

Thus, melasma is chiefly characterized by epidermal hyperpigmentation with or without melanophages. The role of small amount of dermal melanin in the melasma lesional skin remains speculative. Hydroquinone (alone, or as a major component of the triple combination formulation) has been criticized for its ineffectiveness in removing stored melanin in dermal melanophages, its main mechanism being reversible inhibition of melanin synthesis by competitive blocking of tyrosinase. However, at the same time, these conceptual advances lay bare the crux of the paradox of using lasers in melasma, i.e., the twin facts of longer wavelengths penetrating deeper to ostensibly target dermal melanin on one hand, and on the other melanin absorption being better with shorter wavelengths. Most of the light would get absorbed by the increased epidermal melanin in the lesional skin, thus, rendering this technology much less attractive than it originally seemed to be.

Additional discoveries have reinforced the doubts about the chromophore which is practically targeted by lasers opposed to the one which is their theoretical bull's eye. One such important finding is that of modified or degraded melanin molecules in the stratum corneum of lesional skin having significantly different Raman spectra. How effective are the lasers having melanin as chromophore in removing this altered melanin is an open question, as of now.[11]

Another important recent discovery that can adequately explain the phenomenon of PIH, irrespective of the type of laser or the settings in darker skin, is that of the pendulous melanocytes, that are nothing but melanocytes protruding from the basement membrane zone into the dermis in the lesional skin of melasma. Pendulous cells are known to drop down on to the dermis easily in response to phototrauma. Conceivably, such trauma caused by lasers or intense pulsed light (IPL) may either cause their destruction or cause them to be deposited in the dermis, resulting in intense PIH.[12]

All these advances suggest that available evidence must be carefully analyzed for judicious use of lasers in melasma. Tables 1 to 6 summarize the findings from the different studies in melasma with Nd: YAG laser, Q-switched lasers (except Nd:YAG), fractional 1,550 nm erbium (Er) laser, other fractional lasers, IPL, and other lasers, respectively. The grade of recommendations (Table 7) has been summarized according to the GRADE recommendations. There are two levels of strength of recommendation (1 = strong, "we recommend"; and 2 = weak, "we suggest"), and three levels of quality of evidence (A = high; B = moderate; and C = low).[13]

As can be seen from the tables, there is still paucity of trials with a substantial sample size and long-term follow-up. Melasma relapses as a rule and there is no definitive time when it may resurface. There are currently only two trials with longer than 6 months follow-up (Tables 1 and 5). In an evidence based analysis of lasers in melasma, the response to lasers was not consistent and durability of melasma improvement was limited in all cases where laser was used as monotherapy. Moreover, in studies comparing laser to topical treatments, laser based monotherapy failed to show benefit over topical treatments. The analysis suggested that the use of lasers for the treatment of melasma cannot be recommended, due to unpredictable safety and efficacy, time-limited clinical improvement, and no clear benefit over conventional treatments.[14] Three years down the line, we have to recommend the same. To conclude, current evidence and unraveling of melasma pathophysiology warrant great circumspection in the use of lasers and light, particularly in darker skin types, keeping in mind the cost of treatment, inevitable relapse, and the enhanced side effect profile.

EPHELIDES AND SOLAR LENTIGINES

Solar lentigines and ephelides are the most common of all epidermal pigmentary disorders. In spite of their gross similarity, there are clinical and histopathological differences between the two entities. Ephelides are mostly observed in skin phototypes I and II and occur in the background of a genetic predisposition. They are small, light brown, and are more common in adolescence and their pigmentation is directly proportionate to the light exposure. Histopathologically, they are characterized by increased epidermal basal layer pigmentation, increased number, and size of melanocytes with characteristic large melanosomes.[46]

TABLE 1: Neodymium doped yttrium-aluminium-garnet laser

Name of study	Type of study	Number and characteristics of patients	Intervention	Number in each arm	Assessment parameter/tools	Follow-up	Result	Limitations	Grade of recommendation
Moubasher et al. (2014)[15]	Comparative trial	• 65 Egyptian females. Skin III–V, divided into four groups (Three varying concentration of TCA performed every 2 weeks up to eight sessions or clearance of melasma or complications. Q-switched Nd:YAG once monthly sessions till six sessions or melasma clearance or complications)	• Four groups—TCA 20% for epidermal, 25% for epidermal, dermal, mixed, 30% for dermal and mixed • Frequency doubled Nd:YAG (532 nm, 0.8 J/cm^2 for epidermal melasma, 1,064 nm 3–3.8 J/cm^2 for dermal and mixed melasma)	• 20% TCA—15 patients • 25% TCA—20 patients • 30% TCA—15 patients • Nd:YAG—15 patients (7 epidermal melasma 532 nm + 1,064 nm dermal and mixed melasma) • 65 completed Rx	• MASI before and after treatment, digital photograph at each visit. Patient's assessment of improvement after end of treatment	• 3 months after treatment completion, (monthly for patients showing improvement; fortnightly for patients having complications)	• Improvement percentage of MASI score was significantly higher among patients treated with TCA 25% ($p < 0.001$) compared to other three groups • QS Nd:YAG group, mean MASI was higher post-treatment, also showed the highest incidence of post-inflammatory hyperpigmentation (53.3%) • TCA superior to laser in Rx of melasma, 25% being the most effective concentration with least side effects • QS Nd:YAG laser is not effective in the treatment of melasma and is associated with the highest incidence of complications	• Randomization doubtful; no blinding	• 2C
Omi et al. (2012)[16]	Comparative trial (split face)	• Eight Japanese females (41–57 years, mean 52.5 years) with Fitzpatrick skin type III and bilateral melasma	• Nd:YAG 1,064 nm, pulse width: 5–20 ns; spot size: 6 mm diameter; fluence, 3.0 J/cm^2, 5–7 passes, once/week, 4 weeks verses QS ruby 694.3 nm, pulse width 20 ns, spot size 4 mm diameter; fluence 4.0 J/cm^2, one pass with approximately 20% overlap–single session	• Eight patients in each group	• Skin biopsies taken immediately after the 4th Nd:YAG session and the single ruby session, and histopathological comparison was performed with light and TEM	• No long-term follow-up (except 1 case followed up for 2 years). Assessment: just after completion of 4th session • Nd:YAG—just after single session of QS ruby	• Improvement in both but considerably more morphological epidermal and dermal damage in the QS:ruby specimens compared with minimal epidermal disruption and cellular damage in the QS:YAG specimens QS 1,064 nm. Nd:YAG laser toning offered superior results in the treatment of melasma in the Japanese skin type compared with the QS ruby laser	• Randomization doubtful; no long-term follow-up	• 2C

Continued

Continued

Name of study	Type of study	Number and characteristics of patients	Intervention	Number in each arm	Assessment parameter/tools	Follow-up	Result	Limitations	Grade of recommendation
Yun et al. (2014)[17]	Comparative trial, blinded	• 24 Korean females, skin type III and IV	• Fractionated IPL 13–15 J/cm^2 and low fluence QS Nd:YAG 1.5–2 J/cm^2 six sessions vs. fractionated IPL six sessions (13–15 J/cm^2)	• 12 patients in each arm	• Partial MASI score from digital photograph (performed by two dermatologists blinded to treatment), melanin index, erythema index (both measured using spectrophotometer), reporting of adverse effects by patients at each visit, patient satisfaction score using a 5-point rating at 2 months	• At 1 month and 2 months after the treatment	• Decrease in the partial MASI score, melanin index of the combination group was significantly larger than that of the IPL only group $p < 0.05$. In both groups, treatment with IPL-F and LF-QS-Nd:YAG laser was well-tolerated. Single incidence of first degree burn in one patient of combination group which healed without scarring or pigmentary changes	• Randomization doubtful	• 2C
Alsaad et al. (2014)[18]	Split face, comparative	• 10 females with moderate to severe melasma enrolled, seven completed study	• Microdermabrasion followed by QS Nd:YAG 50 ns fluence –1.6 J/cm^2, 5–6 mm spot size (three sessions monthly) + topical (SPF 50 sunscreen, 4% hydroquinone, 0.05% tretinoin cream vs. microdermabrasion followed by QS Nd:YAG 5 ns fluence –1.6 J/cm^2, 5–6 mm spot size (three sessions monthly) + topical (SPF 50 sunscreen, 4% hydroquinone, 0.05% tretinoin cream	• 10 in each arm	• MASI by investigators at baseline and at every treatment, reflectance spectrophotometry for pigmentation. Rating of pain by patients on numerical pain 0–10, rating by three raters on photographs blinded to treatment date and photo sequence	• 1, 3, 6 months after final laser treatment	• At 1 month, both side showed significant decrease from baseline but no significant difference between the two interventions or sides. At 3 months follow-up reduction or improvement in pigment had decreased for both sides (no significant difference between pre-treatment and post-treatment scores). Pain significantly more in shorter pulse duration	• Method of randomization not mentioned, blinding doubtful, small sample size, three patients included did not complete treatment reason not mentioned	• 2C

Continued

Continued

Name of study	Type of study	Number and characteristics of patients	Intervention	Number in each arm	Assessment parameter/tools	Follow-up	Result	Limitations	Grade of recommendation
Fabi et al. (2014)[19]	RCT (split face)	• 20 male + female, moderate to severe, mixed B/L melasma	• Low fluence QS Nd:YAG (1,064 nm) six sessions weekly (8 mm spot size, 1–2 J/cm^2 fluence) vs. low-fluence QSAL (755 nm) six sessions, weekly (effective spot size 8 mm, effective fluence 1.1 J/cm^2)	• 20	• Two independent blinded investigators conducted MMASI evaluations and subjects completed self-assessment questionnaires at baseline, after three treatments and each follow-up visit 2, 12, and 24 weeks after the last treatment. Safety assessment-type, severity of adverse events (erythema, crusting, hypopigmentation, hyperpigmentation noted at each visit	• Follow-up 2, 12, 24 weeks after last Rx	• Both interventions equally effective. No difference in adverse effects	• Blinding doubtful	• 2C
Kar et al. (2012)[20]	Comparative trial	• 75 male + female into three groups	• Group A (low fluence QS Nd:YAG weekly 12 weeks, group B glycolic peel 2 weekly 12 weeks, group C high fluence QS Nd:YAG 12 weeks	• 25 patients randomly into three groups	• MASI on clinical photographs	• 12 weeks (treatment completion) 24 weeks (12 weeks after treatment stoppage)	• The improvement in the MASI score after therapy was maximum in group A (low fluence laser) > group B (glycolic acid peel) > group C (high fluence laser). Recurrence same in all groups. At 12 weeks, mottled confetti like hypopigmentation was seen in 23.8% patients in high fluence group and one patient in low fluence group. Two of the five patients who had mottled hypopigmentation earlier after high fluence laser developed postinflammatory hyperpigmentation.	• Randomization and blinding doubtful	• 2C

Continued

Continued

Name of study	Type of study	Number and characteristics of patients	Intervention	Number in each arm	Assessment parameter/tools	Follow-up	Result	Limitations	Grade of recommendation
							• Postinflammatory pigmentation was seen in only one (5.2%) patient in the glycolic peel group and six (28.5%) in highfluence group. The adverse effects in each study group are given in [Table 5]. No patient in the low fluence group developed postinflammatory hyperpigmentation. Overall, fewer side effects were observed after low fluence QSNYL treatment compared to high-fluence QSNYL		
Wattanakrai et al. (2010)[21]	Split face, comparative	• 22 Asians (21 females,1 male) with mixed and dermal melasma	• 1,064 nm QS Nd:YAG, 6 mm spot size, 3.0–3.8 J/cm^2 fluence for five sessions at 1 week intervals + 2% hydroquinone + sunscreen vs. 2% hydroquinone + sunscreen	• 22	• Lightness index (using colorimeter) , modified MASI by two blinded dermatologists, and treating dermatologist, subjective assessment by patient using 5 point grading	• Assessment before and after each treatment + follow-up at 4, 8, and 12 weeks after treatment completion	• QS Nd:YAG laser treatment significant improvement from baseline and compared to control side. Mottled hypopigmentation developed in three patients. During follow-up, 4 of 22 patients developed rebound hyperpigmentation, and all patients had recurrence of melasma. • Conclusion: QS Nd:YAG laser treatment for melasma in Asians produced only temporary improvement and had side effects	• Randomization doubtful, blinding inadequate	• 2C

Continued

Continued

Name of study	Type of study	Number and characteristics of patients	Intervention	Number in each arm	Assessment parameter/tools	Follow-up	Result	Limitations	Grade of recommendation
Kim et al. (2013)[22]	Comparative, split face study, observer blinded	• 26	• 1,064 nm QSNY (6 mm spot size, 1.2–1.4 J/cm^2 fluence) 10 sessions at 2-week intervals + nonablative fractional photothermolysis (dynamic mode, pulse energy 6–8 mJ/MTZ; total density 300 MTZs/cm^2, 5 sessions at 4-week intervals to the experimental side of the face vs. 1,064 nm QSNY (6 mm spot size, 1.2–1.4 J/cm^2 fluence) 10 sessions at 2-week intervals	• 26	• MMASI, PhGA (two observers not associated with treatment or recruitment of patients), PGA, adverse effect reporting during treatment and follow-up	• Follow-up at 12 weeks after last treatment	• MMASI and patient's subjective assessment show no significant differences in between two sides. Findings do not support the hypothesis of NFP providing a substantial benefit in treating the melasma when compared with the lone treatment of the 1,064 nm QSNY	• Randomization doubtful	• 2C
Bansal et al. (2012)[23]	Comparative trial	• 60 Indian patients male + female	• Three groups: (A) QSNY low fluence weekly, (B) twice daily application of 20% azelaic acid, and (C) both duration, 12 weeks	• 20 patients in each of three groups	• MASI	• Follow-up 0, 6, 12 weeks	• Group C significantly better than A and B , no statistically significant difference between A and B (possibly not blinded)	• Randomization and blinding doubtful	• 2C
Vachiramon et al. (2015)[24]	Comparative, split face study	• 15 male patients, mixed melasma	• Low fluence QS Nd:YAG (1,064 nm) + 30% GA peel five sessions weekly vs. low fluence QS Nd:YAG (1,064 nm)	• 15	• Relative lightness index	• 12 weeks (treatment completion) 24 weeks (12 weeks after treatment stoppage)	• Mean relative lightness index (RLI) of the combined treatment side lowered throughout the study period, with the maximal improvement of 52.3% reduction at the fourth week follow-up ($p = 0.023$). However, the mean RLI increased at 8 and 12 weeks of follow-up. One subject (8.3%) developed guttate hypopigmentation, which did not resolve by the 12-week follow-up. Low-fluence QS Nd:YAG 1,064 nm laser	• Randomization doubtful	• 2C

Continued

Continued

Name of study	Type of study	Number and characteristics of patients	Intervention	Number in each arm	Assessment parameter/tools	Follow-up	Result	Limitations	Grade of recommendation
							combined with GA peeling temporarily reduced melasma in men, but the incidence of side effects does not justify the short-lived benefits of this procedure		
Park et al. (2011)[25]	RCT, observer blinded, split face	• 16 patients (mixed melisma >6 months, not responding to conventional Rx, confirmed by Wood's lamp)	• 1,064 nm QS NDYL (6 mm spot size, 2.0–2.3 J/cm^2 fluence) for six sessions at 1-week intervals + 30% GA–contact time 1–2 min (3 sessions at 2-week intervals) vs. 1,064 nm QS NDYL (6 mm spot size, 2.0–2.3 J/cm^2 fluence) for six sessions at 1-week intervals	• 16	• Melanin index measured instrumentally using mexameter, physician's assessment on 4 point scale and modified MMASI (by two blinded dermatologist not involved in the study and one treating dermatologist), patient satisfaction questionnaire (1–5 scale), adverse effect reporting at each visit	• Evaluation at weeks–0 (baseline), 1, 2, 3, 4, 5, 9, 13, 17, 21, 25	• Significant reduction in pigment from baseline on both sides. Combined treatment significantly superior to 1,064 nm QNYL alone in all assessment parameters in mixed-type melasma	• Nil	• 1A
Jalaly et al. (2014)[26]	RCT, split face	• 40 female patients above the age of 18 years with symmetrical melasma and Fitzpatrick skin types II–IV	• Low-fluence QS 1,064 nm Nd:YAG 1.5-2 J/cm, 7 mm spot size 5 passes vs. low-power fractional CO_2 laser with a power of 1 W and density of 0.7. 1 pass (five sessions 3 weeks interval)	• 40	• Melanin index, MMASI, patients' self-evaluation	• Follow up 1 month, 2 months after last treatment	• Both lasers showed improvement from baseline, low-power fractional CO_2 laser is safe and effective, more effective than low fluence QS Nd:YAG, side effects such as sunburn-like erythema and transient edema with low-fluence Q-switch 1,064 nm Nd:YAG laser treatment and erythema, burning sensation, edema, and scaling, lasting for at least 3 days after low-power fractional CO_2 laser-treatment were seen	• No mention of blinding	• 2C

Continued

Continued

Name of study	Type of study	Number and characteristics of patients	Intervention	Number in each arm	Assessment parameter/tools	Follow-up	Result	Limitations	Grade of recommendation
Jeong et al. (2008)[27]	Case series	• 27	• Q-switched Nd:YAG laser (1,064 nm wavelength, 7 mm spot size,1.6–2.5 J/cm^2 fluence) weekly x 8 weeks	• 27	• Standardized clinical images that used Robo skin analyzer, spectrophotometer, MASI score and general severity		• 17 (58.8%) patients showed 50–75% improvement, partial response in 12/17 patients		• 2C
Suh et al. (2011)[28]	Case series	• 23 Korean female skin type III–V	• 1,064 nm QS Nd:YAG laser, weekly for 10 weeks	• 23	• MASI, patient satisfaction score	• 4, 7, 10 weeks, 1, 2, 3 months after last treatment	• Safe and effective weeks during treatment		• 2C
Zhou (2011)[29]	Case series	• Male + female, skin type IV–VI	• 1,065 nm QS NDYL (low energy weekly, nine sessions)	• 50 (47 females + 3 males)	• MI, MASI, confocal laser microscopy	• Baseline, after each treatment and 3 months after last treatment	• 70% of patients had more than a 50% decrease in their MASI values, and 10% had 100% clearance. Recurrence rate at the 3-month follow-up was 64%, effective and safe treatment for melasma, although recurrence rates remain high		

TCA, trichloroacetic acid; QS, Q-switched; Nd:YAG, neodymium doped yttrium-aluminium-garnet; Rx, reaction; MASI, Melasma Area and Severity Index; TEM, transmission electron microscopy; IPL, intense pulsed light; IPL-F, fractionated IPL; LF, low-fluence; SPF, sun protection factor; RCT, randomized controlled trial; MMASI, modified Melasma Area and Severity Index; QSNYL, Q-switched Nd:YAG laser; QSNY, Q-switched Nd:YAG; MTZ, microthermal zone; PhGA, physician's global assessment; PGA, patient's global assessment; NFP, nonablative fractional photothermolysis; GA, glycolic acid; MI, melanin index; B/L, bilateral.

TABLE 2: Q-switched lasers (except neodymium doped yttrium-aluminium-garnet)

Name of study	Type of study	Number and characteristics of patients	Intervention	Number in each arm	Assessment parameter/tools	Follow-up	Result	Lacking	Grade of recommendation
Fabi et al. (2014)[19]	Split face, comparative trial	20 male + female, moderate to severe, mixed B/L melasma	Low fluence QS Nd:YAG (1,064 nm) six sessions, weekly vs. low-fluence QSAL (755 nm) six sessions, weekly	20	Two independent investigators conducted MMASI evaluations and subjects completed self-assessment questionnaires at baseline, after three treatments and each follow-up visit 2, 12, and 24 weeks after the last treatment	Follow-up visit 2, 12, and 24 weeks after the last treatment	Both equally effective. No difference in adverse effects	Randomization, blinding doubtful	2C
Omi et al. 2012[16]	Comparative trial (split face)	Eight Japanese females (41–57 years, mean 52.5 years) with Fitzpatrick skin type III and bilateral melasma	Nd:YAG 1,064 nm, pulse width 5–20 ns; spot size, 6 mm diameter; fluence, 3.0 J/cm^2, 5–7 passes, once/week, 4 weeks vs. QS ruby 694.3 nm, pulse width 20 ns, spot size 4 mm diameter; fluence 4.0 J/cm^2, one pass with approximately 20% overlap–single session	Eight patients in each group	Skin biopsies taken immediately after the fourth Nd:YAG session and the single ruby session, and histopathological comparison was performed with light and TEM	No long-term follow-up (except 1 case followed up for 2 years). Assessment just after completion of fourth session Nd:YAG, just after single session of QS ruby	Improvement in both but considerably more morphological epidermal and dermal damage in the QS ruby specimens compared with minimal epidermal disruption and cellular damage in the QS YAG specimens Q-switched 1,064 nm Nd:YAG laser toning offered superior results in the treatment of melasma in the Japanese skin type compared with the Q-switched ruby laser	Randomization doubtful, no long-term follow-up	2C
Jang et al. (2011)[31]	Case series	15 Korean female skin type III–IV	Low dose, fractional QS ruby laser six sessions 2 week intervals	15	MASI	4, 16 weeks after last treatment	4, 16 weeks after last treatment, effective		2C
Hilton et al. (2013)[32]	Case series	25 female, skin type I–III	Fractional QS ruby laser	25	MASI by three blinded evaluators	4, 6 weeks and 3 months	Effective and safe, however, significant incidence of recurrence at 3 months		2C

QS, Q-switched; Nd:YAG, neodymium doped yttrium-aluminium-garnet; QSAL, Q-switched alexandrite laser; MMASI, modified Melasma Area and Severity Index; TEM, transmission electron microscopy; MASI, Melasma Area and Severity Index; B/L, bilateral

TABLE 3: Fractional 1,550 nm laser

Name of study	Type of study	Number and characteristics of patients	Intervention	Number in each arm	Assessment parameter/tools	Follow-up	Result	Limitation	Grade of recom-mendation
Kroon et al. (2011)[33]	RCT, observer blinded	10 female >18 years age	Nonablative 1,550 nm erbium glass fractional laser—four sessions 2 week interval vs. triple combination cream (HQ 5%, Tret 0.05%, triamcinolone 0.1%)—8 weeks	10	PGA (VAS 1–10) for improvement, same for laser associated pain, 0–3 for erythema, edema, crusting, melanin index by reflectance spectroscopy, PhGA and MASI by blinded observer from digital photograph (main outcome measurement)	Assessment at 3 weeks, 3 months, 6 months post-treatment	Nonablative 1,550 nm laser at 10 mJ/microbeam safe and comparable in efficacy and recurrence rate to triple combination	Nil	1A
Wind et al. (2010)[34]	RCT, comparative, observer blinded, split face	29 female, >18 years age	Nonablative 1,550 nm erbium glass fractional laser—four sessions for type II skin, five sessions for type IV–VI vs. triple combination cream (HQ 5%, Tret 0.05%, triamcinolone 0.1%)—15 weeks	29	PGA (VAS 1–10) for improvement, same for laser associated pain, 0–3 for erythema, edema, crusting, melanin index by reflectance spectroscopy, PhGA by blinded observer from digital photograph (0–6)	Assessment at 3 weeks, 3 months, 6 months post-treatment	Nonablative 1,550 nm laser not effective using 15 mJ/microbeam, high rate of PIH	Nil	1A
Hong et al. (2012)[35]	Randomized, comparative trial, split face	18 Korean female skin type III–IV, 17 completed follow-up at 4 weeks, 11 completed follow-up at 12 weeks	1,550 nm erbium-doped FP single session (10 mJ/ MTZ, 1,320 MTZ/cm^2) vs. 15% TCA single session	18	MASI (performed on clinical photograph by Robo skin analyzer software), patient self-assessment using VAS 0–100%), evaluation of S/E –persistent erythema, PIH	4 and 12 weeks post-treatment	Both arms equal in all respects, melasma lesions were significantly improved 4 weeks after either treatment, but melasma recurred at 12 weeks. Postinflammatory hyperpigmentation developed in 28% of patients at 4 weeks but resolved in all but one patient by 12 weeks. There was no difference between FP treatment and TCA peeling with respect to any outcome measure. FP laser and	Method of randomization, mechanical evaluation (blinding?)	2C

Continued

Continued

Name of study	Type of study	Number and characteristics of patients	Intervention	Number in each arm	Assessment parameter/tools	Follow-up	Result	Limitation	Grade of recommendation
							TCA peel treatments were equally effective and safe when used to treat moderate-to-severe melasma, but neither treatment was long-lasting		
Kim et al. (2013)[22]	Comparative, split face study, observer blinded	26	1,064 nm QSNY (6 mm spot size, 1.2–1.4 J/cm^2 fluence) 10 sessions at 2-week intervals + non ablative fractional phototherolysis (dynamic mode, pulse energy 6–8 mJ/MTZ; total density 300 MTZs/cm^2 five sessions at 4-week intervals to the experimental side of the face vs. 1,064 QSNY (6 mm spot size, 1.2–1.4 J/cm^2 fluence) 10 sessions at 2-week intervals	26	MMASI, PhGA (two observers not associated with treatment or recruitment of patients), PGA, adverse effect reporting during treatment and follow up	12 weeks after last treatment	MMASI and patient's subjective assessment show no significant differences in between two sides. Findings do not support the hypothesis of NFP providing a substantial benefit in treating the melasma when compared with the lone treatment of the 1,064 nm QSNY	Method of randomization not mentioned	2C
Karsai et al. (2012)[36]	Controlled observer blinded parallel group study	26, male + female, mild melasma MASI <8, skin type I–III	Broad spectrum sunscreen + 1,550 nm nonablative fractional photothermolysis treatment [energy: 15 mJ/ MTZ; total density: 1,048 MTZs/cm^2; density per pass: 131 MTZs/cm^2; number of passes: 8; total coverage: 20%, four treatment at 3 week interval vs. broad spectrum sunscreen	26	Primary—MASI, physicians global assessment, secondary-patients subjective assessment of improvement	24 weeks after start of study	No significant difference between treatment and control arm	Nil (not a randomized trial but details adequate)	2A

Continued

Continued

Name of study	Type of study	Number and characteristics of patients	Intervention	Number in each arm	Assessment parameter/tools	Follow-up	Result	Limitation	Grade of recom-mendation
Rokhsar et al. (2005)[37]	Case series	30 females (skin III–V) with nonresponsive melasma	Fraxel –30 Watt, diode pumped, 1,550 nm erbium fiber laser (1,535–1,550 nm 6–12 mJ/MTZ, 2,000–3,500 MTZ/cm^2, 4–6 treat-ment sessions)	30	Percentage of lightening as rated by two evaluators from photographs and patient	Not known	Effective, 60% achieved 75–100% clearance, 30% had less than 25% response, 1 case of postinflammatory hyperpigmentation		2C
Lee et al. (2009)[38]	Case series	25 Asian	Fractional 1,550 nm laser, four sessions monthly	25	Melanin index, MASI	At 24 weeks from treatment start (?8 weeks after treat-ment completion)	Significant improve-ment in mean MASI in 60% patients after 4 weeks of treatment. However, there was relapse in melanin index and MASI scores at 24 week follow-up visit, and 13% patients reported postinflam-matory hyperpigmen-tation		2C
Goldberg et al. (2008)[39]	Case series	10 patients, skin type III–IV	1,550 nm erbium: glass laser delivering light in a fractional manner (every 2 weeks for four ses-sions)	10	Efficacy as secondary end point, biopsies pretreatment and 3 months after last treatment for light and electron microscopy, inves-tigators assess-ment of pre and post-treatment photograph	Follow-up 3 months after last treatment	Light microscopy on post-treatment specimens showed a relative decrease in melanocytes compared to the pretreatment ones. Post-treatment electron microscopy revealed fewer mela-nocytes and a relative absence of melanin in the surrounding kera-tinocytes compared to pre-treatment speci-mens. In addition, six subjects with skin type III were determined to have good improve-ment, whereas four subjects with skin type IV had fair improve-ment, as assessed by the investigator		2C

RCT, randomized controlled trial; HQ, hydroquinone; PGA, patient's global assessment; PhGA, physician's global assessment; MASI, Melasma Area and Severity Index; PIH, postinflammatory hyperpigmentation; FP, fractional photothermolysis; VAS, Visual Analog Scale; MTZ, microthermal zone; TCA, trichloroacetic acid; QSNY, Q-switched ND:YAG; MMASI, modified Melasma Area and Severity Index; NFP, non-ablative fractional photothermolysis; S/E, side-effects.

TABLE 4: Other fractional lasers

Name of study	Type of study	Number and characteristics of patients	Intervention	Number in each arm	Assessment parameter/tools	Follow-up	Result	Limitation	Grade of recommendation
Hilton et al. (2013)[32]	Case series	25 female, skin type I–III	Fractional QS ruby laser	25	MASI by three blinded assessor	Follow-up 4, 6 weeks and 3 months, after last treatment	Effective and safe, however, significant incidence of recurrence at 3 months		2C
Jang et al. (2011)[31]	Case series	15 Korean female (skin type III–IV)	Low dose, fractional QS ruby laser six sessions 2 week intervals	15	MASI	Follow-up 4, 16 weeks after last treatment	Effective		2C
Polder et al. (2012)[40]	Case series	14	1,927 nm fractional thulium fiber laser, 10–20 mJ. 3–4 sessions monthly	14	MASI by three blinded assessor	Follow-up 1, 3, 6 months after treatment completion	Significant reduction in MASI from baseline. No adverse events		2C
Jalaly et al. (2014)[26]	RCT, split face	40 female patients above the age of 18 years with symmetrical melasma and Fitzpatrick skin types II–IV	Low-fluence QS 1,064 nm Nd:YAG 1.5–2 J/cm, 7 mm spot size five passes vs. low-power fractional CO_2 laser with a power of 1 W and density of 0.7 pass (five sessions 3 weeks interval)	40	Melanin Index, MMASI, patients' self-evaluation	Follow-up 1 month, 2 months after last treatment	Both lasers showed improvement from baseline, low-power fractional CO_2 laser is safe and effective, more effective than low fluence QS Nd:YAG, Side effects such as sunburn-like erythema and transient edema with low-fluence Q-switch 1,064 nm Nd:YAG laser treatment and erythema, burning sensation, edema, and scaling, lasting for at least 3 days after low-power fractional CO_2 laser-treatment were seen	Blinding doubtful	2C
Wanitphakdeedecha et al. (2014)[41]	Comparative trial, split face	30 females skin type III–V, 24 completed study, one withdrawn due to unrelated medical emergency, five could not attend follow-up	1,410 nm fractional laser photothermolysis 20 mJ at 5% coverage five sessions monthly interval vs. 1,410 nm fractional laser photothermolysis 20 mJ at 20% coverage five sessions monthly interval	30, 24 completed study	Melanin index using spectrophotometry, clinical evaluation using VAS, MASI, patient satisfaction at 3 months	Follow-up 1, 2, 3 months after complete treatment	Both parameters effective but 5% coverage is safer with lesser incidence of PIH	Randomization doubtful, no blinding	2C

QS, Q-switched; MASI, Melasma Area and Severity Index; RCT, randomized controlled trial; Nd:YAG, neodymium doped yttrium-aluminium-garnet; MMASI, Modified Melasma Area and Severity Index; VAS, visual analog scale; PIH, post-inflammatory hyperpigmentation

TABLE 5: Intense pulsed light

Name of study	Type of study	Number and characteristics of patients	Intervention	Number in each arm	Assessment parameter/tools	Follow-up	Result	Limitation	Grade of recommendation
Yun et al. (2014)[17]	Comparative, blinded study	24 Korean female, skin type III and IV	Fractionated IPL 13–15 J/cm² and low fluence QS Nd:YAG 1.5–2 J/cm² six sessions vs. fractionated IPL six sessions (13–15 J/cm²)	12 patients in each arm	Partial MASI score from digital photograph (performed by two dermatologists blinded to treatment), melanin index, erythema index (both measured using spectrophotometer), reporting of adverse effects by patients at each visit, patient satisfaction score using a 5 point rating at 2 months	At 1 and 2 months after the treatment	The decrease in the partial MASI score, melanin index, of the combination group was significantly larger than that of the IPL only group ($p < 0.05$). In both groups, treatment with IPL-F and LF-QS Nd:YAG laser was well-tolerated. Single incidence of first degree burn in one patient of combination group which healed without scarring or pigmentary changes	Randomization doubtful	2C
Wang et al. (2004)[42]	Comparative study	33 patients in total (17 Asian patients with dermal or mixed refractory melasma in arm 1, 16 patients in arm 2)	IPL 570 nm filter in first session, 590–615 nm filter in subsequent sessions 26–33 J/cm², (4 weekly x 4 sessions) + 4% HQ + sunscreen vs. 4% HQ + sunscreen	Total 33–17 in arm 1 and 16 in arm 2, 31 patients completed study at 16 weeks (2 patients from control group dropped because of noncompliance), one patient in IPL group failed to complete week-36 follow-up (moved away)	Absolute and relative melanin index using reflectance spectrophotometer and patient satisfaction questionnaire (subjective) in IPL group degree of pain, erythema, blistering was assessed at each visit	Every 4 weeks for 16 weeks in both group and at 36 weeks in IPL group	IPL + HQ more effective than HQ alone; however, the improvement in melanin index decreased at week-36, but still less than baseline. Two patients reported transient postinflammatory hyperpigmentation, no serious adverse effect	Randomization doubtful	2C
Moreno Arias et al. (2001)[43]	Case series	20 (all types of melanocytic disorders), male + female (skin type I–IV	IPL (590 nm, 34 J/cm², 3.8 ms pulse width, double mode, delay of 20 ms, [2 (superficial lesions) - 4 (deep lesions) sessions 4 weeks interval	—	—	—	A clearance of 76–100% (excellent) was obtained for superficial lesions such as ephelides, epidermal melasma, and café au lait macules. Nevus spilus showed good clinical clearance (51–75%); however, deep lesions such as nevus of Becker, epidermal nevus, and mixed melasma		2C

Continued

Continued

Name of study	Type of study	Number and characteristics of patients	Intervention	Number in each arm	Assessment parameter/tools	Follow-up	Result	Limitation	Grade of recommendation
							showed an average clearance of less than 25%. Postinflammatory hyperpigmentation was observed in melasma. 76–100% clearance for superficial lesions, 50–75% for nevus spilus, 25% or less for deeper lesions		
Li et al. (2008)[44]	Case series	89 female, Chinese	IPL (3 weekly x 4 sessions)	89	Colorimeter (mexameter), MASI, global assessment by patient and blinded observer		Effective, more in epidermal than mixed melasma. 77.5% showed 51–100% improvement		2C

IPL, intense pulsed light; QS, Q-switched; Nd:YAG, neodymium doped yttrium-aluminium-garnet; MASI, Melasma Area and Severity Index; IPL-F, fractionated IPL; LF, low-fluence; HQ, hydroquinone.

TABLE 6: Miscellaneous

Name of study	Type of study	Number and characteristics of patients	Intervention	Number in each arm	Assessment parameter/tools	Follow-up	Result	Grade of recommendation
Lee et al. (2010)[45]	Case series	4 Korean females	Copper bromide	4	MASI, physician and patient assessment, immune histopathology		There was a significant improvement in MASI scores post-treatment, decrease in erythema intensity and reduction in the pretreatment raised levels of markers of vascularity	2C

Limitations have been enumerated only in case of comparative trials.

MASI, Melasma Area and Severity Index.

TABLE 7: American College of Chest Physicians grades for recommendations

Grade	Benefit vs risk	Quality of evidence
1A	Benefits clearly outweigh risks, or vice versa; recommendation can apply to most patients in most circumstances	RCTs with no important limitations, or exceptionally strong evidence from obervational studies. Further research is unlikely change our confidence in the estimate of effect
1B		RCTs with important limitations, or strong evidence from obervational studies. Further higher quality research may have an important impact
1C	—	At least one critical outcome from RCTs with serious flaws, observational studies, case series, or indirect evidence. Further higher quality research is likely to have an important impact
2A	Benefits balanced with risks, best action may differ depending on circumstances or patient/society values	RCTs with no important limitations, or exceptionally strong evidence from obervational studies. Further research is unlikely change our confidence in the estimate of effect
2B		RCTs with important limitations, or strong evidence from obervational studies. Further higher-quality research may have an important impact
2C	Benefits balanced with risks, other alternatives may be equally reasonable	At least one critical outcome from RCTs with serious flaws, observational studiesl case series, or indirect evidence. Further highter-quality research is likely to have an important impact

RCT, randomized control trial.

Solar lentigines, on the other hand, are observed in all skin types and in later ages with coexisting photo damage and as such are far more prevalent and of greater cosmetic significance in the Asian population. Histopathologically, the lesions show an increased number of melanocytes with increased mitochondria and more developed endoplasmic reticulum and melanosome complexes in keratinocytes. Basement membrane zone often shows disruption with presence of "pendulous" melanocytes showing microinvaginations into keratinicytes.[46]

The pigmentation being localized to the epidermis, these conditions show good response to treatments with topical agents, chemical peels, cryotherapy, dermabrasion, etc.; various lasers have been used for treatment. Till date, there are only two studies comparing the effects of pulse dye laser and frequency doubled Q-switched Nd:YAG laser, diode laser to cryotherapy.[47,48] Although both of them have found lasers to be more effective and safer than cryotherapy, they are limited by very small sample sizes.

The common lasers that have been used are Nd:YAG (532 nm) Q-switched and long pulse, Q-switched ruby, Q-switched alexandrite, long pulse alexandrite which work on the basis of their selective absorption by epidermal melanin. Long pulse dye laser (LPDL) 595 nm is absorbed very well by melanin and hemoglobin. Addition of a compression handpiece to it compresses the cutaneous blood vessels and removes the blood from the skin in the treatment field and the epidermal melanin can be selectively targeted. Er:YAG laser is an ablative laser which causes controlled ablation of the epidermis to a particular depth, thus causing epidermal resurfacing.

The scarcity of studies assessing the efficacy and safety of these lasers make it impossible to make recommendations regarding use of individual lasers and their relative effectiveness. The few controlled trials that exist are heterogeneous and many of them have limitations of sample size and short follow-up periods. The findings from these studies have been summarized in tables 8–12.

Postinflammatory hyperpigmentation is the most common adverse effect reported. Hypopigmentation, erythema, and textural changes have also been reported.

Nevus of Ota

It is a dermal melanocytic nevus, common among Asians. It shows a distinct female preponderance. The bluish to slate grey macules distributed along the first and second divisions of trigeminal nerve causes cosmetic disfigurement and is resistant to most conventional treatments like topical HQ, cryotherapy, dermabrasion, etc. Over the years, lasers have emerged as the treatment of choice for this condition.[59]

Early treatment of this condition is reported to be associated with better treatment response and chances of complete clearing.[60]

The common lasers used for treatment are Q-switched, Nd:YAG, Q-switched alexandrite. and Q-switched ruby. Due to the paucity of proper large scale randomized studies, it is not possible to assess the superiority of any one of them in terms of relative safety and efficacy. The common adverse effects noted were hypopigmentation, hyperpigmentation, and atrophic scarring. Number of treatment sessions is reported to be an independent risk factor for all complications.[61] The other laser that have been used is picoseconds 755 nm alexandrite in recalcitrant cases not responding to other Q-switched lasers, but there is still not enough evidence to support its use.[62]

Table 13 provides a brief overview of the recent studies on use of lasers in nevus of Ota.

Acquired Bilateral Nevus of Ota-like Macules

This is a dermal melanocytosis which usually appears in the 4th to 5th decade in Asian women as brown to bluish grey macules over the malar area. Histopathology shows melanocytes in the upper dermis. Dermabrasion which was used earlier as a treatment modality leads to unacceptable scarring and postinflammatory pigmentary changes. The similarity with nevus of Ota has led to the use of Q-switched lasers for treating this condition with good results. From the limited number of studies available it is not possible to predict the rate of improvement or recurrence after treatment. Regarding the relative response to laser therapy of ABNOM (acquired, bilateral nevus of Ota-like macule) as compared to nevus of Ota the existing studies provide contradictory results.

The findings of the studies concerned with use of various lasers in treatment of ABNOM are summarized in table 14.

Miscellaneous

Besides the above mentioned conditions, lasers have been used for treatment of numerous other pigmentary disorders. However, hardly any comparative studies exist for such uses and hence no recommendations can be made regarding the use of lasers in such conditions.

TABLE 8: Neodymium doped yttrium-aluminium-garnet

Name of study	Type of study	Number and characteristics of patients	Intervention	Number in each arm	Assessment parameter/tools	Follow-up	Result	Limitation	Grade of recommendation
Vejjabhinanta et al. (2010)[49]	RCT, double blind	17 sets of freckles each arm in patients with skin type I–IV	Arm 1: short pulse 532 nm QS Nd:YAG, 10 ns, 1 J/cm^2 single session vs. arm 2: long pulse 532 nm Nd:YAG, 10 ms, 1 J/cm^2 vs. control (no treatment)	17 sets of freckles	Examiner–subjective scale for pigmentation, vascularity, lesion resolution, and cosmetic appearance by cosmetic VAS. Dermoscopy done at 1 month, surface area measured planometrically	1 day, 1 month, and 3 months after treatment	Short pulse Nd:YAG significantly more effective than long pulse and control group with reference to parameters of vascularity, freckle resolution, and surface area. No difference in parameter of vascularity seen among the three groups. No significant differences between long pulse and control group pain greater in short pulse group but no significant adverse effect in any patient	Nil	1A
Jun et al. (2014)[50]	RCT, split face, evaluator blind	15 Asian patients with light facial lentigines	Q-switched Nd:YAG laser + Er: YAG micropeel (combined therapy) vs. Q-switched Nd:YAG	15	Two blinded evaluators using standard clinical photographs graded the change in pigment severity using a 5 point scale, patients subjective assessment of satisfaction	Baseline, 2 weeks 1 month after treatment	Pigment reduction similar in both groups but significantly higher incidence of PIH in combined group	Small sample size	2B
Jun et al (2014)[51]	RCT, split face, evaluator blind	15 Asian patients with light facial lentigines	Er:YAG micropeel versus Q-switched Nd:YAG	15 out of 17 patients initially enrolled	Two blinded evaluators using standard clinical photographs graded the change in pigment severity using a 5 point scale, patients subjective assessment of satisfaction	Baseline, 2 weeks and 1 month after treatment	Pigmentation reduction was more with QS Nd:YAG at 2 weeks, but similar in both groups at 4 weeks, more PIH in QS Nd:YAG	Small sample size	2B

Continued

Continued

Name of study	Type of study	Number and characteristics of patients	Intervention	Number in each arm	Assessment parameter/tools	Follow-up	Result	Limitation	Grade of recommendation
Negishi et al. (2013)[52]	Comparative study	358 lentigines in 196 female, skin type III–IV, Asian	QS ruby—694 nm, 5 mm spot size, 20 ns • Group 1: QS ruby, aggressive treatment to produce obvious immediate tissue whitening • Group 2: QS ruby, mild treatment parameters to produce slight immediate whitening, QS Nd:YAG 532 nm, 7 ns, 3 mm spot size • Group 3: QS Nd:YAG—aggressive treatment to produce obvious immediate tissue whitening • Group 4: QS Nd:YAG mild treatment parameters to produce slight immediate whitening, sunscreen SPF 30, hydroquinone 5% OD HS for 4 weeks	355 lentigines in 193 cases, 3 cases dropped because of nonadherence • Group 1—120 lesions • Group 2—107 lesions • Group 3—69 lesions • Group 4—59 lesions	• Two blinded observers assessed before and after 4-week photograph improvement on digital photographs (Four grades of pigment clearance) • Complications: erythema, hypopigmentation, hyper pigmentation	4 weeks after treatment	No significant difference in efficacy in all the groups, significantly less PIH in mildly treated group compared to aggressively treated groups. No difference between two mildly treated and between the two aggressively treated group	Nonrandomized	2B
Rashid et al. (2002)[53]	Case series	20 patients (14 freckles, 6 lentigines), skin type IV	QS Nd:YAG (532 nm) 3–8 sessions 4 week interval, till no further improvement occurred/>75% improvement was obvious			Patients showing more than 50% improvement were followed up every 3 months for 24 months	80% showed >50% improvement Complications: hypopigmentation in 25% and mild textural changes 15%, hyperpigmentation–10% which resolved. No long-term adverse effect. 40% recurrence in freckles		2C

RCT, randomized controlled trial; QS, Q-switched; Nd:YAG, neodymium doped yttrium-aluminium-garnet; VAS, Visual Analog Scale; Er: YAG, erbium doped yttrium-aluminium-garnet; PIH, postinflammatory hyperpigmentation; SPF, sun protection factor; OD HS, once daily at bedtime.

TABLE 9: Alexandrite

Name of study	Type of study	Number and characteristics of patients	Intervention	Number in each arm	Assessment parameter/tools	Follow-up	Result	Limitation	Grade of recommendation
Ho et al. (2011)[54]	RCT, split face, single blind	20 Chinese females with freckles or lentigines (skin type III and IV)	Long pulse alexandrite (100 μs), single session vs. QS alexandrite (50 ns) single session	20, 1 was lost to follow up	Two blinded assessor scoring VAS for improvement on pretreatment, post-treatment photographs, investigators global assessment scale. Pain edema erythema subjective scoring by patient, improvement and satisfaction subjective assessment	4, 8, 12 weeks after treatment	Statistically significant improvement in pigmentation ($p < 0.05$) in both groups throughout the study, with no statistical difference found between the groups. Postinflammatory hyperpigmentation was more frequently found after QS treatment (22%), compared to LP treatment (6%). PIH in 11% in QS and 6% in LP. Though no significant difference between these two groups. LP alexandrite is quick and effective, and carries a lower risk of adverse effects than QS alexandrite, for the removal of freckles and lentigines in darker skin types	Nil	1A
Wang et al. (2006)[55]	Comparative trial, split face, physician blinded	Taiwanese women (15 freckles, 17 lentigines)	QSAL (755 nm, 50 n, 3 mm spot size, 6.5–7.5 J/cm^2) single session vs. IPL device (560–1,200 nm, double mode, 3.2/6.0 ms, 26–30 J /cm^2 for session 1, 28–32 J/cm^2 for session 2, interval 4 weeks)	32 (15 freckles, 17 lentigines)	Three independent assessors blinded to study. PSI on digital photographs, subjective grading by patient	Baseline, week 4, 12	All patients experienced improvement. PIH developed in one patient with freckles and nine patients with lentigines after QSAL. No PIH occurred after IPL. Freckles achieved greater improvement after QSAL than IPL ($p = 0.04$). In lentigines, both arms showed equal improvement but QSAL showed more PIH. QSAL was superior to IPL for freckle treatment. IPL should be used for lentigines in Asian persons	Randomization and blinding doubtful	2C
Wang et al. (2012)[56]	Comparative trial, split face, double blinded	36 Taiwanese women (freckles 10, lentigines 18, ABNOM 8)	One session QSAL 3 mm spot size higher fluence vs. one session QSAL 4 mm spot size lower fluence	36 (freckles 10, lentigines 18, ABNOM 8)	Two assessors blinded to study scored PSI, PIH (subjective 4 point score), patient satisfaction score at 12 weeks	Baseline, week 4, 8, 12	Using a larger spot to achieve the same biologic effect at a lower fluence is associated with equal efficacy and less-severe PIH in patients with lentigines. No difference in case of freckles, ABNOM	Randomization and blinding doubtful	2C

RCT, randomized controlled trial; QS, Q-switched; VAS, visual analog scale; LP, long-pulsed; QSAL, Q-switched alexandrite laser; IPL, intense pulsed light; PIH, postinflammatory hyperpigmentation; PSI, Psoriasis Activity and Severity Index; ABNOM, acquired, bilateral nevus of Ota-like macules.

TABLE 10: Q-switched ruby

Name of study	Type of study	Number and characteristics of patients	Intervention	Number in each arm	Assessment parameter/tools	Follow-up	Result	Limitation	*Grade of recommendation*
Kono et al. (2006)[57]	Comparative trial, blinded study	18 patients (36 sites) skin types III–IV, Asian	Long pulse—PDL with compression (595 nm, spot size 7 mm, fluence 10–13 J/cm^2 pulse duration 1.5 ms versus 694 nm QSRL, spot size 4 mm, fluence of 6–7 J/cm^2	18 (1 male, 17 female)	Two blinded observers assessed improvement on digital photographs (four grades), complications–erythema, hypopigmentation, hyperpigmentation and scarring assessed clinically	1, 4, 12 weeks post Rx	LPDL with compression significantly more effective than QSRL. Complication with LPDL treatment were substantially less frequent than after QSRL (erythema in 100% in QSRL, 22% in LPDL, hyperpigmentation in 22% QSRL, nil in LPDL	No randomization, blinding details inadequate	2C
Negishi et al. (2013)[52]	Comparative study	358 lentigines in 196 female, skin type III–IV, Asian	QS ruby 694 nm, 5 mm spot size, 20 ns Group 1—QS ruby, aggressive treatment to produce obvious immediate tissue whitening Group 2—QS ruby, mild treatment parameters to produce slight immediate whitening, QS Nd:YAG 532 nm, 7 ns, 3 mm spot size Group 3—QS Nd:YAG aggressive treatment to produce obvious immediate tissue whitening Group 4—QS Nd:YAG mild treatment parameters to produce slight immediate whitening, sunscreen SPF 30, hydroquinone 5% ODHS for 4 weeks	355 lentigines in 193 cases, 3 cases dropped because of nonadherence, • Group 1—120 lesions • Group 2—107 lesions • Group 3—69 lesions • Group 4—59 lesions	Two blinded observers assessed before and after 4 week photograph improvement on digital photographs (four grades of pigment clearance) Complications: Erythema, hypopigmentation, hyper pigmentation	4 weeks after treatment	No significant difference in efficacy in all the groups, significantly less PIH in mildly treated group compared to aggressively treated groups. No difference between two mildly treated and between the two aggressively treated group	Non randomized	2B
Sadighha et al. (2008)[58]	Case series	91	Patients skin type II–IV	QS ruby 694 nm		6 months	Effective in all. Postinflammatory dyspigmentation occurred in 7.8% patients with Fitzpatrick skin type II, 9.8% patients with type III, and 16.6 patients with type IV ($p = 0.67$); all improved over a 6-month follow-up period	Observational study	2C

PDL, pulsed dye laser; QSRL, Q-switched ruby laser; Rx, reaction; LPDL, long-pulsed dye laser; QS, Q-switched; ND: YAG, neodymium-doped yttrium aluminum garnet; SPF, sun protection factor; PIH, post-inflammatory hyperpigmentation; ODHS, once daily at bedtime.

TABLE 11: Intense pulsed light

Name of study	Type of study	Number and characteristics of patients	Intervention	Number in each arm	Assessment parameter/tools	Follow-up	Result	Limitation	Grade of recommendation
Wang et al. (2006)[55]	Comparative trial, split face, physician blinded	Taiwanese women (15 freckles, 17 lentigines)	QSAL (755 nm, 50 ns, 3 mm spot size, 6.5–7.5 J/cm^2) single session vs. IPL device (560–1,200 nm, double mode, 3.2/6.0 ms, 26–30 J/cm^2 for session 1, 28–32 J/cm^2 for session 2, interval 4 weeks)	32 (15 freckles, 17 lentigines)	Three independent assessors blinded to study. PSI on digital photographs, subjective grading by patient	Baseline, week 4, 12	All patients experienced improvement. PIH developed in one patient with freckles and nine patients with lentigines after QSAL. No PIH occurred after IPL. Freckles achieved greater improvement after QSAL than IPL ($p = 0.04$). In lentigines, both arms showed equal improvement but QSAL showed more PIH. QSAL was superior to IPL for freckle treatment. IPL should be used for lentigines in Asian persons	Randomization doubtful, blinding details not adequate	2C

QSAL, Q-switched alexandrite laser; IPL, intense pulsed light; PSI, Psoriasis Activity and Severity Index; PIH, post-inflammatory hyperpigmentation.

TABLE 12: Erbium doped yttrium-aluminium-garnet

Name of study	Type of study	Number and characteristics of patients	Intervention	Number in each arm	Assessment parameter/tools	Follow-up	Result	Limitation	Grade of recommendation
Jun et al. (2014)[50]	RCT, split face, evaluator blind	15 Asian patients with light facial lentigines	Q-switched Nd:YAG laser + Er:YAG micropeel (combined therapy) vs. Q-switched Nd:YAG	15	Two blinded evaluators using standard clinical photographs graded the change in pigment severity using a 5 point scale, patients subjective assessment of satisfaction	Baseline, 2 weeks 1 month after treatment	Pigment reduction similar in both groups but significantly higher incidence of PIH in combined group	Small sample size	2B
Jun et al. (2014)[51]	RCT, split face, evaluator blind	15 Asian patients with light facial lentigines	Er:YAG micropeel vs. Q-switched Nd:YAG	15 out of 17 patients initially enrolled	Two blinded evaluators using standard clinical photographs graded the change in pigment severity using a 5 point scale, patients subjective assessment of satisfaction	Baseline, 2 weeks1 month after treatment	Pigmentation reduction was more with QS Nd:YAG at 2 weeks, but similar in both groups at 4 weeks, more PIH in QS Nd:YAG	Small sample size	2B

RCT, randomized controlled trial; Nd:YAG, neodymium doped yttrium-aluminium-garnet; Er:YAG, erbium doped yttrium-aluminium-garnet: YAG; PIH, post-inflammatory hyperpigmentation; QS, Q-switched

TABLE 13: Nevus of Ota

Name of study	Type of study	Number and characteristics of patients	Intervention	Number in each arm	Assessment parameter/tools	Follow-up	Result	Limitation	Grade of recommendation
Wen et al. (2015)[63]	Comparative trial, split face	17 B/L nevus of Ota	QSAL vs. QS Nd:YAG	17	Subjective assessment patient, two blinded dermatologist grading using 5 point scale	12 weeks after last treatment	Nd:YAG laser were equally effective at improving bilateral nevus of Ota. Patients tolerate QS Nd:YAG laser better than QS alex laser	Randomization doubtful	2C
Chan et al. (2000)[61]	Retrospective study	Nevus of Ota (171 patients with 211 treatment sites)	QS alex laser only (n = 58), QS Nd:YAG laser (n = 105) only, or a combination of both systems (n = 48)	—	Patients graded the clearance of lesion into six grades, two independent clinicians examined for complications	Period of study—6 years	No significant difference amongst the three groups. Hypopigmentation most common S/E (in some cases permanent) more in combined treatment group. Number of Rx sessions is an independent risk factor for hypopigmentation and all complications. Hyperpigmentation seen in skin type V only but skin type otherwise not associated with any other complication. Recurrence seen in 13 patients (5 in Nd:YAG and 8 in combined Rx; however, not to baseline level). Recurrence at 13–60 months and not associated with number of treatment sessions. 3% had hypopigmentation, 2.9% had hyperpigmentation, and texture changes and scarring were seen in 2.9% and 1.9%, respectively. The combined treatment group was associated with a significantly higher risk of complications		2C
Chan et al. (1999)[64]	Comparative trial	Nevus of Ota, 32 patients, 42 treatment session, half of each lesion	QSAL vs. QS Nd:YAG	33 patients 45 treatment session	Patient assessment using VAS for scoring, pain, swelling, discomfort, lightening and bleeding, and question regarding laser preference	Immediate post-treatment and 1 week after treatment	Immediate pain after treatment was more severe for QS alexandrite than for QS Nd:YAG laser. However, 1 week after laser therapy, most patients found QS alex to be superior	Details about randomization and blinding not available	2C

Continued

Continued

Name of study	Type of study	Number and characteristics of patients	Intervention	Number in each arm	Assessment parameter/tools	Follow-up	Result	Limitation	Grade of recommendation
Chan et al. (2000)[65]	Comparative trial, evaluator blinded	Nevus of Ota, 44 patients, 45 treatment session, half of each lesion	QS 755 nm alex (3–6 session at interval, 3–9 months, for half lesion) vs. QS Nd:YAG (3–6 session at interval, 3–9 months, for half lesion)	40 completed study, 4 defaulters	Degree of lightening—subjective assessment by patient using VAS and objective assessment by two blinded clinicians using VAS and assessment of complications (hypo and hyperpigmentation, textural change, scarring)	1–15 months	In terms of subjective degree of lightening, QS 1,064 nm ND: YAG laser was found to be significantly more efficacious than QS alex ($p = 0.018$). Both clinicians also found QS 1,064 nm ND: YAG laser to be more effective, but statistical significance was only seen for one observer. Four QS alex laser treatment sites developed complications; one developed texture change, another hyperpigmentation, and for the remaining two, one had hypopigmentation and the other had atrophic scarring. For QS Nd:YAG laser, one treatment site developed hypopigmentation and another hyperpigmentation and texture change. The difference in the overall complication rate was not significant	Randomization doubtful	2C
Chang et al. (2011)[66]	Retrospective study	94 Asian patients, 3–64 years age	QS ruby (694 nm) 7–10 J/cm², 1–8 sessions vs. QS Nd:YAG, number of treatment ranged from 1–8, duration of treatment–6 months to 3 years and 10 months (mean 14 months)	47	Clearing and fading response using derma spectrometer		QS ruby laser resulted in better clearing and fading as compared with QS Nd:YAG laser. No long-term adverse effect in any group	—	2C
Seo et al. (2015)[60]	Retrospective study	31 Korean patients, skin type IV	A low-fluence 1,064 nm QS Nd:YAG, 6–32 treatment sessions at 2–3 weeks intervals, 7 or 8 mm spot, 1.9–5.0 J/cm² mean fluence				QSAL tends to be more efficient than the QS Nd:YAG laser		2C

Continued

Continued

Name of study	Type of study	Number and characteristics of patients	Intervention	Number in each arm	Assessment parameter/tools	Follow-up	Result	Limitation	Grade of recommendation
Choi et al. (2015)[67]	Retro-spective, multicenter study	31 patients (QSAL) + 45 patients (QS Nd:YAG)	QSAL 5.5–8.0 J/cm^2, 4 mm spot size vs. QS Nd:YAG 6.0–12.0 J/cm^2, 2 mm spot size	31 and 45	—	—	QSAL treatment was more likely to achieve a better response compared with that with QSNY laser treatment. The odds ratio of achieving an excellent response, compared with the odds ratio of having a poor response, was 12 to 13-times more likely when a QSAL was used than when a QSNY laser was used ($p = 0.026$) —	—	2C
Kono et al. (2001)[68]	Retrospective study	101	QS ruby	101	—	—	Hypopigmentation was the most common complication affecting 16.8% of the patients and 5.9% had hyperpigmentation. Recurrence is rare, but hypopigmentation can be permanent	—	2C
Moreno-Arias et al. (2001)[69]	Case series	13	QSAL 6–8 J/cm^2,1–15 sessions interval 8 weeks	13	—	—	More than 75% lightening was achieved in seven patients, between 51 and 75% in three, less than 50% in one, and less than 25% in one. No recurrence	—	2C
Lu et al. (2003)[70]	Case series	522	QSAL	522	—	—	QSAL is an ideal method for treating nevus of Ota without injury. The number of treatment sessions is more important than interval or fluence	—	2C
Kar et al. (2011)[71]	Case series (open label prospective)	50 Indian patients, skin type IV, V	QSNY 3.5–8.5 J, 5–15 sessions (2007–2009)	50	Clinical examination using quartile grading scale	Till 6 months after last treatment	Near total improvement was seen in 8%, marked improvement in 22%, moderate improvement in 38% and 32% patients reported less than 25% clearing of the lesion. Transient post-inflammatory hyperpigmentation was observed in four (8%) patients, which cleared with the use of sunscreens and bleaching agents within 2 months. No textural change or scarring was observed in any patient	—	2C

Continued

Continued

Name of study	Type of study	Number and characteristics of patients	Intervention	Number in each arm	Assessment parameter/tools	Follow-up	Result	Limitation	Grade of recommendation
Aurangabadkar (2008)[72]	Case series	50 Indian patients	QSNY 3.5–3.5 J (7–8.5 J/cm^2 in seven cases), six sessions	50	Physicians global assessment	Till 1 year after last treatment	Greater than 60% improvement was seen in 66% of the patients. The remaining patients had moderate clearing of pigmentation (30–60% improvement). No significant adverse effects were seen immediately after the treatments and on long-term follow-up. Transient post-inflammatory hyperpigmentation was observed in five (10%) patients, which cleared with use of sunscreens and bleaching agents within 2 months. No textural change or scarring was seen. Hypopigmentation (guttate type) was observed in one (2%) patient, which resolved within 3 months. No recurrence was observed after 1 year of follow-up	—	2C

Limitations have been enumerated for comparative trials only.

QSAL, Q-switched alexandrite laser; QS, Q-switched; Nd:YAG, neodymium doped yttrium-aluminium-garnet; Rx, reaction; VAS, visual analog scale; QSNY, Q-switched Nd:YAG; B/L, bilateral; S/E,side-effects.

TABLE 14: Acquired bilateral nevus of Ota-like macules

Name of study	Type of study	Number and characteristics of patients	Intervention	Number in each arm	Assessment parameter/ tools	Follow-up	Result	Grade of recommendation
Cho et al. (2009)[73]	Case series	15 ABNOM	QS Nd:YAG 2.2–2.6 J/cm^2 using a 6 mm spot size, followed by 4–6 J/cm^2 using a 4 mm spot size	15	—	2 months after treatment	7 of the 15 patients (46.7%) demonstrated clinical improvement of 76–100%, and 5 (33.3%) of 51–75%	2C
Polnikorn et al. (2000)[74]	Case series	66 ABNOM	QS Nd:YAG 3 mm spot size, 4–6 J/cm^2	66	—	3–44 months	Effective but results are not as good as those seen with nevus of Ota	2C
Kunachak et al. (1999)[75]	Case series	140 ABNOM	QS ruby 7–10 J/cm^2, repetition rate of 1 Hz, spot size of 2–4 mm. The number of treatment sessions 1–6 (mean 2.3)	140	—	6 months–4.3 years (mean 2.5 years)	131 showed complete clearance, no recurrence, post-inflammatory hypopigmentation in 3	2C

Continued

Continued

Name of study	Type of study	Number and characteristics of patients	Intervention	Number in each arm	Assessment parameter/ tools	Follow-up	Result	Grade of recommendation
Ee et al. (2006)[76]	Split face, comparative study	10 B/L Hori's nevus	Combination of the QS 532 nm and 1,064 nm Nd:YAG lasers on the right cheek, single session vs. QS 1,064 nm Nd:YAG laser alone on the left cheek	10	Mexameter assessment, patient's assessment, two blinded dermatologists' assessment	6 months	QS 532 nm Nd:YAG laser in combination with the 1,064 nm laser is more effective in pigment clearance than the QS 1,064 nm Nd:YAG laser alone	2C
Manuskiatti et al. (2003)[77]	Comparative study, split face	13 female patients, Thai; B/L Hori's nevus, skin type III–V	Scanned CO_2 laser followed by QSRL vs. QSRL alone	13	Mexameter assessment of melanin index, HPE at 3 months after treatment(only from one patient)	1, 3, 4, and 16 months	The response rate, defined as "the percentage of reduction in melanin index," was significantly higher on the sides treated with scanned CO_2 laser followed by QSRL, compared with the sides irradiated with QSRL alone at both follow-up visits. At the 3-month follow-up, the most common adverse effect was hypopigmentation, found in 15% (2 of 13) of the patients on the sites treated with QSRL alone, and on the sites treated with scanned CO_2 laser followed by QSRL (8%, 1/13). Erythema was observed in 15% (2/13) of the patients only on the sites that received combination treatment. However, no adverse sequelae were observed at the 16-month post-treatment	2C
Lee et al. (2009)[78]	Case series	29	1,064 nm QS Nd:YAG (a pulse duration of 5–7 ns, a spot size of 3 mm, and a fluence of 8–9.5 J/cm^2), up to 10 sessions ,interval of 4 -12 weeks	29	Percentage of pigment clearing by two blinded observers, observation for erythema, hyperpigmentation and hypopigmentation	At each visit	Of the 29 treated patients, 19 (66%) showed excellent or good results; 76% who were treated more than three times had good or excellent result (Table 3). Of patients who were treated more than six times, 90% demonstrated good or excellent results. The average number of treatment sessions for patients with excellent results was 6.5, compared with 2.0 for patients with moderate results. There was a statistically significant correlation between the number of treatments and therapeutic outcomes	2C

ABNOM, acquired, bilateral nevus of Ota-like macules; QS, Q-switched; Nd:YAG, neodymium yttrium-aluminium-garnet; QSRL, Q-switched ruby laser; B/L, bilateral; HPE, histopathological examination.

Congenital melanocytic nevi have been treated using CO_2 laser and Er:YAG lasers, but adverse effects like scarring and repigmentation have occurred especially with CO_2 laser.[79] Acquired melanocytic nevi have been safely removed using Er:YAG laser and Q-switched pigment lasers but such a treatment prevents a histopathological evaluation of the lesion which is a cause for concern.[80,81]

Becker's nevus has been treated using nonselective CO_2 and Er:YAG lasers, ablative fractional 10,600 nm laser, and also using pigment selective lasers like Q-switched ruby and Q-switched Nd:YAG with variable response.[82-84]

Nevus spilus has been reported to show good response to Q-switched Nd:YAG laser, Q-switched ruby, and Q-switched alexandrite laser. However, there have been instances of worsening of lesions.[85,86] Café au lait macules have been reported to show variable response to the Q-switched ruby and frequency doubled Nd:YAG laser with chances of recurrence and darkening of the lesions.[87]

Not much is known about use of lasers in treatment of lichen planus pigmentosus and postinflammatory hyperpigmentation. Fractional 1,550 nm laser therapy has been shown to be ineffective in treating these conditions.[88] There have been case reports of LPP responding to Q-switched Nd:YAG laser therapy.[89,90]

CONCLUSION

Over the last decade or two, a large body of work has found place in the literature regarding the use of lasers in hyperpigmentary disorders. While in some of these conditions, e.g., nevus of Ota, black tattoos, or even lentigines, there is evidence of a degree of success with lasers, and light-based therapies, while in some conditions, like melasma, such use is fraught with problems such as lack of effectiveness and serious side-effects such as persistent postinflammatory pigmentation. The evidence, in most cases, is inadequate, with studies lacking proper power, randomization, control, and follow-up period. Thus, evidence dictates that we use lasers with circumspection in such conditions in the skin phototypes prevalent in our population.

REFERENCES

1. Li YT, Yang KC. Comparison of the frequency-doubled Q-switched Nd:YAG laser and 35% trichloroacetic acid for the treatment of face lentigines. Dermatol Surg. 1999;25:202-4.
2. Kunachak S, Leelaudomlipi P, Wongwaisayawan S. Dermabrasion: a curative treatment for melasma. Aesthetic Plast Surg 2001;25:114-7.
3. Goldman L, Rockwell RJ, Meyer R, Otten R, Wilson RG, Kitzmiller KW. Laser treatment of tatoos: A preliminary survey of three year's clinical experience. JAMA. 1967;201:841-4.
4. Stratigos AJ, Dover JS, Arndt KA. Laser treatment of pigmented lesions-2000: how far have we gone? Arch Dermatol 2000; 136:915-21.
5. Anderson RR, Parish JA. Selective photothermolysis. precise microsurgery by selective absorption of pulsed radiation. Science. 1983;220:524-7.
6. Brazzini B, Hautmann G, Ghersetich I, Hercogova J, Lotti T. Laser tissue interaction in epidermal pigmented lesions. J Eur Acad Dermatol Venereol. 2001;15:388-91.
7. Briganti S, Camera E, Picardo M. Chemical and instrumental approaches to treat hyperpigmentation. Pigment Cell Res. 2003;16:101-10.
8. Aurangabadkar S, Panda S. Debate on The use of Lasers for Melasma. Pigment Bulletin. 2014;2:18-23.
9. Sanchez NP, Pathak MA, Sato S, Fitzpatrick TB, Sanchez JL, Mihm MC Jr. Melasma: a clinical, light microscopic, ultrastructural, and immunofluorescence study. J Am Acad Dermatol. 1981;4:698-710.
10. Panda S. Recent trends and future treatment paradigms of melasma based on current understanding of pathophysiology. In: Lahiri K, Chatterjee M, Sarkar R, editors. Pigmentary Disorders: A Comprehensive Compendium. Jaypee Brothers Medical Publisher (P) Ltd.: New Delhi, 2014. pp. 349-60.
11. Moncada B, Sahagún-Sánchez LK, Torres-Alvarez B Castanedo-Cázares JP, Martínez-Ramírez JD, González FJ. Molecular structure and concentration of melanin in the stratum corneum of patients with melasma. Photodermatol Photoimmunol Photomed. 2009;25:159-60.
12. Lee DJ, Park KC, Ortonne JP Kang HY.Pendulous melanocytes: a characteristic feature of melasma and how it may occur. Br J Dermatol. 2012;166:684-6.
13. Guyatt GH, Cook DJ, Jaeschke R, Pauker SG, Schünemann HJ. Grades of recommendation for antithrombotic agents: American College of Chest Physicians Evidence-Based Clinical Practice Guidelines (8th Edition). Chest. 2008;133:123S-31S.
14. Rivas S, Pandya AG. Treatment of melasma with topical agents, peels and lasers: an evidence-based review. Am J Clin Dermatol. 2013;14: 359-76.
15. Moubasher AE, Youssef EM, Abou-Taleb DA. Q-switched Nd: YAG laser versus trichloroacetic acid peeling in the treatment of melasma among Egyptian patients. Dermatol Surg. 2014;40(8):874-82.
16. Omi T, Yamashita R, Kawana S, Sato S, Naito Z. Low Fluence Q-Switched Nd: YAG Laser Toning and Q-Switched Ruby Laser in the Treatment of Melasma: A Comparative Split-Face Ultrastructural Study. Laser Ther. 2012;21(1):15-21.
17. Yun WJ, Moon HR, Lee MW, Choi JH, Chang SE. Combination treatment of low-fluence 1,064-nm Q-switched Nd: YAG laser with novel intense pulse light in Korean melasma patients: a prospective, randomized, controlled trial. Dermatol Surg. 2014;40(8):842-50.
18. Alsaad SM, Ross EV, Mishra V, Miller L. A split face study to document the safety and efficacy of clearance of melasma with a 5 ns Q switched Nd YAG laser versus a 50 ns q switched Nd YAG laser. Lasers Surg Med. 2014;46:736-40.
19. Fabi SG, Friedmann DP, Niwa Massaki AB, Goldman MP. A randomized, split-face clinical trial of low-fluence Q-switched neodymium-doped yttrium aluminum garnet (1,064 nm) laser versus low-fluence Q-switched alexandrite laser (755 nm) for the treatment of facial melasma. Lasers Surg Med. 2014;46(7):531-7.
20. Kar HK, Gupta L, Chauhan A. A comparative study on efficacy of high and low fluence Q-switched Nd:YAG laser and glycolic acid peel in melasma. Indian J Dermatol Venereol Leprol. 2012;78(2):165-71.
21. Wattanakrai P, Mornchan R, EimpunthS. Low-fluence Q-switched neodymium-doped yttrium aluminum garnet (1,064 nm) laser for the treatment of facial melasma in Asians. Dermatol Surg. 2010;36(1):76-87.
22. Kim HS, Kim EK, Jung KE, Park YM, Kim HO, Lee JY.A split-face comparison of low-fluence Q-switched Nd: YAG laser plus 1550 nm

fractional photothermolysis vs. Q-switched Nd: YAG monotherapy for facial melasma in Asian skin. J Cosmet Laser Ther. 2013;15(3):143-9.
23. Bansal C, Naik H, Kar HK, Chauhan A. A Comparison of Low-Fluence 1064-nm Q-Switched Nd: YAG Laser with Topical 20% Azelaic Acid Cream and their Combination in Melasma in Indian Patients. J Cutan Aesthet Surg. 2012;5(4):266-72.
24. Vachiramon V, Sahawatwong S, Sirithanabadeekul P. Treatment of melasma in men with low-fluence Q-switched neodymium-doped yttrium-aluminum-garnet laser versus combined laser and glycolic acid peeling. Dermatol Surg. 2015;41(4):457-65.
25. Park KY, Kim DH, Kim HK, Li K, Seo SJ, Hong CK. A randomized, observer-blinded, comparison of combined 1064-nm Q-switched neodymium-doped yttrium-aluminium-garnet laser plus 30% glycolic acid peel vs. laser monotherapy to treat melasma. Clin Exp Dermatol. 2011;36(8):864-70.
26. Jalaly NY, Valizadeh N, Barikbin B, Yousefi M. Low-power fractional CO_2 laser versus low-fluence Q-switch 1,064 nm Nd:YAG laser for treatment of melasma: a randomized, controlled, split-face study. Am J Clin Dermatol. 2014;15(4):357-63.
27. Jeong SY, Chang SE, Bak H. New melasma treatment by collimated low fluence Q-switched Nd:YAG laser. Korean J Dermatol. 2008;46:1163-70.
28. Suh KS, Sung JY, Roh HJ, Jeon YS, Kim YC, Kim ST. Efficacy of the 1064-nm Q-switched Nd:YAG laser in melasma. J Dermatolog Treat. 2011;22(4):233-8.
29. Zhou X, Gold MH, Lu Z, Li Y. Efficacy and safety of Q-switched 1,064-nm neodymium-doped yttrium aluminum garnet laser treatment of melasma. Dermatol Surg. 2011;37(7):962-70.
30. Fabi SG, Friedmann DP, Niwa Massaki AB, Goldman MP. A randomized, split-face clinical trial of low-fluence Q-switched neodymium-doped yttrium aluminum garnet (1,064 nm) laser versus low-fluence Q-switched alexandrite laser (755 nm) for the treatment of facial melasma. Lasers Surg Med. 2014;46(7):531-7.
31. Jang WS, Lee CK, Kim BJ, Kim MN. Efficacy of 694-nm Q-switched ruby fractional laser treatment of melasma in female Korean patients. Dermatol Surg. 2011;37(8):1133-40.
32. Hilton S, Heise H, Buhren BA, Schrumpf H, Bölke E, Gerber PA. Treatment of melasma in Caucasian patients using a novel 694-nm Q-switched ruby fractional laser. Eur J Med Res. 2013;18:43.
33. Kroon MW, Wind BS, Beek JF, van der Veen JP, Nieuweboer-Krobotová L, Bos JD, et al. Nonablative 1550-nm fractional laser therapy versus triple topical therapy for the treatment of melasma: a randomized controlled pilot study. J Am Acad Dermatol. 2011;64(3):516-23.
34. Wind BS, Kroon MW, Meesters AA, Beek JF, van der Veen JP, Nieuweboer-Krobotová L, et al. Non-ablative 1,550 nm fractional laser therapy versus triple topical therapy for the treatment of melasma: a randomized controlled split-face study. Lasers Surg Med. 2010;42(7):607-12.
35. Hong SP, Han SS, Choi SJ, Kim MS, Won CH, Lee MW, et al. Split-face comparative study of 1550 nm fractional photothermolysis and trichloroacetic acid 15% chemical peeling for facial melasma in Asian skin. J Cosmet Laser Ther. 2012;14(2):81-6.
36. Karsai S, Fischer T, Pohl L, Schmitt L, Buhck H, Jünger M, et al. Is non-ablative 1550-nm fractional photothermolysis an effective modality to treat melasma? Results from a prospective controlled single-blinded trial in 51 patients. J Eur Acad Dermatol Venereol. 2012;26(4):470-6.
37. Rokhsar CK, Fitzpatrick RE. The treatment of melasma with fractional photothermolysis: a pilot study. DermatolSurg. 2005;31:1645-50.
38. Lee HS, Won CH, Lee DH, An JS, Chang HW, Lee JH, et al. Treatment of melasma in Asian skin using a fractional 1,550-nm laser: an open clinical study. Dermatol Surg. 2009;35(10):1499-504.
39. Goldberg DJ, Berlin AL, Phelps R. Histologic and ultrastructural analysis of melasma after fractional resurfacing. Lasers Surg Med. 2008;40(2):134-8.
40. Polder KD, Bruce S. Treatment of melasma using a novel 1,927-nm fractional thulium fiber laser: a pilot study. Dermatol Surg. 2012;38(2):199-206.
41. Wanitphakdeedecha R, Keoprasom N, Eimpunth S, Manuskiatti W. The efficacy in melasma treatment using a 1410 nm fractional photothermolysis laser. J Eur Acad Dermatol Venereol. 2014;28(3):293-7.
42. Wang CC, Hui CY, Sue YM, Wong WR, Hong HS. Intense pulsed light for the treatment of refractory melasma in Asian persons. Dermatol Surg. 2004;30(9):1196-200.
43. Moreno Arias GA, Ferrando J. Intense pulsed light for melanocytic lesions. Dermatol Surg. 2001;27:397-400.
44. Li YH, Chen JZ, Wei HC, Wu Y, Liu M, Xu YY, et al. Efficacy and safety of intense pulsed light in treatment of melasma in Chinese patients. Dermatol Surg. 2008;34:693-700.
45. Lee HI, Lim YY, Kim BJ, Kim MN, Min HJ, Hwang JH, et al. Clinicopathologic efficacy of copper bromide plus/yellow laser (578 nm with 511 nm) for treatment of melasma in Asian patients. Dermatol Surg. 2010;36: 885-93.
46. Praetorius C, Sturm AR, Steingrimsson E. Sun-induced freckling: ephelides and solar lentigines. Pigment Cell Melanoma Res. 2014;27;339-50.
47. Seirafi H, Fateh S, Farnaghi F, Ehsani AH, Noormohammadpour P. Efficacy and safety of long-pulse pulsed dye laser delivered with compression versus cryotherapy for treatment of solar lentigines. Indian J Dermatol. 2011;56(1):48-51.
48. Todd MM, Rallis TM, Gerwels JW, Hata TR. A comparison of 3 lasers and liquid nitrogen in the treatment of solar lentigines: a randomized, controlled, comparative trial. Arch Dermatol. 2000;136:841-6.
49. Vejjabhinanta V, Elsaie ML, Patel SS, Patel A, Caperton C, Nouri K. Comparison of short-pulsed and long-pulsed 532 nm lasers in the removal of freckles. Lasers Med Sci. 2010;25:901-6.
50. Jun HJ, Cho SH, Lee JD, Kim HS. A split-face, evaluator-blind randomized study on the early effects of Q-switched Nd:YAG laser versus Er:YAG micropeel (combined therapy) versus Q-switched Nd:YAG alone in light solar lentigines in Asians. Lasers Med Sci. 2014;29(3):1153-8.
51. Jun HJ, Kim SM, Choi WJ, Cho SH, Lee JD, Kim HS.A split-face, evaluator-blind randomized study on the early effects of Q-switched Nd:YAG laser versus Er:YAG micropeel in light solar lentigines in Asians. J Cosmet Laser Ther. 2014;16(2):83-8.
52. Negishi K, Akita H, Tanaka S, Yokoyama Y, Wakamatsu S, Matsunaga K. Comparative study of treatment efficacy and the incidence of post-inflammatory hyperpigmentation with different degrees of irradiation using two different quality-switched lasers for removing solar lentigenes on Asian skin. J Eur Acad Dermatol Venereol. 2013;27(3):307-12.
53. Rashid T, Hussain I, Haider M, Haroon TS. Laser therapy of freckles and lentigines with quasi-continuous, frequency-doubled, Nd:YAG (532 nm) laser in Fitzpatrick skin type IV: a 24-month follow-up. J Cosmet Laser Ther. 2002;4(3-4):81-5.
54. Ho SG, Yeung CK, Chan NP, Shek SY, Chan HH.A comparison of Q-switched and long-pulsed alexandrite laser for the treatment of freckles and lentigines in oriental patients. Lasers Surg Med. 2011;43(2):108-13.
55. Wang CC, Sue YM, Yang CH, Chen CK. A comparison of Q-switched alexandrite laser and intense pulsed light for the treatment of freckles and lentigines in Asian persons: a randomized, physician-blinded, split-face comparative trial. J Am Acad Dermatol. 2006; 54(5):804-10.
56. Wang CC, Chen CK. Effect of spot size and fluence on Q-switched alexandrite laser treatment for pigmentation in Asians: a randomized, double-blinded, split-face comparative trial. J Dermatolog Treat.2012;23:333-8.
57. Kono T, Manstein D, Chan HH, Nozaki M, Anderson RR. Q-switched ruby versus long-pulsed dye laser delivered with compression for treatment of facial lentigines in Asians. Lasers Surg Med. 2006;38(2):94-7.

58. Sadighha A, Saatee S, Muhaghegh-Zahed G. Efficacy and adverse effects of Q-switched ruby laser on solar lentigines: a prospective study of 91 patients with Fitzpatrick skin type II, III, and IV. Dermatol Surg. 2008;34(11):1465-8.
59. Shah VV, Bray FN, Aldahan AS, Mlacker S, Nouri K. Lasers and nevus of Ota: a comprehensive review. Lasers Med Sci. 2016;31:179-85.
60. Seo HM, Choi CW, Kim WS. Beneficial effects of early treatment of nevus of Ota with low-fluence 1,064-nm Q-switched Nd:YAG laser. Dermatol Surg. 2015;41(1):142-8.
61. Chan HH, Leung RS, Ying SY, Lai CF, Kono T, Chua JK, et al. A retrospective analysis of complications in the treatment of nevus of Ota with the Q-switched alexandrite and Q-switched Nd:YAG lasers. Dermatol Surg. 2000;26(11):1000-6.
62. Chestnut C, Diehl J, Lask G. Treatment of nevus of ota with a picoseconds 755-nm alexandrite laser. Dermatol Surg. 2015;41(4):508-10.
63. Wen X, Li Y, Jiang X. A randomized, split-face clinical trial of Q-switched alexandrite laser versus Q-switched Nd:YAG laser in the treatment of bilateral nevus of Ota. J Cosmet Laser Ther. 2015;6:1-4.
64. Chan HH, King WW, Chan ES, Mok CO, Ho WS, Van Krevel C, Lau WY. In vivo trial comparing patients' tolerance of Q-switched Alexandrite (QS Alex) and Q-switched neodymium: yttrium-aluminum-garnet (QS Nd:YAG) lasers in the treatment of nevus of Ota. Lasers Surg Med. 1999;24(1):24-8.
65. Chan HH, Ying SY, Ho WS, Kono T, King WW. An in vivo trial comparing the clinical efficacy and complications of Q-switched 755 nm alexandrite and Q-switched 1064 nm Nd:YAG lasers in the treatment of nevus of Ota. Dermatol Surg. 2000;26(10):919-22.
66. Chang CJ, Kou CS. Comparing the effectiveness of Q-switched Ruby laser treatment with that of Q-switched Nd:YAG laser for oculodermal melanosis (Nevus of Ota). J Plast Reconstr Aesthet Surg. 2011;64(3):339-45.
67. Choi JE, Lee JB, Park KB, Kim BS, Yeo UC, Huh CH, et al. A retrospective analysis of the clinical efficacies of Q-switched Alexandrite and Q-switched Nd:YAG lasers in the treatment of nevus of Ota in Korean patients. J Dermatolog Treat. 2015;26(3):240-5.
68. Kono T, Nozaki M, Chan HH, Mikashima Y.A retrospective study looking at the long-term complications of Q-switched ruby laser in the treatment of nevus of Ota. Lasers Surg Med. 2001;29(2):156-9.
69. Moreno-Arias GA, Camps-Fresneda A. Treatment of nevus of Ota with the Q-switched alexandrite laser. Lasers Surg Med. 2001;28(5):451-5.
70. Lu Z, Fang L, Jiao S, Huang W, Chen J, Wang X. Treatment of 522 patients with Nevus of Ota with Q-switched Alexandrite laser. Chin Med J (Engl). 2003;116(2):226-30.
71. Kar HK, Gupta L. 1064 nm Q switched Nd: YAG laser treatment of nevus of Ota: an Indian open label prospective study of 50 patients. Indian J Dermatol Venereol Leprol. 2011;77:565-70.
72. Aurangabadkar S. QYAG5 Q-switched Nd:YAG Laser Treatment of Nevus of Ota: An Indian Study of 50 Patients. J Cutan Aesthet Surg. 2008;1(2):80-4.
73. Cho SB, Park SJ, Kim MJ, Bu TS. Treatment of acquired bilateral nevus of Ota-like macules (Hori's nevus) using 1064-nm Q-switched Nd:YAG laser with low fluence. Int J Dermatol. 2009;48(12):1308-12.
74. Polnikorn N, Tanrattanakorn S, Goldberg DJ. Treatment of Hori's nevus with the Q-switched Nd:YAG laser. Dermatol Surg. 2000;26(5):477-80.
75. Kunachak S, Leelaudomlipi P, Sirikulchayanonta V. Q-Switched ruby laser therapy of acquired bilateral nevus of Ota-like macules. Dermatol Surg. 1999;25(12):938-41.
76. Ee HL, Goh CL, Khoo LS, Chan ES, Ang P. Treatment of acquired bilateral nevus of ota-like macules (Hori's nevus) with a combination of the 532 nm Q-Switched Nd:YAG laser followed by the 1,064 nm Q-switched Nd:YAG is more effective: prospective study. Dermatol Surg. 2006;32(1):34-40.
77. Manuskiatti W, Sivayathorn A, Leelaudomlipi P, Fitzpatrick RE. Treatment of acquired bilateral nevus of Ota-like macules (Hori's nevus) using a combination of scanned carbon dioxide laser followed by Q-switched ruby laser. J Am Acad Dermatol. 2003;48(4):584-91.
78. Lee WJ, Han SS, Chang SE, Lee MW, Choi JH, Moon KC, et al. Q-Switched Nd:YAG Laser Therapy of Acquired Bilateral Nevus of Ota-like Macules. Ann Dermatol. 2009;21(3):255-60.
79. Arora H, Falto-Aizpurua L, Chacon A, Griffith RD, Nouri K. Lasers for nevi: a review. Lasers Med Sci. 2015;30(7):1991-2001.
80. Baba M, Bal N. Efficacy and safety of the short-pulse erbium:YAG laser in the treatment of acquired melanocytic nevi. Dermatol Surg. 2006;32(2):256-60.
81. Sardana K, Chakravarty P, Goel K. Optimal management of common acquired melanocytic nevi (moles): current perspectives. Clin Cosmet Investig Dermatol. 2014;7:89-103.
82. Trelles MA, Allones I, Moreno-Arias GA, Vélez M. Becker's naevus: a comparative study between erbium: YAG and Q-switched neodymium:YAG; clinical and histopathological findings. Br J Dermatol. 2005;152(2):308-13.
83. Tse Y, Levine VJ, McClain SA, Ashinoff R. The removal of cutaneous pigmented lesions with the Q-switched ruby laser and the Q-switched neodymium: yttrium-aluminum-garnet laser. A comparative study. J Dermatol Surg Oncol. 1994;20(12):795-800.
84. Meesters AA, Wind BS, Kroon MW, Wolkerstorfer A, van der Veen JP, Nieuweboer-Krobotová L, van der Wal AC, Bos JD, Beek JF. Ablative fractional laser therapy as treatment for Becker nevus: a randomized controlled pilot study. J Am Acad Dermatol. 2011;65(6):1173-9.
85. Kar H, Gupta L. Treatment of nevus spilus with Q switched Nd:YAG laser. Indian J Dermatol Venereol Leprol. 2013;79:243-5.
86. Grevelink JM, González S, Bonoan R, Vibhagool C, Gonzalez E. Treatment of nevus spilus with the Q-switched ruby laser. Dermatol Surg. 1997;23:365-9.
87. Grossman MC, Anderson RR, Farinelli W, Flotte TJ, Grevelink JM. Treatment of cafe au lait macules with lasers. A clinicopathologic correlation. Arch Dermatol. 1995;131(12):1416-20.
88. Kroon MW, Wind BS, Meesters AA, Wolkerstorfer A, van der Veen JP, Bos JD, et al. Non-ablative 1,550 nm fractional laser therapy not effective for erythema dyschromicum perstans and postinflammatory hyperpigmentation: a pilot study. J Dermatolog Treat. 2012;23(5):339-44.
89. Han XD, Goh CL. A case of lichen planus pigmentosus that was recalcitrant to topical treatment responding to pigment laser treatment. Dermatol Ther, 2014;27:264-7.
90. Kim JE, Won CH, Chang S, Lee MW, Choi JH, Moon KC. Linear lichen planus pigmentosus of the forehead treated by neodymium:yttrium-aluminum-garnet laser and topical tacrolimus. J Dermatol. 2012;39(2):189-91.

CHAPTER 17

Lasers for Tattoo Removal

Chee-Leok Goh, Stephanie G Ho

INTRODUCTION

Tattooing is an ancient procedure and has been identified in different societies for centuries. It has been estimated that up to a quarter of young to middle-aged adults in the United States have at least one tattoo.[1] Results from an online survey group, Harris Interactive, reported a rise in the United States adult tattoo prevalence from 16% in 2003 to 21% in 2012.[2] As more tattoos are being acquired, increasing numbers of people are also seeking to have them removed. The American Society of Dermatologic Surgery reported carrying out 100,000 tattoo removal procedures in 2011, up from 86,000 in 2010.[3] Motivation for tattoo removal includes new jobs or careers, the need to portray a certain image at work or in new social circles, and new negative feelings towards old tattoos.[4] Unfortunately, the removal of tattoos is generally more costly and time consuming than acquiring them.

CLASSIFICATION OF TATTOOS

Tattooing is a process where exogenous pigments are introduced into the dermis and epidermis. Tattoos consist of thousands of particles of tattoo pigment suspended in the skin. While normal human growth and healing processes will remove small foreign particles from the skin, tattoo pigment particles are permanent because they are too big to be removed. Such pigment can be introduced into the skin intentionally to decorate or mark the skin, or as a result of accidents and trauma. Tattoos can broadly be divided into professional, amateur, cosmetic, traumatic, or medical tattoos depending on who performs the tattooing or what the intent of the tattoo is for.

- Professional tattoos are applied with a tattoo machine into the deeper layer of the dermis, and are intended to be permanent in nature. The pigments are generally darker, deeper, and often require repeated treatments to remove
- Amateur tattoos are usually smaller using diluted pigments with lighter colors applied more superficially in the epidermis or upper dermis, often with hand held needles or homemade machines, which are generally easier to remove[5]
- Cosmetic tattoos are often referred to as permanent makeup, and are increasingly popular. Permanent eyeliners, eyebrows, and lip liners are examples. The cosmetic pigments are commonly applied using micropigmentation technique to save time (of having to apply cosmetics daily) and enhance facial features. These cosmetic pigments often contain pigments which are red, brown, white, or flesh colored (containing titanium dioxide and iron oxide)[6] which are difficult to remove
- Traumatic tattoos are deposited in the skin following abrasion, laceration, or explosive injuries. Such pressurized penetration of dark particles into the deep

dermis give rise to black or blue tattoos, depending on the type and depth of the pigment.[7] Tattoos have also been used in the field of medicine, from corneal tattooing, and radiotherapy field marking to medical alert tattoos, where tattoos etched into skin replaces medical alert jewellery for the purpose of alerting medical personnel during emergency situations.[8]

TATTOO REMOVAL

Before the introduction of selective photothermolysis, removal of unwanted tattoos is carried out by physical destruction and removal of the tattooed epidermis and dermis including full thickness dermabrasion, salabrasion, chemical destruction, cryosurgery, electrosurgery, and surgical excision.[9-11] Such nonselective destructive modalities often result in incomplete removal, and varying degrees of scarring and dyspigmentation. The introduction of selective photothermolysis,[12] which targets specific chromophores (tattoo pigments) has enabled dermatologists to remove tattoos fully or partially. Various wavelengths of light energy can be used to target different colored pigments more effectively with much less complications than before.

Q-switched lasers with very short pulsed width (in nanoseconds) have long been the traditional workhorse for the removal of tattoos. The laser treatment of tattoos is based on the concept of selective photothermolysis, where laser light of different wavelengths is preferentially absorbed by different chromophores. If the target chromophore is heated for no longer than its thermal relaxation time (time required for target to lose 50% of its heat), selective destruction of these chromophores can be achieved.[12] In the case of tattoos, the chromophore is exogenously placed ink, which is found in membrane bound granules in macrophages, fibroblasts, or mast cells.[13] Such tattoo pigment is very small, and can reach its thermal relaxation time very quickly. Rapid heating with very short pulse durations, in the nanosecond or picosecond range is, therefore, required to cause photoacoustic injury and rupture of these pigment-containing cells. Laser treatment causes tattoo pigment particles to heat up and fragment into smaller pieces. These smaller pieces are then removed by normal body processes by phagocytosis and the tattoo fragments are packaged for lymphatic drainage and further scavenged by dermal macrophages, fibroblasts, and mast cells, leading to lightening of the tattoo.

Patient Evaluation and Pretreatment Counseling

A thorough history and examination are essential in establishing the type of tattoo and the skin type of patient prior to treatment. Previous oral isotretinoin treatment, systemic gold therapy, herpes infection, keloidal tendencies, and sun exposure habits should be enquired as additional precautionary measures may be needed. Standardized digital photography is helpful in recording the baseline appearance, and any subsequent improvement. The patient's treatment objective and expectation should be counseled, and treatment options, expected outcome, potential risks, downtime, and postoperative care discussed. There should be adequate opportunity for patients to have all their questions answered. Obtaining informed consent with a clear outline of risks and benefits prior to tattoo removal is essential and protects both the clinician and patient. Establishing realistic patient expectations through good rapport is helpful in achieving a satisfactory outcome.

Number of Treatment Sessions Needed for Laser Tattoo Removal

Multiple laser treatments are usually required to remove a tattoo via selective photothermolysis. An average number of seven to ten treatments are often needed. Kirby et al. published a scale (Table 1) to better help clinicians estimate the number of treatment sessions needed, which can be a useful aid during patient counseling.[14] In the scale, numerical values are assigned to six parameters—Fitzpatrick skin phototype, location, color, amount of ink used in tattoo, scarring or tissue change, and ink layering. Parameter scores can then be added up to give a combined score that will show the approximate number of treatment sessions needed for successful tattoo removal, plus or minus 2.5.

Typically, laser treatment sessions are spaced at least 8 weeks apart. Treating more frequently than 8 weeks increases the risk of adverse effects and does not necessarily accelerate the rate of tattoo ink removal. Anecdotal reports of treatments sessions at 4 weeks leads to more scarring and dyschromia. At each session, some but not all of the tattoo pigment particles are effectively fragmented, and the body removes the smallest fragments over the course of several weeks. The result is that the tattoo is lightened over time.

TABLE 1: Kirby-Desai Scale for estimating number of treatment sessions needed for tattoo removal*

Phototype	Location	Color	Ink amount	Scarring	Layering
1 point	Head and neck—1 point	Black only—1 point	Amateur—1 point	No scar—0 points	None—0 points
2 points	Upper trunk—2 points	Mostly black with some red—2 points	Minimal—2 points	Minimal—1 point	Layering—2 points
3 points	Lower trunk—3 points	Mostly black and red with some other colors—3 points	Moderate—3 points	Moderate—3 points	–
4 points	Proximal extremity—4 points	Multiple colors—4 points	Significant—4 points	Significant—5 points	–
5 points	Distal extremity—5 points	–	–	–	–
6 points	–	–	–	–	–

*The points for each column can be added up for individual tattoos to arrive at the estimated number of treatment sessions needed for laser removal, plus or minus 2.5.

The number of sessions and spacing between treatments depends on several parameters, including the tattoo color, area of the body treated, skin color, and the type of lasers wavelengths and pulse width used. Tattoos located on the extremities and on bony surfaces such as the ankle, generally take longest to clear and are often associated with textural changes post-treatment. As tattoos fade, clinicians may recommend that patients wait many months between treatments to facilitate ink resolution and minimize side effects.

Patient Preparation

The area to be treated should be cleansed thoroughly and free from any residual cosmetics or skin care products with sterile noninflammable solution, e.g., normal saline. Avoid using potentially flammable cleansing agents such as isopropyl alcohol.

Pain Management during Laser Tattoo Removal

Laser tattoo removal is uncomfortable and often worse than the tattooing procedure. The pain is often described to be similar to "snapping" from an elastic band. Most patients will require topical and sometimes local anesthesia. Topical anesthetic cream, e.g., 5% lidocaine cream and 2.5% lidocaine and 2.5% prilocaine cream is applied under occlusion for 45–90 minutes prior to the laser treatment. The topical anesthetics should be completely removed prior to treatment. Other methods of reducing discomfort for the patient include the use of cool air during treatment.

Occasionally, local anesthesia or regional nerve block or a combination of both may be necessary to abrogate the pain completely using 1–2% lidocaine.

Personnel Protection

All medical personnel in the laser room must wear wavelength-specific protective goggles during the laser procedure. The patient must also be provided with protective goggles or external metal eye shields. If the area treated is on the eyelid or near the orbit, intraocular metal eye shields should be applied to the cornea or conjunctiva for the patient.

Test Patch

In darkly pigmented patients or those with unfamiliar multicolored pigments or those at risk of developing burns or postinflammatory hyperpigmentation, test spots can be carried out and evaluated at 4–6 weeks for efficacy and side effects. Test spots should be considered for cosmetic tattoos where paradoxical darkening is likely to be encountered.[6] When performing test spots, always start with a low fluence. Similarly, when treating dark tattoos, always start with lower fluence than the normal therapeutic fluence.

Laser Treatment

The desired endpoint of Q-switched laser treatment [neodymium doped yttrium-aluminium-garnet (Nd:YAG), alexandrite, or ruby] is immediate tissue whitening, although this may not occur if the tattoo has faded significantly. Such whitening can last approximately 20 minutes, and is a result of rapid heating of the chromophore leading to gas bubble formation.[15] The optimal fluence is the lowest possible setting that elicits this endpoint in order to minimize the risk of thermal injury, such as blister formation and scarring. A low starting fluence should be used to attain this desired endpoint during initial tattoo treatment especially when treating dark and densely pigmented tattoos. The fluence can be increased as the tattoo becomes lighter. Different wavelengths of laser can be used, depending on tattoo color treated, previous response to laser treatment, and also skin phototype of the patient. Laser spots (3–4 mm spot sizes are used usually) are applied with approximately 10–20% overlap, aiming for immediate whitening, and minimizing pinpoint bleeding. Laser treatments can be repeated approximately every 8 weeks.

Post-treatment Concerns

Patients should be advised on wound care to the laser treated sites. Immediately postlaser treatment, patients should expect the treated area to become red and swollen and painful. Cold compresses can be used to minimize any discomfort. Antibiotic ointment or simple ointment-based emollients can be applied for 10–14 days after. Patients should be counseled that blisters and crusting may occur. If large blisters occur, these can be pricked with a sterile needle and dressed. Prevention of secondary bacterial infection is important to prevent morbidity and scarring. Patients should be taught sterile techniques of dressing the laser wound till complete healing has occurred. Possible longer term adverse effects such as scarring, hyper- or hypopigmentation, and color change of tattoo pigment should also be discussed with patients.

Selection of Types of Lasers

The Q-switched ruby laser (694 nm) was the first commercially available Q-switched laser for tattoo removal in 1983,[16] followed by Q-switched Nd:YAG laser (532 nm, 1,064 nm) and Q-switched alexandrite laser (755 nm). These are all still used today in dermatology practices. The tattoo color and patient skin type should be taken into consideration when selecting the appropriate laser for tattoo removal. A summary of the different lasers used for treating different tattoo colors are shown in table 2.

- Q-switched frequency-doubled Nd:YAG: 532 nm creates a green light which is highly absorbed by red and orange targets. It is used for removing red and orange tattoo pigments. As this wavelength is highly absorbed by melanin, there is an increased risk of superficial burns. In addition, such a short wavelength only allows superficial penetration of the laser beam up to the upper dermis rendering it ineffective for deeper dermal pigments
- Q-switched ruby: 694 nm laser creates a red light which is highly absorbed by green and dark tattoo pigments. Because it is more highly absorbed by melanin this laser may produce undesirable side effects such as pigmentary changes for patients of all but white skin. This is the best wavelength for blue ink. Post-treatment burn and blisters followed by hypopigmentation is not uncommon if used on darkly pigmented skin.
- Q-switched alexandrite: 755 nm emits a red light which is highly absorbed by green and dark tattoo pigments. However, the alexandrite laser color is slightly less absorbed by melanin, so this laser has a slightly lower incidence of unwanted pigmentary changes than a ruby laser. This laser works well on green tattoos but because of its weaker peak power it works only moderately well on black and blue ink
- Q-switched Nd:YAG 1,064 nm: this laser creates a near-infrared light (invisible to humans) which is poorly absorbed by melanin, making this the only laser suitable for darker skin type. This laser wavelength is also absorbed by all dark tattoo pigments and is the safest wavelength to use on the tissue due to the low melanin absorption and low hemoglobin absorption. This is the wavelength of choice for tattoo removal in darker skin types and for black ink.

TABLE 2: Tattoo pigment response to different laser wavelengths (tick indicate positive response)

Q-switched laser	Black	Blue	Green	Red	Orange	Purple
Ruby 694 nm	√	√	√			√
Alexandrite 755 nm	√	√	√			
Nd:YAG 1,064 nm	√	√				
Nd:YAG 532 nm				√	√	

Nd:YAG, neodymium doped yttrium-aluminium-garnet

Laser Treatment Parameters for Tattoo Removal

Laser pulse width or pulse duration is a critical laser parameter. All Q-switched lasers have nanosecond pulse width, which is the appropriate pulse width for tattoo removal. Lasers with shorter pulse widths are a safer and more efficient removal method because the peak power of the pulse is greater and has less photothermal effects.

Spot size of the laser beam also affects treatment. Light is optically scattered in the skin. Larger spot sizes slightly increase the effective penetration depth of the laser light, thus enabling more effective targeting of deeper tattoo pigments. Larger spot sizes also help make treatments faster.

Fluence or energy density is another important consideration. Fluence is measured in joules per square centimeter (J/cm^2). It is important to be treated at high enough settings to fragment tattoo particles.

Repetition rate helps make treatments faster but is not associated with any treatment effect.

TATTOO COLOR AND TREATMENT RESPONSE

Certain pigment colors are more difficult to remove than others. Hence, the choice of laser type (wavelength) is particularly important in ensuring efficacy. If you look at green ink in particular, some have postulated that the reason for slow resolution is due to the molecular size of the green ink particles being significantly smaller than other colours.[17] Consequently, green ink tattoos response best with 755 nm light but they may also respond to 694 nm, 650 nm, and 1,064 nm. Multiple wavelengths of light may be needed to remove multicolored tattoo inks (Fig. 1).

Blue or Black Tattoos

Darkly pigmented black or blue tattoos can be effectively treated by Q-switched ruby, Q-switched Nd:YAG (1,064 nm) or Q-switched alexandrite laser.[18,19] Leuenberger et al. compared the three different lasers and found that Q-switched ruby laser showed more significant tattoo clearing after four to six treatments compared to the Q-switched Nd:YAG and Q-switched alexandrite laser. The authors attributed it to the use of a larger spot size in the Q-switched ruby laser, which would afford greater depth of thermal injury to the targeted chromophore. The smaller spot sizes used in the Q-switched Nd:YAG and Q-switched alexandrite lasers may have led to more scatter and more rapid decrease in fluence, and hence less effectiveness. Treatment with Q-switched ruby laser, however, resulted in the highest incidence of hypopigmentation (38% for ruby, 0% for Nd:YAG and 2% for alexandrite, respectively) in the Asian study cohort. This is due to increased absorption by epidermal melanin at this shorter wavelength, and their

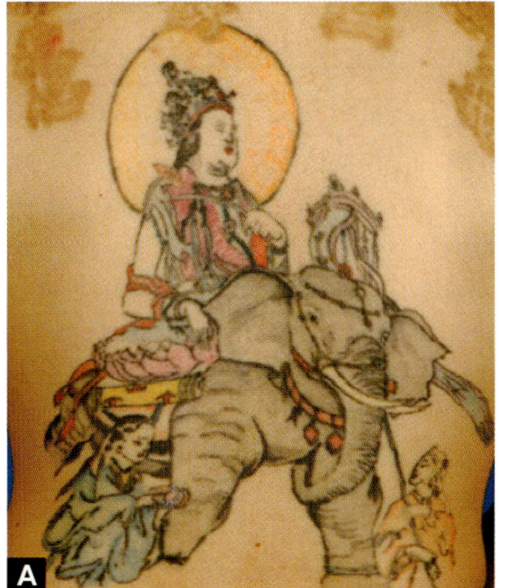

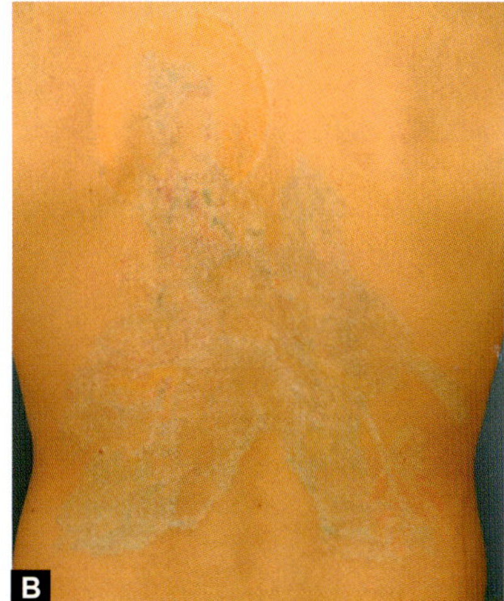

FIG. 1: Difficult to treat multicolored tattoo on back before and 30 treatments with Q-switched neodymium doped yttrium-aluminium-garnet 1,064 nm, 532 nm, and Q-switched alexandrite 755 nm lasers. Note good clearance after multiple treatment and hypopigmentation from the laser treatment in skin type IV patient.

Photo courtesy: National Skin Centre, Singapore.

resultant destruction. Treatment with the longer 1,064 nm wavelength results in minimal absorption by epidermal melanin and allows light to penetrate greater than 2 mm in skin, making it ideal for the treatment of dermal chromophores such as tattoo pigments.[18] In darker skin types where there is heavy epidermal melanin content, the Nd:YAG 1064 nm laser is the laser of choice to reduce the risks of postinflammatory hyper and hypopigmentation.[20] The importance of a homogenous beam profile and large spot size in attaining better tattoo removal was further highlighted in another study by Karsai et al.[21]

Jones et al. carried out a study on 8 skin type VI patients with 15 amateur tattoos treated with the 1,064 nm Q-switched Nd:YAG laser at 8 week intervals. Eight of the 15 tattoos were rated as 75–95% cleared, and 5 tattoos 50% cleared after an average of 3–4 treatments. Only two of the tattoos were associated with slight lightening of the skin. None of the other tattoos had any pigmentary or textural changes.[20] Lapidoth et al. treated 404 Ethiopian patients (skin types V and VI) with blue or black tattoos with the 1,064 nm Q-switched Nd:YAG (380 patients) or Q-switched ruby laser (24 patients), and reported a clearance of 75–100% in 92% of patients after three to six laser treatments (average 3.6) at intervals of at least 8 weeks. Most of these tattoos were carbon based and located on the face or neck. Transient mild hyperpigmentation lasting 2–4 months was noted in 44% of patients and mild textural changes in two patients. There were no cases of scarring or permanent pigmentary changes.[22]

Q-switched alexandrite laser has also been found to be safe and effective for tattoo removal in darker skin types. Burkhari et al. treated 20 Arabic women with skin type III-IV and achieved more than 95% lightening in five patients, and more than 75% lightening in 10 patients. These patients were given three to six treatments at 6–12 weeks intervals. Pinpoint bleeding was observed in one case but no pigmentary alteration or scarring was seen.[23]

Red Tattoos

The light emitted from the 1,064 nm Q-switched Nd:YAG laser may be frequency doubled to produce light with a wavelength of 532 nm. Red, orange, and red-brown pigments respond well to this wavelength.[19,24] Studies comparing the Q-switched 532 nm Nd:YAG have also found it to be superior to the Q-switched ruby and Q-switched 1,064 nm Nd:YAG in the removal of red colors in professional tattoos.[25,26]

Green Tattoos

Both the Q-switched alexandrite and Q-switched ruby laser are effective for the treatment of green tattoos, although the Q-switched alexandrite laser is considered the modality of choice.[19,24] Q-switched alexandrite can, therefore, be used effectively for the treatment of black, blue, or green tattoos. In addition to black, blue, and green tattoos, Q-switched ruby also works well for purple and violet pigments.[19]

Light Colored Tattoos

Cosmetic tattoos or pale colored tattoos can be more difficult to treat as they often contain red, brown, flesh-colored, and white pigment inks which may contain iron oxides and titanium dioxide, which may irreversibly turn black after Q-switched laser irradiation (Fig. 2).[27] Chemical reduction of ferric to ferrous oxide is thought to be responsible for such a phenomenon. Such paradoxical darkening has been successfully treated with further Q-switched laser treatments, sometimes requiring up to 20 sessions.[28,29] Ablative laser resurfacing with pulsed CO_2 and Er:YAG lasers have also been successfully used in cosmetic tattoos.[30,31]

Figures 3 to 5 demonstrate lightening of different colored tattoos with different laser wavelengths. Q-switched Nd:YAG lasers are effective for the treatment of black (with the 1,064 nm wavelength) and red tattoos (with frequency doubled 532 nm wavelength). Multicolored tattoos are more resistant to treatment.

COMPLICATIONS OF LASER TATTOO REMOVAL

It is important to highlight the potential side effects of tattoo removal to patients. Patients should be counseled that tattoo clearance is often incomplete and a residual tattoo outline and textural changes may often be seen. An online questionnaire with 157 participants post-tattoo removal showed that only 38% achieved complete tattoo removal.[32]

Immediate local reactions following tattoo removal occurred in 97% of participants. Melanin in the epidermis especially in darker skin types can compete for the absorption of laser light intended for tattoo removal. This can cause destruction of the melanin containing cells and manifest as burn, blistering (Fig. 6), erythema, edema, crusting, and pain.

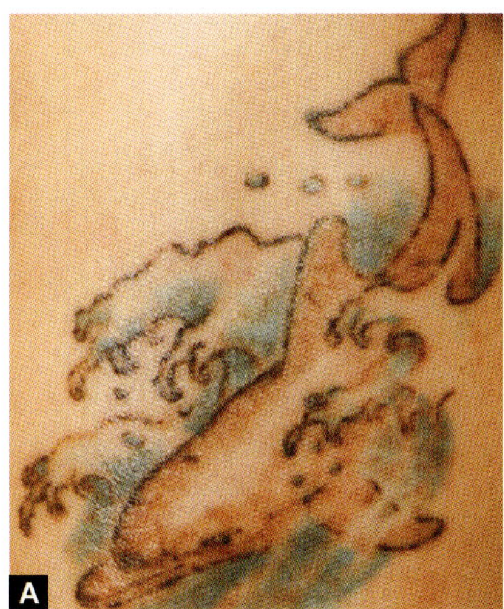
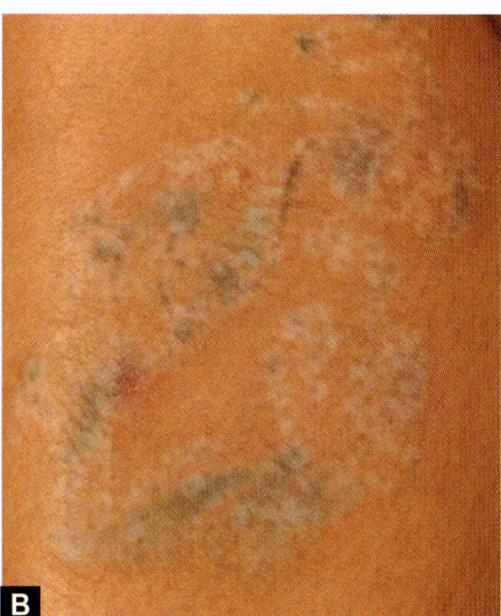

FIG. 2: Multicolored tattoo partially removed with the Q-switched neodymium doped yttrium-aluminium-garnet laser. Note the persistence of green pigment removed with the Q-switched alexandrite 755 nm laser and hypopigmentation commonly seen in darker skin type as complications of Q-switched laser treatment
Photo courtesy: National Skin Centre, Singapore.

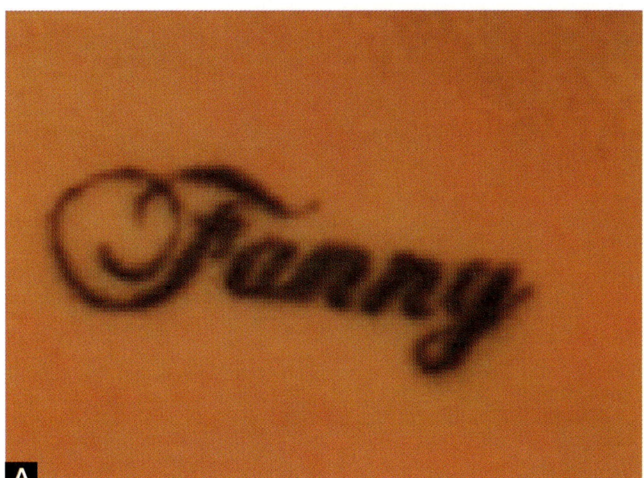

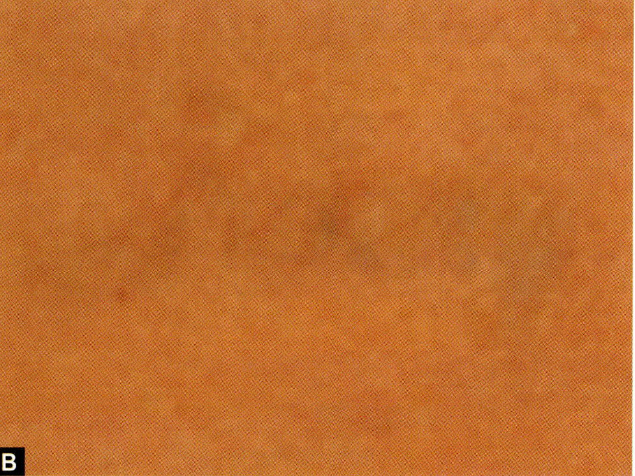

FIG. 3: Dark blue tattoo readily removed with the Q-switched neodymium doped yttrium-aluminium-garnet laser 1,064 nm after 6 treatments.
Photo courtesy: National Skin Centre, Singapore.

Late complications include hyperpigmentation, hypopigmentation (Figs 1, 2, and 7), scarring, and color change of tattoo pigment (Fig. 8). Patients with darker skin type are at a higher risk of complications.[15] Twice daily treatment with topical hydroquinones and broad-spectrum sunscreens usually resolve the hyperpigmentation within a few months, although, in some patients, resolution can be prolonged.[23] Strict sun protection measures must be emphasized to all patients to prevent postinflammary hyperpigmentation. Treatment with longer wavelengths lasers such as the Q-switched Nd:YAG (1,064 nm) in patients with darker skin type and those with a tan can reduce the risk of complications. Hyperpigmentation is related to the patient's skin type with skin types IV, V, and VI more prone regardless of the wavelength used.

Transient textural changes are often noted but may resolve after a few months; however, permanent textural changes and scarring may occur. If a patient is prone to pigmentary or textural changes, lower treatment fluence and longer treatment intervals resulting in more treatment

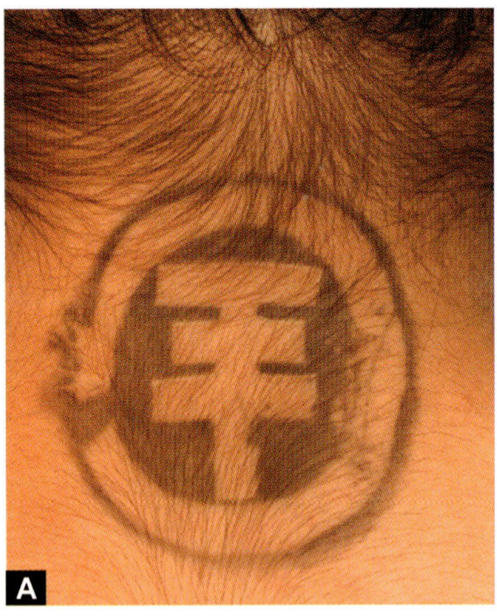
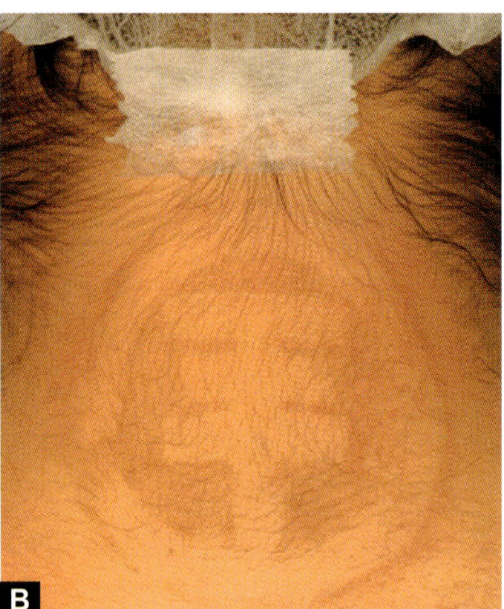

FIG. 4: Black amateur tattoo on nape of neck before and after two treatments with 1,064 nm Q-switched neodymium doped yttrium-aluminium-garnet laser
Photo courtesy: National Skin Centre, Singapore.

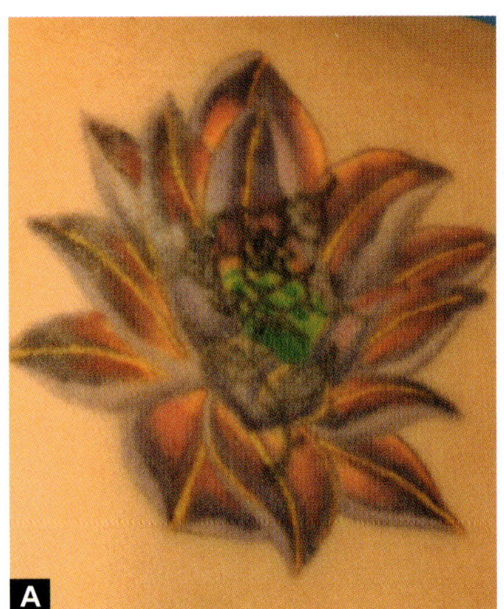
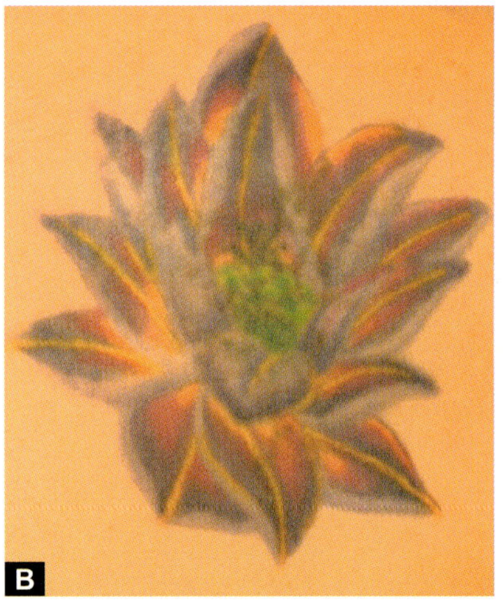

FIG. 5: Difficult to treat multicolored tattoo on back before and after 4 treatments with 755 nm Q-switched alexandrite laser. Note the poor clearance of tattoo pigment in multicolored tattoos.
Photo courtesy: National Skin Centre, Singapore.

sessions are recommended. Additionally, patients with a history of hypertrophic or keloidal scarring need to be warned of their increased risk of scarring.

Local allergic responses to tattoo pigments have been reported, and allergic reactions to tattoo pigment after Q-switched laser treatment are also possible. Photoallergic reactions may occur, when yellow cadmium sulfide is used to "brighten" the red or yellow portion of a tattoo. Such reactions may also be seen with red tattoo ink, which may contain cinnabar (mercuric sulfide). Erythema, pruritus, and even inflamed nodules, verrucous papules, or granulomas may manifest in tattoos as a result of an allergic reaction.

NEW STRATEGIES IN TATTOO REMOVAL

A novel method for laser tattoo removal using a fractionated CO_2 or Er:YAG laser, alone or in combination with Q-switched lasers was reported by Ibrahimi and coworkers from the Wellman Center of Photomedicine at the Massachusetts General Hospital.[33] This new approach to laser tattoo removal may afford the ability to remove

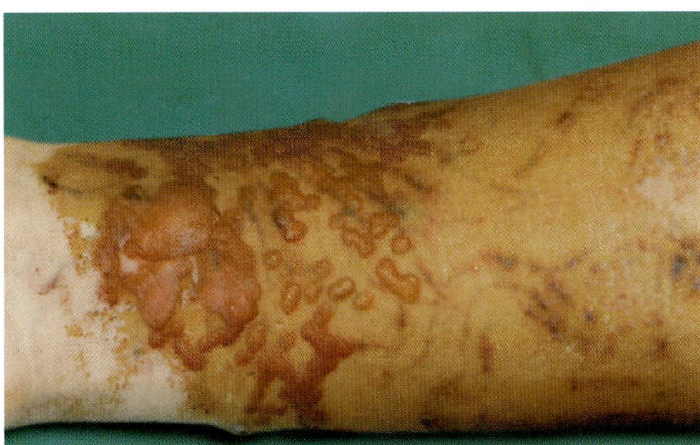

FIG. 6: Blistering eruptions from Q-switched neodymium doped yttrium-aluminium-garnet laser removal of tattoo, may occur especially in dark skin type

Photo courtesy: National Skin Centre, Singapore.

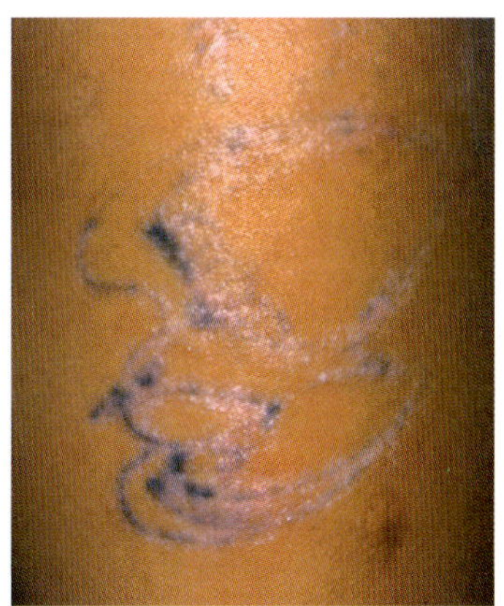

FIG. 7: Hypopigmentation following multiple Q-switched neodymium doped yttrium-aluminium-garnet laser treatment for tattoo removal, a common complications in dark skin type

Photo courtesy: National Skin Centre, Singapore.

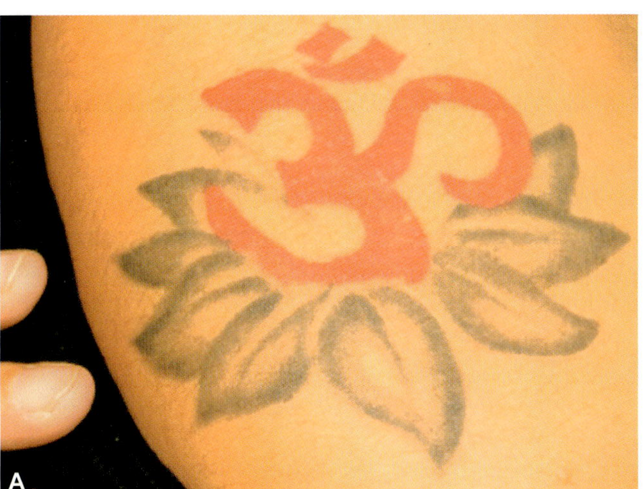

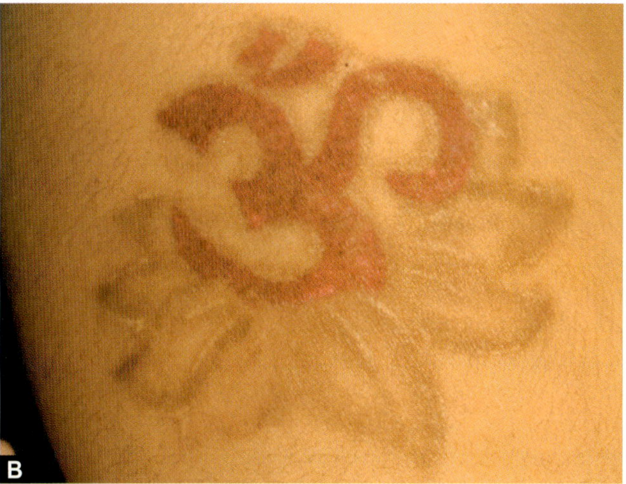

FIG. 8: Red and black tattoo on right deltoid before and after four treatments with 532 nm and 1,064 nm Q-switched neodymium doped yttrium-aluminium-garnet laser. Note the darkening of the red pigment postlaser treatment

Photo courtesy: National Skin Centre, Singapore.

colors such as yellow and white, which have proven to be resistant to traditional Q-switched laser therapy.

Combination Laser Treatment

Nonablative or ablative fractional resurfacing has been reported to be effective for tattoo removal, when combined with Q-switched ruby laser treatment, or as monotherapy.[34,35] It appears to enhance pigment clearance, prevent blistering, shorten recovery, and diminish treatment induced hypopigmentation.[32] It has also been reported to be effective for the treatment of traumatic, allergic, and multicolored tattoos.[33,35] Animal models with cosmetic tattoos treated with nonablative and ablative fractional lasers have demonstrated tattoo pigments in the microscopic coagulation zones migrating to the epidermis and becoming part of the microscopic exudative necrotic debris that can be exfoliated after 5 days.[36,37] Such fractional resurfacing can be combined with the traditional Q-switched lasers for a synergistic effect.

Multipass Treatments

The use of multipass treatments to reduce the number of treatment sessions has been explored. Kossida et al. first described the R20 method of tattoo removal, where accelerated lightening can be achieved by using four laser passes in one treatment session, with an interval of 20 minutes between the passes.[38] The 20 minutes waiting time allows for the postlaser immediate whitening to resolve completely before a second pass is given. The authors hypothesize that such repeated passes allow for treatment of pigment in successively deeper layers of the dermis. One patient developed transient hypopigmentation. Reddy et al. then demonstrated that application of topical perfluorodecalin prior to Q-switched laser treatment allows for immediate treatment of the tattoo with repeated passes, thereby improving results while decreasing overall treatment time (R0 method).[39] Topical perfluorodecalin is a highly gas soluble liquid fluorocarbon that can resolve the whitening reaction within seconds. These studies reported superior tattoo clearance with both the R20 and R0 methods compared to traditional single pass laser treatment.

Picosecond Lasers

The first commercially available picosecond laser was launched in 2013 and recently published studies have confirmed its efficacy. Saedi et al. reported 12 patients with darkly pigmented tattoos who completed treatment with the 755 nm picosecond alexandrite laser obtaining greater than 75% clearance. Nine of the patients obtained 75% clearance after just two to four treatments.[42] Brauer et al. also reported rapid and successful treatment with the picosecond alexandrite laser for multicolored or recalcitrant tattoos. Seventy five percent clearance of 12 blue or green tattoos was obtained after one or two treatments, with more than two-thirds of these tattoos approaching 100% clearance.[43]

A recently presented but unpublished study by Tanghetti and Tanghetti demonstrated significant tattoo clearing in 17 patients using the picosecond 755 nm alexandrite laser at fluences in the 1.3–2.0 J/cm^2 range. Gradual dose escalation of fluence based on previous responses, skin type, tanning, and melanin index increased safety by minimizing downtime and blistering. They noted that blue and green inks are often eliminated in one treatment.[44] Kilmer and Custis treated 26 tattoos with a picosecond laser, treating each half with R20 or single pass treatment. After one session, the mulitpass R20 method showed a 3.4-fold improvement from baseline, compared to 2.1-fold improvement with the single pass treatment. They concluded that the R20 method may further improve the efficacy of the new picosecond laser technology.[45]

Microencapsulated Tattoo Ink

Kitzman previously presented his unpublished data on microencapsulated tattoo ink. Such designer inks are made by microencapsulation of water soluble dye in polymethylmethacrylate beads. Removal can then be accomplished by targeting the encapsulating shell instead of more extensive disruption of the entire pigment particle. Preclinical studies in hairless rats and guinea pigs showed significantly increased ease of removal. One laser treatment effectively removed 80% of tattoo intensity, while only 20% of conventional ink was removed in a single identical laser treatment.[46] Further studies are needed to establish the safety and efficacy of such microencapsulated tattoo inks in human clinical studies.

CONCLUSION

As the trend for tattoo acquisition increases, the demand for tattoo removal will similarly rise. The Q-switched ruby, alexandrite, and Nd:YAG lasers are established armamentarium against blue, black, red, and green tattoos with varying degrees of effectiveness. Other colors can be challenging to treat, although outcomes using fractional resurfacing and picosecond lasers are promising. Multipass treatments and picosecond technology are new strategies for faster and more effective removal of tattoo pigments. Regulation of tattoo inks and pigments can help ensure safe application and ease of removal but are currently lacking.

REFERENCES

1. Laumann AE, Derick AJ. Tattoos and body piercings in the United States: a national data set. J Am Acad Dermatol. 2006;55(3):413-21.
2. Harris Interactive. One in five US adults now has a tattoo. [online]. Available from: http://www.harrisinteractive.com/NewsRoom/HarrisPolls/tabid/447/ctl/ReadCustom%20Default/mid/1508/ArticleId/970/Default.aspx. [Accessed February, 2016].
3. American Society for Dermatologic Surgery.Unwanted tattoos. [online]. Available from: https://www.asds.net/TattooRemovalInformation.aspx [Accessed February, 2016].
4. Armstrong ML, Roberts AE, Koch JR, Saunders JC, Owen DC, Anderson RR. Motivation for contemporary tattoo removal: a shift in identity. Arch Dermatol. 2008;144(7):879-84
5. Alster TS. Q-switched alexandrite laser treatment (755 nm) of professional and amateur tattoos. J Am Acad Dermatol. 1995;33(1):69-73.
6. Ortiz AE, Alster TS. Rising concern over cosmetic tattoos. Dermatol Surg. 2012;38(3):424-9.
7. Moreno-Arias GA, Casals-Andreu M, Camps-Fresneda A. Use of Q-switched alexandrite laser (755 nm, 100 nsec) for removal of traumatic tattoo of different origins. Lasers Surg Med. 1999;25(5):445-50.

8. Kluger N, Aldasouqi S. A new purpose for tattoos: medical alert tattoos. Presse Med. 2013;42(2):134-7.
9. McDowell F. Plastic surgery: removal of commercial tattoos of the skin. West J Med. 1976;125(2):143.
10. Dvir E, Hirshowitz B. Tattoo removal by cryosurgery. Plast Reconstr Surg. 1980;66(3):373-9.
11. Groot DW, Arlette JP, Johnston PA. Comparison of the infrared coagulator and the carbon dioxide laser in the removal of decorative tattoos. J Am Acad Dermatol. 1986;15(3):518-22.
12. Anderson R, Parrish J. Selective photothermolysis: precise microsurgery by selective absorption of pulsed radiation. Science. 1983;220(4596):524-7.
13. Taylor CR, Anderson RR, Gange W, Michaud NA, Flotte TJ. Light and electron microscopic analysis of tattoos by Q-switched ruby laser. J Invest Dermatol. 1991; 97(1):131-6.
14. Kirby W, Desai A, Desai T, Kartono F, Geeta P. The Kirby-Desai Scale: A Proposed Scale to Assess Tattoo-removal Treatments. J Clin Aesthet Dermatol. 2009;2(3):32-7.
15. Taylor CR, Gange RW, Dover JS, Flotte TJ, Gonzalez E, Michaud N, et al. Treatment of tattoos by Q-switched ruby laser. A dose-response study. Arch Dermatol. 1990;126(7):893-9.
16. Reid WH, McLeod PJ, Ritchie A, Ferguson-Pell M. Q-switched Ruby laser treatment of black tattoos. Br J Plast Surg. 1983; 36(4):455-9.
17. Siomos K, Bailey RT, Cruickshank FR, Murphy M. Q-switched laser removal of tattoos: a clinical and spectroscopic investigation of the mechanism. Proc SPIE. 1996;40:2623.
18. Leuenberger ML, Mulas MW, Hata TR, Goldman MP, Fitzpatrick RE, Grevelink JM. Comparison of the Q-switched alexandrite, Nd:YAG, and ruby lasers in treating blue-black tattoos. Dermatol Surg. 1999;25(1):10-4.
19. Zelickson BD, Mehregan DA, Zarrin AA, Coles C, Hartwig P, Olson S, et al. Clinical, histologic, and ultrastructural evaluation of tattoos treated with three laser systems. Lasers Surg Med. 1994;15(4):364-72.
20. Jones A, Roddey P, Orengo I, Rosen T. The Q-switched ND: YAG laser effectively treats tattoos in darkly pigmented skin. Dermatol Surg. 1996;22(12):999-1001.
21. Karsai S, Pfirrmann G, Hammes S, Raulin C. Treatment of resistant tattoos using a new generation Q-switched Nd:YAG laser: influence of beam profile and spot size on clearance success. Lasers Surg Med. 2008;40(2): 139-45.
22. Lapidoth M, Aharonowitz G. Tattoo removal among Ethiopian Jews in Israel: tradition faces technology. J Am Acad Dermatol. 51(6):906-9.
23. Bukhari IA. Removal of amateur blue-black tattoos in Arabic women of skin type (III-IV) with Q-switched alexandrite laser. J Cosmet Dermatol. 2005;4(2):107-10.
24. Guedes R, Leite L. Removal of orange eyebrow tattoo in a single session with the Q-switched Nd:YAG 532-nm laser. Lasers Med Sci. 2010;25(3):465-6.
25. Levine VJ, Geronemus RG. Tattoo removal with the Q-switched ruby laser and the Q-switched Nd:YAG laser: a comparative study. Cutis. 1995;55(5): 291-6.
26. Ferguson JE, August PJ. Evaluation of the Nd/YAG laser for treatment of amateur and professional tattoos. Br J Dermatol 1996;135(4):586-91.
27. Anderson RR, Geronemus R, Kilmer SL, Farinelli W, Fitzpatrick RE. Cosmetic tattoo ink darkening. A complication of Q-switched and pulsed-laser treatment. Arch Dermatol. 1993;129(8):1010-4.
28. Fitzpatrick RE, Lupton JR. Successful treatment of treatment-resistant laser-induced pigment darkening of a cosmetic tattoo. Lasers Surg Med. 2000;27(4):358-61.
29. Kirby W, Kaur RR, Desai A. Paradoxical darkening and removal of pink tattoo ink. J Cosmet Dermatol. 2010;9(2):149-51.
30. Mafong EA, Kauvar AN, Geronemus RG. Surgical pearl: removal of cosmetic lip-liner tattoo with the pulsed carbon dioxide laser. J Am Acad Dermatol. 2003;48(2):271-2.
31. Wang CC, Huang CL, Yang AH, Chen CK, Lee SC, Leu FJ. Comparison of two Q-switched lasers and a short-pulse erbium-doped yttrium aluminum garnet laser for treatment of cosmetic tattoos containing titanium and iron in an animal model. Dermatol Surg. 2010;36(11):1656-63.
32. Klein A, Rittmann I, Hiller KA, Landthaler M, Bäumler W. An internet-based survey on characteristics of laser tattoo removal and associated side effects. Lasers Med Sci. 2014;29(2):729-38.
33. Ibrahimi OA, Syed Z, Sakamoto FH, Avram MM, Anderson RR. Treatment of tattoo allergy with ablative fractional resurfacing: a novel paradigm for tattoo removal. J Am Acad Dermatol. 2011;64(6):1111-4.
34. Weiss ET, Geronemus RG. Combining fractional resurfacing and Q-switched ruby laser for tattoo removal. Dermatol Surg. 2011;37(1):97-9.
35. Seitz AT, Grunewald S, Wagner J, Simon JC, Paasch U. Fractional CO2-laser are as effective as Q-switched ruby laser for the initial treatment of a traumatic tattoo. J Cosmet Laser Ther. 2014;16(6):303-5.
36. Wang CC, Huang CL, Lee SC, Sue YM, Leu FJ. Treatment of cosmetic tattoos with non-ablative fractional laser in an animal model: a novel method with histopathologic evidence. Lasers Surg Med. 2013;45(2):116-22.
37. Wang CC, Huang CL, Sue YM, Lee SC, Leu FJ. Treatment of cosmetic tattoos using carbon dioxide ablative fractional resurfacing in an animal model: a novel method confirmed histopathologically. Dermatol Surg. 2013;39(4):571-7.
38. Kossida T, Rigopoulos D, Katsambas A, Anderson RR. Optimal tattoo removal in a single laser session based on the method of repeated exposures. J Am Acad Dermatol. 2012;66(2):271-7.
39. Reddy KK, Brauer JA, Anolik R, Bernstein L, Brightman L, Hale E, et al. Topical perfluorodecalin resolves immediate whitening reactions and allows rapid effective multiple pass treatment of tattoos. Lasers Surg Med. 2013;45(2):76-80.
40. Ross V, Naseef G, Lin G, Kelly M, Michaud N, Flotte TJ, et al. Comparison of responses of tattoos to picosecond and nanosecond Q-switched neodymium: YAG lasers. Arch Dermatol. 1998;134(2):167-71.
41. Izikson L, Farinelli W, Sakamoto F, Tannous Z, Anderson RR. Safety and effectiveness of black tattoo clearance in a pig model after a single treatment with a novel 758 nm 500 picosecond laser: a pilot study. Lasers Surg Med. 2010;42(7):640-6.
42. Saedi N, Metelitsa A, Petrell K, Arndt KA, Dover JS. Treatment of tattoos with a picosecond alexandrite laser: a prospective trial. Arch Dermatol. 2012;148(12):1360-3.
43. Brauer JA, Reddy KK, Anolik R, Weiss ET, Karen JK, Hale EK, et al. Successful and rapid treatment of blue and green tattoo pigment with a novel picosecond laser. Arch Dermatol. 2012;148(7):820-3.
44. Tanghetti EA, Tanghetti M. Dose optimization with a picosecond 755 nm alexandrite laser for tattoo removal. 34thAmerican Society for Laser Medicine and Surgery (ASLMS) annual conference. Phoenix: Arizona; 2014.
45. Kilmer S, Custis T. Single vs repeat exposure tattoo removal during single sessions with picosecond pulse duration laser technology. 34th American Society for Laser Medicine and Surgery (ASLMS) annual conference. Phoenix: Arizona; 2014.
46. Klitzman B. Development of permanent but removable tattoos. First international conference on tattoo safety. Berlin: BfR-Symposium; 2013.

CHAPTER 18

Laser and Light Treatment of Acne

Shehnaz Z Arsiwala

INTRODUCTION

Acne has a multifactorial and complex etiology making therapies a challenge. Multimodality approach with oral topical retinoid and hormonal therapies constitutes the main framework of treating acne. Partial remission, incompliance, and adverse effects of medical therapies often increase demands of safe and fast therapies, especially, interventional therapies for acne.

Interventional procedures comprising chemical peels and laser and light based devices constitute adjunctive treatments for acne and have gained some importance in the recent years. Recent literature evidences focus on laser and light devices to benefit of acne, though data is insufficient to conclude that the optical systems can be used as monotherapy and are often recommended in combination with medical modalities to facilitate longer resolution of existing acne lesions.

Multiple laser and light based devices are now evidenced to improve acne, and certain short duration studies report promising improvement up to 50–70%. However, standardization of parameters, frequencies, and settings need to be optimized. This chapter gives and insight into rationale, efficacy, and limitations of laser and light based devices for acne with a comprehensive literature review.

The available laser and light based devices for targeting acne are known to function either by targeting the *Propionibacerium acne* or by targeting the sebaceous glands. The mechanism of action of this is not exactly known. The regulatory approval process for devices is less stringent than drugs so a large number of devices are commercially available to reduce acne. However, both safety and efficacy requires clinical expertize and studies and regulatory approvals do not mean efficacy and safety, especially, in dark skin types. Treating acne which is multifactorial with intrinsic and extrinsic triggering influences is a challenge as the squeal includes pigmentary changes, so caution needs to be exerted in selection of right wavelength, fluence, parameters, and number of sessions while treating acne with these devices.

RATIONALE FOR LASERS AND LIGHT THERAPIES IN ACNE

Rationale for using an optical or laser based device for acne may include facilitate faster clearance of acne lesions, reduce inflammation and prevent precursor lesions and always used as an adjunct to medical therapy or in cases where patient cannot use or tolerate medical therapies.

The mechanisms by which optical devices can act on acne are described as photomechanical, photothermal, or combination of both. Ultraviolet (UV) light and visible (blue) light kill the bacterium and/or sebaceous cells through activated mechanisms of endogenous porphyrins and in turn cause a reduction in acne lesions.[1,2] Porphyrins produced by *P. acne* are light sensitive and absorb light between 400 and 700 nm wavelengths, this evokes porphyrins excitation. A study by freedman shows lights combined with medical treatments speed up acne clearance and prevents microcomedones.[3] Thus, the visible light, specific narrow band light, intense pulse light, pulse dye laser, and photodynamic therapy (PDT) with or without photosensitizing agents are absorbed by either the *P. acnes* or by the sebaceous glands or both and are useful to reduce acne (Table 1).

Propionibacerium acne is known to produce porphyrins protoporphyrin, uroporphyrin, and copro-porphyrin III which are light sensitive and are responsible for inflammatory acne.[4,5]

TABLE 1: Action of lasers on *Propionibacerium acne*

Devices tragetting *P. acnes*	• UVA/UVB, blue light, blue/red light combination • Narrowband light sources, IPL devices (broadband light), KTP lasers (532 nm), PDLs (585–595 nm), and various orange/red light lasers or light sources (610–635 nm)
Devices targetting sebaceus glands	• ALA and photodynamic therapy • Infrared lasers (1,320–1,540 nm), long pulsed/quasi-Nd:YAG lasers (1,064 nm)
Devices targetting both *P. acnes* and sebaceus glands	• Pulsed dye laser *P acnes*/sebaceaous gland • KTP laser *P acnes*/sebaceous gland

UVA, ultraviolet light A; UVB, ultraviolet light B; IPL, intense pulsed light; KTP, potassium-titanyl-phosphate; PDLs, pulsed dye lasers; ALA, aminolevulinic acid; Nd:YAG, neodymium doped yttrium-aluminium-garnet.

The porphyrins can absorb visible spectrum of light between 400 and 700 nm also called as the soret band, which includes the red light (630 nm) and blue light (415 nm). The porphyrin compound is excited by light absorption, releasing single oxygen and reactive free radicals. The free radicals damage the *P. acne* cell membrane, thus causing bacterial lyses, improving acne lesions (Fig. 1). In addition, light may also have action on inflammatory cytokines and help to bring down inflammation may affect *Propionibacerium acnes*. *Propionibacerium acnes* has affinity for narrowband light sources, intense pulsed light (IPL) devices (broadband light), potassium-titanyl-phosphate lasers (532 nm), pulsed dye laser (PDLs) (585–595 nm), and various orange or red light lasers or light sources (610–635 nm). Shorter wavelengths peak absorption by porphyrins whereas longer wavelengths are less effective.[4,6]

Photosensitizing agents with PDT to lyse *P. acne* add interesting dimension to therapies with optical systems (Figs 2–4). Optical devices that lyse *P. acne* often need to be combined with topical agents like retinoids that inhibit and alleviate precursor lesions and comedones since with monotherapy using lasers and lights for acne relapses are a rule. Relapse occurs soon after cessation and clearance to whatever degree needs to be maintained with topical therapy.

Enhancing bacterial lysis can be achieved by usage of concurrent photosensitizing agents like 5-aminolevulinic acid (ALA) and indocyanine green (ICG) and has paved way for concept of PDT.[7]

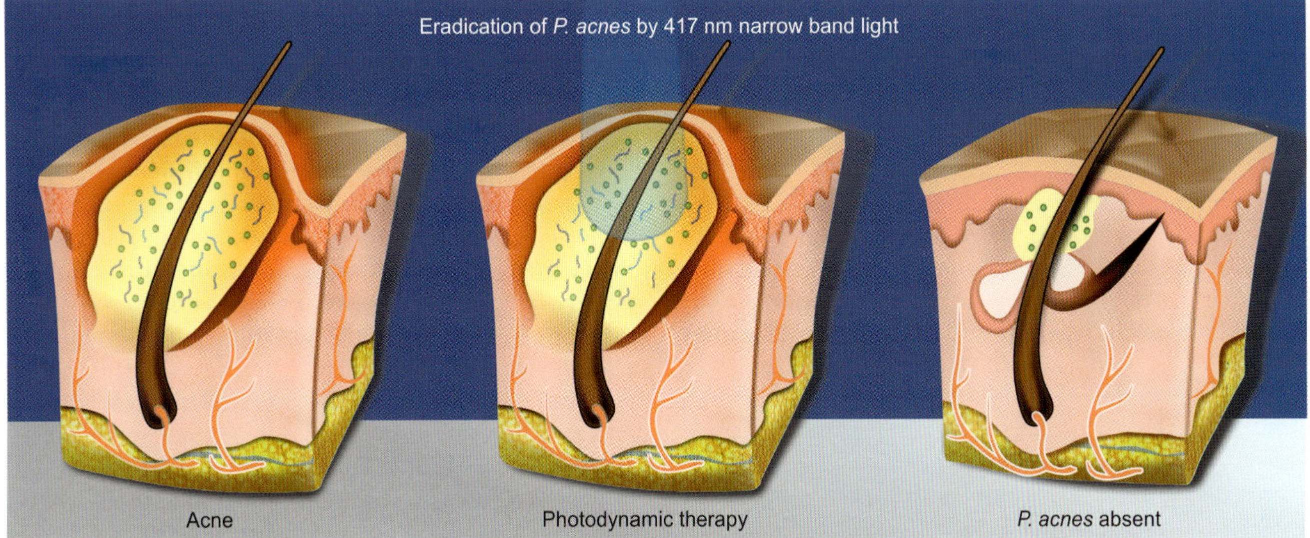

FIG. 1: Action of light device on *P. acnes*

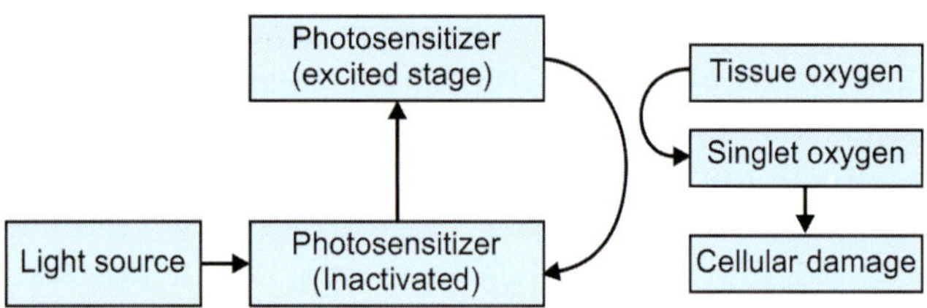

FIG. 2: Cellular damage by light source in presence of photosensitizer

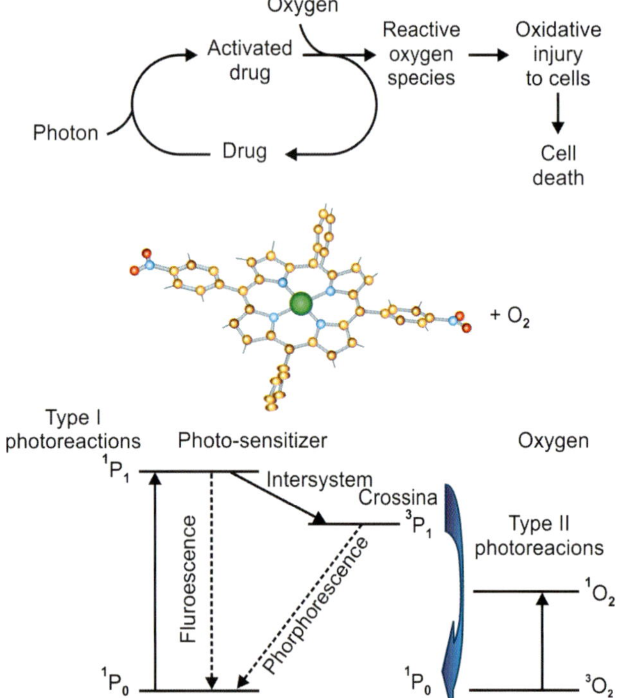

FIG. 3: Photoreactions with photosensitizers

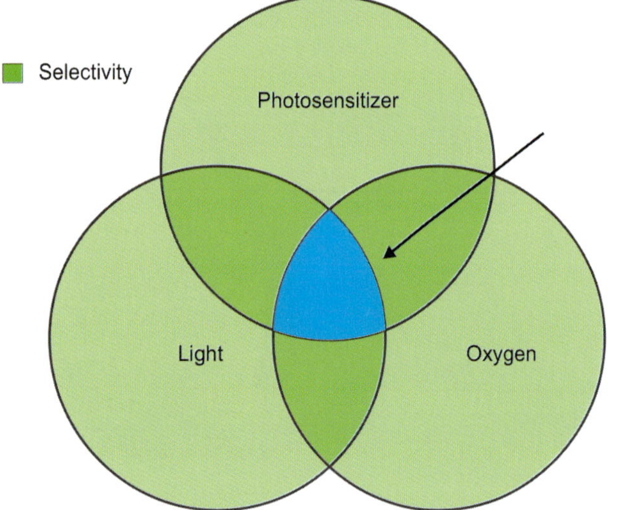

FIG. 4: Interaction of photosensitizer with light sources

Agents like ALA markedly reduce viability of *P. acnes in vitro* as shown by Ashkenazi et al.[8] On contrary some reports also indicate no effect on *P. acnes* after PDT therapy.[9] Transient reduction, however, in *P. acne* colonies have been reported with single application of methyl aminolevulinate (MAL) or hexyl aminolevulinate plus light by Yung et al., found that a PDT may have a mechanism of action in acne other than eradication of *P. acnes* and may be bacterostatic and antimicrobial effect as demonstrated in vitro but not in vivo.[10] Thus, light devices for *P. acne* may be useful only while they are used.

According to global alliance update, laser and light therapy may not be very useful for dark skin type cases as the UV penetration is partly filtered by melanin. Further Asian patients tend to reflect postinflammatory hyperpigmentation after topical ALA-PDT treatment secondary to accumulation of protoporphyrin in the epidermis. However, a few case reports and studies have reported clearance of acne in dark skin types with optical devices.[11]

DISRUPTION OF SEBACEOUS GLAND FUNCTION

Thermal destruction of sebocytes and sebaceous glands by optical devices is another concept used for clearing up acne lesions and may be a transient phenomenon.

Damaging the sebocytes, elimination of sebum, or reduction of sebum excretion are various means by which the free oxygen radicals generated by application of photosensitizers may work and more studies are required. Concerns regarding thermal sebolysis include detriment to normal skin function if destruction is permanent and pain during the procedure often limit the application of these systems.[12]

The 810 diode laser can cause selective necrosis of sebaceous glands when used with topical photosensitizers that accumulate in the sebaceous gland like ICG. Consequent to reduced sebum excretion, a secondary reduction in *P. acne* concentrations is facilitated too.[13] Bhardwaj et al. suggest the photosensitizers with laser therapy generates destruction by both photodynamic and photothermal effects.[14]

Heat generated by long wavelength near-infrared and mid-infrared lasers (e.g., 1,320–1,540 nm) heat the sebaceous gland thus decreasing the gland output, i.e., sebum and create a thermal destruction and also target water in surrounding tissues which cannot be achieved by safe pulses which can heat the glands suboptimally. Near-infrared light 1,064 nm laser preservation of epidermis is another advantage achieved with longer wavelengths. The long wavelengths may also be associated with some pain while treating facial areas. Devices that resolve acne lesions by sebaceous gland destruction have longer duration of effect than those which target *P. acnes*. Randomized trials of infrared lasers for acne report some clearances ranging from 54–76% clearance.[3,15,16] The infrared lasers are more beneficial for inflamed lesions. No clinical trials to date have compared the devices and its long-term efficacy in a split face trial and, hence, clinical data is lacking.

EFFICACY OF VARIOUS LIGHT SOURCES FOR ACNE (TABLE 2)

Blue Light for Acne

Since porphyrins absorb optimum light at 400–420 nm, the blue light (415 nm) when used repeatedly is reported to improve acne, especially, for mild to moderate variety. The available studies use different regimens so optimal duration of exposure and number of treatments is not standardized. It is often used as an adjunct and biweekly treatments are given for a series of 8–10 sessions. Reports claim this works on inflammatory acne and often shows no effect on comedones. A session typically consists of 5–7 mins duration of exposure. The clearance achieved is comparable to topical clindamycin or benzoyl peroxide (BPO).[8,17] Blue light is best used in combination with topical therapy retinoids, BPO, and red light; combined red light and blue light have a superior effect on acne clearance as reported in literature and never used as a monotherapy.[8,18]

Since shorter absorption peaks by porphyrins are also seen at 500–700 nm, the red light is also useful similarly for acne improvement. Reports of combined blue light and red light which has absorption peak of 415–660 nm is found to be synergistically effective for inflammatory acne lesions.[19]

However, acne clearing is variable among patients and relapse rates are high after therapy discontinues. Various studies do report response to acne but with different treatment regimens thus duration of light exposure and frequency of treatments are not standardized.

A comparison of red light and blue light versus BPO reported better results with light combinations though modest.

TABLE 2: Studies on lasers and lights for acne[7,13,16,19-35]

Study, number of patients	Treatment interval	Duration of study-weeks	Response
Blue light			
Kawada et al.[20] N = 30	Biweekly	5	64% decrease acne lesions
Shalita et al.[21] N = 35	Biweekly	4	80% had significant clearance
Gold[22] N = 40	Biweekly	12	43% decrease in inflammatory lesions
Goldman et al.[23] N = 12	Biweekly	24	40% decrease in papules, 65% decrease in pustules, 62% decrease in comedones
Taub[7] N = 18	Biweekly	16	11 out of 18 patients showed 50% improvement, and 5 exhibited >75% improvement.
Green light, 532/ 1,064 nm			
Bowes et al.[24] N = 11	Weekly	12	Acne lesions decreased 35.9% (control group–11.8%), sebum excretion rate decreased by 28.1% (control group–6.4%)
Blue and red light combined, 415–660 nm			
Papageorgiou et al.[19] N = 20	Daily 15 mins	12	Combination of blue light and red light reduced inflammatory acne vulgaris lesions by 76% vs. 58% in the blue light only group

Continued

Continued

Study, number of patients	Treatment interval	Duration of study-weeks	Response
Blue light and ultraviolet A, 410–420 nm			
Meffert et al.,[25]	Weekly	10	Marked improvement in pustular acne at 10 sessions
Pulsed dye laser, 585–595 nm			
Seaton et al.[26] N = 41	Weekly	4	Acne severity score decreased from 3.9–1.9 vs. 3.6–3.5 in placebo group; 49% reduction in inflammatory lesions was seen
Orringer et al.[27] N = 40	Weekly	4	No significant difference
Intense pulsed light			
Elman et al.[28] N = 19	Biweekly	4	85% patients had >50% clearance
Dierickx[29] N = 14	2–4 weekly	6–12	72–73% clearance of inflammatory and non-inflammatory lesions
1,450 nm lasers for acne			
Paithankar et al.[16] N = 27 Acne on back	3 weeks	6–12	98% reduction
Friedman et al.[30] N = 19 Acne on face	3 weeks	9	One treatment 37% reduction after two treatments 58% and 83% after three treatments
Nd: YAG laser, 532/1,064 nm			
Hongcharu et al.[31] N = 22	Multiple	12	Moderate reduction in inflammatory lesions
ALA-PDT			
Itoh et al.[32] 695 PDL + ALA N = 1	Single	8 months	
600 nm halogen lamp + ALA			
Itoh et al.[33] N = 13	Monthly	7 months	Reduction in inflammatory lesions
ICG + diode laser, 810–900 nm			
Lloyd et al.[13] N = 22 Face and back	Monthly	6	60% reduction in inflammatory acne
Santos et al.[34] ALA + PDT, split face N = 13	Monthly	3	10 out of 13 patients showed a marked response in the ALA-IPL treated side vs. the IPL side alone after a single treatment
Rojanamatin et al.[35] ALA – PDT split face, N = 14	Monthly	3	ALA- IPL combination reported superior results

Nd:YAG, neodymium doped yttrium-aluminium-garnet; ALA, aminolevulinic acid; PDT, photodynamic therapy; PDL, pulsed dye laser; ICG, indocyanine green

Lasers for Acne (Table 2)

Lasers can benefit acne with or without photosensitizing agents.

Photosensitizing molecules when used externally along with laser or light therapies have an additive and synergistic effect constituting the photodynamic therapy PDT.

Diode Lasers

The 1,450 nm diode laser has a low level of evidence for acne imrpovement. While treatments on face showed improvement in inflammatory acne but associated with pain while therapy, study on back acne have reflected prolonged improvement for up to 24 weeks.[3]

Erythema and hyperpigmentation is an adverse effect of this laser seen more in skin of color. Optimum regimens have not been standardized due to varied results with different settings and frequencies in studies and cotherapies with topical treatment modalities. Most studies have conducted an average of 8–10 sessions weekly over 3–4 months with treatment duration of 7–15 minutes.[15,16,30]

Neodymium Doped Yttrium-aluminium -garnet Lasers

Inconclusive evidence is reported with treatment of acne lesions can be targeted by 1,320 nm neodymium doped yttrium-aluminium-garnet (Nd:YAG) laser to reduce open comedones with transient response.[27]

Qausi-long Pulse 1,064 nm Neodymium Doped Yttrium-aluminium-garnet Laser (Figs 5–11)

The high energy Nd:YAG laser treatment enables destruction of sebaceous glands as well as lysis of *P. acnes,* thus helpful for active acne lesions and also reducing seborrhea. The resultant effects show a long period of latency and treatments are best recommended softer gentle expression of acne lesions with expressor or alcohol swipes. The two randomized trials by Jung et al. and Cho et al. report clinical and histopathological benefits of combining long quasipulse diode along with Q-switched Nd:YAG assisted with topical carbon suspension added as a photodynamic agent.[36,37] The author finds great reduction in acne lesions, especially inflamed acne lesions by using quasi long pulsed Nd:YAG laser and the 595 nm wavelength in an unpublished data

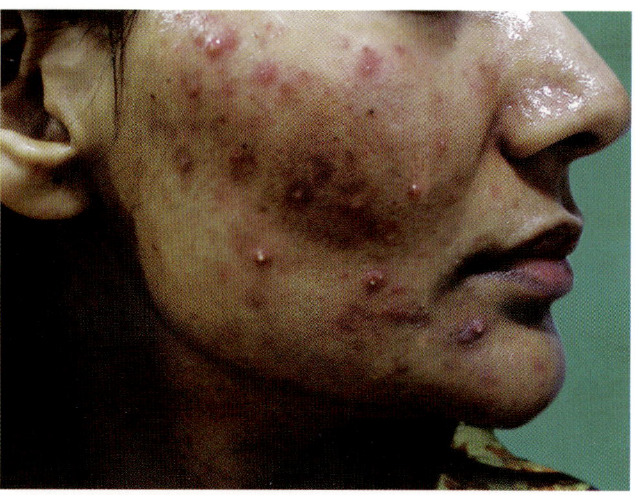

FIG. 5: Inflammatory acne—before.

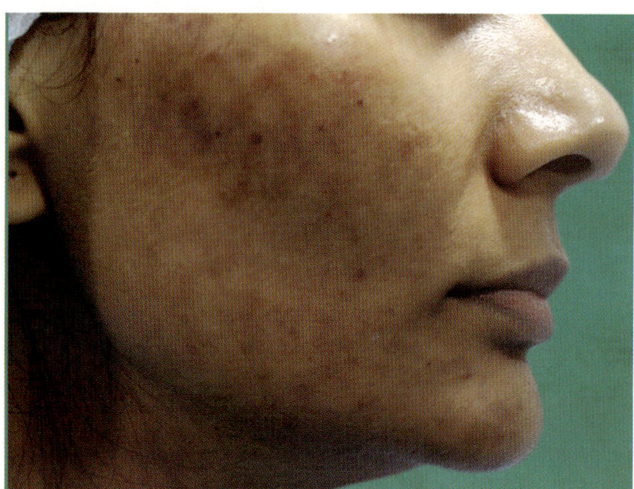

FIG. 6: Inflammatory acne—after 1,064 nm combined with 595 nm wavelength lasers

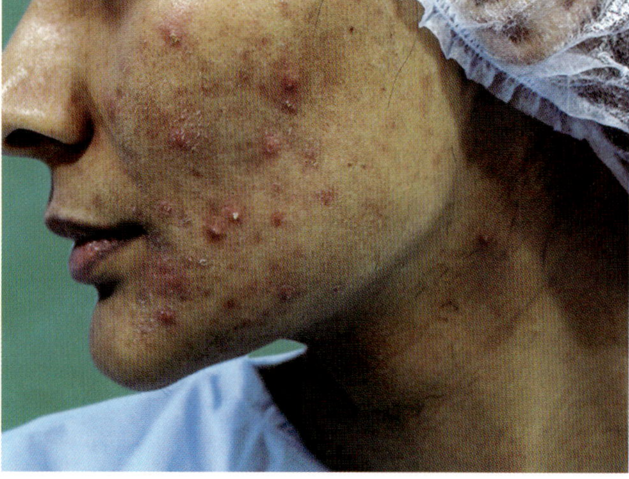

FIG. 7: Inflammatory acne

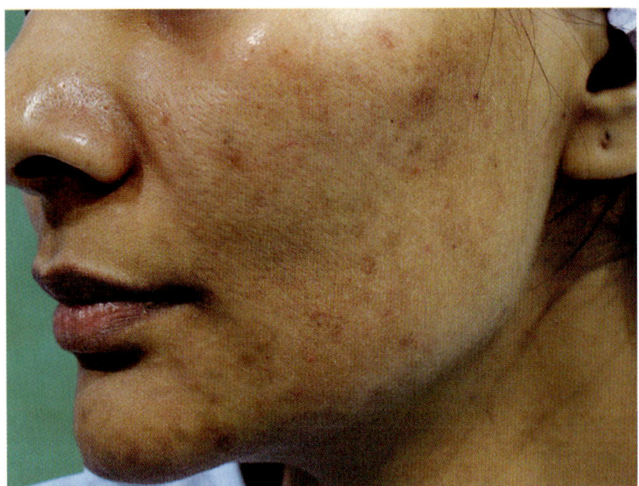

FIG. 8: Inflammatory acne—after 1,064 nm combined with 595 nm wavelength lasers

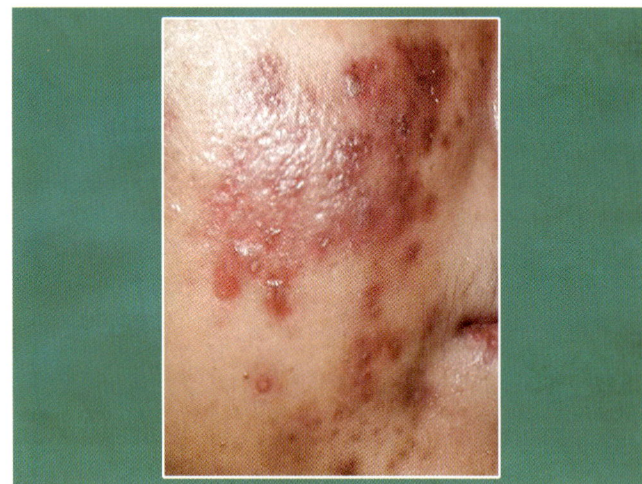

FIG. 10: Inflammatory acne—after 1064 nm combined with 595 nm wavelength lasers
Photo courtesy: Dr Swapnil Shah.

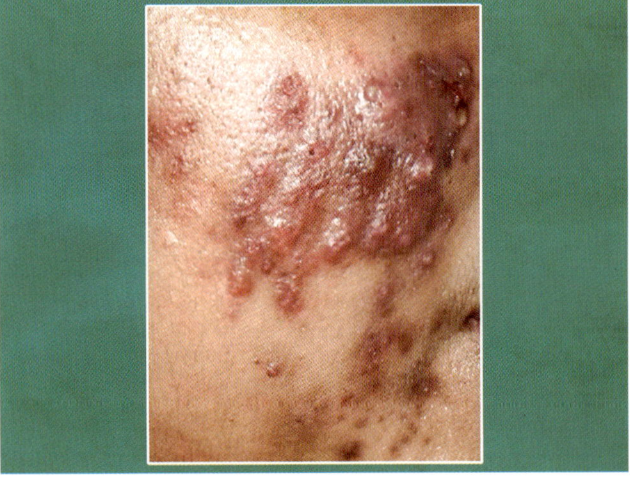

FIG. 9: Inflammatory acne
Photo courtesy: Dr Swapnil Shah.

FIG. 11: Inflammatory acne—after1064 nm combined with 595 nm wavelength lasers
Photo courtesy: Dr Swapnil Shah.

of 15 patients. Combination of these at the same sessions has synergistic effects on treatment.

Pulsed Dye Lasers

Oxyhemoglobin as a target chromophore to improve acne has been a concept studied with use of the 585 nm PDL in randomized controlled trials. Reduction of 49% in acne lesions were reported by Seaton et al., but concomitant use of BPO was a protocol of this study thus reducing its validity.[26] The studies reported mild improvement but good tolerance and minimal adverse effects in treated cases.[26,27]

Light therapy plus photosensitizers: exogenous photosensitizing agents when used in synergy with lasers and lights constitute PDT. Aminolevulinic acid, MAL, and ICG are used for PDT. They act by photochemical mechanism and they are metabolized to the porphyrins which are photoexcited by laser sources.

Blue, red, and green lights can activate ALA and convert it to protoporphyrin IX.[13,31-33] However, the hydrophilic ALA can penetrate with limited efficacy through cell membranes and interstitial spaces.[33] Thus, its esterified form MAL, which is lipophilic than ALA, is used as a photosensitizer for its better penetration in acne lesions.[34,35]

After application, 3–4 hours are required for absorption of ALA and MAL into the sebaceous glands. Photodynamic therapy is conducted with light sources of continuous waveform like IPL or PDL after this contact time. The vehicle used and contact time of application determines the accumulation of the dye in the lesions in adequate amounts.[35] This is followed by exposure to the continuous wave light sources, IPL and PDL. Multiple studies reveal acne lesions treated with PDT show decrease in severity of acne, significant decrease in *P. acne* populations, and sebum secretion compared to controls.[13,31-35] The longevity of this clearance is reported around 10 weeks after a single treatment and up to 20 weeks with multiple treatments. Pain while treatment, flare of acne, itching, erythema, edema, hyperpigmentation, and exfoliation are the reported side effects.[34] Indocyanine green dye has the ability to concentrate selectively in the sebaceous glands in a micro-emulsified form and can absorb at 800 nm wavelength making it a strong photosensitizer for PDT. Occlusion facilitates active accumulation of the dye in sebaceous glands and not only in the epidermis.[34]

While conducting PDT, the patient has to avoid sun exposure for about 48 hours afterward and thorough counseling is required.[33-35]

Further studies on the standard protocol of technique, strength, and contact time of formulations and duration of exposure of light sources are needed.

COMBINATIONS OF LASERS AND LIGHTS WITH MEDICAL THERAPIES

As is crucial to long-term management of acne, the optical interventions in acne are used as an adjuvant and need concomitant medical therapies before, during, and after laser and light therapies to induce and maintain remission of acne lesions.

The therapy comminuting topical and laser devices showed superior results in a shorter time interval than monotherapy with topical or lasers. Relapses were faster with monotherapy and maintenance of results were for more than 3 months in more than 50% patients.[3,30]

To effectively target comedones, topical retinoids and salicylic acid and cleansers are used with noticeable improvement reported in 80–90% of patients after the second treatment, with significant improvement in lesion counts after the fourth treatment (70–80% reduction in inflammatory lesions) (Box 1).[7,17,30]

Postprocedure care revolves around adequate sun protection and anti-inflammatory agents. Topical anti-comedogenic and antiacne therapies can be continued. Lightening agents form a mainstay along with sun protection to prevent and alleviate the important squeal of postacne hyperpigmentation seen more abundantly in skin of color.

Box 1: Tips for optimizing optical therapies for acne

- Medical therapy forms first line
- Optical interventions are adjuvant therapies
- Remissions may be incomplete
- Recurrence is a rule when optical interventions are used as monotherapy
- Combinations are used synergistically to optimize acne clearance
- Maintenance with topical agents are mandatory
- Inflammatory acne responds best to optical interventions
- Poor response is seen in comedogenic acne
- Multiple sessions weekly or biweekly depending on device used
- Optimum reduction may be achieved in 8-10 sessions

Complications of optical therapies for lasers are few and include pain during therapy, transient flare, postinflammatory hyperpigmentation, and generally do not limit the use of laser applications.

CONCLUSION

Optical interventions with laser and light based devices are indicated as an adjuvant therapy along with medical therapy and are sought when one seeks faster clearance of inflammatory lesions which were unresponsive to medical therapies alone. The optical interventions for acne should always be followed by maintenance with topical therapies. Broadband lights, such as blue, red, and green lights, yield good response in multiple sittings and are safe to use even in dark skin types. Combinations of red light and blue light give better clearance of acne lesions. Though evidences are limited and no standard protocols are available from the various randomized controlled trials, it is clear that the light therapies need multiple sessions to maintain the destruction of *P. acnes* and sebocytes. Treatment that target sebocytes offers better efficacy and long-term results than those which target only the bacteria. Laser based therapies work synergistically when treated with photosensitizing agents and are promising then broadband light sources in terms of efficacy and longer period of remission. However, use of laser based devices with photosensitizers has increased potential for side effects like pain while treating and allergic reactions to the dyes, which are more than seen with broadband light sources. While inflammatory acne responds adequately, the comedogenic acne shows poor response to optical interventions and, hence, need for combination with topical retinoid, BPO, or clindamycin as reflected in the studies. In dark skin types, the optical devices yield moderate results and responses to photosensitizers and absorption of light source is filtered by the high melanin content in this skin types raises potential question on their efficacy. Though some data is available on definite role of lasers and light therapies in acne, lack of standardization makes them less significant and, hence, well-designed clinical trials are required, especially in skin of color to view these as standard technologies in clinical practice.

REFERENCES

1. Haedersdal M, Togsverd-Bo K, Wulf HC. Evidence-based review of lasers, light sources and photodynamic therapy in the treatment of acne vulgaris. J Eur Acad Dermatol Venereol. 2008;22:267-78.
2. Munavalli GS, Weiss RA. Evidence for laser-and light-based treatment of acne vulgaris. Semin Cutan Med Surg. 2008;27(3):207-11.
3. Jih MH, Friedman PM , Goldberg LH, Robles M, Glaich AS, Kimyai-Asadi A. The 1450-nm diode laser for facial inflammatory acne vulgaris: dose-response and 12-month follow up study. J Am Acad Dermatol. 2006;55(1):80-7.
4. Gold MH. Efficacy of lasers and PDT for the treatment of acne vulgaris. Skin Therapy Lett. 2007;12(10):1-6.
5. Gold MH. Acne and PDT: new techniques with lasers and light sources. Lasers Med Sci. 2007;22(2):67-72.
6. Sigurdsson V, Knulst AC, van Weelden H. Phototherapy of acne vulgaris with visible light. Dermatology. 1997;194(3):256-60.
7. Taub AF. Photodynamic therapy in dermatology: history and horizons. J Drugs Dermatol. 2004;3(1 Suppl):S8-25.
8. Ashkenazi H, Malik Z, Harth Y, Nitzan Y. Eradication of Propionibacterium acnes by its endogenic porphyrins after illumination with high intensity blue light. FEMS Immunol Med Microbiol. 2003;35:17-24.
9. Hörfelt C, Funk J, Frohm-Nilsson M, Wiegleb Edström D, Wennberg AM. Topical methyl aminolevulinate photodynamic therapy for treatment of facial acne vulgaris: results of a randomized, controlled study. Br J Dermatol. 2006;155:608-13.
10. Yung A, Stables GI, Fernandez C, Williams J, Bojar RA, Goulden V. Microbiological effect of photodynamic therapy (PDT) in healthy volunteers: a comparative using methyl aminolevulinate and hexyl aminolevulinate cream. Clin Exp Dermatol. 2007;32:716-21.
11. Gollnick H, Cunliffe W, Berson D, Dreno B, Finlay A, Leyden JJ, et al. Management of acne:a report from a Global Alliance to Improve Outcomes in Acne. J Am Acad Dermatol. 2003;49(suppl):S1-37.
12. Katsambas AD, Stefanaki C, Cunliffe WJ. Guidelines for treating acne. Clin Dermatol. 2004;22:439-44.
13. Lloyd JR, Mirkov M. Selective photothermolysis of the sebaceous glands for acne treatment. Lasers Surg Med. 2002;31(2):115-20.
14. Bhardwaj SS, Rohrer TE, Arndt K. Laser and light therapy for acne vulgaris. Semin Cutan Med Surg. 2005;24:107-12.
15. Wang SQ, Counters JT, Flor ME, Zelickson BD. Treatment of inflammatory facial acne with the 1,450 nm diode laser alone versus microdermaabrasion plus the 1,450 nm laser: a randomized, split-face trial. Dermatol Surg. 2006;32:249-55.
16. Paithankar DY, Ross EV, Saleh BA, Blair MA, Graham BS. Acne treatment with a 1450 nm wavelength laser and cryogen spray cooling. Laser Surg Med. 2002;31:106-14.
17. Gold MH, Rao J, Goldman MP, Bridges TM, Bradshaw VL, Boring MM, et al. A multicenter clinical evalution of the treatment of mild to moderate inflammatory acne vulgaris of the face with visible blue light in comparison to topical 1% clindamycin antibiotic solution. J Drugs Dermatol. 2005;4:64-70.
18. Tzung TY, Wu KH, Huang ML. Blue light phototherapy in the treatment of acne. Photodermatol Photoimmunol Photomed. 2004;20:266-9.
19. Papageorgiou P, Katsambas A, Chu A. Phototherapy with blue (415 nm) and red (660 nm) light in the treatment of acne vulgaris. Br J Dermatol. 2000;142(5):973-8.
20. Kawada A, Aragane Y, Kameyama H, Sangen Y, Tezuka T. Acne phototherapy with a high-intensity, enhanced narrow-band, blue light source: an open study and in vitro investigation. J Dermatol Sci. 2002;30(2):129-35.
21. Shalita AR, Harth Y, Elman M. Acne photoclearing using a novel, high-intensity, enhanced, narrow-band, blue light source. Clin Application Notes. 2001;9(1):1-4.
22. Gold MH. The utilization of ALA-PDT and a new photoclearing device for the treatment of severe inflammatory acne vulgaris–results of an initial clinical trial. J Lasers Surg Med. 2003;15(S):46.
23. Goldman MP, Boyce SM. A single-center study of aminolevulinic acid and 417 NM photodynamic therapy in the treatment of moderate to severe acne vulgaris. J Drugs Dermatol. 2003;2(4):393-6.
24. Bowes LE, Manstein D, Anderson RR. Effect of 532 nm KTP laser exposure on acne and sebaceous glands. Lasers Med Sci. 2003; 18(Suppl 1):S6-7.
25. Meffert H, Gaunitz K, Gutewort T, Amlong UJ. Therapy of acne with visible light: Decreased irradiation time by using a blue-light high energy lamp. Dermatol Monatsschr. 1990; 176(10):597-603.
26. Seaton ED, Charakida A, Mouser PE, Grace I, Clement RM, Chu AC. Pulsed-dye laser treatment for inflammatory acne vulgaris: randomized controlled trial. Lancet. 2003;362(9393):1347-52.
27. Orringer JS, Kang S, Hamilton T, Schumacher W, Cho S, Hammerberg C, et al. Treatment of acne vulgaris with a pulsed dye laser: a randomized controlled trial. JAMA. 2004;291(23):2834-9.
28. Elman M, Lask G. The role of pulsed light and heat energy (LHE) in acne clearance. J Cosmet Laser Ther. 2004;6(2):91-5.
29. Dierickx CC. Treatment of acne vulgaris with a variable-filtration IPL system. Lasers Surg Med. 2004;34(S16):66.
30. Friedman PM, Jih MH, Kimyai-Asadi A, Goldberg LH. Treatment of inflammatory facial acne vulgaris with the 1450-nm diode laser: a pilot study. Dermatol Surg. 2004;30:147-51.
31. Hongcharu W, Taylor CR, Chang Y, Aghassi D, Suthamjariya K, Anderson RR. Topical ALA-photodynamic therapy for the treatment of acne vulgaris. J Invest Dermatol. 2000;115(2):183-92.
32. Itoh Y, Ninomiya Y, Tajima S, Ishibashi A. Photodynamic therapy for acne vulgaris with topical 5-aminolevulinic acid. Arch Dermatol. 2000;136(9):1093-5.
33. Itoh Y, Ninomiya Y, Tajima S, Ishibashi A. Photodynamic therapy of acne vulgaris with topical delta-aminolaevulinic acid and incoherent light in Japanese patients. Br J Dermatol. 2001;144(3):575-9.
34. Santos MA, Belo VG, Santos G. Effectiveness of photodynamic therapy with topical 5-aminolevulinic acid and intense pulsed light versus intense pulsed light alone in the treatment of acne vulgaris: comparative study. Dermatol Surg. 2005;31:910-5.
35. Rojanamatin J, Choawawanich P. Treatment of inflammatory facial acne vulgaris with intense pulsed light and short contact of topical 5-aminolevulinc acid: a pilot study. Dermatol Surg. 2006;32(8):991-7.
36. Jung JY, DH Suh. Prospective randomized controlled clinical and histopathological study of acne vulgaris treated with dual mode of quasi-long pulse and Q-switched 1064-nm Nd:YAG laser assisted with topically applied carbon suspension. J Am Acad Dermatol. 2012;66:626-33.
37. Chun SI, Calderhead RG. Carbon assisted Q-switched Nd:YAG laser treatment with two different sets of pulse width parameters offers a useful treatment modality for severe inflammatory acne: a case report. Photomed Laser Surg. 2011;29:131-5.
38. Fabbrocini G, Cacciapuoti S, De Vita V, Fardella N, Pastore F, Monfrecola G. The effect of aminolevulinic acid photodynamic therapy on microcomedones and macrocomedones. Dermatology. 2009;219: 322-8.

CHAPTER 19

Principles of Vascular Lasers

Abhishek De, Manmit K Hora

INTRODUCTION

Vascular lesions were one of the first indication for which lasers were used. In 1963, Goldman used ruby, neodymium doped yttrium-aluminium-garnet (Nd:YAG), and argon lasers to treat vascular lesions like hemangioma and port wine stain at the Children's Hospital Research Foundation, Cincinnati, United States. Initially, lasers were used only for the congenital lesions but later, the indications were extended to the acquired vascular lesions also.

Vascular anomalies are one of the most common indications for laser surgeries. If not treated, vascular lesions can often result in disfiguring scars, hemorrhagic episodes and infections, apart from the severe psychological impact it can cause. The advent and evolution of vascular lasers have tremendous impact in the management of vascular lesions including hemangiomas, port wine stain, telangiectasia, erythema, rosacea, and leg veins.

The initial argon or ruby lasers though gave a satisfactory color change in many cases, these were often pledged with unacceptable high rate of complications including disfiguring scarring. With better understanding of mechanism of action through selective photothermolysis, more emphasis was given, selective destruction of target tissue and minimizing collateral damage; this led to the advent of pulsed laser.

Even though present day vascular lasers are considered effective and safe modality of treatment, it is important to follow proper guidelines and safe practices to achieve satisfactory results and to avoid any untoward reaction. This chapter focuses on the principles of vascular lasers and the guidelines for patient selection and treatment protocol required for providing safe and effective treatment.

CLASSIFICATION OF VASCULAR ANOMALIES[2]

The International Society for Study of Vascular Anomalies have classified vascular anomalies into mainly two groups: vascular tumor and malformation. Hemangiomas are vascular tumors that are rarely apparent at birth, grow rapidly during the first 6 months of life, involute with time, and do not necessarily infiltrate, but can sometimes be destructive. Vascular malformations are irregular vascular networks defined by their particular blood vessel type. In contrast to hemangiomas, they are present at birth, slow growing, infiltrative, and destructive. Almost all vascular malformations and nearly 40% of hemangiomas eventually require intervention. Hemangiomas are categorized into two types: "infantile" and "congenital". The rare congenital hemangioma is less understood and is present since birth. Congenital hemangiomas either rapidly involute and are called rapidly involuting

TABLE 1: Difference between hemangioma and port wine stain

	Hemangioma	Port wine stain
Onset	Can be present at birth or in early infancy	Present at birth
Progression	Can be involuting or noninvoluting	Persists
Tissue marker	Glucose transporter 1 positive	Glucose transporter 1 negative

congenital hemangiomas or never involute and are called the noninvoluting congenital hemangioma. Rapidly involuting congenital hemangiomas do not require any treatment. Port wine stains are a type of capillary vascular malformations, appear as congenital pink to erythematous patches affecting 0.3–0.5% of the population. They do not resolve. There is no sex predilection, and the inheritance pattern is generally sporadic (Table 1).

PRINCIPLES OF LASERS FOR VASCULAR LESIONS

Laser Physiology

The treatment of various cutaneous lesions by lasers is based on the principle of selective photothermolysis. In 1983, Anderson and Parrish postulated that selective thermal damage can be predicted by choosing the appropriate wavelength, pulse duration, and energy for a particular target. The target chromophore of vascular lesions is the oxyhemoglobin which is present in the red blood cells in the blood vessels. Oxyhemoglobin shows three major absorption peaks at 418, 542, and 577 nm (Fig. 1). The optimal absorption being in the range of 577–600 nm.[2] The ideal pulse duration is either equal to or shorter than the thermal relaxation time of the target vessels. A pulse duration, which is too short, may not be effective and a pulse duration, which is too long, may cause increase dissipation of heat causing excess thermal damage to the surrounding tissue and therefore, may result in complications.

Once the laser is absorbed by the oxyhemoglobin, the light energy gets converted to thermal energy. This thermal energy then diffuses rapidly within the blood vessel causing photocoagulation and mechanical injury which leads to selective microvascular damage causing thrombosis of the blood vessels. This is known as the theory of selective photothermolysis. Recently, other types of hemoglobin have been recognized as possible chromophore.

Factors Involved in Vascular Laser Treatment

The factors determining the outcome of treatment, such as site, size, color and depth of the lesion, the age, the

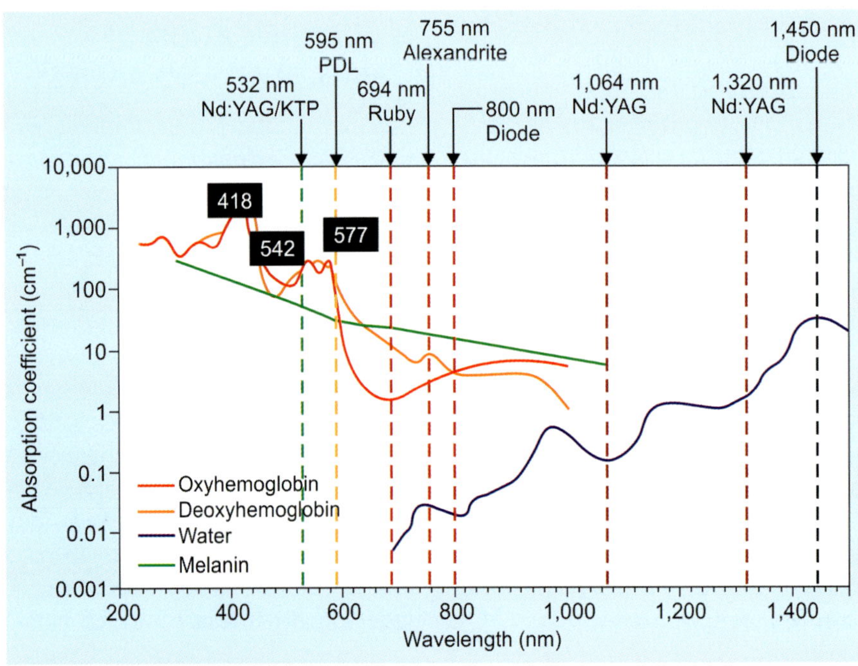

Nd:YAG: neodymium doped yttrium-aluminium-garnet; KTP, potassium titanyl phosphate; PDL, pulsed dye laser.

FIG. 1: Oxyhemoglobin has three major absorption peaks at 418, 542, and 577 nm

Box 1: Factors determining the outcome of treatment

Factors involving laser
- Wavelength of laser
- Spot size
- Fluence

Factors involving tissue
- Diameter of vessels
- Depth of vessel
- Site of lesions
- Age of patients
- Skin type

TABLE 2: Most commonly used lasers and light devices for vascular pathology

Laser	Wavelength (nm)
Potassium titanyl phosphate	532
Pulsed dye laser	585, 595
Alexandrite	755
Diode	800, 810
Long-pulsed Nd:YAG laser	1,064
Dual energy laser	595 pulsed dye laser + 1,064 Nd:YAG
Intense pulsed light	Using an appropriate filter

Nd:YAG, neodymium doped yttrium-aluminium-garnet.

Fitzpatrick skin type of the patient, and the spot size of the laser, are discussed below (Box 1).

Wavelength of Laser

Three components are essential for selective photothermolysis of vascular laser:

1. A wavelength with preferential absorption by hemoglobin
2. An appropriate pulse duration to match the target vessel size
3. A fluence with maximum efficacy and minimum collateral damage.

Pulsed dye laser (PDL), which has become available from 1986, is often considered as a gold standard of treatment. Initial PDL was at 577 nm, but soon it was understood that for selective photothermolysis to occur, the wavelength might not have to be in the exact absorption peak for oxyhemoglobin, as long as there is preferential absorption the laser would still work. Next generation PDL was shifted to much higher wavelength of 585–595 nm, achieving greater depth of penetration. With longer and variable pulse duration from 0.45 to 40 ms second generation PDLs are able to treat vascular anomalies of different diameters purpurically or sub-purpurically.[3]

Though still considered a gold standard, efficacy of PDL is often limited by its inability to penetrate a depth beyond 2 mm. So, other lasers with longer wavelength, especially alexandrite (755 nm) and long-pulsed Nd:YAG (1,064 nm) are being tried for different vascular anomalies. As absolute absorption of hemoglobin are lower for these wavelength, higher fluence is required.[4]

Nonlaser light device like intense pulsed light (IPL) are also being used increasingly using a cut off filter suiting vascular pathology. Table 2 sums up the most commonly used lasers and light devices for vascular pathology.

Spot Size

Spot size for the laser helps to control the amount of energy being delivered into the desired target. Lasers with larger spot size penetrate deeper into the tissue as they cause less scattering of energy and deliver more heat to the target tissue leading to thermocoagulation. Similarly, laser with smaller spot size cause more scattering of energy and is, therefore, not very effective in thermocoagulation of deeper vessels.[4] Also, increase in spot size may cause a dramatic increase in the amount of energy delivered to the target tissue if the fluence is not adjusted. Smaller spot sizes are recommended if in doubt, with manipulation of the fluence to achieve the desired energy at the target level.

Fluence

Fluence is defined as the energy delivered per unit area. It is measured in J/cm^2. It is important to manipulate the fluence according to the type of lesion and the area of body being treated as delivering excessive energy may lead to tissue damage. Various parameters, like vessel color, size and depth of vessel, and spot size of the laser, should be taken into account while selecting the appropriate fluence.[5] Smaller vessels absorb less energy as they have less amount of chromophore, hence, require a higher fluence. Vessels that are blue and purple require less fluence as compared to pink and red vessels, as they absorb more light energy.[6] Vessels in areas of greater intravascular pressure like that of nose or legs, require higher fluences than those with less intravascular pressure.

Diameter of Vessels

The pulse duration required depends on the diameter of the underlying vessel. Vessels with a diameter of 10–100 μm usually have a thermal relaxation time of 1–10 ms and will require a shorter pulse duration whereas vessels with a larger diameter, that is more than 100 μm will have a higher thermal relaxation time and hence, will require a longer pulse duration.[6]

Depth of Vessel

The depth of the underlying blood vessels must be taken into account while choosing the parameters for treatment. Vessels that are located superficially usually respond well to the wavelengths of 577 and 585 nm whereas the vessels lying deeper need lasers with longer wavelength usually up to 600 nm.[7] Longer the wavelength of a laser, deeper is its penetration.[6]

Site of Lesions

The response to treatment also depends on the site of location of the lesion. Lesions located on the head, neck, and upper half of the body show a good response as compared to the lesions on the lower half.[6]

Age of Patients

Children, adolescents, and young adults show a better response to treatment than the people in older age group. The earlier the lesion is treated, better is the response seen. This is due to the fact that the blood vessels are smaller and more superficially located in children and become deeper as the age advances.[6]

Skin Type

Epidermal melanin selectively absorbs the laser energy, hence, patients with darker skin types (Fitzpatrick skin type IV and V) require lasers with longer wavelength, longer pulse width, and a higher fluence as compared to the fairer skin people.[4]

Epidermal Cooling

A pre- and postoperative cooling is of utmost importance to prevent tissue damage and scarring. The epidermal melanocytes and keratinocytes tend to absorb some amount of the high light energy needed to coagulate the deeper vessels, appropriate cooling of the epidermis can protect its temperature from exceeding it threshold for thermal injury. Various methods have been used to achieve epidermal cooling. Devices, such as a cryogen spray, cool dry air blower, or cold sapphire contact handpiece that promote rapid and selective cooling, can be used.[4] While cooling may minimize epidermal damage, it paradoxically reduces the efficacy of lasers, by blanching of the underlying blood vessels.

Patient Selection and Counseling

Patient selection should be done carefully. Thorough examination and evaluation of the patient should be done before enrolling them for treatment. Patients should be counseled in detail about the nature of lesion, the different treatment options available, and their possible outcome and complications. A detailed information brochure should be provided to the patients for their understanding of the disease.

Patients who have any history of photosensitivity disorder, epilepsy, keloidal tendencies, and patients on photosensitive drug, pregnant females, and uncooperative patients with an unrealistic expectation should not be enrolled for treatment. Patients with port wine stain on the face in the distribution of V1 dermatome should be evaluated for possible glaucoma. Magnetic resonance imaging scan of the head and neck should be done in relevant cases. Doppler study of the vascular lesions should be done to rule out arterial and venous ectasia.[8]

The patient must sign an informed consent form. In case of minors, the consent should be obtained from any one of the parents. Photographs of the lesions should be taken on each session to compare the treatment outcome.

Preoperative Anesthesia

Laser treatment causes mild discomfort rather than pain. Most of the patients usually tolerate the discomfort well. Anesthesia may be required in patients who are apprehensive and also in children.

General anesthesia can be considered in children who are having large lesions and those who are very uncooperative. This is sometimes difficult for dermatologists as it require a huge setup. Topical anesthesia like EMLA (eutectic mixture of local anesthetics) or local anesthesia like 1% lignocaine is more convenient and is also effective in reducing the discomfort to the patient. In children below the age of 6 months, EMLA should not be used as it may get absorbed and may cause methemoglobinemia leading to cerebral hypoxemia.[8]

Preoperative Care

Broad spectrum sunscreen should be started 4 weeks prior to treatment wherever applicable. Preoperative photographs should be taken at the beginning of each session. Treating doctors should wear protective goggles provided by the laser company. Eye shield should be used to protect the patients. Cooling of the skin should be done immediate prior to starting the treatment.[9]

Postoperative Care

Postoperative epidermal cooling should be done immediately after the laser treatment. Patients should be advised to use topical antibiotic ointment for a few days at the treated site to prevent infections. Patients should continue to use broad spectrum sunscreen daily wherever applicable. The patients should avoid exercising and swimming during the healing period.[8]

INDICATIONS OF VASCULAR LASERS

Port wine stain and hemangioma are the most common anomalies that are treated with laser, however, there are many indications for vascular lasers (Box 2).[8]

The absolute and relative contraindications for vascular lasers have been listed below (Box 3).

Box 2: Indications for vascular lasers[8]

Congenital vascular lesions
- Port wine stain
- Hemangioma

Acquired vascular lesions
- Facial telangiectasia
- Rosacea
- Spider angioma
- Poikiloderma of Civatte
- Pyogenic granuloma
- Venous lakes
- Cherry angioma
- Leg telangiectasia
- Angiofibroma
- Blue rubber bleb nevus syndrome
- Cutaneous lesions of Kaposi's sarcoma

Box 3: Contraindications for vascular lasers

Absolute contraindications
- Active local infection
- Photoaggravated skin diseases and medical conditions

Relative contraindications
- Unstable vitiligo
- Psoriasis
- Keloid and keloidal tendencies
- Patient on isotretinoin

Port Wine Stain[9,10]

Port wine stain are composed of ectatic capillaries and postcapillary venules in the superficial venous plexus. Port wine stain are congenital in most cases, but may appear after birth in rare instances. Approximately 0.03% of the newborn babies are affected by port wine stain and they tend to persist throughout life and increase in thickness with time. A study showed that by 3rd–5th decade of life, majority of port wine stain become thickened and at times, nodular. Port wine stain is often complicated with soft tissue overgrowth causing functional impairment and also may cause recurrent bleeding episodes and infection. The vessel size varies considerably from 7 to 300 µm, with older lesion tending to have larger vessel diameter. Port wine stain can be associated with various syndromes, and before starting laser treatment, one should always eliminate the possibility of associated artery venous malformation.

The treatment of port wine stain with lasers effectively diminishes redness, thickness, general appearance, possibility of bleb formation, and psychosocial discomfort. Pulsed dye lasers is often considered the gold standard of treatment for port wine stain, and usually successful in improving 80% of the patients. However, only 20% of the patients show complete clearance after requisite number of sessions. Studies confirm that predictors for good response are early age of treatment, small size, and location over bony prominences. Huikeshoven et al. showed that port wine stain can redarken even after successful laser treatment, either due to revascularization happening as a result of injury or hypoxia or due to dilatation of the residual blood vessels caused by diminished autonomic supply. Treatment of port wine stain with PDL usually needs ten sessions or more at an interval of 4–6 weeks. An ideal fluence of PDL is determined by appearance of instant purpura, but higher fluence leading to confluent grey color may lead to unforgiving complications. It is always advisable to learn the best fluence by trusting the desired clinical end point rather than going by preset parameters. Use of larger spot size, lower fluence, and longer pulse duration in darker patients can save from complications like scar, postinflammatory pigmentation, and hypopigmentation.

Other lasers, which were used for port wine stain, are long-pulsed Nd:YAG, alexandrite, and IPL. Pulsed dye laser resistant port wine stain are often treated with alexandrite with good effect. Though long-pulsed Nd:YAG can also be used, and ensures deeper penetration, need good amount of expertise to minimize the chances of scarring, due to narrow safety window. An ablative laser like carbon dioxide or erbium doped yttrium-aluminium-garnet can be used to treat associated vascular nodules.

Hemangioma[11]

Infantile hemangiomas appear in the first 4 weeks of birth. It is seen in 4–10% of the neonates with a girl child being more commonly affected. Hemangioma is benign endothelial cell proliferation arising possibly as a response to tissue hypoxia. Hemangioma can be superficial (cherry red), deep (bluish), or mixed. As high as 90% of the hemangioma regress by 10th years of age, often leaving residual fibrofatty tissue, atrophy, or telangiectasia. Since majority of the hemangioma may regress, it was considered prudent to "masterly observe without intervention" as the first line of management for hemangioma. However, recent studies indicate that laser treatment can minimize scarring. Other indications for treating hemangioma are cosmetic, nondisappearances even after long observations, and possibility of functional impairment. Treatment modalities include topical corticosteroid, topical timolol, and oral propranolol. Though laser treatment as first line therapy for hemangioma is controversial, recent randomized controlled trial shows early clearance and lesser chance of scarring and atrophy with laser treatment.

For treatment of hemangiomas with PDL, pulse duration of 0.45–1.5 ms and spot size of 7–10 mm are commonly used with appropriate fluence and cooling system. Multiple sessions at the interval of 4–6 weeks are generally required for treating hemangiomas. Complications are uncommon, may include hemorrhage, ulceration, infections, and scarring. Apart from PDL, long-pulsed Nd:YAG, potassium titanyl phosphate (KTP) lasers, and IPL are used to treat hemangiomas.

Other Indications

Telangiectasia can be present in rosacea, and also in other diseases like connective tissue diseases and many genodermatoses. Lasers like PDL or KTP and IPL are commonly used, once in 3–4 months, for a good result in telangiectasia. Though purpuric fluence may be more effective, subpurpuric energy is generally recommended for the darker skin type.[12] Other vascular indications for which lasers are being extensively used are venous malformation, venous lakes, poikiloderma of Civatte, angiokeratoma, and cherry angiomas.[8]

CONCLUSION

Lasers have revolutionized the treatment of vascular malformations. Though pulsed dye laser still remained the gold standard; other lasers and light devices are also gaining popularity. The surgeon needs thorough understanding of the type of the lesion, and its expected prognosis before choosing a laser as a treatment modality.

REFERENCES

1. Tanzi EL, Lupton JR, Alster TS. Lasers in dermatology: four decades of progress. J Am Acad Dermatol. 2003;49(1):1-31.
2. Wassef M, Blei F, Adams D, Alomari A, Baselga E, Berenstein A, et al; ISSVA Board and Scientific Committee. Vascular anomalies classification: recommendations from the International Society for the Study of Vascular Anomalies. Pediatrics. 2015;136(1):e203-14.
3. Adamic M, Troilius A, Adatto M, Drosner M, Dahmane R. Vascular lasers and IPLS: guidelines for care from the European Society for Laser Dermatology. J Cosmet Laser Ther. 2007;9:113-24.
4. Garden JM, Bakus AD. Laser treatment of port-wine stains and hemangiomas. Dermatol Clin. 1997;15(3):373-83.
5. Woo WK, Handley JM. Does fluence matter in the laser treatment of port-wine stains? Clin Exp Dermatol. 2003;28:556-7.
6. Rothfleisch JE, Kosmann MK, Levine VJ, Ashinoff R. Laser treatment of congenital and acquired vascular lesions: update on lasers: a review. Dermatol Clin. 2002;20(1):1-18.
7. Nymann P, Hedelund L, Hædersdal M. Long-pulsed dye laser vs. intense pulsed light for the treatment of facial telangiectasias: A randomized controlled trial. J Eur Acad Dermatol Venereol. 2010;24(2):143-6.
8. Srinivas CR, Kumaresan M. Lasers for vascular lesions: standard guidelines of care. Indian J Dermatol Venereol Leprol. 2011;77(3):349-68.
9. Smit JM, Bauland CG, Wijnberg DS, Spauwen PH. Pulsed dye laser treatment, a review of indications and outcome based on published trials. Br J Plast Surg. 2005;58:981-7.
10. Sharma VK, Khandpur S. Efficacy of pulsed dye laser in facial port-wine stains in Indian patients. Dermatol Surg. 2007;33(5):560-6.
11. Kono T, Sakurai H, Groff WF, Chan HH, Takeuchi M, Yamaki T, et al. Comparison study of a traditional pulsed dye laser versus a long-pulsed dye laser in the treatment of early childhood hemangiomas. Lasers Surg Med. 2006;38(2):112-5.
12. Clark SM, Lanigan SW, Marks R. Laser treatment of erythema and telangiectasia associated with rosacea. Lasers Med Sci. 2002;17(1):26-33.

CHAPTER 20

Pulsed Dye Laser for Vascular Lesions

Marisa Pongprutthipan

INTRODUCTION

Since the first tunable dye laser was developed in 1966 by Schäfer and his colleagues using dye as a lasing medium, following studies showed the advantages of dye laser that demonstrated broad tuning range of wavelength up to 100 nm and wide range of applications.[1] The dye used as a lasing medium for dermatology laser is usually a liquid solution, which also provides flexibility of wavelength but degrades over time.[2] An external high energy source such as a flashlamp is needed to pump (stimulate emission) the liquid beyond its lasing threshold. The initial pulsed dye laser (PDL) for vascular lesion emitted 577 nm which corresponded to the peak absorption of oxygenated hemoglobin. Later, the available PDLs in the market deliver 585 and 595 nm for better penetration of laser and they have been combined dual wavelength 595 nm PDL with 1,064 nm neodymium doped yttrium-aluminium-garnet (Nd:YAG) laser. Nowadays, the applications of these PDLs are not limited to vascular lesions but also nonvascular indications including wound healing process.

BASIC CONCEPT AND MECHANISM OF ACTION

The principle of laser treatment in vascular lesion employs the theories of selective[3] and extended selective photothermolysis (photosclerotherapy).[4] The selective photothermolysis demonstrates the correlation between selected wavelength, well-absorbed by target chromophore (hemoglobin), appropriate pulse duration, and energy that last sufficiently enough resulting in specific damage to the target without excessive heating to the surrounding tissue. Target chromophore for vascular lesion is mainly hemoglobin. Oxygenated hemoglobin strongly absorbs visible light at 418, 542, and 577 nm. Deoxygenated hemoglobin (venous blood) selectivity is maximal at 694 nm, and significant at 595, 600, 633, and 755 nm. Methemoglobin is relatively strongly absorbed at 633 nm,[5] which corresponds to the wavelength of PDL available in the market, as shown in figure 1.

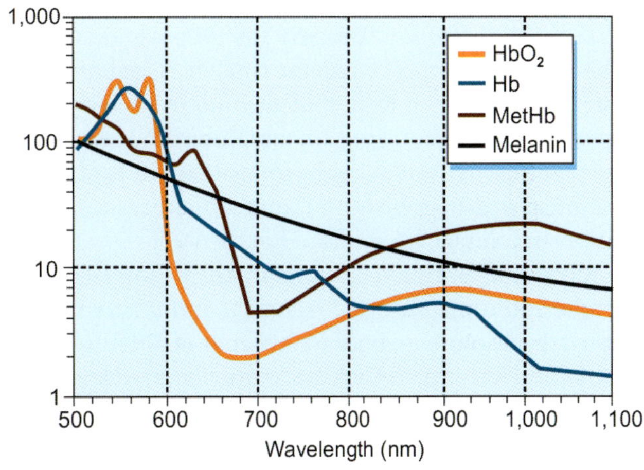

HbO_2, oxyhemoglobin; Hb, hemoglobin; MetHb, methemoglobin.

FIG. 1: Absorption coefficients for chromophores in the blood and epidermis

The initial model of PDL used 577 nm wavelength, which utilized the weaker oxyhemoglobin absorption peak to avoid melanin absorption, when compared with the other two hemoglobin absorption peaks (418 and 542 nm) where melanin absorption is still higher than oxyhemoglobin. The benefit was that the longer wavelength (577 nm) also provided deeper penetration. The wavelengths that were later selected, i.e., 585 and 595 nm are strongly absorbed by oxygenated hemoglobin and also provide deeper penetration (1.0–1.5 mm depth, mean 1.45 mm for 590 nm laser),[6] enough to reach deeper target vessels. Besides the ability to be absorbed by the hemoglobin, desired effects also depend on the appropriate heating time to damage the target. Selective photothermolysis describes the time interval required for the target to deliver 50% of heat to surrounding tissue, so called thermal relaxation time (TRT). The appropriate pulse duration to optimize thermal damage should be limited to shorter or equal to the TRT of target. Studies on port wine stains (PWS) showed that optimum permanent vessel closure can be achieved by denaturation of the endothelium (when core vessel temperature reaches 70°C) leading to coagulation of vessel wall and vessel wall necrosis,[3,7,8] despite the fact that endothelium lacks any chromophore. The extended theory of selective photothermolysis proposed photosclerosis by diffusion of energy from the heated chromophore to reach and damage the target. The time required for the outermost part of the target to be damaged from heat diffusion, leading to irreversible target damage with sparing of the surrounding tissue, is called the thermal damage time (TDT). The suggestion from this 577 nm laser study on vein is pulse width should be made shorter than or equal to the TDT while the TDT can be longer than the TRT of the target. Different laser pulse durations must take into account the blood flow and the different diameters of the vessels, shorter pulses for smaller vessel and vice versa. Altshuler et al. reported technique to success in large vessel is to blocking of the blood flow is crucial for optimum treatment with super-long pulse.[4] Pulse durations in the millisecond domain are optimal for intradermal vessel treatment. The available laser units provide pulse durations between 0.4–40 milliseconds. Study by Suthamjariya et al.[9] using 532 and 1,064 nm laser showed the sequence of vascular change at different pulse duration including coagulation, constriction, thread-like appearance (splitting and retraction of the intravascular thermal coagulum), vessel disappearance, cavitation, bubble formation, hemorrhage, and collagen damage, respectively. The inappropriately short pulse widths cause erythrocyte and water vaporization (temperature above 100°C), rapid thermal expansion, and may be followed by mechanical rupture with hemorrhage while the long pulse-widths appear to cause thermal denaturation conforming to the vessel lumen with less violent vessel damage.[9-11] The required endpoint for permanent vascular closure is immediate vessel disappearance, so the amount of energy must be sufficient to reach the target temperature to achieve this reaction. The potential for recanalization survival depends on other variables including skin pigmentation, vessel size, depth of target, and hemoglobin concentration.[9] Another factors that affect the outcomes are cooling methods and the new pulse form that provides slow heating the target. Adequate epidermal cooling, e.g., dynamic cooling device (DCD)or air-cooled, is beneficial for successful outcome, especially in the high setting, and prevent adverse events. In the new innovative mode, each pulse is divided into multiple mini-pulses or pulselets; which helps in gradually increasing the temperature to the target temperature; so that the possibility of vascular rupture is minimized but the success rate of vascular closure is increased.

The spot size also plays a role in the successful vascular therapy. Larger spot size has less scattering and more efficient delivery of the laser into the deep tissue than smaller spot size.[12] The other variable that affects the outcome is the overlapped pulses demonstrated by Dinehart et al.[13] From their study, the beam intensity decreases from the center toward the rim of the beam (Gaussian beam) explaining a rationale for the degree of overlap (18%) is essential to homogenously cover the lesion completely while still minimizing adverse reactions (Fig. 2). Table 1 illustrates the commonly used PDL systems.

CLINICAL APPLICATION

Vascular Lesions

Facial Telangiectasia and Small Vessel Disorders

Pulsed dye laser represents an excellent modalities for facial small telangiectasia and facial skin conditions which presence of telangiectasia; for example, diffuse facial erythema, rosacea, inflammatory acne, angioma serpiginosum, and discoid lupus erythematosus. New European guideline in 2015 classifies facial telangiectasia into four categories, which are:

1. Simple or linear
2. Arborizing, spider, or star
3. Punctiform
4. Papular.

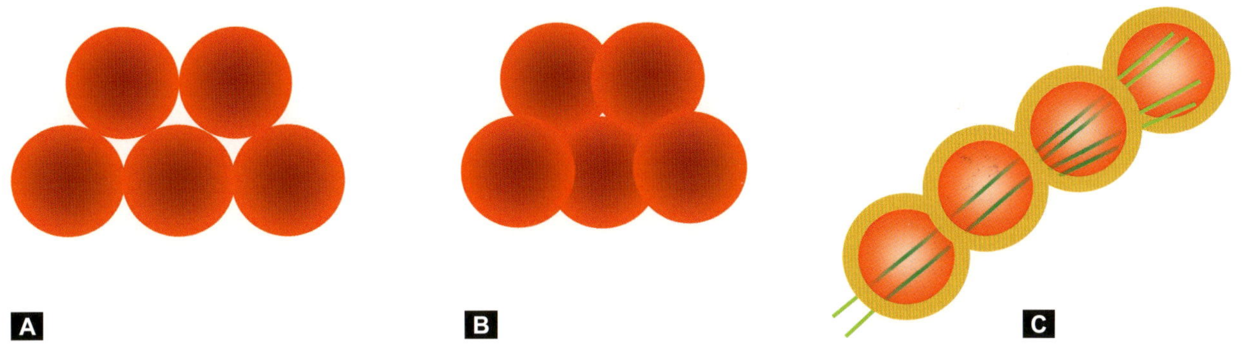

FIG. 2: **A,** 10% not treated; **B,** 18% treated twice; **C,** 18% overlapped pulse allows the least overlap while covering the lesion completely

TABLE 1: Commonly used pulsed dye laser systems

Wavelength, brand name (manufacturer)	Pulse duration	Spot size and maximum energy setting	Cooling
595 nm PDL (V-Beam Perfecta,® Syneron Candela Medical Ltd., Irvine, CA, USA)	0.45–40 ms	• 3 mm; 40 J/cm^2 • 5 mm; 30 J/cm^2 • 7 mm; 20 J/cm^2 • 10 mm; 10 J/cm^2 • 12 mm; 7 J/cm^2 • 3 x 10 mm; 25 J/cm^2 • 7 mm.PL*; 15 J/cm^2 • 10 mm.PL*; 10 J/cm^2	Dynamic cooling device
585-597 nm PDL and MultiPlex 585-597 nm + 1,064 nm Nd:YAG (Cynergy®, Cynosure, Inc., Westford, MA, USA)	0.5-40 ms (PDL) and 0.3-300 ms (1,064 nm Nd:YAG)	• PDL: ○ 5 mm; 40 J/cm^2 ○ 7 mm; 20 J/cm^2 ○ 10 mm; 10 J/cm^2 ○ 12 mm; 7 J/cm^2 • MultiPlex: ○ 7 mm; 20 J/cm^2 PDL and 160 J/cm^2 1,064 nm Nd:YAG ○ 10 mm; 10 J/cm^2 PDL and 80 J/cm^2 1,064 nm Nd:YAG	Air-cooled

*PL; pigmented lesion handpiece (compression tip).
PDL, pulsed dye laser; Nd:YAG; neodymium doped yttrium-aluminium-garnet.

Red linear and arborizing facial telangiectases are usually 0.1–1.0 mm in diameter and represent a dilate arteriole, venule, and capillary. Guidelines suggest 595 nm PDL as the first line laser treatment with evidence grade 1A.[14] The common parameter setting for the facial telangiectasia ranges from 10 to 40 milliseconds pulse width, fluence range from 8.0 to 14.5 J/cm^2 with either 10 or 7 mm spot size[15] (Fig. 3). Large veins need significantly lower fluences, power density, and longer pulse widths than small veins.[4] Madan et al. reported treatment for resistant nasal telangiectasia with 3 mm × 10 mm elliptical spot size, 40 milliseconds, 10–12 J/cm^2, double pulse, DCD open spray 30 milliseconds, and 20 milliseconds delay after laser with 80% improvement in 80% of patient without purpura.[16] Increased number of passes or stacking pulses has been reported to treat larger vessel (600–10,000 μ)[17] and sebaceous gland hyperplasia. The other new PDL model (V-beam Perfecta®, Syneron Candela Medical Ltd., USA), dividing each pulse into eight minipulses or "pulselets", has the better outcome due to multiple pulse-train technology allowing target to cool and prevent purpura when using high energy setting.[16-18] Weiss et al. demonstrated much lower temperature in the eight-pulselets comparing with one-pulse PDL in the ratio 0.2:1,[18] therefore, the new PDL model treatment endpoint aim for subpurpuric instead of purpuric change.[17] From

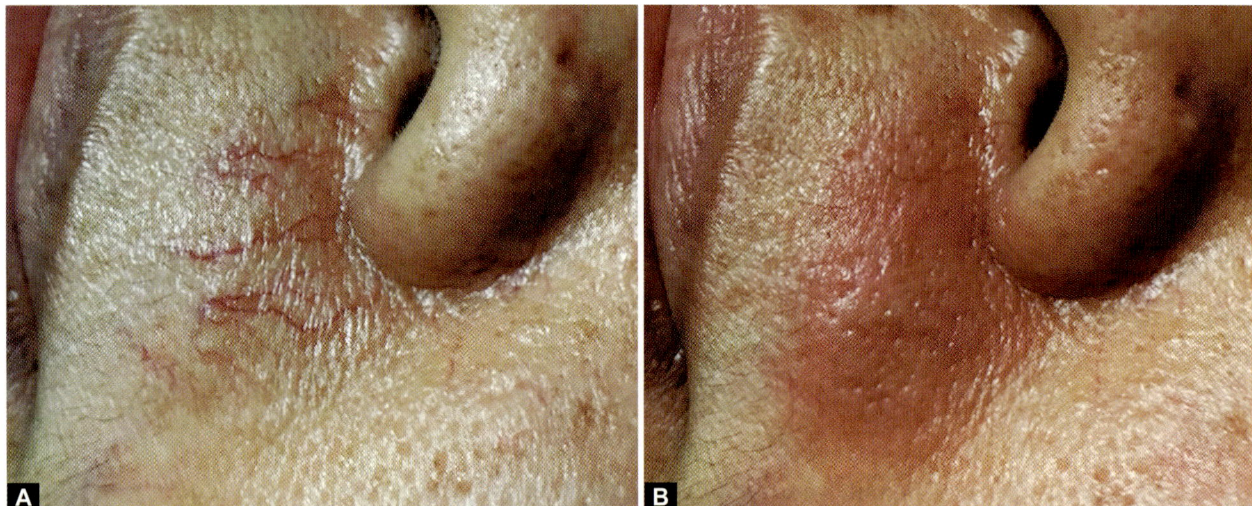

FIG. 3: Facial telangiectasia treatment with 595 nm pulsed dye laser (V-Beam Perfecta, Syneron Candela Medical Ltd., Irvine, CA, USA), with parameter setting; 7 mm spot size, pulse duration 20 ms, fluence 13 J/cm^2 with dynamic cooling device open spray 30 ms before laser and 10 ms postlaser delay. **A,** Before; **B,** immediately after laser, immediate blanching and swelling is noted.

the author experience, recurrence is between 10–20%, second treatment with different parameter setting or multiple passes will achieve further improvement.

Port Wine Stains

Port wine stain is a capillary malformation which comprise of variety of distribution (300–600 μm in depth) and sizes of blood vessels (10–150 μm) involved in individual PWS.[19] The color of PWS may determine the depth of the vessel, pink and purple vessels signify deeper lesion than red. The mean vessel diameter is also different, namely smaller diameter in pink lesions (mean 16.5 μm) and larger diameter in purple lesions (mean 51.2 μm).[20] Port wine stain is generally best treated with PDL but less than 20 μm vessels, as well as deeper vessels greater than 400 μm from dermoepidermal junction,[21] turn out to respond less to PDL than moderately enlarged vessels and more superficial vessels.[20,22,23] Poor prognostic outcome post-PDL treatment included deeper vessels, purple PWS, hypertrophic type, skin thickness relates with age,[24] and location on leg.[22,25] The face and back PWS showed to have better response to PDL.[26] In the new multivariate analysis, increased age, a newly described type III capillaroscopic pattern (combined feature of red globular structure; 0.3–0.4 mm in diameter, ectatic dermal papillary loop) and ring and arch-like (0.08–0.1 mm in diameter, horizontal deeper subpapillary vessels), and presence of lesions in dermatome V2 were all associated with a reduced clinical response to treatment.[27] Parameters used in PWS are varied, the tips for successful treatment are:

- Pulsed dye laser 585–597 nm (Cynergy®): 7 mm spot size, 2 milliseconds pulse width, 11 J/cm^2 pulse width with cold-air cooling system of level 3[23]
- Pulsed dye laser 595 nm (V-Beam Perfecta®): 7 mm spot size, 1.5–20 milliseconds pulse width and 9–11 J/cm fluence with cryogen spray cooling (DCD 30 milliseconds of cooling with a 20 milliseconds postlaser delay).[23] Since the capillary is the main structure in the PWS, the use of 1.5 milliseconds pulse width has more supporting evidence of benefit over the others[28]
- Stacking of pulses and increase, number of passes (2–3 passes) have been reported to improve resistant PWS[29]
- Multiple treatment sessions in skin of color patient increase the risk of prolong hyperpigmentation and scarring.[30] The combination of PDL with other modalities, e.g., topical sirolimus,[31] timolol gel,[32] and photodynamic therapy,[33] has been reported to improve outcome.

Leg Vein

Pulsed dye laser has some limitations from penetration depth and larger diameter of leg veins, i.e., treatment of leg veins has variable results, with PDL being usually effective.[34-36] The treatment usually showed effective against blue and red spider vein which diameter less than

0.2-1.5 mm.[34,37,38] The treatment usually need multiple passes (1-3 passes),[1-3] one to two treatment sessions with 4-8 weeks interval for vessel clearance.[34,39] The common PDL setting for treatment of leg vein are:

- Spot sizes of 7 mm, 10-40 milliseconds, and 9-25 J/cm.[2,34,39] With 1.5 milliseconds showed variable results in the studies,[35,40,41] which may be related to the variety of leg vessel diameter. Bernstein et al. suggested that 1.5 milliseconds is benefit for the vessel less than 1.5 mm diameter[40]
- Spot size of 3 × 10 mm, 40 milliseconds, and 17.5-25 J/cm^2.[34,38]

The appropriate setting for each patient is tailor-made which should vary pulse-width and spot size during the treatment course. Factors that contributed for energy setting include vessel diameter, depth, and patient skin type (most studies reported in patient skin type I-II). The benefit of the combination of PDL and 1,064 nm Nd:YAG laser is significant when applied on leg vein telangiectases in terms of the effectiveness for treating large diameter vein (2-4 mm) and deeper vein.[42] Trelles et al. reported setting of 7 mm spot size, 10 milliseconds, and 9 J/cm^2 of PDL, and pulses of 30 milliseconds and, 80 J/cm^2 of 1,064 nm Nd:YAG with time delays between sequential PDL and Nd:YAG pulses were 125, 250, and 500 milliseconds for vein diameter of 4, 3, and 2 mm, respectively, with cold-air, demonstrated good to very good improvement in 47 by photograph evaluation and 49 of 60 patients by computer edge detection data with 1-2 treatment sessions.[42] Common adverse events post laser are purpura and hyperpigmentation. Scarring has also been reported following crusting and blistering.[36]

Hemangioma

Hemangioma is benign proliferation of vascular tumor which occurs in children. In general, they usually present at the first week of life and rapidly develop to plaque and nodule in the following months. The regression usually begins after 1-2 years and left the residual lesion afterward. Pulsed dye laser should be used to treat hemangioma in the proliferative phase to induce growth arrest and accelerate the epithelialization in ulcerated hemangioma. Parameter setting reported in the study are 7 and 10 mm spot size, 3-20 milliseconds, and 9-15 J/cm^2 with surface cooling or DCD open spray 30 milliseconds and 10 milliseconds delay after laser.[43] Pulse dye laser can also combine with other treatment modalities, e.g., oral and intralesional corticosteroids.[44]

At present, as oral propanolol is the mainstay treatment for infantile hemangioma, the use of laser is declining.[45] Combination of PDL with topical propanolol demonstrate, the better clinical responses than PDL alone.[46] For involuted hemangioma, PDL is still considered the treatment of choice with high patient satisfaction (Fig. 4).

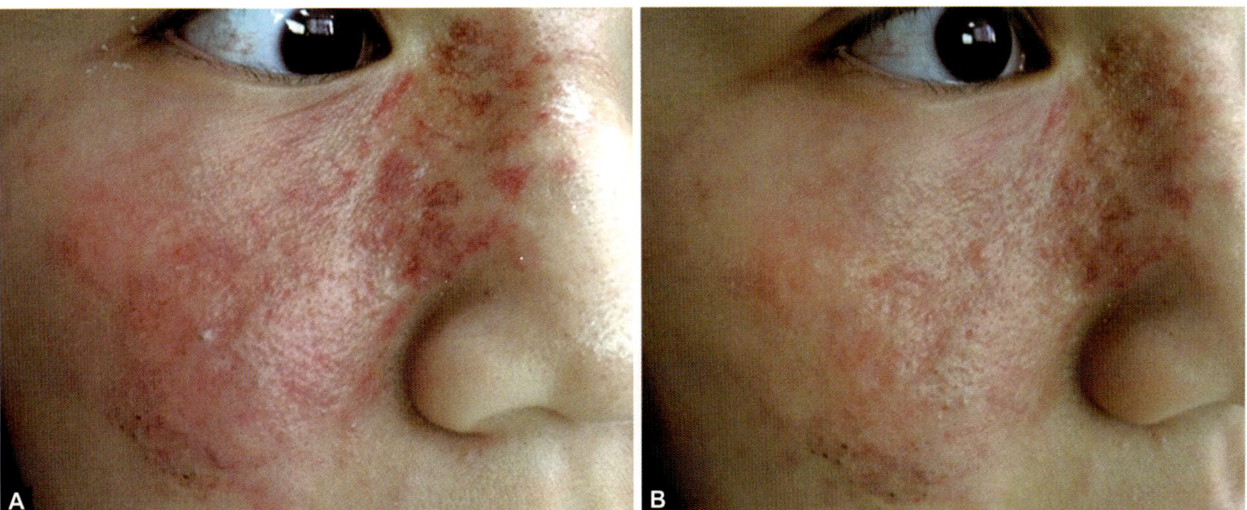

FIG. 4: Residual telangiectasia and scarring in involuted hemangioma. **A,** Before; **B,** 6 months after 2 sessions of 595 nm PDL (V-Beam Perfecta), parameter setting; 7 mm spot size, pulse duration 10–20 ms, fluence 10.5–11 J/cm^2 with dynamic cooling device open spray 30 ms and 20 ms delay after laser.

Other vascular lesions that have been reported with high successive result are hereditary hemorrhagic telangiectasia,[47] angioma serpiginosum,[48,49] erythemato-telangiectatic rosacea,[50] tufted angioma,[51] poikiloderma of civatte,[52,53] and angiokeratoma.[54]

Connective Tissue Disease

Chronic cutaneous lupus erythematosus (CCLE) is a heterogeneous autoimmune disorder with a wide range of skin manifestations including the classical chronic discoid lupus erythematosus lesions and other uncommon variants such as lupus tumidus, hypertrophic or verrucous lupus erythematosus, mucosal lupus erythematosus, palmar and plantar lupus erythematosus, lupus erythematosus panniculitis, and chilblain. Current treatment options comprise of oral and topical medication but some features cannot be improved such as atrophic skin and telangiectases. Pulsed dye laser has been reported to treat telangiectatic chronic erythema in systemic lupus erythematosus patient since 1996 with 585 nm PDL (SPTL-1). Possible mechanism of PDL apart from selective photothermolysis include its thermal effect on the inflammatory cells leading to regression of CCLE lesions. Averaged clinical improvement have been report of 60% on lesion clearance.[55] Parameter setting for 595 nm PDL reported in the literatures range from 5 to 10 mm spot sizes pulse width of 1.5–10 milliseconds and fluences range from 3 to 13 J/cm^2.[56] Beside the appearance of chronic lupus erythematosus scarring improvement, patient symptoms of CCLE, e.g., burning and stinging has been improved after 1 session of laser treatment (Fig. 5). The other form of CCLE that has been effective treated with PDL is lupus tumidus, 10 mm spot size at 0.5 milliseconds pulse-width and a fluence of 8 J/cm^2. Significant reduction of the dermal lymphocytic infiltrate, an important reduction of the basal damage and decrease in intercellular adhesion molecule and vascular cell adhesion molecule expression have been demonstrated.[57]

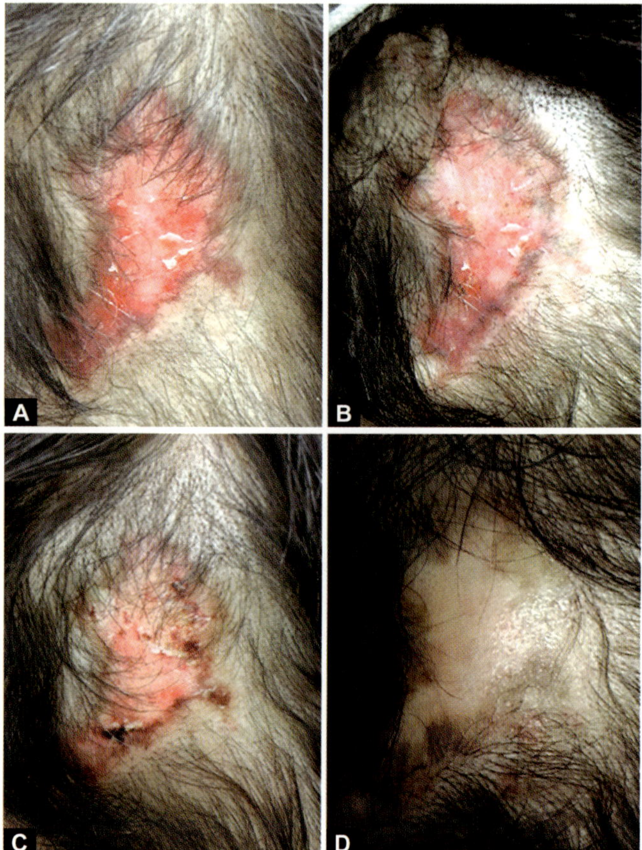

FIG. 5: Discoid lupus erythematosus treated with one session of 595 nm pulsed dye laser (V Beam) with parameter setting; 7 mm spot size, pulse duration 10 m, fluence 10 J/cm^2 with dynamic cooling device open spray 30 ms before laser/10 ms postlaser delay. **A,** Before; **B,** immediately after laser; **C,** 1 week after laser; **D,** 2 months after laser.

Note: Chloroquine and prednisolone were used for several months prior to the start of laser therapy.

Inflammatory Dermatoses

Acne vulgaris and acne erythema is one of the most common PDL indications in real-life practice. The mechanism of action is through transforming growth factor-β, which is known to be a potent stimulus for neocollagenesis and immunosuppressive cytokine which promotes inflammation resolution. Its upregulation after PDL treatment results in the stimulation of dermal remodeling with inhibition of acne inflammation.[58] The effectiveness demonstrated in the studies showed significant improvement of acne but there was no significant difference between other treatment modalities.[58-61] Pulsed dye laser is also safe to use in conjunction with other acne treatments.[60] The effects of PDL on blood vessels has shown to improve multiple inflammatory dermatoses, e.g., angiolymphoid hyperplasia with eosinophilia,[62,63] granuloma annulare (localized),[64-66] granuloma faciale,[67,68] poikilodermatous erythema, Gottron papules and telangiectasia of dermatomyositis,[69,70] sarcoidosis (study mainly on lupus pernio),[71-74] and lichen sclerosus (PDL alone or combined with methylaminolevulinic acid).[75,76]

Pigmentary Condition

For pigment diseases, PDL have some effectiveness on melasma, solar lentigo, photorejuvenation, and postinflammatory hyperpigmentation. For melasma, the role of PDL is incompletely understood. The mechanism of action is unclear. Vascular endothelial growth factor receptor on melanocyte may play a role. Passeron et al. reported combination treatment of triple combination cream (hydroquinone, 4%; tretinoin, 0.05%; and fluocinolone acetonide, 0.01%) and PDL (compression handpiece of 10 mm, 1.5 ms, fluence 7 J/cm^2) with significantly improvement on Melasma Area and Severity Index score.[32] The author preferred setting is 7 mm spot size, 1.5 milliseconds, fluence 5–6.5 J/cm^2, off cryogen spray cooling. The compression handpiece is specially design for purpura-free treatment of lentigo, the parameter setting is compression handpiece of 7–10 mm, 9–13 J/cm^2, 1.5 milliseconds and off cryogen spray cooling. Majority of the patient in the studies obtained excellent results.[77-80]

Superficial Basal Cell Carcinoma

The 595 nm PDL and combination of 585 nm PDL and 1,064 nm Nd:YAG lasers have been used in superficial basal cell carcinoma (BCC) at low risk anatomical sites,[81] superficial and nodular type,[82] and high risk BCC group.[83] The mechanism of action is through selective destruction of the supporting vascular network and stimulation of inflammatory processes secondary to vascular injury. Pulsed dye laser treatment may be considered as alternative treatment or add-on treatment for reduction of tumor burden (Table 2).

Other Skin Conditions

Pulsed dye laser is also widely used to treat several nonvascular conditions including scar/burn scar/hypertrophic scar,[84-88] red striae,[89] plane warts,[90] angiofibroma,[91-93] and pyogenic granulomas.[94]

Treatment Considerations

- Correct diagnosis is essential particularly in the skin of color
- Topical anesthetic may be applied in patients who could not tolerate the pain of treatment
- Pulsed dye laser can accidentally cause hair loss; hair bearing areas should be covered, e.g., eyebrows and beard
- Patient and doctor should wear eye goggles throughout the procedure. An optical density of at least 4 (light transmittance 0.01%) is required for a laser goggle which protects against a specific laser wavelength.
- If the treatment is close to the eyelid, corneal eye shield should be placed (metallic corneal eye shield provides better protection)[95]

TABLE 2: Evidence of efficacy and safety of use of pulsed dye laser in basal cell cancer

Authors	Type of BCC	Laser	Energy setting	Results
Karsai et al.[81]	56 treated/44 control superficial type BCC	595 nm PDL (Multiplex Cynergy®; Cynosure Inc., Langen, Germany)	Fluence 8 J/cm^2; pulse width 0.5 ms; spot size 10 mm with 5-10 mm margin	Complete remission in 44 of 56 cases (78.6%) in the laser and in two of 44 cases (4.5%) in the sham treatment arm
Alonso-Castro et al.[83]	7 high risk BCC with varying diameters	595 nm PDL (Cynergy®, Cynosure, Inc., Westford, MA, USA)	Fluence 15 J/cm^2, pulse duration of 2 ms, and a spot size 7 mm with 2 stacked pulses, 4 mm margin for three session	Complete clinical response was achieved in 5/7 patients. One patient who did not undergo MMS showed a recurrence after 14 months
Jalian et al.[82]	13 superficial and nodular subtypes BCC with varying diameters	Combined 585–597 nm + 1,064 nm Nd:YAG lasers (Cynergy,® Cynosure, Inc., Westford, MA, USA)	Fluence 8 J/cm^2, pulse width 2 ms; spot size 7 mm with 4 mm margin followed by a 250 ms delay and 1,064 nm Nd:YAG laser, fluence 40 J/cm^2, pulse width 15 ms with 10% overlap. 2-4 weeks intervals.	Complete clinical response was achieved in 75% (n = 6/8) of all tumors <1 cm in diameter. Tumor types among the complete responders included superficial and nodular BCCs

BCC, basal cell carcinoma; PDL, pulsed dye laser; MMS, Mohs micrographic surgery; Nd:YAG, neodymium doped yttrium-aluminium-garnet..

- Post-treatment, ice pack or air-cooling applied on the treated area alleviates the discomfort from laser treatment
- Sun protection in the treated area is recommended to reduce the risk of postprocedural dyspigmentation[96]

Adverse Events

Adverse events from PDL treatment are generally considered minor and reversible when using recommended setting. Pain is tolerable and can be reduced by cooling system, infrequently required topical anesthetic. Redness, swelling, stinging, and itching are normal reactions which immediately appeared after the procedure. Pain, redness, and swelling can be relieved with ice pack and resolve in a few hours (may last for a few days). Purpura can develop in a high energy setting, up to 10% of patient, but easily fades in the following days. Burn and blistering can be predicted when grayish (epidermal necrosis) or whitish discoloration appears immediately or in a few minutes after laser (especially ones that do not fade away in a few minutes), indicating inappropriately high energy setting. Adequate pretreatment and/or parallel epidermal coolings (dynamic cooling) is key to reducing burning and blistering.[97-99] The pigmentary change, i.e., hyperpigmentation or hypopigmentation, may follow bruising and blistering, especially in darker skin types which possess significant amount of melanin to absorb laser light. Hypopigmentation is more common when treating on the trunk and extremities. Scarring has been reported after high energy setting and repeated treatments. Seukeran et al. reported that incidence of atrophic and hypertrophic scarring following PDL treatment for PWSs are 4.3 and 0.7%, respectively. Atrophic scars are predisposed in younger patients and hypertrophic scars are predisposed when the neck is treated.[100] Infection rarely occurs but herpes reactivation is a precaution in patients who has herpes recurrence in the treatment area. Recommendation from guidelines suggested antiviral therapy the day before laser treatment.[14]

CONCLUSION

Long term studies in PDL showed its high efficacy and safety PDL in the treatment of vascular malformation, hemangiomas, and a variety of acquired cutaneous vascular lesions including telangiectases, cherry angiomas, and poikiloderma of Civatte. Pulsed dye laser was also used to treat nonvascular lesions like melasma, scars, lentigo, basal cell carcinoma and various inflammatory skin disorders.

REFERENCES

1. Schäfer FP. Dye lasers. In: Schäfer, editor. 3rd ed. Germany: Springer; 1990. pp. 1-2.
2. Kilck D. Industrial applications of dye laser. In: Duarte FJ, Hillman LW, editors. Dye Laser Principles: With Applications. San Diego: Academic Press, Inc.; 1990. p. 345.
3. Anderson RR, Parrish JA. Selective photothermolysis: precise microsurgery by selective absorption of pulsed radiation. Science. 1983;220(4596): 524-7.
4. Altshuler GB, Anderson RR, Manstein D, Zenzie HH, Smirnov MZ. Extended theory of selective photothermolysis. Lasers Surg Med. 2001;29(5):416-32.
5. Rubin IK, Farinelli WA, Doukas A, Anderson RR. Optimal wavelengths for vein-selective photothermolysis. Lasers Surg Med. 2012;44(2):152-7.
6. Aihara H, Tanino R, Osada M, Osamura RY. Attempt to obtain greater dermal depth of vascular injury using dye-enhanced laser technique: a new approach. Lasers Surg Med. 1996;18(3):260-4.
7. van Gemert MJ, Welch AJ, Amin AP. Is there an optimal laser treatment for port wine stains? Lasers Surg Med. 1986;6(1):76-83.
8. Anderson RR, Parrish JA. Microvasculature can be selectively damaged using dye lasers: a basic theory and experimental evidence in human skin. Lasers Surg Med. 1981;1(3):263-76.
9. Suthamjariya K, Farinelli WA, Koh W, Anderson RR. Mechanisms of microvascular response to laser pulses. J Invest Dermatol. 2004;122(2):518-25.
10. Garden JM, Tan OT, Kerschmann R, Boll J, Furumoto H, Anderson RR, et al. Effect of dye laser pulse duration on selective cutaneous vascular injury. J Invest Dermatol. 1986;87(5):653-7.
11. Borges da Costa J, Boixeda P, Moreno C, Santiago J. Treatment of resistant port-wine stains with a pulsed dual wavelength 595 and 1064 nm laser: a histochemical evaluation of the vessel wall destruction and selectivity. Photomed Laser Surg. 2009;27(4):599-605.
12. Grekin RC, Flynn TC, Cooper D, Geisse J. Efficacy of a 2-mm spot size lens for the treatment of superficial vascular lesions with a flashlamp-pumped dye laser. Int J Dermatol. 1997;36(11):865-9.
13. Dinehart SM, Flock S, Waner M. Beam profile of the flashlamp pumped pulsed dye laser: support for overlap of exposure spots. Lasers Surg Med. 1994;15(3):277-80.
14. Adamič M, Pavlović MD, Troilius Rubin A, Palmetun-Ekback M, Boixeda P. Guidelines of care for vascular lasers and intense pulse light sources from the European Society for Laser Dermatology. J Eur Acad Dermatol Venereol. 2015;29(9):1661-78.
15. Tanghetti EA. Split-face randomized treatment of facial telangiectasia comparing pulsed dye laser and an intense pulsed light handpiece. Lasers Surg Med. 2012;44(2):97-102.
16. Madan V, Ferguson J. Using the ultra-long pulse width pulsed dye laser and elliptical spot to treat resistant nasal telangiectasia. Lasers Med Sci. 2010;25(1):151-4.
17. Ross EV, Uebelhoer NS, Domankevitz Y. Use of a novel pulse dye laser for rapid single-pass purpura-free treatment of telangiectases. Dermatol Surg. 2007;33(12):1466-9.
18. Weiss RA, Ross EV, Tanghetti EA, Vasily DB, Childs JJ, Smirnov MZ, et al. Characterization of an optimized light source and comparison to pulsed dye laser for superficial and deep vessel clearance. Lasers Surg Med. 2011;43(2):92-8.
19. Shafirstein G, Baumler W, Lapidoth M, Ferguson S, North PE, Waner M. A new mathematical approach to the diffusion approximation theory for selective photothermolysis modeling and its implication in laser treatment of port-wine stains. Lasers Surg Med. 2004;34(4):335-47.
20. Fiskerstrand EJ, Svaasand LO, Kopstad G, Dalaker M, Norvang LT, Volden G. Laser treatment of port wine stains: therapeutic outcome in relation to morphological parameters. Br J Dermatol. 1996;134(6):1039-43.

21. Fiskerstrand EJ, Svaasand LO, Kopstad G, Ryggen K, Aase S. Photothermally induced vessel-wall necrosis after pulsed dye laser treatment: lack of response in port-wine stains with small sized or deeply located vessels. J Invest Dermatol. 1996;107(5):671-5.
22. Katugampola GA, Lanigan SW. Five years' experience of treating port wine stains with the flashlamp-pumped pulsed dye laser. Br J Dermatol. 1997;137(5):750-4.
23. Yu W, Ma G, Qiu Y, Chen H, Jin Y, Yang X, et al. Prospective comparison treatment of 595-nm pulsed-dye lasers for virgin port-wine stain. Br J Dermatol. 2015;172(3):684-91.
24. Nagore E, Requena C, Sevila A, Coll J, Costa D, Botella-Estrada R, et al. Thickness of healthy and affected skin of children with port wine stains: potential repercussions on response to pulsed dye laser treatment. Dermatol Surg. 2004;30(12 Pt 1):1457-61.
25. Shi W, Wang J, Lin Y, Geng J, Wang H, Gong Y, et al. Treatment of port wine stains with pulsed dye laser: a retrospective study of 848 cases in Shandong Province, People's Republic of China. Drug Des Devel Ther. 2014;8:2531-8.
26. Yu W, Ma G, Qiu Y, Chen H, Jin Y, Yang X, et al. Why do port-wine stains (PWS) on the lateral face respond better to pulsed dye laser (PDL) than those located on the central face? J Am Acad Dermatol. 2016;74(3):527-35.
27. Bencini PL, Cazzaniga S, Galimberti MG, Zane C, Naldi L. Variables affecting clinical response to treatment of facial port-wine stains by flash lamp-pumped pulsed dye laser: the importance of looking beyond the skin. Lasers Med Sci. 2014;29(4):1365-70.
28. Yamauchi PS, Soriano TT, Lask GP. Treatment of port wine stains using the pulsed-dye laser at 585 nm with the dynamic cooling device. J Cutan Laser Ther. 2000;2(1):33-6.
29. Rajaratnam R, Laughlin SA, Dudley D. Pulsed dye laser double-pass treatment of patients with resistant capillary malformations. Lasers Med Sci. 2011;26(4):487-92.
30. Thajudheen CP, Jyothy K, Priyadarshini A. Treatment of port-wine stains with flash lamp pumped pulsed dye laser on Indian skin: a six year study. J Cutan Aesthet Surg. 2014;7(1):32-6.
31. Griffin TD Jr, Foshee JP, Finney R, Saedi N. Port wine stain treated with a combination of pulsed dye laser and topical rapamycin ointment. Lasers Surg Med. 2016; 48(2):193-6.
32. Passeron T, Maza A, Fontas E, Toubel G, Vabres P, Livideanu C, et al. Treatment of port wine stains with pulsed dye laser and topical timolol: a multicenter randomized controlled trial. Br J Dermatol. 2014;170(6):1350-3.
33. Zhang B, Zhang TH, Huang Z, Li Q, Yuan KH, Hu ZQ. Comparison of pulsed dye laser (PDL) and photodynamic therapy (PDT) for treatment of facial port-wine stain (PWS) birthmarks in pediatric patients. Photodiagnosis Photodyn Ther. 2014;11(4):491-7.
34. Woo WK, Jasim ZF, Handley JM. 532-nm Nd:YAG and 595-nm pulsed dye laser treatment of leg telangiectasia using ultralong pulse duration. Dermatol Surg. 2003;29(12):1176-80.
35. Alora MB, Stern RS, Arndt KA, Dover JS. Comparison of the 595 nm long-pulse (1.5 msec) and ultralong-pulse (4 msec) lasers in the treatment of leg veins. Dermatol Surg. 1999;25(6):445-9.
36. Buscher BA, McMeekin TO, Goodwin D. Treatment of leg telangiectasia by using a long-pulse dye laser at 595 nm with and without dynamic cooling device. Lasers Surg Med. 2000;27(2):171-5.
37. Kono T, Yamaki T, Erçöçen AR, Fujiwara O, Nozaki M. Treatment of leg veins with the long pulse dye laser using variable pulse durations and energy fluences. Lasers Surg Med. 2004;35(1):62-7.
38. Bernstein EF. The new-generation, high-energy, 595 nm, long pulse-duration, pulsed-dye laser effectively removes spider veins of the lower extremity. Lasers Surg Med. 2007;39(3):218-24.
39. Tanghetti E, Sherr E. Treatment of telangiectasia using the multi-pass technique with the extended pulse width, pulsed dye laser (Cynosure V-Star). J Cosmet Laser Ther. 2003;5(2):71-5.
40. Bernstein EF, Lee J, Lowery J, Brown DB, Geronemus R, Lask G, et al. Treatment of spider veins with the 595 nm pulsed-dye laser. J Am Acad Dermatol. 1998;39(5 Pt 1):746-50.
41. Hsia J, Lowery JA, Zelickson B. Treatment of leg telangiectasia using a long-pulse dye laser at 595 nm. Lasers Surg Med. 1997;20(1):1-5.
42. Trelles MA, Weiss R, Moreno-Moragas J, Romero C, Velez M, Alvarez X. Treatment of leg veins with combined pulsed dye and Nd:YAG lasers: 60 patients assessed at 6 months. Lasers Surg Med. 2010;42(9):609-14.
43. Kwon SH, Choi JW, Byun SY, Kim BR, Park KC, Youn SW, et al. Effect of early long-pulse pulsed dye laser treatment in infantile hemangiomas. Dermatol Surg. 2014;40(4):405-11.
44. Gorst CM, Munnoch DA, Hancock K. Combined treatment of a proliferative peri-orbital haemangioma with a tuneable dye laser and intra-lesional steroids to prevent deprivation amblyopia. J R Coll Surg Edinb. 2001;46(4):234-6.
45. Katona G, Csákányi Z, Gács E, Szalai Z, Ráth G,, Gerlinger I. Propranolol for infantile haemangioma: striking effect in the first weeks. Int J Pediatr Otorhinolaryngol. 2012;76(12):1746-50.
46. Ehsani AH, Noormohammadpoor P, Abdolreza M, Balighi K, Arianian Z, Daklan S. Combination therapy of infantile hemangioma with pulsed dye laser with topical propranolol: a randomized clinical trial. Archives of Iranian medicine. 2014;17(10):657-60.
47. Halachmi S, Israeli H, Ben-Amitai D, Lapidoth M. Treatment of the skin manifestations of hereditary hemorrhagic telangiectasia with pulsed dye laser. Lasers Med Sci. 2014;29(1):321-4.
48. Madan V, August PJ, Ferguson JE. Pulsed-dye laser treatment of angioma serpiginosum. Clin Exp Dermatol. 2009;34(5):e186-8.
49. Long CC, Lanigan SW. Treatment of angioma serpiginosum using a pulsed tunable dye laser. Br J Dermatol. 1997;136(4):631-2.
50. Neuhaus IM, Zane LT, Tope WD. Comparative efficacy of nonpurpuragenic pulsed dye laser and intense pulsed light for erythematotelangiectatic rosacea. Dermatol Surg. 2009;35(6):920-8.
51. Robati RM, Hejazi S, Shakoei S, Bidari F. Late-onset tufted angioma with remarkable response to pulse dye laser. Indian J Dermatol. 2014;59(6):635.
52. Meijs MM, Blok FA, de Rie MA. Treatment of poikiloderma of Civatte with the pulsed dye laser: a series of patients with severe depigmentation. J Eur Acad Dermatol Venereol. 2006;20(10):1248-51.
53. Wheeland RG, Applebaum J. Flashlamp-pumped pulsed dye laser therapy for poikiloderma of Civatte. J Dermatol Surg Oncol. 1990;16(1):12-6.
54. Su Q, Lin T, Wu Q, Wu Y, Guo L, Ge Y. Efficacy of 595nm pulsed dye laser therapy for Mibelli angiokeratoma. J Cosmet Laser Ther. 2015;17(4):209-12.
55. Diez MT, Boixeda P, Moreno C, Gonzalez JA, Zamorano ML, Olasolo PJ. Histopathology and immunohistochemistry of cutaneous lupus erythematosus after pulsed dye laser treatment. Dermatol Surg. 2011;37(7):971-81.
56. Baniandrés O, Boixeda P, Belmar P, Pérez A. Treatment of lupus erythematosus with pulsed dye laser. Lasers Surg Med. 2003;32(4):327-30.
57. Truchuelo MT, Boixeda P, Alcantara J, Moreno C, de las Heras E, Olasolo PJ. Pulsed dye laser as an excellent choice of treatment for lupus tumidus: a prospective study. J Eur Acad Dermatol Venereol. 2012;26(10):1272-9.
58. Seaton ED, Mouser PE, Charakida A, Alam S, Seldon PM, Chu AC. Investigation of the mechanism of action of nonablative pulsed-dye laser therapy in photorejuvenation and inflammatory acne vulgaris. Br J Dermatol. 2006;155(4):748-55.
59. Karsai S, Schmitt L, Raulin C. The pulsed-dye laser as an adjuvant treatment modality in acne vulgaris: a randomized controlled single-blinded trial. Br J Dermatol. 2010;163(2):395-401.
60. Shariff A, Keck L, Zlotoff B. Acne vulgaris in the context of complex medical co-morbities: the management of severe acne vulgaris in a female with retinitis pigmentosa - utilizing pulse dye laser in conjunction with medical therapy. Dermatol Online J. 2014;20(3).

61. Leheta TM. Role of the 585-nm pulsed dye laser in the treatment of acne in comparison with other topical therapeutic modalities. J Cosmet Laser Ther. 2009;11(2):118-24.
62. Rohrer TE, Allan AE. Angiolymphoid hyperplasia with eosinophilia successfully treated with a long-pulsed tunable dye laser. Dermatol Surg. 2000;26(3):211-4.
63. Angel CA, Lewis AT, Griffin T, Levy EJ, Benedetto AV. Angiolymphoid hyperplasia successfully treated with an ultralong pulsed dye laser. Dermatol Surg. 2005;31(6):713-6.
64. Sniezek PJ, DeBloom JR 2nd, Arpey CJ. Treatment of granuloma annulare with the 585 nm pulsed dye laser. Dermatol Surg. 2005;31(10):1370-3.
65. Sliger BN, Burk CJ, Alvarez-Connelly E. Treatment of granuloma annulare with the 595 nm pulsed dye laser in a pediatric patient. Pediatr Dermatol. 2008;25(2):196-7.
66. Passeron T, Fusade T, Vabres P, Bousquet-Rouaud R, Collet-Vilette AM, Dahan S, et al. Treatment of granuloma annulare with the 595-nm pulsed dye laser, a multicentre retrospective study with long-term follow-up. J Eur Acad Dermatol Venereol. 2013;27(6):785-8.
67. Fikrle T, Pizinger K. Granuloma Faciale treated with 595-nm pulsed dye laser. Dermatol Surg. 2011;37(1):102-4.
68. Hruza GJ, Ammirati CT. Granuloma faciale treated with 595-nm pulsed dye laser. Dermatol Surg. 2011;37(7):1060-1.
69. Yanagi T, Sawamura D, Shibaki A, Shimizu H. Treatment for poikilodermatous erythema of dermatomyositis with the pulsed dye laser. Br J Dermatol. 2005;153(4):862-4.
70. Calvo Pulido M, Boixeda De Miquel P, Martin Saez E, Fernandez Guarino M, García-Millán C.. Treatment of Gottron papules of dermatomyositis with pulsed dye laser. Eur J Dermatol. 2006;16(6):702-3.
71. Emer J, Uslu U, Waldorf H. Improvement in lupus pernio with the successive use of pulsed dye laser and nonablative fractional resurfacing. Dermatol Surg. 2014;40(2):201-2.
72. Roos S, Raulin C, Ockenfels HM, Karsai S. Successful treatment of cutaneous sarcoidosis lesions with the flashlamp pumped pulsed dye laser: a case report. Dermatol Surg. 2009;35(7):1139-40.
73. Cliff S, Felix RH, Singh L, Harland CC. The successful treatment of lupus pernio with the flashlamp pulsed dye laser. J Cutan Laser Ther. 1999;1(1):49-52.
74. Goodman MM, Alpern K. Treatment of lupus pernio with the flashlamp pulsed dye laser. Lasers Surg Med. 1992;12(5):549-51.
75. Passeron T, Lacour JP, Ortonne JP. Comparative treatment of extragenital lichen sclerosus with methylaminolevulinic Acid pulsed dye laser-mediated photodynamic therapy or pulsed dye laser alone. Dermatol Surg. 2009;35(5):878-80.
76. Rabinowitz LG. Lichen sclerosus et atrophicus treatment with the 585-nm flashlamp-pumped pulsed dye laser. Arch Dermatol. 1993;129(3):381-2.
77. Galeckas KJ, Ross EV, Uebelhoer NS. A pulsed dye laser with a 10-mm beam diameter and a pigmented lesion window for purpura-free photorejuvenation. Dermatol Surg. 2008;34(3):308-13.
78. Kono T, Chan HH, Groff WF, Sakurai H, Takeuchi M, Yamaki T, et al. Long-pulse pulsed dye laser delivered with compression for treatment of facial lentigines. Dermatol Surg. 2007;33(8):945-50.
79. Pootongkam S, Asawanonda P. Purpura-free treatment of lentigines using a long-pulsed 595 nm pulsed dye laser with compression handpiece: a randomized, controlled study. J Drugs Dermatol. 2009;8(11 Suppl):s18-24.
80. Seirafi H, Fateh S, Farnaghi F, Ehsani AH, Noormohammadpour P. Efficacy and safety of long-pulse pulsed dye laser delivered with compression versus cryotherapy for treatment of solar lentigines. Indian J Dermatol. 2011;56(1):48-51.
81. Karsai S, Friedl H, Buhck H, Jünger M,, Podda M. The role of the 595-nm pulsed dye laser in treating superficial basal cell carcinoma: outcome of a double-blind randomized placebo-controlled trial. Br J Dermatol. 2015;172(3):677-83.
82. Jalian HR, Avram MM, Stankiewicz KJ, Shofner JD, Tannous Z. Combined 585 nm pulsed-dye and 1,064 nm Nd:YAG lasers for the treatment of basal cell carcinoma. Lasers Surg Med. 2014;46(1):1-7.
83. Alonso-Castro L, Rios-Buceta L, Boixeda P, Paoli J, Moreno C, Jaén P.. The effect of pulsed dye laser on high-risk basal cell carcinomas with response control by Mohs micrographic surgery. Lasers Med Sci. 2015;30(7):2009-14.
84. Allison KP, Kiernan MN, Waters RA, Clement RM. Pulsed dye laser treatment of burn scars. Alleviation or irritation? Burns. 2003;29(3):207-13.
85. Brewin MP, Lister TS. Prevention or treatment of hypertrophic burn scarring: a review of when and how to treat with the pulsed dye laser. Burns. 2014;40(5):797-804.
86. Donelan MB, Parrett BM, Sheridan RL. Pulsed dye laser therapy and z-plasty for facial burn scars: the alternative to excision. Ann Plast Surg. 2008;60(5):480-6.
87. Kono T, Erçöçen AR, Nakazawa H, Nozaki M. Treatment of hypertrophic scars using a long-pulsed dye laser with cryogen-spray cooling. Ann Plast Surg. 2005;54(5):487-93.
88. Parrett BM, Donelan MB. Pulsed dye laser in burn scars: current concepts and future directions. Burns. 2010;36(4):443-9.
89. McDaniel DH, Ash K, Zukowski M. Treatment of stretch marks with the 585-nm flashlamp-pumped pulsed dye laser. Dermatol Surg. 1996;22(4):332-7.
90. Grillo E, Boixeda P, Ballester A, Miguel-Morrondo A, Truchuelo T, Jaén P. Pulsed dye laser treatment for facial flat warts. Dermatol Ther. 2014;27(1):31-5.
91. Boixeda P, Sánchez-Miralles E, Azaña JM, Arrazola JM, Moreno R, Ledo A. C02, argon, and pulsed dye laser treatment of angiofibromas. J Dermatol Surg Oncol. 1994;20(12):808-12.
92. Hoffman SJ, Walsh P, Morelli JG. Treatment of angiofibroma with the pulsed tunable dye laser. J Am Acad Dermatol. 1993;29(5 Pt 1):790-1.
93. Weiss ET, Geronemus RG. New technique using combined pulsed dye laser and fractional resurfacing for treating facial angiofibromas in tuberous sclerosis. Lasers Surg Med. 2010;42(5):357-60.
94. Abd-el-Raheem TA, Hohenleutner U, Landthaler M. Granuloma pyogenicum as a complication of flashlamp-pumped pulsed dye laser. Dermatology. 1994;189(3):283-5.
95. Russell SW, Dinehart SM, Davis I, Flock ST. Efficacy of corneal eye shields in protecting patients' eyes from laser irradiation. Dermatol Surg. 1996;22(7):613-6.
96. Haedersdal M. Cutaneous side effects from laser treatment of the skin: skin cancer, scars, wounds, pigmentary changes, and purpura--use of pulsed dye laser, copper vapor laser, and argon laser. Acta Derm Venereol Suppl (Stockh). 1999;207:1-32.
97. Nelson JS, Milner TE, Anvari B, Tanenbaum BS, Kimel S, Svaasand LO, et al. Dynamic epidermal cooling during pulsed laser treatment of port-wine stain. A new methodology with preliminary clinical evaluation. Arch Dermatol. 1995;131(6):695-700.
98. Chang CJ, Kelly KM, Nelson JS. Cryogen spray cooling and pulsed dye laser treatment of cutaneous hemangiomas. Ann Plast Surg. 2001;46(6):577-83.
99. Chang CJ, Nelson JS. Cryogen spray cooling and higher fluence pulsed dye laser treatment improve port-wine stain clearance while minimizing epidermal damage. Dermatol Surg. 1999;25(10):767-72.
100. Seukeran DC, Collins P, Sheehan-Dare RA. Adverse reactions following pulsed tunable dye laser treatment of port wine stains in 701 patients. Br J Dermatol. 1997;136(5):725-9.

CHAPTER 21

Intense Pulsed Light for Vascular Lesions

Dhepe Niteen Vishwanath

INTRODUCTION

Vascular lesions can be congenital or acquired. They can be superficial or deep or mixed. Superficial vascular lesions are easily targeted by intense pulsed light (IPL), while thicker lesions usually require lasers with deeper penetration.

LASERS AND LIGHTS IN VASCULAR LESIONS TREATMENT[1,2]

Author has summarized the currently available and commonly used technologies and devices for vascular lesions (Box 1).

Box 1: Currently available and commonly used technologies and devices for vascular lesions

- Energies with hemoglobin as chromophore
  - IPL (540, 570, 590, 610, and 650 nm on various devices with upper filter as water at 1000 nm)
  - Sandwich filter of duel filter IPL like Dye VL with lower filter at 500 or 550 nm and upper filter at 600 nm
  - Long-pulsed neodymium doped yttrium-aluminium-garnet 1064 nm
  - Long-pulsed alexandrite
- Lasers with water as chromophores used in hypertrophic lesions
  - Erbium doped yttrium-aluminium-garnet lasers
  - Ultrapulse carbon dioxide laser

It is interesting to note that there is not a single wavelength specified as vascular in IPL. All wavelengths (530–650 nm) can act as vascular in different clinical scenario. Fair patients respond to 540 nm as vascular wavelength while Indian patients need 570–590 nm. Very dark patients even respond to 650 nm safely.

Adult vascular lesions have an element of fibrosis and may need carbon dioxide (CO_2) or neodymium doped yttrium-aluminium-garnet (Nd:YAG) 106 nm as an adjuvant. In authors experience, many lesions like lymphohemangioma or angiokeratoma respond better to long-pulsed 1,064 nm Nd:YAG laser or ultrapulse CO_2 laser than pulsed dye laser (PDL) or IPL 550–590 nm.

PRINCIPLES OF TREATMENTS OF VASCULAR LESIONS

Lasers and light work in vascular lesion by principle of selective photothermolysis. It considers three main parameters of laser light to make selective for vascular lesions.

1. Wavelength: oxyhemoglobin is the target chromophore that absorbs 545 and 577 nm as preferential peak absorption. One needs to target capillaries with lasers and light at the same time sparing melanin-containing epidermis. The peak absorption wavelength is 532 nm for melanin in epidermis. Lasers and lights matching wavelengths around peak absorption of hemoglobin, but avoiding peak near melanin absorption are useful for vascular lesions (Fig. 1).

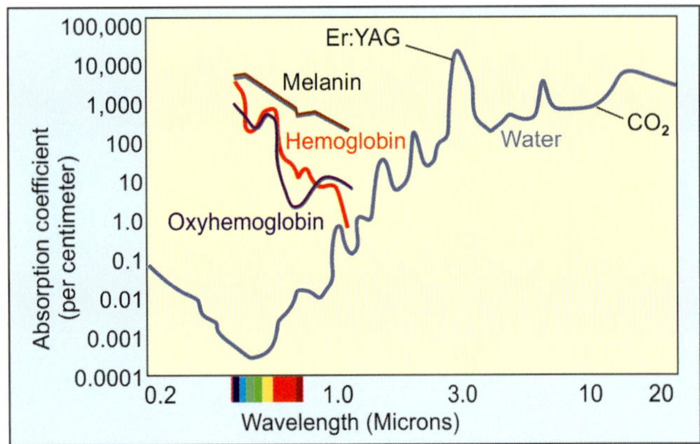

Er:YAG: erbium doped yttrium-aluminium-garnet; CO_2, carbon dioxide.

FIG. 1: Absorption coefficient of various tissue chromophores

Ideal peak of absorption by oxyhemeoglobin was at 577 nm. It caused a lot of purpura in initial devices, so manufacturers changed the device wavelength to 585 nm. It was still causing purpura so third-generation vascular laser devices used wavelength of 595 nm[3]

2. Pulse duration: pulse duration (pulse width) less than thermal relaxation of capillaries is used to ablate those. It is wider than thermal relaxation time (TRT) of red blood cells (RBC). It is found that very short pulse width will target RBC, but not capillary endothelium. Therefore, in small capillaries of port wine stain (PWS), the TRT is in microseconds, while thick capillaries of hemangioma it is in milliseconds. Initial pulsed dye lasers (PDLs) had a pulsed width of 0.45 ms that has caused a lot of purpura. This pulse width is not enough to coagulate the endothelium. Then the next version of vascular lasers evolves at pulse width of 1.5 milliseconds. Current vascular protocols have a pulse width range of 2–10 milliseconds.[4]
3. Fluence: a sufficient fluence is required to ablate the target chromophore as per theory of selective photothermolysis.

INTENSE PULSED LIGHT

Introduction

Intense pulsed light is by definition intense and pulsed-like lasers, but is polychromatic and noncoherent unlike lasers. Light source is flashlamp that emits a range of wavelengths. Infrared wavelengths beyond 1,000 nm are erythemogenic and not therapeutically required. The upper filter in IPL is at 1,000 nm. The IPL light is passed through a thin layer of water that absorbs and hence filters wavelengths beyond 1,000 nm. Special glass filters are used to filter cutoff wavelengths that are ultraviolet and those which are not required. If a special glass filter absorbs wavelengths below 530 nm, the output beam will have rays at 530–1,000 nm and suitable for pigmentary lesions. Similarly, a filter at 570 nm will cutoff lower wavelengths and make the IPL output vascular specific.

Therefore, IPL remained broadband and polychromatic though various handpieces with different lower filters are promoted for clinical indications.

Narrow Band Vascular Specific Intense Pulsed Light Wavelengths (Dye VL)

It was possible to cutoff lower wavelengths, but upper filter remained water at 1,000 nm and beyond. A real breakthrough came when outer filters were developed in glass that filters wavelengths beyond certain limit. Dye VL was one such IPL handpiece on Harmony XL, which used 500 nm as lower filter and 600 nm (Fig. 2) as upper one. Another handpiece used 550 nm as lower and 650 nm as upper filter.

LASER TISSUE INTERACTION OF VASCULAR LASERS AND LIGHT

Red colored oxyhemoglobin is the primary target of vascular lasers and lights. It is interesting to note that the actual target i.e., endothelium of the capillaries in vascular tumors is colorless (Fig. 3). Here, hemoglobin acts as a primary heater and pass on the heat to secondary heater i.e., endothelim. That is why, though the thermal

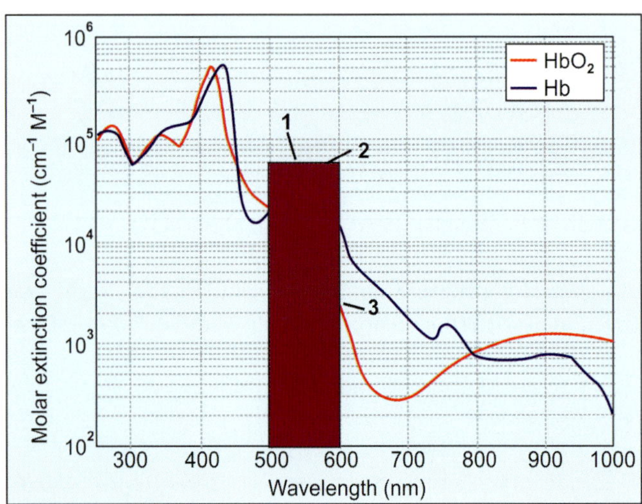

HbO_2, oxyhemoglobin; Hb, hemoglobin.

FIG. 2: Dye VL using 500 nm as lower filter and 600 nm as upper filter

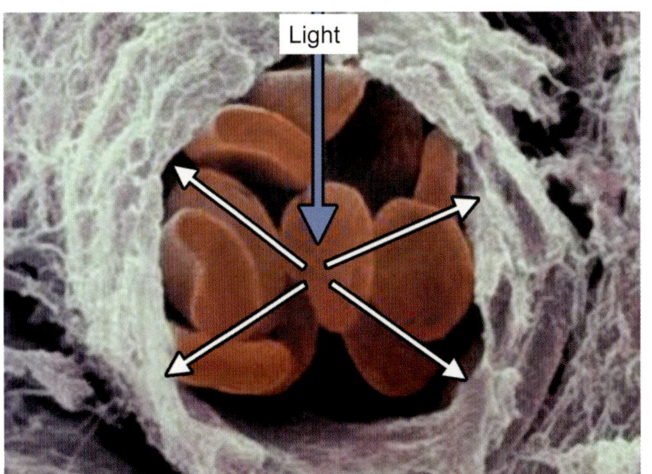

FIG. 3: Electron micrograph of capillary showing colored red blood cells versus colorless endothelium

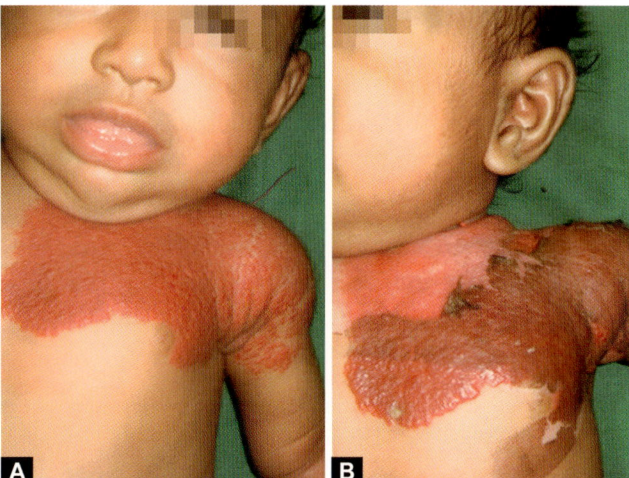

FIG. 4: **A,** Area affected with port wine stain; **B,** improvements shown after one treatment

relaxation time of RBCs is in microseconds, the actual effective pulse width is 1-10 milliseconds.

- Port wine stain
  - Childhood type
  - Adult type
- Port wine stain of arteriovenous malformation (AVM)
- Rosacea
- Telangiectasia
  - Hereditary/poikiloderma
  - Steroid induced
- Red scars
- Angiokeratoma
- Lymphangioma
- Lymphohemangioma
- Infantile hemangioma.

PROTOCOLS FOR SPECIFIC VASCULAR LESION TREATMENT WITH AUTHOR'S EXPERIENCE

Port Wine Stain: Childhood Type (Fig. 4)

Preoperative protocol includes careful examination and investigation to rule out internal extension of lesion in form of AVM. Anesthesia is usually not required. Vascular nature of the lesion may lead to significant and rapid systemic absorption of local anesthetic. Intraoperative cooling is not recommended as it may reduce the chromophore density because of capillary vasoconstriction. Position preferred is trendelenburg position to induce hyperemia of the part to be treated (Fig. 5).

Intense pulse, light with pulse width lowest available (usually 10 ms or less) with energy density 20-30 J/cm^2 is selected. Without much pressure and with little gel as optical coupler, IPL light is fired with overlap of 10%. The author prefers stacking of two pulses at each location till significant bleaching is observed as immediate end point.

Postoperatively, moisturizers or white petroleum jelly is applied three times a day. Peeling off of skin above the lesion is an expected sequel. Treatment can be repeated at an interval of 4-6 weeks for 4-10 sittings till resolution of the PWS lesion is achieved.

Predictive Indicators

Blanchability will determine outcome. Blanchable and early lesions respond best to vascular IPL. Indian skin requires more than 10 sitting with partial outcome. Treatment at very early age will have better clearance.[5,6]

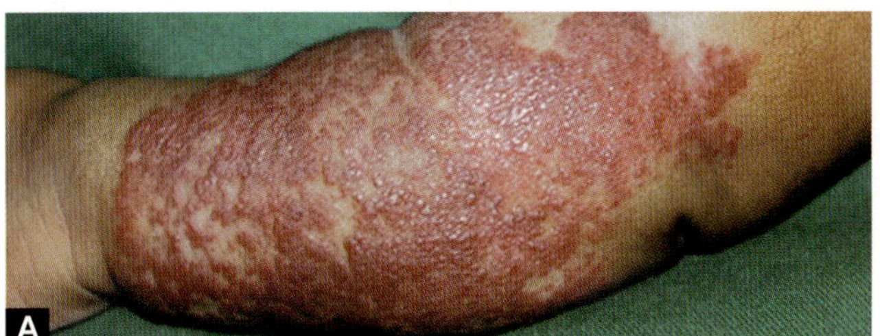

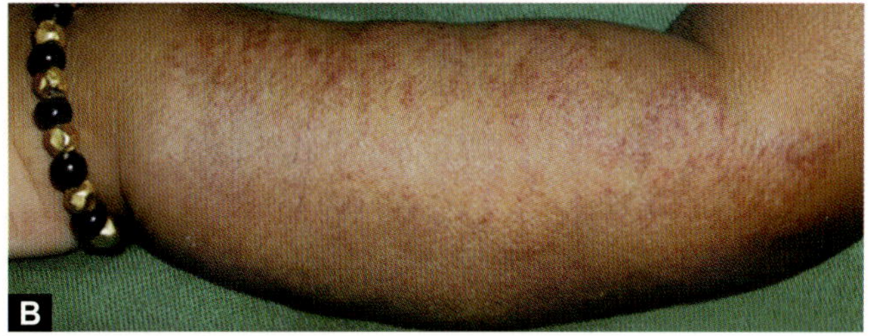

FIG. 5: **A,** Port wine stain lesions; **B,** resolution of port wine stain lesion after several treatments

Adjuvant Treatment

Topical potent steroids are recommended by many, but without established efficacy. Role of oral or intralesional steroids and propranolol is not well established in case of PWS. Rapamycin is a recent adjuvant in treatment of PWS. It is angiogenesis factor inhibitor and used topically after laser or IPL treatment of PWS. It prevents neoangiogenesis and hence recur. Currently, this drug is under trial for prevention of recurrence after vascular laser therapy.

Port Wine Stain: Adult Type

Adult type PWS have a significant element of fibrous tissue. These types of PWS are notoriously known as no responders to lasers and light. Resurfacing lasers like UltraPulse carbon dioxide (CO_2) (Fig. 6) and long-pulsed neodymiumdoped yttrium-aluminum-garnet (Nd:YAG) lasers (Fig. 7) are tried with scarring and partial outcome. Therefore, it is highly recommended that PWS has to be treated at earliest to prevent its progression into more resistant adult type.

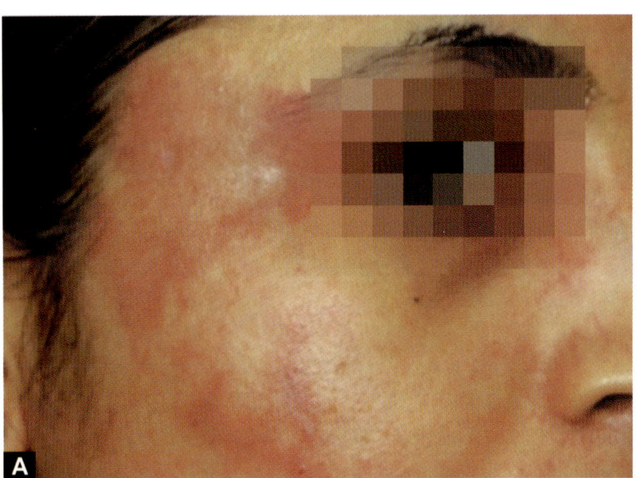

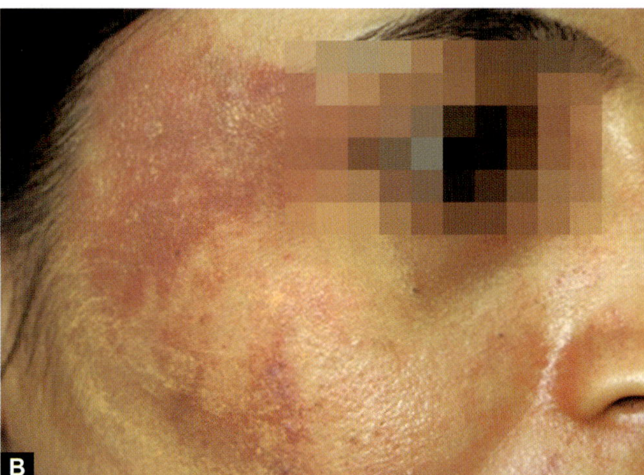

FIG. 6: Partial outcome with intense pulsed light in adult port wine stain without hypertrophy

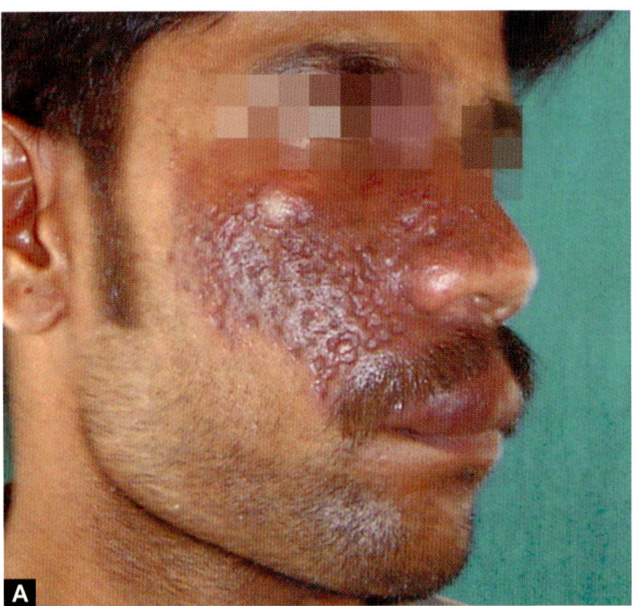

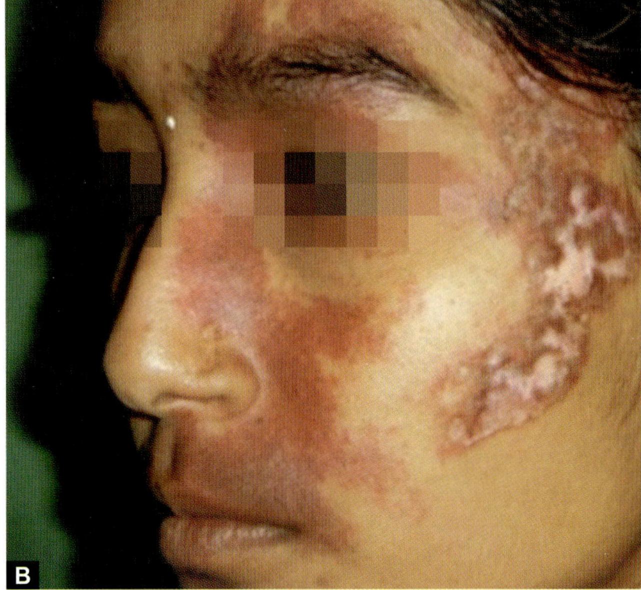

FIG. 7: Atrophic scars with long-pulsed neodymium doped yttrium-aluminum-garnet laser used in adult type of port wine stain. Pulse stacking was the technical culprit

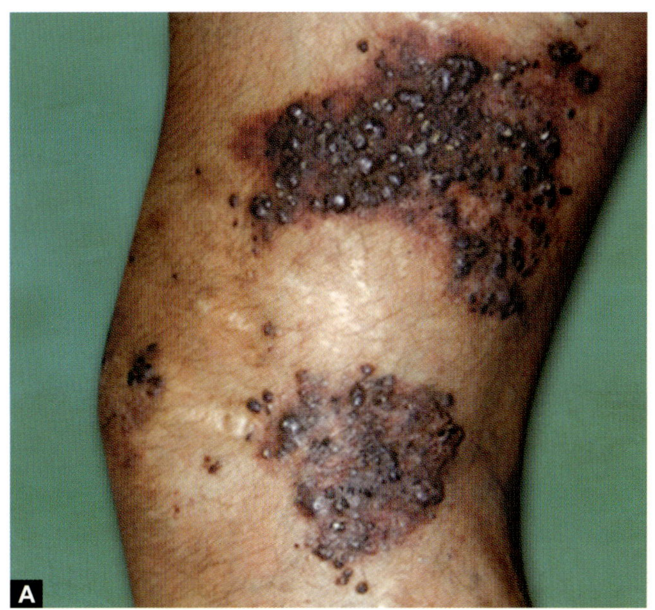

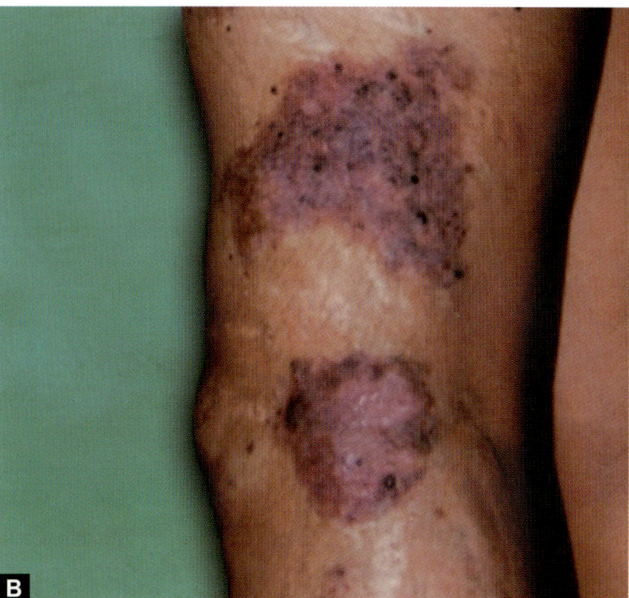

FIG. 8: **A,** Angiokeratoma lesions; **B,** treatment of angiokeratoma lesions with high density UltraPulse carbon dioxide laser

Port Wine Stain of Arteriovenous Malformation

Port wine stain as a part of complex AVM can arise at birth or several years after birth. They can evolve over a long-standing subcutaneous AVM, suddenly as an indicator of activity in the lesion. The PWS can evolve to adult type or angiokeratoma type lesions over the time. Early PWS lesions can partially respond to vascular specific IPL or PDL. But adult type and angiokeratoma type lesions may require resurfacing with Ultrapulse CO_2 laser or long-pulsed Nd:YAG lasers with variable possibility of scarring.

Intralesional or oral steroids are tried in early AVM with variable success, but its role in long-standing AVM is not known.

This case of AVM had an element of PWS on surface that evolved to angiokeratoma lesions. Responded very well to resurfacing with high density UltraPulse CO_2 fractional resurfacing two sessions (Fig. 8).

Same patient treated with aggressive parameter to target deeper vessels ended up in large wound healed over months (Fig. 9).

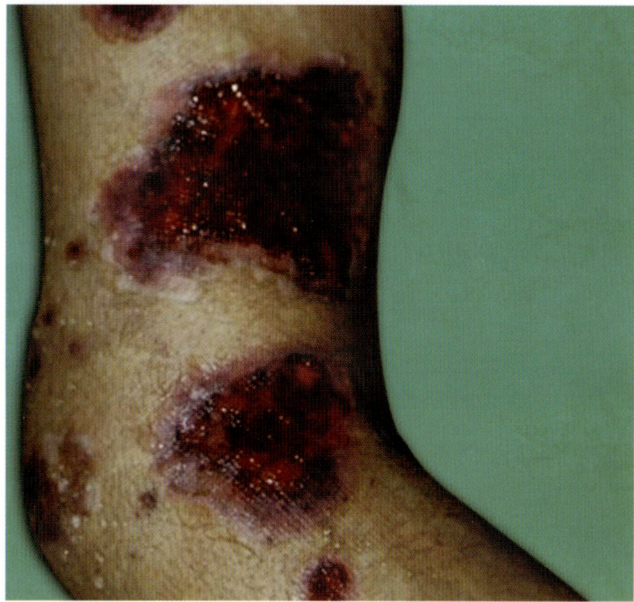

FIG. 9: Angiokeratoma lesions treated with aggressive parameter resulting in large wounds

Angiokeratoma

Angiokeratoma at various site are best treated with LP Nd:YAG laser are not amenable to IPL. The author has experienced good clearance without scarring or angiokeratoma lesions with long-pulsed Nd:YAG laser, but not found any improvement with IPL. The same is true with lymphangioma and lymphohemangioma.

Infantile Hemangioma

Ideal treatment for infantile hemangioma is PDL of long-pulsed Nd:YAG laser. Intense pulsed light may give partial clearance in selected cases of smaller hemangiomas.

Rosacea[7]

Telangiectasia of rosacea responds well to vascular specific IPL. Filter 570–600 nm is used in IPL devices with an interval of 4–8 weeks in between for 6–10 sessions. Regular treatments may prevent formation of phymas (Fig. 10).

Telangiectasia[8]

Telangiectasia is the most commonly topical steroid induced or hereditary. They respond well to IPL within 3–4 sessions at an interval of 6 weeks (Fig. 11).

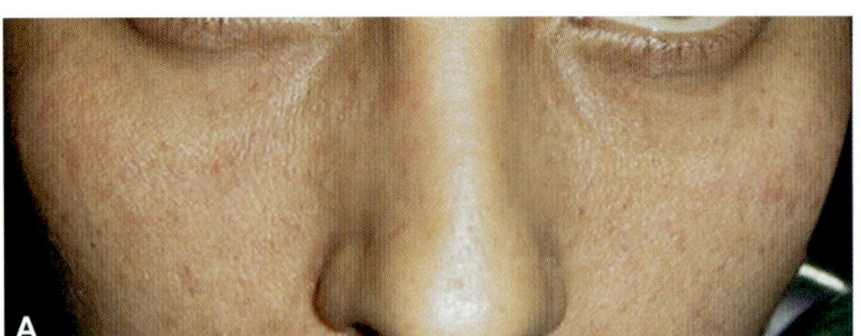

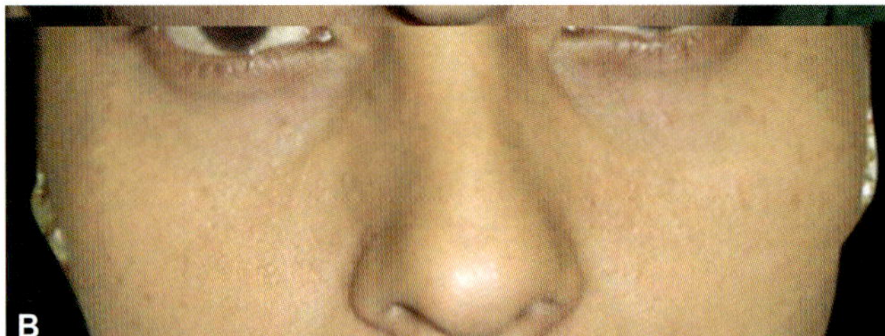

FIG. 10: **A,** Case of rosacea; **B,** after treatment with vascular specific intense pulsed light

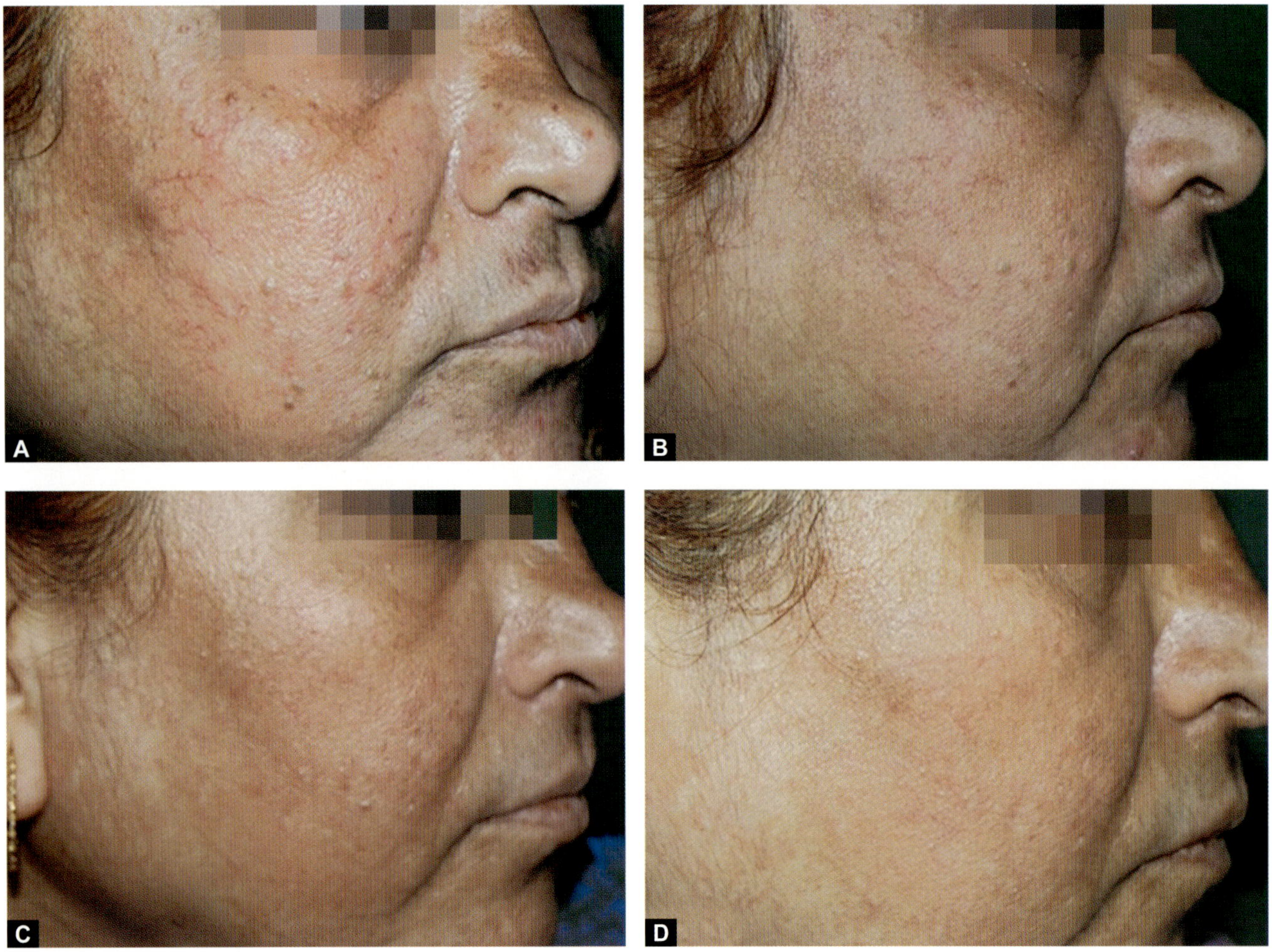

FIG. 11: Case of telangiectasia responding well to intense pulsed light within 3–4 sessions

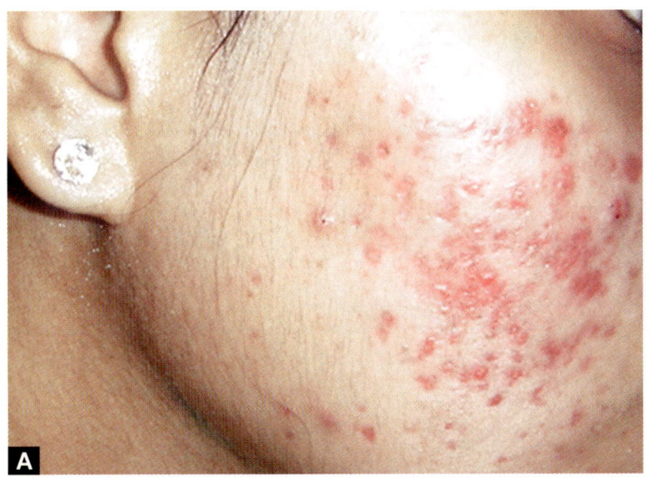

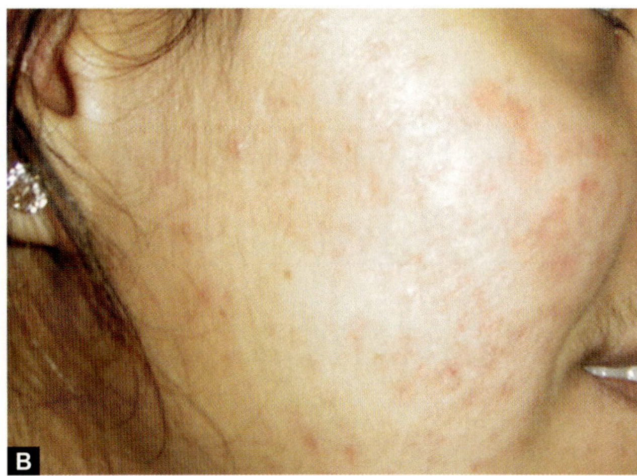

FIG. 12: Red scars treated with vascular specific narrow band or broad band intense pulsed light

Red Scars

Red scars are treated with vascular specific narrow band or broad band IPL with regular protocols.[9] Red acne scars, young red postoperative scars, and early hypertrophic scars are best treated with vascular IPLs (Fig. 12).

COMPLICATIONS

Crusting, peeling off of skin, postinflammatory hypo- and hyperpigmentation, and rarely scarring are complications of IPL. Reliable device, thorough understanding of laser tissue interactions, and safe protocols will give safe and excellent results.

CONCLUSION

Intense pulse light with capsular specific filters are effective tools for treatment of variety of vascular conditions. Newer "sandwich filter" or narrow band IPL are more effective and safer devices. Port wine stain, telangiectasia, and red scars are common indications. Proper understanding of laser tissue interactions is necessary to achieve excellent results without side effects.

REFERENCES

1. Babilas P, Schreml S, Szeimies RM, Landthaler M. Intense pulsed light (IPL): a review. Lasers Surg Med. 2010;42(2):93-104.
2. Bahmer F, Drosner M, Hohenleutner U, Kaufmann R, Kautz G, Kimmig W, et al. Recommendation for laser and intense pulsed light (IPL) therapy in dermatology. J Dtsch Dermatol Ges. 2007;5(11):1036-42.
3. Levine VJ, Geronemus RG. Adverse effects associated with the 577-and 585-nanometer pulsed dye laser in the treatment of cutaneous vascular lesions: a study of 500 patients. J Am Acad Dermatol. 1995;32(4):613-7.
4. Dover JS, Arndt KA. New approaches to the treatment of vascular lesions. Lasers Surg Med. 2000;26:158-63.
5. Raulin C, Schroeter CA, Weiss RA, Keiner M, Werner S. Treatment of port-wine stains with a noncoherent pulsed light source: a retrospective study. Arch Dermatol. 1999;135(6):679-83.
6. Ho WS, Ying SY, Chan PC, Chan HH. Treatment of port wine stains with intense pulsed light: a prospective study. Dermatol Surg. 2004;30(6):887-90.
7. Clementoni MT, Gilardino P, Muti GF, Signorini M, Pistorale A, Morselli PG, et al. Facial telangiectasias: our experience in treatment with IPL. Lasers Surg Med. 2005;37(1):9-13.
8. Schroeter CA, Haaf-von Below S, Neumann HA. Effective treatment of rosacea using intense pulsed light systems. Dermatol Surg. 2005;31(10):1285-9.
9. Cartier H. Use of intense pulsed light in the treatment of scars. J Cosmet Dermatol. 2005;4(1):34-40.

CHAPTER 22

Long-pulsed Neodymium Doped Yttrium-aluminium-garnet Laser for Treatment of Vascular Malformations

Abhishek De, Manmit K Hora

INTRODUCTION

Lasers are good therapeutic tool for both congenital and acquired vascular lesions. Technological advances in lasers have reduced adverse effects and increased efficacy. Though various lasers are used for treating vascular lesions, pulsed dye laser (PDL) is widely considered as the gold standard of treatment and has best efficacy and safety data. However, PDL also have certain limitations. Post-treatment purpura is common after PDL, which can last for 7–14 days and cosmetically, may be unacceptable for some patients. Other side effects, like hyperpigmentation, hypopigmentation, scarring, and atrophy, are also quite common. Use of PDL is also limited by its high purchasing and maintenance cost. Moreover, often incomplete and unsatisfactory result, especially in lesions involving deeper vessels, encourages laser surgeons to look beyond PDL. A good amount of clinical data are also accumulating in other devices including pulsed potassium titanyl phosphate (KTP) laser, alexandrite laser, long-pulsed neodymium doped yttrium-aluminium-garnet (Nd:YAG) laser, and intense pulsed light (IPL). Amongst these lasers and light devices, long-pulsed Nd:YAG have the benefit of wider availability, vast experience in use of darker skin, and longer wavelength allowing to treat deeper blood vessels.[1]

Neodymium Doped Yttrium-aluminium-garnet Laser

Long-pulsed Nd:YAG laser has a wavelength of 1,064 nm. This laser has a deeper penetration when compared to PDL. However, it also has lower absorption by hemoglobin limiting its efficacy. Possibly, Nd:YAG has a better absorption by the deep spider veins than the traditionally used lasers with shorter wavelength.[2] The 1,064 nm Nd:YAG laser produces a coagulation effect at a depth of 5–6 mm. This is much deeper than the 1–2 mm depth of coagulation achieved by PDL. So, long-pulsed Nd:YAG is capable of treating moderately deep and larger blood vessels, and also the feeding reticular veins.[3]

The wavelength 1,064 nm is well beyond the three absorption peaks of oxyhemoglobin which are at 418, 542, and 577 nm. However, beyond 1,000 nm, the relative absorption curves of oxyhemoglobin and melanin run close. So, though the absolute values of absorption and scattering coefficients of Nd:YAG are much lower when compared to that of PDL, the ratio of melanin to blood absorption is similar to that of PDL. This allows long-pulsed Nd:YAG to work as a vascular laser with relative safety. The absorption coefficient of blood at 1,064 nm is found to be 0.4/mm, which is much higher to that of the surrounding dermal tissue (0.05/mm) at the same wavelength. The treatment selectivity of the deep blood vessels is due to this difference in absorption coefficient. The relative safety of the epidermis is ensured by the fact, the longer wavelength ensure deeper penetration and at this wavelength, the absorption of light by melanin is also low.[4]

Conventionally, it is advisable to limit the use of Nd:YAG lasers to deeper and blue vessels, but increasingly Nd:YAG laser is being used for hemangioma and port wine stain. Neodymium doped yttrium-aluminium-garnet can be used to treat both superficial and deep vascular lesions by controlling the depth of penetration through appropriate spot size selection (3, 5, 7, and 10 mm), variable pulse duration (0.1–300 ms), and high fluences (up to 300 J/cm^2). Optimal cooling system should be used to prevent pain, burning, and dyschromia. However, if the Nd:YAG laser devices have limitation as per choice of parameter combinations, their use in vascular condition should be very restricted.[5]

PARAMETERS FOR LONG-PULSED NEODYMIUM DOPED YTTRIUM-ALUMINIUM-GARNET LASER

Neodymium doped yttrium-aluminium-garnet lasers can be used to treat superficial vascular lesions such as rosacea, facial telangiectasia, poikiloderma of Civatte, and flat hemangiomas with spot sizes of 3–5 mm. The larger spot sizes between 5 and 7 mm are required for thicker and deeper lesions such as tuberous hemangiomas or port wine stain and leg veins.[6] Pulse duration should be selected according to the estimated vessel size of the target lesion; 1–5 ms for thin, 10–25 ms for medium, and 25–50 ms for thick vessels. Choice of fluences may vary from 10–100 J/cm^2 according to the depth of the lesion and patients skin type. There should be no fixed fluence for any vascular laser. It is advisable that the laser surgeon should adjust the parameters for individual patient depending on the clinical signs like immediate reaction and color change on the vessel, on each treatment.[5]

INDICATIONS FOR VASCULAR LASERS[7]

Vascular lasers are indicated for the following vascular lesions:

Congenital vascular lesions:
- Port wine stain
- Hemangioma

Acquired vascular lesions:
- Facial telangiectasia
- Rosacea associated telangiectasia
- Spider angioma
- Poikiloderma associated telangiectasia and erythema
- Pyogenic granuloma
- Venous lake
- Leg telangiectasia
- Angiofibroma
- Blue rubber bleb nevus syndrome
- Cherry angioma.

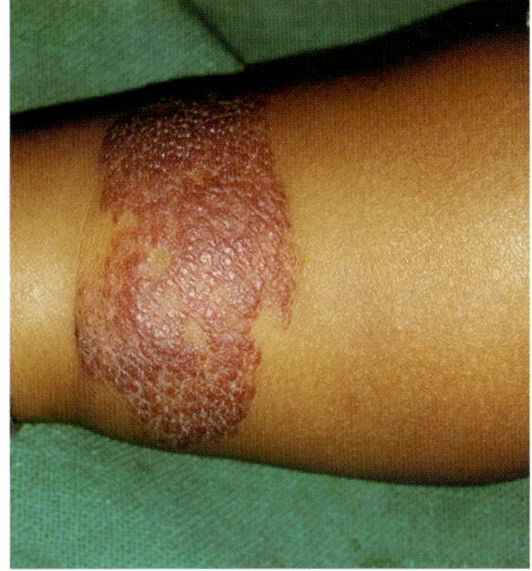

FIG. 1: Vascular lesion before neodymium doped yttrium-aluminium-garnet laser treatment.

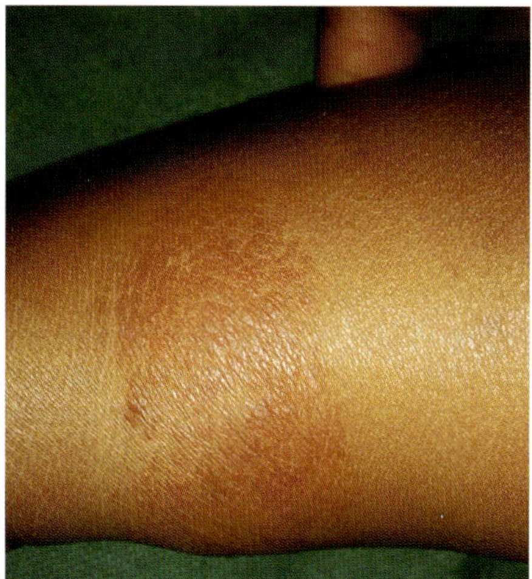

FIG. 2: Vascular lesion after three sessions of long-pulsed neodymium doped yttrium-aluminium-garnet laser treatment.

Congenital Vascular Lesions

Hemangioma

Hemangioma is the most common vascular anomaly, affecting up to 12% of all children by 1 year of age. Based on the depth of the lesion, hemangioma may be superficial, subcutaneous, or mixed tumor.

Majority of hemangioma appear shortly after birth and undergo rapid growth during the first year of life, while some involute spontaneously. These hemangiomas do not require treatment. However, even after complete involution, 40–50% of children are still left with residual fibrofatty tissue. Some lesions can be life-threatening (lesions over the head and neck) or function-threatening (periorbital lesions) or cosmetically disfiguring.[8]

Laser treatment can be considered in the following conditions:

- Ulcerated hemangioma, which may bleed on mildest trauma and can become secondarily infected
- Hemangiomas which are function-threatening, for example, lesions located over the lip, can cause difficultly in feeding. Lesion in periorbital area can lead to obstruction of vision
- Superficial hemangioma which is cosmetically disfiguring
- Residual telangiectasia after complete involution.[8]

Long-pulsed PDL has been reported to be safer and more effective than PDL for childhood hemangioma in one study.[9] In a recent study, Zhong et al. treated 794 Chinese patients with infantile hemangiomas and found that the efficacy of long-pulsed 1,064 nm Nd:YAG laser was 87.57%. Efficacy of laser did not depend on sex or the location of the lesion. Older age and superficial hemangioma were the primary factors contributing to greater efficacy of long-pulsed 1,064 nm Nd:YAG laser treatment for infantile hemangiomas. The most common side effects were pigment changes, skin atrophy, and wrinkled redundant skin, which usually resolved spontaneously within 1-3 years.[10] Though the superficial hemangiomas are usually treated uneventfully with long-pulsed laser, while treating the deep components of hemangiomas, this laser carries the risk of scarring, blistering, crusting, pigmentation, and textural abnormalities. These complications are due to deep thermal injury from intensely penetrating near infrared light. Neodymium doped yttrium-aluminium-garnet laser has a narrow band of safety and efficacy.[11] Ulcerated lesions are painful and require local anesthesia (1% lignocaine).

Long-pulsed Nd:YAG is available as continuous or pulsed beams and can penetrate to a depth of 4–6 mm and coagulate the deeper and large vessels. Thermal energy diffuses rapidly within the blood vessels leading to selective microvascular damage, through photocoagulation and mechanical injury. The end result is thrombosis of the blood vessels. There is always an inherent risk of scarring. The parameters for the treatment of hemangioma are spot size 3–10 mm, pulse duration of 0.1–300 ms, and maximum fluence of up to 300 J/cm^2. The most common side effect of Nd:YAG laser is ulceration, scarring, and hypopigmentation.[12]

Port Wine Stain

Histologically, port wine stain is composed of elastic vessels in the papillary dermis. They can vary from a few millimeters in size to up to 50% of the body surface area. They persist throughout the life, and are usually located on the face, commonly on the V2 distribution. As the child grows, the initial flat pink macules and patches turn into "cobblestoned" purple plaques and nodules due to progressive vascular ectasia. Therefore, it is advisable to start laser treatment in early stages to prevent complications.

Pulsed dye laser is considered as the gold standard treatment for port wine stain. There is paucity of literature in efficacy and safety of long-pulsed Nd:YAG in port wine stain. Groot et al. demonstrated good efficacy and safety with long-pulsed Nd:YAG lasers in deeper vessel anomalies.[5] In another study, long-pulsed Nd:YAG laser is shown to provide better efficacy in the treatment of hypertrophic and nodular port wine stain, as longer wavelength provides deeper penetration.[6] Treatment must be started at a low fluence and overlapping pulses should be avoided. Care must be taken to provide

Box 1: Tips for using neodymium doped yttrium-aluminium-garnet laser for vascular lesions[7,8]

- Increase pulse duration with larger blood vessels and higher vascular volume
- For deeper and large diameter blood vessels, use larger spot size and for superficial and smaller diameter blood vessels, use smaller spot size
- Purple or blue blood vessels absorb more light than pink or red blood vessels, so, use less fluence
- Fluence has to be adjusted as per vessel type; it should increase in smaller diameter, deeper, and high pressure blood vessels

adequate surface cooling to prevent scarring and hypopigmentation. Port wine stain on the temple, around the eye, forehead, lateral cheek, and chin respond better to treatment than those on the central cheek and nose.[5]

While treating port wine stain, it is important to mark the border of the lesion beforehand with a skin-marking pen and start the treatment from the edge of the lesion and slowly move towards the center. This is because the reactive erythema often masks the lesional border. Authors' experience and available data suggest that early onset of treatment gives better result. Treatment should ideally begin in early infancy, and the first three sessions give most effective results. Likely, factors contributing for the better results in infancy could be thinner skin, smaller and more superficial vessels, and smaller affected surface area. It is mandatory to use intraocular shield for treating port wine stain close to eyes. We noticed that the degree of clearance might be site dependent. The neck, forehead, and lateral cheek areas respond better than central face.

Acquired Vascular Lesions

Facial Telangiectasia

Telangiectasia is seen in at least 10–15% of adults and children. Facial telangiectasia is commonly located over the midface region as small, dilated vessels of about 0.1–1.0 mm in diameter. It can be seen in both children and adults. Many exogenous factors, like alcohol, estrogen, corticosteroids, and chronic sun exposure, can lead to telangiectasia.

Prior to the advances in lasers, the treatment of facial telangiectasia was limited to sclerotherapy and electrocautery, which had a high risk of ulceration, atrophy, or hyperpigmentation. Pulsed dye laser and IPL have been widely used for facial telangiectasia. However, long-pulsed Nd:YAG laser can be considered as another modality to treat telangiectasias of the face.

In a prospective study of a variable pulse 1,064 nm Nd:YAG laser with 6 mm spot size on facial telangiectasias, clearance of 75% of telangiectasias was found at 1 month in 97% of the sites that were treated.[13] In another study, moderate-to-significant improvement in 80% of patients treated for telangiectasias of the face was demonstrated.[14] Safety of long-pulsed Nd:YAG was also studied by Major et al. who reported swelling and crusting that lasted for a few days in every 1 of 25 patients treated with the 1,064 nm Nd:YAG laser for facial telangiectasias.[15]

A small spot size (1.5 mm) Nd:YAG laser using a pulse width of 20 ms or higher reported clearing in 50–75% of facial ectasias with a single pass with minimal side effects.

The limited available evidence suggests long-pulsed 1,064 nm Nd:YAG laser is safe and effective for the treatment of facial telangiectasia and satisfactory results were achieved with a single treatment with minimal side effects like transient erythema and some very mild swelling and crusting that lasts for a few days. Facial telangiectasia is treated at a fluence of 100 J/cm^2, pulse duration of 10 ms, and 2 Hz repetition rate.

Rosacea Associated Telangiectasia

Rosacea is a chronic skin disorder that is characterized by flushing, persistent erythema, telangiectasia, papules, and pustules affecting the central face. It is often mistaken for other skin disorders like acne vulgaris, steroid induced acne, or lupus. Even though it is a common skin condition, the treatment modalities available are not satisfactory.

According to a study, smaller spot sizes with moderate fluences (100–400 J/cm^2) and longer pulse durations (10–100 ms) were effective and well-tolerated by the patients. Neodymium doped yttrium-aluminium-garnet laser due to its deeper depth of penetration, low absorption in melanin, and relatively good absorption in oxyhemoglobin[16] has been used effectively for the treatment of telangiectatic blood vessels less than 1 and up to 2 mm in diameter with minimal side effects.

Fluence of 160–210 J/cm^2 can be used. A lower fluence is preferred for shallow vessels whereas higher fluence is used for deeper vessels. Based on the thermal relaxation time of the treated vessels, pulse durations can be between 10 and 15 ms.

Leg Telangiectasia

Leg telangiectasia is more difficult to treat as the vessels are deeper and larger than those of the facial telangiectasia. In 1999, Weiss and Weiss for the first time reported the use of a 1,064 nm long-pulsed laser on leg telangiectasia.[17] They demonstrated that the 1,064 nm wavelength laser gave more satisfactory results in the treatment of dilated leg vessels (0.5–3.0 mm) than lasers with shorter wavelength. The long wavelength facilitates deeper penetration into the skin and targets the deep vessels. The Nd:YAG laser has a maximum penetration of 3 mm, thus destroying the large vessels in the deep dermis. It is safer in patients with darker skin as there is scanty absorption by melanin. The 1,064 nm Nd:YAG laser allows treatment of leg telangiectasia using a fluence ranging from 100 to 200 J/cm^2, using a spot size of 2.5–3 mm and a pulse width of 10–30 ms.

Cherry Angiomas

Cherry angiomas are well-circumscribed, small red papules composed of vascular telangiectasia that typically present in the 3rd or 4th decades of life. The lesions may be found anywhere on the body, especially on the trunk and proximal extremities, but usually, the mucous membranes are spared.

The treatment options for cherry angiomas include electrocautery, shave excision, and laser therapy. A variety of lasers like KTP, PDL, argon, and Nd:YAG has been used for its treatment. Long-pulsed Nd:YAG laser provides effective treatment of the lesions. The only side effect is crusting of the lesions which can be treated with topical antibiotics.[18]

Venous Lakes

Venous lakes are dilated vessels which result due to weakening of preexisting vessel walls due to photodamage. They usually present as blue papules on the face in older people. The lesions respond well to laser therapy. Long-pulsed Nd:YAG laser has an excellent response to treatment.

CONCLUSION

Though Pulsed dye laser is considered as the gold standard of vascular lasers; Nd:YAG lasers which is more widely available, has come up as a cost effective alternative. A thorough knowledge of patient's condition and understanding of basic laser physics will help the doctor in selecting appropriate pulse duration, spot size, and fluence. However, more quality data is awaited in establishing the efficacy and safety of Nd:YAG laser in various vascular malformations, especially in context of darker skin type.

REFERENCES

1. Tanzi EL, Lupton JR, Alster TS. Lasers in dermatology: four decades of progress. J Am Acad Dermatol. 2003;49(1):1-31.
2. Adamic M, Troilius A, Adatto M, Drosner M, Dahmane R. Vascular lasers and IPLS: guidelines for care from the European Society for Laser Dermatology (ESLD). J Cosmet Laser Ther. 2007;9(2):113-24.
3. Landthaler M, Hohenleutner U, Abd el Raheem TA. Therpy of vascular lesions in the head and neck area by means of argon, Nd:YAG, and flashlamp-pumped pulsed dye lasers. Adv Otorhinolaryngol. 1995;49:81-6.
4. Landthaler M, Haina D, Brunner R, Waidelich W, Braun-Falco O. Neodymium-YAG laser therapy for vascular lesions. J Am Acad Dermatol. 1986;14:107-17.
5. Groot D, Rao J, Johnston P, Nakatsui T. Algorithm for using a long-pulsed Nd:YAG laser in the treatment of deep cutaneous vascular lesions. Dermatol Surg. 2003;29(1):35-42.
6. Yang MU, Yaroslavsky AN, Farinelli WA, Flotte TJ, Rius-Diaz F, Tsao SS, et al. Long-pulsed neodymium: yttrium-aluminum-garnet laser treatment for port-wine stains. J Am Acad Dermatol. 2005;52:480-90.
7. Srinivas CR, Kumaresan M. Lasers for vascular lesions: standard guidelines of care. Indian J Dermatol Venereol Leprol. 2011;77(3):349-68.
8. Garden JM, Bakus AD. Laser treatment of port-wine stains and hemangiomas. Dermatol Clin. 1997;15(3):373-83.
9. Kono T, Sakurai H, Groff WF, Chan HH, Takeuchi M, Yamaki T, et al. Comparison study of a traditional pulsed dye laser versus a long-pulsed dye laser in the treatment of early childhood hemangiomas. Lasers Surg Med. 2006;38:112-5.
10. Zheng JW, Wang YA, Zhou GY, Zhu HG, Ye WM, Zhang ZY. Head and neck hemangiomas: how and when to treat. Shanghai Kou Qiang Yi Xue. 2007;16(4):337-42.
11. Galeckas KJ. Update on lasers and light devices for the treatment of vascular lesions. Semin Cutan Med Surg. 2008;27(4):276-84.
12. Willey A, Anderson RR, Azpiazu JL, Bakus AD, Barlow RJ, Dover JS, et al. Complications of laser dermatologic surgery. Lasers Surg Med. 2006;38:1-15.
13. Eremia S, Li CY. Treatment of face veins with a cryogen spray variable pulse width 1064 nm Nd:YAG laser: a prospective study of 17 patients. Dermatol Surg. 2002;28(3):244-7.
14. Sarradet DM, Hussain M, Goldberg DJ. Millisecond 1064-nm neodymium:YAG laser treatment of facial telangiectases. Dermatol Surg. 2003;29(1):56-8.
15. Major A, Brazzini ÀB, Campolmi P, Bona P, Mavilia L, Ghersetich I, et al. Nd:YAG 1064 nm laser in the treatment of facial and leg telangiectasias. J Eur Acad Dermatol Venereol. 2001;15(6):559-65.
16. Laube S, Lanigan SW. Laser treatment of rosacea. J Cosmet Dermatol. 2002;1(4):188-95.
17. Weiss RA, Weiss MA. Early clinical results with a multiple synchronized pulse: 1064 nm laser for leg telangiectasias and reticular veins. Dermatol Surg. 1999;25(5):399-402.
18. Pancar GS, Aydin F, Senturk N, Bek Y, Canturk MT, Turanli AY. Comparison of the 532-nm KTP and 1064-nm Nd:YAG lasers for the treatment of cherry angiomas. J Cosmet Laser Ther. 2011;13(4):138-41.

CHAPTER 23

Evidence Based Vascular Laser Treatment

Imran Majid

INTRODUCTION

Cutaneous vascular lesions are one of the major causes of psychosocial morbidity among dermatology patients. Even though most of these lesions are benign, the effect these lesions have on the patient's self-esteem is considerable. Moreover, some of these lesions, like hemangiomas are associated with severe and life-threatening complications. This necessitates a timely diagnosis and a proper treatment. A number of treatment modalities have been tried with variable success rates. But the advent of lasers has revolutionized the treatment of this group of cutaneous lesions.

PROPERTIES OF VASCULAR LASERS

Most of the lasers used for the treatment or ablation of vascular lesions utilize the principle of selective photothermolysis as proposed by Anderson and Parish.[1] Once photons of light from the laser source fall upon the target site, this incident light gets converted into heat after being absorbed by the specific chromophore. In turn, the heat generated is dissipated by conduction. However, if the rate of heat production exceeds the rate of loss, the heat causes selective damage to the target chromophore.

In case of cutaneous vascular lesions, the target chromophores are two molecules: oxyhemoglobin and deoxyhemoglobin. Oxyhemoglobin molecule has absorption peaks at 418 nm, 542 nm, and 577 nm for blue, green, and yellow light, respectively.[2] The largest peak at 418 nm does not allow adequate penetration in the skin. However, the longer 542 nm, 577 nm peaks, and a broad 800–1,100 nm band form the basis of most of the vascular lasers.

PROPERTIES OF VASCULAR LASERS

Wavelength

Penetration into the skin is governed by the wavelength of the incident light. Longer wavelength penetrates the skin more than shorter wavelength.[3] The maximum absorption peak of oxyhemoglobin within superficial vessels (e.g., those of the face and neck) is at 542 nm (α peak) and 577 nm (β peak). Arteries and veins being deeper vessels have more deoxyhemoglobin which in turn has a longer absorption peak. Venous malformations like portwine stains can be treated more selectively with approximately 630–780 nm laser sources, whereas 1,064 nm [neodymium doped yttrium-aluminium-garnet (Nd:YAG) lasers] tend to affect arterial more than venous blood.[4] So, the nature and depth of the target vessel, i.e., the type of vascular malformation should be taken into consideration when deciding the type of the laser to be used for a vascular malformation or disease.

Fluence

Based on the concept of selective photothermolysis, a defined value of fluence, also called as the energy density is required to achieve the desired temperature for ablation of the target vessel.[1] Too high fluence can cause damage to the adjoining tissues with increased incidence of side effects, like scarring and pigmentary disturbances.

Pulse Frequency

The pulse frequency of the laser is another important property that should be considered. Usually, higher frequencies need to be avoided to minimize thermal damage to the surrounding skin.[5] However, higher pulse frequency yields good results in some situations if used by an experienced operator. Studies have shown that stacked pulses of a lower fluence (energy density) may have a similar effect on the target as a single pulse at a higher fluence.[6-8]

Pulse Duration

The concept of thermal relaxation time (TRT) is pertinent in the context of laser pulse duration. Thermal relaxation time is the time interval required for the target to deliver 50% of heat to the surrounding tissues. Thermal damage to the adjoining tissues can be minimized if the laser pulse duration is equal or less than the TRT of the target.[9] Pulse duration is thus governed by the type of vessel to be ablated. In case of larger diameter vessels, more heat is required to dissipate thermal energy from red blood cells to the adjoining vessel wall to cause thrombosis. Accordingly, larger pulse duration is needed for such vessels to achieve the desired therapeutic effect.[10,11]

Spot Size

Spot size or the diameter of the laser beam governs the energy density (fluence). If a larger spot size is selected, only a small amount of energy is scattered outside the target site, with resultant greater energy being directed at the target site and hence a greater damage to the deeper dermal tissue.[12]

Skin Cooling

Laser beams produce sufficient energy to ablate the target tissue. So there is a higher risk of damage to the superficial tissues especially the epidermis. This is minimized by using cooling techniques. This includes a number of techniques like contact cooling, e.g., the use of ice packs, cold gel, and sapphire window. Other methods include cold air convection and dynamic cooling wherein a liquid cryogen is sprayed immediately before the laser pulse.[13]

CLASSIFICATION OF VASCULAR ANOMALIES

A large number of lesions are included within the spectrum of vascular anomalies. Many of these anomalies are highly amenable to laser treatment with excellent clinical results, while others respond poorly. So, a proper knowledge of these lesions is required to make a proper diagnosis, decide whether laser treatment is useful or not and then choose which laser would be the most appropriate.

Boxes 1 and 2, respectively, list the classification of congenital and acquired cutaneous vascular anomalies that can be treated by laser treatment.

Box 1: Vascular anomalies which may be treated by transcutaneous vascular lasers[14,15]

Benign vascular tumors
- Infantile hemangioma
  - Pattern: focal, multifocal, segmental, and indeterminate
  - Types: superficial, deep, mixed, reticular/abortive/minimal growth, others
  - Within complex anomalies: PHACE and SACRAL and PELVIS syndromes
- Congenital hemangioma
  - RICH
  - NICH
  - PICH
- Pyogenic granuloma (lobular capillary hemangioma)
- Angiokeratoma

Vascular malformations
- Capillary malformations
  - Cutaneous and/or mucosal CM (PWS)
  - PWS associated with other anomalies (e.g., Klippel-Trennaunay)
  - Telangiectasia
  - Hereditary hemorrhagic telangiectasia (various subtypes)
  - Nevus simplex (salmon patch, stork bite)
- Venous malformations
  - Common venous malformations
  - Familial venous malformations cutaneomucosal
  - Glomuvenous malformation
  - Blue rubber bleb nevus syndrome
- Combined malformations

CM, capillary malformations; NICH, noninvoluting congenital hemangioma; PHACE, posterior fossa malformations–hemangiomas–arterial anomalies–cardiac defects–eye abnormalities–sternal cleft and supraumbilical raphe; PELVIS, perineal hemangiomas with the following congenital abnormalities: external genitalia malformations, lipomyelomeningocele, vesicorenal abnormalities, imperforate anus and skin tags; SACRAL syndrome, perineal hemangiomas and spinal dysraphism, anogenital anomalies, cutaneous anomalies, renal and urologic anomalies, associated with angioma of lumbosacral localization; PICH, partially involuting congenital hemangioma; PWS, port-wine syndrome; RICH, rapidly involuting congenital hemangioma; VM, vascular malformation.

Box 2: Acquired vascular malformations that can be treated by laser therapy[5]

- Facial telangiectasia
- Rosacea
- Nevus araneus (spider angioma)
- Venous angiomas
- Venous lake
- Senile angioma
- Poikiloderma of Civatte
- Granuloma telangiectaticum (pyogenic granuloma)
- Angiofibroma
- Cutaneous lesions of Kaposi sarcoma
- Leg telangiectasias

PREPROCEDURE EVALUATION

Success of the treatment depends on a number of factors which include the following preprocedure parameters.

History and clinical examination:

- A complete medical history
- A detailed drug history
- Duration of the lesion or lesions and progression
- Treatments taken till now
- History of any similar procedure done previously; if yes, whether any complication occurred; whether improvement occurred or not?
- Proper clinical examination:
  - Skin type of patient
  - Nature and extent of lesion
  - Whether lesion is amenable to treatment
  - Whether there are any associated pigmentary changes, scarring, or any sequelae of previous treatment seen; if yes, explaining their effect on treatment to the patient.

Also, the nature of the procedure to be done, the approximate number of sittings required, the interval between the sittings, possible side effects that can occur, and how to manage them should all be explained to the patient before taking up any patient for vascular laser therapy.

Finally, a patient with realistic expectations is an ideal candidate and only such patients should be taken up for laser treatment.

PREPROCEDURE STEPS

Once a patient is selected for laser treatment, the following steps need to be followed:

- A written consent should be taken from the patient
- The patient should be instructed to start applying sunscreen with a high sun protection factor, at least 4 weeks prior to the procedure.[16]

OVERVIEW OF VASCULAR LASERS

Since the introduction of the first vascular laser—the flashlamp-pumped pulsed dye laser (PDL) in 1989,[17] a large number of lasers have been developed since then which are more selective for vascular pathologies. A brief overview of these lasers is summarized in table 1.

TABLE 1: Different types of lasers with their properties and indication

Laser type	Absorption peaks and penetration depth	Major indications
KTP (532 nm; green)	Oxyhemoglobin > melanin; ~1 mm	Facial telangiectasias and diffuse erythema, rosacea, cherry and spider angiomata, poikiloderma of Civatte, thin leg telangiectasias (<1 mm), PWS
PDL (585–595 nm; yellow)	Oxyhemoglobin > melanin; 1–1.5 mm	PWS, infantile hemangioma, facial telangiectasias, rosacea, cherry and spider angiomata, poikiloderma of Civatte, thin leg telangiectasias
Alexandrite laser (755 nm; infrared)	Melanin > deoxyhemoglobin > oxyhemoglobin; 2.5–3 mm	PWS, wider leg telangiectasias
Diode lasers (800–983 nm; infrared)	Oxyhemoglobin ≥ melanin; above 900 nm low melanin absorption; 3–5 mm	Facial telangiectasia, PWS, leg telangiectasia, venous lakes
Nd:YAG laser (1,064 nm; infrared)	Ratio of melanin to blood absorption is similar to PDL, but due to generally low absorption, higher energies are needed; 5–6 mm	PWS, larger leg telangiectasia, infantile hemangiomas, venous malformations, pyogenic granuloma
Intense pulsed light sources (IPLS) (500–1,200 nm)	For vascular lesions cutoff filters at 550 nm and 570 nm are used (deliver mainly yellow and red light)	Facial telangiectasia and diffuse erythema; rosacea, PWS, fine leg telangiectasia, poikiloderma of Civatte.

KTP, potassium titanyl phosphate; Nd:YAG, neodymium dope yttrium-aluminum-garnet; PDL, pulsed dye laser; PWS, port wine stain.

TREATMENT OF SOME COMMON VASCULAR ANOMALIES

As explained previously, the type of laser to be used for a particular lesion is governed by many factors including the laser specifications as well as patient related factors. Various guidelines have been proposed by different authorities in different centers. However, the latest guidelines and recommendations put forth by the European Society for Laser Dermatology[5] are highlighted in this chapter.

Facial Telangiectasias and Diffuse Facial Erythema

The use of lasers and intense pulsed light sources have been recommended for both these conditions.[18-20] Among the various lasers, the short wavelength lasers, like PDL (595 nm), potassium titanyl phosphate (KTP) laser (532 nm) and intense pulsed light sources (IPLS) have been advocated as the first choice. Various studies have shown response rates in the range of 50–90% with these lasers for various variants of facial telangiectasias. If good results are not obtained, millisecond or microsecond Nd:YAG (1,064 nm) or diode (940 or 980 nm) are used as second line treatment choices. Long-pulse, alexandrite (755 nm) and copper vapor (510 and 578 nm) can be used as lasers, but extreme caution needs to be exercised while using them.[21-23] However, adequate cooling measures are recommended to protect the epidermis from thermal damage.

Rosacea

European Society for Laser Dermatology proposes that the erythema and telangiectasia of rosacea are effectively reduced by the use of LPDL (595 nm), KTP (532 nm), and IPLS, thus causing a marked improvement in the clinical symptoms.[22,24] However, little evidence is available for millisecond and microsecond Nd:YAG lasers. Moreover, it has been seen that the use of topical niacin enhances the use of PDL in this condition, especially in dark skinned individuals.[25]

Port Wine Stain

It is a commonly seen capillary malformation, causing severe cosmetic disfigurement to the patient. The treatment becomes important as most of the lesions turn darker and thicker with age. Usually, the lesion is more amenable to treatment at an early stage.[5]

European Society for Laser Dermatology recommends early onset of laser treatment in case of PWS and flashlamp-pumped dye laser (FPDL) (585 nm) or LPDL (595 nm) as the first choice treatment. In case of flatter lesions, large spot KTP (532 nm) and IPLS may also be tried with varying success.[26,27] However, in treatment resistant cases, millisecond Nd:YAG laser (1,064 nm), alexandrite (755 nm), diode lasers, and IPLS have been tried at some centers.[28,29]

Spider Angioma

This lesion shows a central feeding arteriole associated with fine, red telangiectasia radiating from it.[10] Millisecond Nd:YAG (1,064 nm), KTP (532 nm), and LPDL lasers and IPLS have been recommended as effective for rapid ablation of spider angiomas.[10,30] Argon or copper vapor lasers have been used as second line lasers in case of refractory lesions or at places where the first group of lasers is not available or contraindicated.

Pyogenic Granuloma

A friable benign vascular tumor that bleeds with the slightest trauma, pyogenic granuloma, is treated by a number of therapeutic options. Laser treatment is one such modality giving satisfactory results. Long-pulsed dye laser (595 nm), carbon dioxide (10,600 nm), and millisecond Nd:YAG lasers (1,064 nm) have been successfully used for treating small and superficial cutaneous pyogenic granulomas.[31,32]

Venous Lakes

These represent cutaneous vascular anomalies which are formed from dilated venules in the upper dermis. Among the various lasers available, millisecond Nd:YAG (1,064 nm), dual PDL-Nd:YAG laser, alexandrite (755 nm), and diode (800, 808, and 980 nm) lasers are used as a first-line therapeutic option.[33,34]

Cherry Angioma

It is a commonly found vascular tumor mostly found in elderly people and presents as a circumscribed bright red papule. Histologically, it is composed of interconnected vascular dilations, ranging from 10 μm to 50 μm in diameter, are closely packed within the papillary dermis.[35] Potassium titanyl phosphate (532 nm), millisecond Nd:YAG (1,064 nm), LPDL (595 nm) lasers, and IPLS are considered to be suitable for the successful removal of this lesion.[36,37]

Poikiloderma of Civatte

It is believed to be induced by sun exposure and often found unresponsive to standard treatment options.[38] Laser therapy has been found to be safe with the IPLS, KTP (532 nm), and LPDL (595 nm) lasers being useful treatment options.[39,40]

Telangiectatic Leg Veins

These dilated vessels are usually treated effectively by ambulatory phlebectomy and sclerotherapy. Lasers are not usually effective due to wide variation in the size, depth, flow, and nature of the vessel to be targeted. However, lasers become pertinent in patients who have some contraindication to phlebectomy and sclerotherapy like needle phobia, allergies to components of sclerosants, popliteal fossa or ankle telangiectasias, and telangiectatic matting or have failed to respond to sclerotherapy.[3]

Accordingly, KTP (532 nm) or LPDL (595 nm) lasers are recommended for leg telangiectasia with a diameter less than 1 mm.[41,42] Among lasers, millisecond Nd:YAG (1,064 nm) laser is a first-line laser, while alexandrite (755 nm) and various diode lasers (800, 810, 940, and 983 nm) are used as second line lasers for large vessels.[43,44]

TREATMENT ENDPOINT

With every vascular laser treatment, the endpoint is signaled by the development of bluish or grayish discoloration of the targeted skin surface due to coagulation of the intradermal vessels or rupturing of the specific vessel. Large vessels, like veins of the legs and blanching of the vessel, indicates treatment endpoint.[10,45]

Postprocedure Care[45,46]

The dermatologist as well as the patient need to take some precautions, following are the procedure to achieve good results. These include:

- Proper cooling of the treated site should be done using ice packs to reduce edema and erythema
- Sun exposure immediately following the procedure should be avoided and the patient advised to use a broad spectrum sunscreen
- A mild moisturizer can be applied by the patient to reduce dryness and scaling
- The patient should be instructed to avoid use of makeup on erythematous or crusted skin
- In case of blistering or crusting, petrolatum jelly can be applied.

SIDE EFFECTS[45,46]

The common side effects that can be seen with laser treatment include:

- Burning sensation and pain
- Bruising and purpura
- Blister formation
- Edema
- Postinflammatory hyperpigmentation or hypopigmentation
- Postprocedure crusts and scabs
- Infection, especially reactivation of latent herpes virus infection
- Change in the texture of skin
- Scarring.

CONCLUSION

A large number of cutaneous and mucosal vascular lesions are commonly encountered by the dermatologist in his/her daily practice. These lesions not only cause disfigurement but also can cause serious and at times, lethal complications. Nowadays many of these anomalies are amenable to laser treatment. The type of the lesion, its anatomical location, age of the patient, and the side effect profile associated with each laser govern the type to be used for a particular patient.

REFERENCES

1. Anderson RR, Parish JA. Selective photothermolysis: precise microsurgery by selective absorption of pulsed radiation. Science. 1983;220: 524-7.
2. van Gemert MJ, Henning JP. A model approach to laser coagulation of dermal vascular lesions. Arch Dermatol Res. 1981;270:429-39.
3. Meesters AA, Pitassi LH, Campos V, Wolkerstorfer A, Dierickx CC. Transcutaneous laser treatment of leg veins. Lasers Med Sci. 2014;29:481-92.
4. Rubin IK, Farinelli WA, Doukas A, Anderson RR. Optimal wavelengths for vein-selective photothermolysis. Lasers Surg Med. 2012;44:152-7.
5. Adamic M, Pavlovic MD, Troilius Rubin A, Palmetun –Ecback M, Boixeda P. Guidelines of care for vascular lasers and intense pulse light sources from the European Society for Laser Dermatology. J Eur Acad Dermatol Venereol. 2015;29(9):1661-78.
6. Anderson RR, Dierickx CC. Have millisecond–domain lasers changed the approach to treatment of vascular anomalies and ectasia? In: Arndt K, Dover J, editors. Controversies and Conversations in Cutaneous Laser Surgery. Chicago: AMA Press; 2002. pp. 159-61.
7. Aldanondo I, Boixeda P, Fernandez-Lorente M, Marquet A, Calvo M, Jaén P, et al. [Selectivity of photothermolysis in the treatment of port wine

stains using multiple pulses with a pulsed dye laser]. Actas Dermosifiliogr. 2008;99:546-54.
8. Boixeda P. Treatment with millisecond domain lasers of port wine stains and facial telangiectasia. In: Arndt K, Dover J, editors. Controversies and Conversations in Cutaneous Laser Surgery. Chicago: AMA press; 2002. pp. 125-43.
9. Altshuler GB, Anderson RR, Manstein D, Zenzie HH. Smirnov MZ Extended theory of selective photothermolysis. Lasers Surg Med. 2001;29:416-32.
10. Bencini PL, Tourlaki A, De Giorgi V, Galimberti M. Laser use for cutaneous vascular alterations of cosmetic interest. Dermatol Ther. 2012;25:340-51.
11. Cameron H, Ibbotson SH, Ferguson J, Dawe RS, Moseley H. A randomized, blinded, controlled study of the clinical relevance of matching pulse duration to thermal relaxation time when treating facial telangiectasia. Lasers Med Sci. 2005;20:117-21.
12. Keijzer M, Pickering JW, van Germert MJ. Laser beam diameter for port-wine stain treatment. Laser Surg Med. 1991;11:601-5.
13. Chang CJ, Nelson JS. Cryogen spray cooling and higher fluence pulsed dye laser treatment improve port-wine stain clearance while minimizing epidermal damage. Dermatol Surg. 1999;25:767-72.
14. International Society for the Study of Vascular Anomalies. (2014). ISSVA Classification of Vascular Anomalies 2014 International Society for the Study of Vascular Anomalies. [online] Available from: www.issva.org/classification. (Accessed Feb, 2016).
15. Hoeger PH, Colmenero I. Vascular tumours in infants. Part I: benign vascular tumours other than infantile haemangioma. Br J Dermatol. 2014;171:446-73.
16. Fourtanier A, Moyal D, Seite S. Sunscreens containing the broad-spectrum UVA absorber, Mexoryl SX, prevent the cutaneous detrimental effects of UV exposure: a review of clinical study results. Photodermatol Photoimmunol Photomed. 2008;24:164-74.
17. Bucci J, Goldberg D. Past, present, and future: Vascular lasers/light devices. J Cosmet Laser Ther. 2006;8(3):149-53.
18. Nymann P, Hedelund L, Haedersdal M. Long-pulsed dye laser vs. intense pulsed light for the treatment of facial telangiectasias: a randomized controlled trial. J Eur Acad Dermatol Venereol. 2010;24:143-6.
19. Uebelhoer NS, Bogle MA, Stewart B, Arndt KA, Dover JS. A split-face comparison study of pulsed 532-nm KTP laser and 595-nm pulsed dye laser in the treatment of facial telangiectasias and diffuse telangiectatic facial erythema. Dermatol Surg. 2007;33:441-8.
20. Karsai S, Roos S, Raulin C. Treatment of facial telangiectasia using a dual-wavelength laser system (595 and 1,064 nm): a randomized controlled trial with blinded response evaluation. Dermatol Surg. 2008;34:702-8.
21. Tierney E, Hanke CW. Randomized controlled trial: comparative efficacy for the treatment of facial telangiectasias with 532 nm versus 940 nm diode laser. Laser Surg Med. 2009;41:555-62.
22. Alam M, Voravutinon N, Warycha M, Whiting D, Nodzenski M, Yoo S, et al. Comparative effectiveness of nonpurpuragenic 595-nm pulsed dye laser and microsecond 1064-nm neodymium:yttrium-aluminum-garnet laser for treatment of diffuse facial erythema: a double-blind randomized controlled trial. J Am Acad Dermatol. 2013;69:438-43.
23. Carniol PJ, Price J, Olive A. Treatment of telangiectasias with the 532-nm and the 532/940-nm diode laser. Facial Plast Surg. 2005;21:117-9.
24. Tan SR, Tope WD. Pulsed dye laser treatment of rosacea improves erythema, symptomatology, and quality of life. J Am Acad Dermatol. 2004;51:592-9.
25. Kim TG, Roh HJ, Cho SB, Lee JH, Lee SJ, Oh SH. Enhancing effect of pretreatment with topical niacin in the treatment of rosacea-associated erythema by 585-nm pulsed dye laser in Koreans: a randomized, prospective, split-face trial. Br J Dermatol. 2011;164:573-5.
26. Renfro L, Geronemus RG. Anatomical differences of portwine stains in response to treatment with the pulsed dye laser. Arch Dermatol. 1993;129:182-8.
27. Bjerring P, Christiansen K, Troilius A. Intense pulsed light source for the treatment of dye laser resistant port-wine stains. J Cosmet Laser Ther. 2003;5:7-13.
28. Izikon L, Nelson JS, Anderson RR. Treatment of hypertrophic and resistant port wine stain with 755 nm laser: a case series of 20 patients. Lasers Surg Med. 2009;41:427-32.
29. Faurschou A, Togsverd-Bo K, Zachariae C, Haedersdal M. Pulsed dye laser vs. intense pulsed light for port-wine stains: a randomized side-by-side trial with blinded response evaluation. Br J Dermatol. 2009;160:359-64.
30. Becher GL, Cameron H, Moseley H. Treatment of superficial vascular lesions with the KTP532-nm laser: experience with 647 patients. Lasers Med Sci. 2014;29:267-71.
31. Lee J, Sinno H, Tahiri Y, Gilardino MS. Treatment options for cutaneous pyogenic granulomas: a review. J Plast Reconstr Aesthet Surg. 2011;64:1216-20.
32. Pohl L, Karsai S, Raulin C. [Recurrent pyogenic granuloma: treatment at difficult anatomic sites with the long-pulsed Nd:YAG laser (1064 nm)]. Hautarzt. 2011;62:46-50.
33. Roncero M, Cañueto J, Blanco S, Unamuno P, Boixeda P. Multiwavelength laser treatment of venous lakes. Dermatol Surg. 2009;35:1942-6.
34. Weiss J, Weiss KD, Ross AL, Weiss E. A simplified minimally invasive technique for the treatment of venous lakes. Dermatol Online J. 2014;20:21257.
35. Aghassi D, Anderson RR, Gonzalez S. Time-sequence histologic imaging of laser-treated cherry angiomas with in vivo confocal microscopy. J Am Acad Dermatol. 2000;43:37-41.
36. Pancar GS, Aydin F, Senturk N, Bek Y, Canturk MT, Turanli AY. Comparison of the 532-nm KTP and 1064-nm Nd:YAG lasers for the treatment of cherry angiomas. J Cosmet Laser Ther. 2011;13:138-41.
37. Fodor L, Ramon Y, Fodor A, Carmi N, Peled IJ, Ullmann Y. A side-by-side prospective study of intense pulsed light and Nd:YAG laser treatment for vascular lesions. Ann Plast Surg. 2006;56:164-70.
38. Nofal A, Salah E. Acquired poikiloderma: proposed classification and diagnostic approach. J Am Acad Dermatol. 2013;69:e129-40.
39. Batta K, Hindson C, Cotterlll JA, Foulds IS. Treatment of poikiloderma of Civatte with the potassium titanyl phosphate (KTP) laser. Br J Dermatol. 1999;140:1191-2.
40. Rusciani A, Motta A, Fino P, Menichini G. Treatment of poikiloderma of Civatte using intense pulsed light source: 7 years of experience. Dermatol Surg. 2008;34:314-9.
41. Bernstein EF, Noyaner-Turley A, Renton B. Treatment of spider veins of the lower extremity with a novel 532 nm KTP laser. Lasers Surg Med. 2014;46:81-8.
42. Fournier N, Brisot D, Mordon S. Treatment of leg telangiectases with a 532 nm KTP laser in multipulse mode. Dermatol Surg. 2002;28:564-71.
43. Trelles MA, Allones I, Martın-Vazquez MJ, Trelles O, Velez M, Mordon S. Long pulse Nd:YAG laser for treatment of leg veins in 40 patients with assessments at 6 and 12 months. Lasers Surg Med. 2004;35:68-76.
44. Ross EV, Meehan KJ, Gilbert S, Domankevitz Y. Optimal pulse durations for the treatment of leg telangiectasias with an alexandrite laser. Lasers Surg Med. 2009;41:104-9.
45. Adamic M, Troilius A, Adatto M, Drosner M, Dahmane R. Vascular lasers and IPLS: guidelines for care from the European Society for Laser Dermatology (ESLD). J Cosmet Laser Ther. 2007;9:113-24.
46. Alam M, Warycha M. Complications of lasers and light treatments. Dermatol Ther. 2011;24:571-80.

CHAPTER 24

Scar Reduction: The Principles and The Options

Dhepe Niteen Vishwanath

INTRODUCTION

Any wound in human is healed by three mechanisms. First, genesis where entire damaged tissue is regenerated through pluripotent stem cells and is found in embryo below age of 5 weeks.[1] Second, repair where the wound is healed by migration of similar tissue from the surrounding. Third is replacement, when tissue injury is too large for repair with functional tissue and the defect is replaced by nonfunctional collagen.[2-5]

Scars are usually flat or atrophic. They become hypertrophic when balance between collagen production and collagen degradation (through matrix metalloproteinase) is disturbed. The quantity, alignment of collagen, and its proportion in tissue is progressively disturbed as a spectrum from atrophic scar to hypertrophic scars and is most abnormal in keloids.

Most common scar conditions dermatosurgeons treat in their practice are acne scars, hypertrophic scars, and keloids. Burn scars previously treated by surgeons mainly with skin grafting surgeries is increasingly handled by dermatosurgeons after advent of breakthrough fractional UltraPulse carbon dioxide (CO_2) lasers.

Layton et al.[6] reported that 95% of acne vulgaris cases can have at least some degree of scarring while prevalence of acne scarring in population was reported 1–11%.[7] As per the American Burn Association, 70% of burn cases were male, while in rest of the world including India, 80% cases were women and children. Out of all burn scars, 32–72% cases were hypertrophic.[8]

Treatment of acne scars has evolved from potentially risky full face dermabrasion or very deep chemical peels to safer fractional laser resurfacing. In similar evolution in hypertrophic scar treatment, fractional lasers and nonsurgical interventions are increasingly becoming common than surgeries.

With wider availability of lasers and energy based devices, many conditions where quality, alignment or proportion of collagen, and elastin in tissue is disturbed and where selective dermal ablation leading to its renewal may alter the pathology, are treated using same protocols. The author has proposed a classification of "laser treatable" conditions where subdermal collagen remodeling is common treatment principle.

CLASSIFICATIONS OF SCARS

Scars are classified by various authors on various parameters. Thickness was a prime parameter to classify scars into atrophic, hypertrophic, and flat. Elasticity or pliability was considered in hypertrophic scars while stretch ability in acne scars. Erythema is important parameter in young scars and keloids. Two commonly used classifications are Vancouver Scar Scale[9] (Table 1) and Goodman Baron Scale[10] (Table 2) qualitative for acne scar.

TABLE 1: Vancouver Scar Scale

	Scar characteristic	Score
Vascularity	Noraml	0
	Pink	1
	Red	2
	Purple	3
Pigmentation	Normal	0
	Hypopigmentation	1
	Hyperpigmentation	2
Pliability	Normal	0
	Supple	1
	Yielding	2
	Firm	3
	Ropes	4
	Contracture	5
Hight	Flat	0
	<2 mm	1
	2–5 mm	2
	>5 mm	3
	Total score	13

The Vancouver Scar Scale (VSS), first described by Sullivan in 1990, is perhaps the most recognized burn scar assessment method. It assesses 4 variable: vascularity, height/thickness, pliability, and pigmentation. Patient perception of his or her respective scars is not factored in to the overall score. Lye et al. compared the pliability sore from the VSS to measurements obtained through tonometry, noting moderate correlation in scores. The VSS remains widely applicable to evaluate therapy and as a measure of outcome in burn studies.

ROLE OF LASERS IN SCAR TREATMENT

Laser and lights have profound effect on all the stages of life cycle of scars. A low-level laser therapy is useful in early resolution of any surgical or traumatic wound, active acne, and hence preventing or minimizing chances and severity of acne. A vascular laser or vascular specific wavelength of intense pulsed light (IPL) will control vascularity of young red scar and prevent hypertrophy. Laser can resurface the skin to the scar base or just shoulder the scar edge for smooth transition from skin to scar base. Also, ablative lasers can debulk a hypertrophic scar as horizontal slicing or shrink the bulk in fractional mode. A very strong fractional laser beam can break tough fibrous septa at scar base. A blanket fractional laser treatment of entire face will induce skin tightening with resultant vertical vector lifting the scar base. Fractional lasers are shown to be effective in repigmenting hypopigmented scars. While fractional Q-switched neodymium doped yttrium-aluminium-garnet lasers dilute hyperpigmentation of old scars.

A careful knowledge of mechanism of action of each laser in scar life cycle is necessary to choose appropriate laser in a given patient. The author proposes a classification for scar lasers based on mechanism (Table 3). A combination or sequencing of various lasers addressing thickness, depth profile, vascularity and pigment should be practiced.

TABLE 2: Goodman Barron classification (qualitative approach)

Grade	Level of disease	Characteristics	Example
1	Macular disease	Erythematous, hyper- or hypopigmented flat marks visible to patient or observer irrespective of distance	Erythematous, hyper- or hypopigmented flat marks
2	Mild	Mild atrophy or hypertrophy that may not be obvious at social distances of 50 cm or greater and may be covered adequately by makeup or the normal shadow of shaved beard hair in males or normal body hair if extrafacial	Mild rolling, small soft popular
3	Moderate	Moderate atrophic or hypertrophic scarring that is obvious at social distances of 50 cm or greater and is not covered easily by makeup or the normal shadow of shaved beard hair but is still able to be flattened by manual stretching of the skin	More significant rolling, shallow "boxscar", mild to moderate hypertrophic or popular scars
4	Severe	Severe atrophic or hypertrophic scarring that is obvious at social distances of 50 cm or greater and is not covered easily by makeup or the normal shadow of shaved beard hair in males or body hair (if extrafacial) and is not able to be flattened by manual stretching of the skin	Punched out atrophic (deep "boxscar"), "ice pick", bridges and tunnels, gross atrophy, dystrophic scars, significant hypertrophy, or keloid

TABLE 3: Scar lasers—classification by mechanism

Desired mechanism	Devices available
Wound healing and minimizing scarring	LLLT, blue light, red light, LED
Debulking of hypertrophic scar	Er:YAG, UltraPulse CO_2
Vascularity of young red scar	PDL, Dye VL vascular IPL, LP Nd:YAG
Scar shouldering	Er:YAG, UltraPulse CO_2 surgical 1 mm tip
Dermal collagen neogenesis and lateral vector of skin tightening and vertical vector of skin lift	Fractional CO_2, fractional Er:YAG, nonablative lasers
Loosen the scar base and induce thickness of collagen	Subcision, high fluence narrow deep fractional CO_2 (Deep FX) laser

LLLT, low level laser therapy; LED, light emitting diode; Er:YAG, erbium doped yttrium-aluminium-garnet; PDL, pulsed dye laser; LP, long pulsed; Nd:YAG, neodymium doped yttrium-aluminium-garnet.

Box 1: Morphological classification of laser treatable scar conditions

- Macular (pigmented or erythematous) scars
- Atrophic scars
  - Ice pick scars
  - Boxcar scars
    - Chickenpox scars
    - Acne scars
  - Rolling scars (valley scars)
  - Shallow atrophic scars
    - Stretchable
    - Nonstretchable
- Hypertrophic scars
  - Popular acne scars
  - Phymas
  - Surgical scars
  - Postaccidental scars
  - Postburn scars
- Contractures
  - Postburn contractures
- Keloids
- Stretch marks
  - Striae rubra
  - Striae nigra
  - Striae alba
- Morphea
- Wrinkles, lines, and solar elastosis

Box 2: Principles of atrophic and acne scar treatments

- Anticipation and prevention: treat the original wound promptly and prevent or minimize scarring. Identify scar prone individuals
- Control excess vascularity in young scars
- Take out the scar tissue
  - Punch excision and suturing (ice pick scars)
- Level the scar base to surrounding skin (resurfacing)
  - Resurface the normal skin to the scar level
  - Shoulder the scar edge to make it rolling
  - Lift the scar base by subcision
  - Lift the scar base by punch float, punch graft
  - Lift the scar base by fillers, platelet rich plasma
- Match the color to the surrounding skin
  - Red scar treated with vascular specific lights and lasers
  - Hyperpigmentation treated with pigmentary lasers and light
  - Hypopigmentation treated with fractional carbon dioxide or excimer laser/light
  - Blue green color: traumatic tattoo treated with Q-switched neodymium doped yttrium-aluminium-garnet laser and fractional lasers
- Replace abnormal collagen/elastin with normal one. Restore elasticity.

Laser Treatment of Acne Scars: Protocols and Approaches

Each morphological type of acne scar need individualized approach to match that to the surrounding skin. The author proposes a working classifications of all laser treatable scars and 'scar-like' conditions where laser-induced collagen and elastin remodeling plays a key role. (Boxes 1 and 2). Author has proposed a working classifications of all lasers treatable scars and 'scar like' conditions where lasers induced collagen and elastin remodeling plays a key role. One has to note that the author does not aim at reversing the skin anatomy to the preacne status, but camouflaging with normal skin in parameters of depth, thickness, redness, texture, and color (Table 3).

Approaches to Individual Scars

- Macular (pigmented): though these scars are flat and pigmented, only pigmentary lasers are less useful. One should aim at pigment dilution and collagen remodeling also. A better protocol is combination of fractional Q-switched and YAG lasers with fractional ablative or nonablative lasers.
- Atrophic scars:
  - Ice pick scars: though the ideal treatment for ice pick scar is punch excision with or without suturing, a scar shouldering with 1 mm surgical tip of UltraPulse CO_2 laser or Er:YAG laser will reduce the depth of the scar. Repeated shouldering eliminates the need of excision in many if not all the cases of ice picks scars
  - Boxcar scars:
    - Chickenpox scars: scar shouldering with 1 mm surgical tip of UltraPulse CO_2 laser or Er:YAG laser will make the scar more rolling. A low-density very high-power fractional beam at the base of the scar will induce collagenesis at the base. Additional subcision is always helpful in the same session or another session (Fig. 1)
    - Acne scars: boxcar acne scars are best treated with punch excision or punch grafting. Equally good results are achieved with combination of subcision, scar shouldering and deep narrow fractional CO_2 laser at high fluence and low density
  - Rolling scars (valley scars): same principle of boxcar scar management applied here, additionally, rolling scars are mainly a volume loss; only focused treatment for the scar will not work. The surrounding skin need to be treated to greater depth in factional or nonfractional way.
  - Shallow atrophic scars:
    - Stretchable: subcision followed by deep fractional CO_2 laser with high fluence and low density shall be enough to treat these scars in 3–4 sessions separated 6–8 weeks apart
    - Nonstretchable: treating entire skin with fractional lasers will not suffice in these scars. Scar shouldering on individual scar will yield better results.

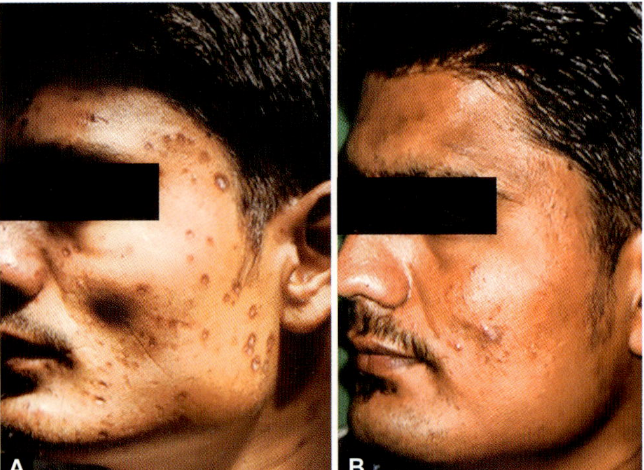

FIG. 1: Hyperpigmented chicken pox scars treated with combination of superficial wide and narrow deep fractional CO_2 laser (Total FX on ultrapulse)

Global Approaches

Mild Scarring (Mainly Rolling)

Subcision followed by two-layered fractional laser works well in this case. Low density fractional CO_2 laser with very high fluence (35 mJ on Deep FX) followed by superficial resurfacing with low density low fluence Active FX is called two-layered technique or more popularly Total FX protocol.

Severe Scarring

Individual scars are tried with punch replacement or punch grafting at an initial sitting followed by laser session after couple of weeks. Scar shouldering is combined with multiple passes of variable depth fractional laser.

TECHNIQUES OF LASER SCAR REDUCTION

Fractional Laser Dermabrasion (Total FX)

Full face dermabrasion with ablative lasers like surgical CO_2 or Er:YAG was a popular surgical treatment among dermatosurgeons and plastic surgeons for acne scar management. It was largely unsafe in darker patients and is rarely followed now. A safer version of this is practiced by many including the author in form of Total FX treatment protocol at high density. Dermabrasion of entire facial skin to the level below papillary dermis is largely unnecessary with the advent of fractional laser beams.

After topical anesthesia under occlusion, the area with scars is treated with two passes of narrow deep fractional CO_2, i.e. Deep FX one with very high power 35 mJ and another pass at 15 mJ and at 45° to initial pass. Superficial dermabrasion of entire facial skin is achieved with Active FX at higher density. Ablated tissue is removed with wet gauge after each pass. Maneksha's manual dermabrader may be used to remove ablated tissue in between. One more pass of Deep FX on this dermabraded skin will reach a greater depth inducing deep dermal collagen remodeling. A last pass with low density Active FX is used to cover entire face to match the skin. This time the ablated tissue is not removed and will remain behind as biological dressing.

Scar Shouldering (Authors Technique)

Active FX on UltraPulse device is chosen with very narrow spot size and very high density. This becomes a 1–2 mm surgical beam. Deep scars are marked at its base with the marking ink. 1 mm laser beam at higher repetition rate (Hz) is applied to the border of the scar. One may repeat the same procedure twice or thrice for deeper scars. In authors experience on Active FX, spot size 2 works better than spot size 1.

Five-tier Technique with UltraPulse Carbon Dioxide Laser under Tumescent Anesthesia (Authors Technique) (Box 3)

Acne scars need intervention at various depths of epidermis and dermis. Traditional approach was laser dermabrasion to plane down normal skin to the level of scar base. Fractional CO_2 laser beam at various parameters can selective reach various depths. This multilevel approach eliminates need of aggressive resurfacing. The author has evolved a comprehensive protocol that addresses all aspects of moderate to severe acne scars with fractional CO_2 device in ultrapulse pulse mode, and two beam profile deep narrow fractional called Deep FX and wide superficial called Active FX on UltraPulse device.

After standardized photography, acne scars are marked with water proof surgical marker at the base.

Entire face is infiltrated with tumescent fluid made up of 500 mL Ringer lactate mixed with 40 mL of 2% lignocaine, 1 mL of 1:100,000 adrenaline, 10 mL of sodium bicarbonate and 5 units of triamcinolone; 100 mL on each side is usually enough. Additionally, nerve block may be given. If scars are extensive, procedure may take longer.

Subcision of the scarred area is performed using 18 G needle in same session or another. The author prefers subcision in islands of small areas with few scars leaving normal skin in between.

Active FX on UltraPulse device is chosen for scar shouldering. Spot size 1 or 2 with density 6 or more to make it surgical, fluence 175–200 mm and at power 60 Watt will make this beam as good as a surgical knife. Pass this beam around the edge of the scar in free hand mode. Ablated tissue removed with wet gauge in between the passes. A total of 3–5 passes are needed to plane down the edge.

Deep FX mode with density 5% and very small spot size at 35 mJ fluence is used to target the base of the scar. This is believed to break fibrous band retracing the scar base.

Deep FX beam at maximum size and 20 mJ is passed on entire facial skin in to passes. Second pass is taken 45° to the first pass at 15 mJ. This induces generalized neocollagenesis in entire regional skin. Like lifting in facial skin sagging, this pass will help most of the rolling and stretchable scars.

Last pass in this protocol is Active FX, i.e., superficial wide fractional laser with low density and low fluence (80 mJ at density 3) to match the color and texture to surrounding skin. If patient is ready for downtime of 3–5 days, this protocol can achieve 60–80% global scar improvement in two sessions in mild to moderate scars and three sessions in sever scarring.

Box 3: Components of 5-tier technique

- Subcision
- Scar shouldering with 1–2 mm surgical tip
- Low density high fluence factional at base of scar to break tough collagen
- Regional skin lifting with deep narrow fractional
  - Direct volume loss in ablation columns
  - Lateral stretch of new collagen with vertical vector of skin lift
- Superficial resurfacing with wide narrow fractional at low dose low density

Preoperative and Postoperative Protocols

Preoperatively, recent sun exposure and active herpes simplex are excluded. The author usually does not exclude patients on isotretinoin for this treatment. A recent metacentric study in India has established safety of laser treatment in patients on isotretinoin.[11] Preoperative bleaching protocols are not useful to avoid postinflammatory pigmentation. A valacyclovir 500 mg twice a day prophylactic course starting 48 hour in advance is recommended in treatment of face and in prone individuals.

Postoperatively, antibiotics like cefadroxil and anti-inflammatory like nonsteroidal anti-inflammatory drugs are prescribed for 5 days. The treated area is cleansed several times a day with white vinegar diluted 1:30 with water to maintain acidic pH of skin and hence preventing infections. Bland ointment like white petroleum jelly, aquaphor, or cicabio is preferred over antibiotic ointments to be applied for several times a day. Sunscreens are started after third day. Scabs are allowed to fall on its own and not picked up.

LASER SCAR REDUCTION VERSUS LASER WRINKLE REDUCTION

The author believed that pathology and treatment principles of scars and wrinkles are overlapping. So techniques and protocols of scar treatment and wrinkle treatment are shared. That is why the author has classified solar elastolysis and wrinkles in laser treatable scar-like conditions.

The principles of treatments are:

- Subcision for collagen build up below base
- Low density high-fluence fractional at base of scar to break tough collagen scar/wrinkle shouldering with 1–2 mm surgical tip
- Regional skin lifting with deep narrow fractional
  - Direct volume loss in ablation columns
  - Lateral stretch of new collagen with vertical vector of skin lift
- Superficial resurfacing with wide narrow fractional at low dose low density for color match and textural improvement.

HYPERTROPHIC SCARS

These are surgical, postaccidental, or postburn scars. Debulking of hypertrophic scar was achieved with surgical debulking (vertical slicing) or horizontal slicing with manual or laser dermabrasion. Surgical excision is more invasive while dermabrasion is always associated with risk of worsening of the scar. Concept of laser debulking has been greatly changed from horizontal slicing to vertical fractional shrinking after advent of deep narrow fractional lasers. The limiting factor in hypertrophic scar treatment with lasers was the width to depth ratio. One was not able to reach the depth of more than 1 mm without a significant lateral thermal damage. It was SCAAR FX or very deep narrow fractional CO_2 on UltraPulse device that achieved an extraordinary ablation column profile with width of ablation 100 μ and depth 4,000 μ, i.e., 4 mm with significantly less lateral thermal damage (Fig. 2).

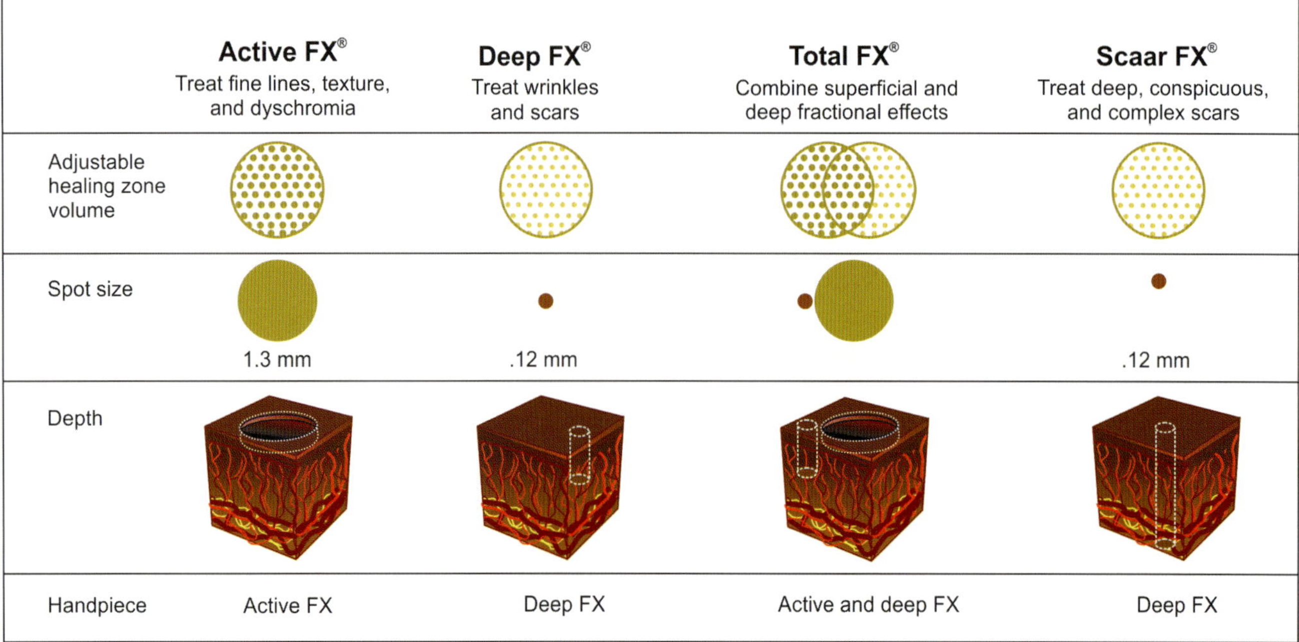

FIG. 2: Beam profiles in ultrapulse laser. Wide superficial mode is 1.3 mm vs narrow deep mode has 0.12 mm width. The penetration depth in Active Fx vs Deep FX vs SCAAR FX is 100u vs 1.5 mm vs 4 mm

Authors Protocol for Hypertrophic and Burn Scar Treatment with Ultrapulse

Tumescent anesthesia is infiltrated around and below the scar. SCAAR FX on UltraPulse at density 3-5% maximum and fluence 60-120 mJ per pulse is applied. Three or more passes of 3% density is preferred to 10% of single pass. For scars thinner than 1.5-2 mm, Deep FX at fluence 25-40 mJ is useful; while scars thicker than 2 mm SCAAR FX is recommended.

One may rub in injection Kenalog for fractional drug delivery. Three to four sessions at an interval of 6-8 weeks is recommended. This treatment can be combined with pressure, silicone gel sheets, and intralesional injections.

The author has conducted a study and presented it at the American Society for Laser Medicine and Surgery annula meeting in 2008,[12] in which 24 patients with postburn scars of average 6 year duration were treated with UltraPulse Deep FX fractional CO_2 laser. Typical protocol is three treatments at an interval of 2-3 months in between and used 0.12 mm spots with density 5%, single stacking, and pulse fluence of 20-35 mJ/pulse as per thickness of scar after topical anesthesia with tetracaine 7% and lignocaine 7%. The scars are assessed for thickness, surface wrinkling, color and match with surrounding at the time of each treatment, 1, 2, and 3 months postoperatively after last sitting by two independent dermatologists on Visual Analog Scale (VAS) of 4. Pain during treatment is scored by patient on a VAS of 4.

Three months after three sessions of fractional CO_2 treatment reduced the scar thickness to a mean VAS score of 3.47 out of 4. The score increased from 2.14 before second sitting to 3.47 at third month follow-up of last sitting. Reduction in scar surface wrinkling was 3.85, and color match to surrounding was 2.89 on a VAS scale of 4. Pain during procedure scored by patient was 1.12 on scale of 4 using topical anesthesia.

The author concluded that fractional CO_2 laser with Deep FX scanner is a well tolerated and effective treatment of hypertrophic postburn scars in Indian patients (Figs 3 and 4).

After introduction of SCAAR FX laser, the maximum fluence used has gone up to 120-140 mJ per pulse and penetration depth up to 3-4 mm. Similar protocol using SCAAR FX has improved efficacy and reduced total number of sessions significantly (Box 4).

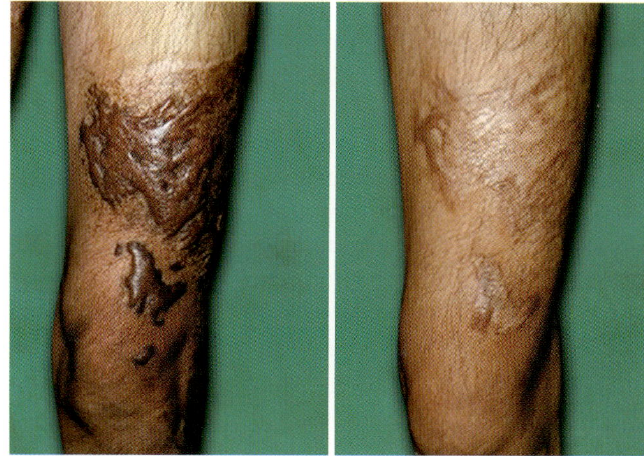

FIG. 3: Patient with regeneration of hair follicle after flattening of hypertrophic scar

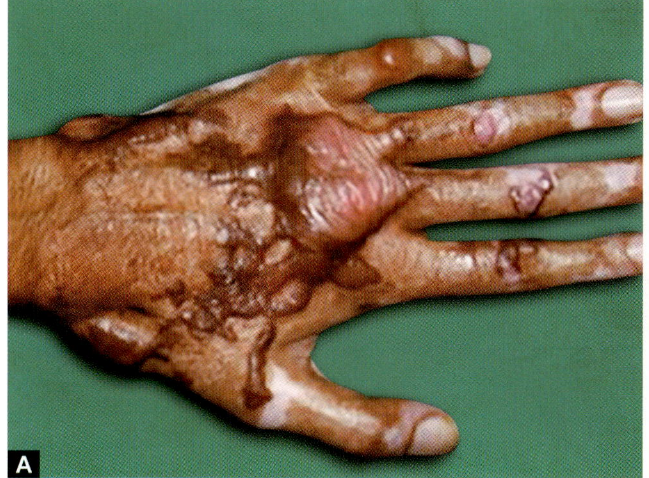

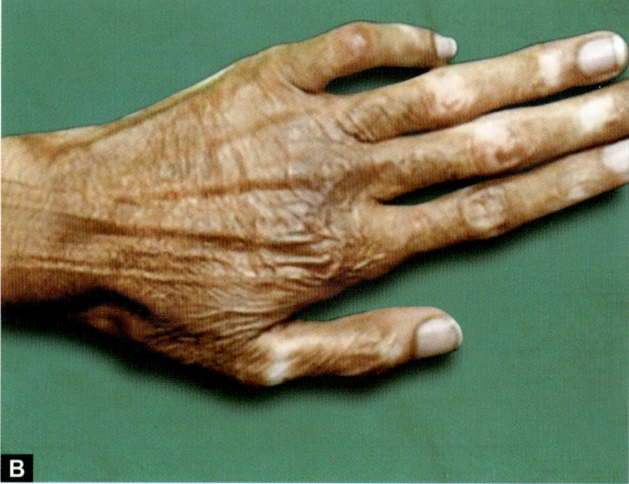

FIG. 4: Hypertrophic burn scar due to chemical burn was treated with Ultrapulse SCAAR FX and fractional drug delivery and intralesional injection of trimcinolone

Box 4: Principles of hypertrophic scars treatments

- Prompt wound care and vascular lasers in early phase
- Reduce the thickness—debulking
- Downregulate collagen synthesis by pressure, interleukin injections
- Improve surface irregularity, texture
- Improve pliability/elasticity
- Match color with surrounding

Principles of Laser Treatments of Keloids

Keloids are different than hypertrophic scars due to their potential for spread beyond the original limit of injury. This drive for growth in keloids is influenced by genetic factors, traction on keloids, recurrent infections, and poor wound care. Debulking alone is not effective in keloid management. Pressure therapy and intralesional injections of antiproliferative agents are indispensible. Lasers and lights can influence all stages in life cycle of keloid from early formation till recurrence. In keloid prone patients, addition of low level lasers or light emitting diodes will improve healing profile and possibly a keloid. Prolonged erythema is another etiological factor in keloids. Hence vascular specific IPL (Dye VL) or pulsed dye laser can cut down vascularity in granulation phase or erythematous phase of a scar. Deep fractional lasers can debulk the volume of the keloids. While laser hair removal of area in and around the keloid will minimize the recurrence rate (author's personal experience) (Box 5).

Box 5: Principles in treatments of keloids

- Prevent by early and clean wound healing: low level laser therapy
- Target the vascularity: Vascular intense pulsed lights, pulsed dye laser
- Reduce thickness (debulking)
  - Fractional lasers
  - Silicone
  - Pressure
- Arrest progression
  - Injections of steroids
  - Cytotoxic drugs
- Control trigger factors
  - Hair follicles
  - Recurrent infection
  - Sebaceous activity
  - Stretch and tension

CONTRACTURE

Contractures primarily need a surgical intervention if they are limiting movement across a joint. In case of limited restriction, a combination of fractional CO_2 laser with intralesional triamcinolone in contracture and scar bands can extend the length of the scar band and decrease the tension in contracture. Clementoni[13] demonstrated contracture release as 15–25° more freedom in joint mobility (Fig. 5).

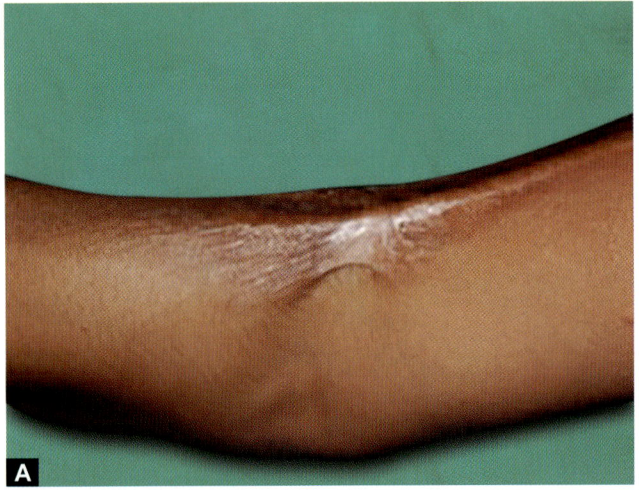

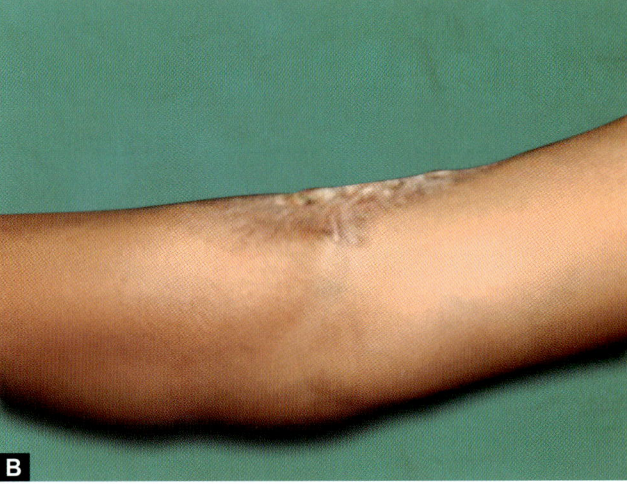

FIG. 5: Post burn contracture on forearm treated with SCAAR FX laser and fractional delivery of steroid

MISCELLANEOUS SCAR TYPES

Hypopigmented Scars

Friedman[14] reported improvement in hypopigmented scars with fractional CO_2 laser resurfacing. Using 308 excimer laser or light applied only to the hypopigmented scar base and sparing the surrounding skin with a mold will significantly improve hypopigmented scars.[15]

Stretch Marks

Stretch marks are irreversible damage to structure and alignment of collagen and elastin fibers in prone skin.[16,17] Stretch marks are red and erythematous in early phase (striae rubra) that matures to become either darker than surrounding skin (striae nigricans) or lighter than surrounding skin (striae alba).[17-19]

In darker skin, deep narrow fractional laser in low density and high fluence will induce both improved surface profile and better color match with surrounding.

Protocol for Treatment of Stretch Marks

Topical anesthesia is used. Fractional laser Deep FX 15–25 mJ at 5% density on stretch marks and normal skin around. Very high dose 35 mJ at 3% density only on stretch mark as an additional pass will be helpful. Preoperative and postoperative protocols have been described above.

Technique and Protocols for Morphea

Morphea is an inflammatory skin condition leading to scarring changed in dermis and subcutaneous structure. The author had an experience of treating morphea combining anti-inflammatory treatments like excimer or ultraviolet B phototherapy, collagen remodeling therapy like fractional CO_2 laser, and collagen stimulating therapy like platelet rich plasma.

COMPLICATIONS OF LASER SCAR REDUCTION

The common complications of laser treatments with fractional CO_2 lasers are given in table 4. This is to be noted that after advent of fractional lasers, most serious complications of laser resurfacing are quiet rare. Other complications are easily manageable and reversible.

CONCLUSION

Thickness or depth, contour, vascularity, and pigment are key parameters targeted in laser scar reduction. Lasers have role in all the phases of life cycle of scar from formation till recurrence. Deep FX CO_2 lasers have evolved as superior and safer option to surgical debulking by dermabrasion and safer than surgical excision. While generalized collagen tightening of scar affected skin is achieved by most of fractional devices, scar shouldering

TABLE 4: Common complications in fractional carbon dioxide laser[20]

Complications	Frequency	Severity
Postinflammatory hyperpigmentation	Common	–
Postinflammatory hypopigmentation	Uncommon	Temporary
Erythema	Common	Temporary
Worsening of scar	Uncommon	Severe
Nonhealing ulcer	Common in contractures	Severe
Keloid formation	Uncommon	In susceptible individuals
Injury to deeper structure like panniculitis	Common with SCAAR FX	–
Infection	Uncommon	–
Reactivation of herpes simplex	Uncommon	–
Reactivation of vitiligo	Common in prone patient	–
Reactivation of inflammatory disorders	Uncommon	–
Contact dermatitis	Uncommon	–
Pain	Common	–
Syncope	Common	–

is required for deeper scars like ice pick scars and boxcar scars. Skillful manipulation of parameters will allow us to reach various levels into skin and hence 3-tier or 5-tier techniques can eliminate the need of surgical intervention in many cases if not all.

This chapter aims at sharing authors experience on protocols using certain devices. These protocols can be modified using other alternative devices working on same principles with variable success. One should remember that lasers are one of the adjuvant therapies for scars and must be combined with established therapies like pressure and intralesional injections for superior results.

Understanding of collagen remodeling has opened possibilities of using these devices in related conditions like morphea, keloids, and stretch marks.

ACKNOWLEDGMENT

The author thanks Dr Vibhor Goyal, Postgraduate Fellow in lasers at Skin City Postgraduate Institute of Dermatology, for his kind help in writing this chapter.

REFERENCES

1. Nichols J, Zevnik B, Anastassiadis K, Niwa H, Klewe-Nebenius D, Chambers I, et al. Formation of Pluripotent Stem Cells in the Mammalian Embryo Depends on the POU Transcription Factor. Cell Volume. 1998;95(3)379-91.
2. Chen J, Jia-Han W, Hong-Xing Z. "Inhibitory effects of local pretreated epidermis on wound scarring: a feasible method to minimize surgical scars". Burns. 2005;31(6):758-64.
3. Wipff PJ, Rifkin DB, Meister JJ, Hinz B. "Myofibroblast contraction activates latent TGF-beta1 from the extracellular matrix". J Cell Biol. 2007;179(6):1311-23.
4. Lay summary – Ecole Polytechnique Fédérale de Lausanne (December 17, 2007).
5. Parlange, Mary (17 December 2007). "New mechanical insights into wound healing and scar tissue formation". Ecole Polytechnique Fédérale de Lausanne. Available from: eurekalert.org. Retrieved 28 August 2010. The matrix grows stiffer and, at a certain point, the fibroblasts stop migrating and, like Popeye, change into powerful contractile cells, anchoring themselves to the matrix and pulling the edges of the wound together.
6. Layton AM, Henderson CA, Cunliffe WJ. A clinical evaluation of acne scarring and its incidence. Clin Exp Dermatol. 1994;19:303-8.
7. Cunliffe WJ, Gould DJ. Prevalence of facial acne vulgaris in late adolescence and in adults. Br Med J. 1979;1(6171):1109-10.
8. Lawrence JW, Mason ST, Schomer K, Klein MB. Epidemiology and impact of scarring after burn injury: a systematic review of the literature. J Burn Care Res. 2012;33(1):136-46.
9. Goodman GJ, Baron JA. Postacne scarring: a qualitative global scarring grading system. Dermatol Surg. 2006;32(12):1458-66.
10. Nedelec B, Shankowsky HA, Tredget EE. Rating the resolving hypertrophic scar: comparison of the Vancouver Scar Scale and scar volume. J Burn Care Rehabil. 2000;21(3):205-12.
11. Chandrashekar BS, Varsha DV, Vasanth V, Jagadish P, Madura C, Rajashekar ML. Safety of performing invasive acne scar treatment and laser hair removal in patients on oral isotretinoin: a retrospective study of 110 patients. Int J Dermatol. 2014;53(10):1281-5.
12. Dhepe N, et al. Successful treatment of post burn scars with fractional CO_2 laser in Indian skin. Lasers in Surgery and Medicine. vol. 43. USA:Wiley-Blackwell, 2011.
13. Tapan Patel, Matteo Tretti Clementoni. A new treatment for severe burn and post-traumatic scars: a preliminary report. Available from: http://www.laserplast.org/wp-content/uploads/2013/01/A-New-Treatment-for-Severe-Burn-and-Post-traumatic-Scars-A-Preliminary-Report-Treatment-Strategies-Dermatology-Volume-2-Issue-2.pdf.
14. Glaich AS, Rahman Z, Goldberg LH, Friedman PM. Fractional Resurfacing for the Treatment of Hypopigmented Scars: A pilot study Dermatol Surg. 2007;33(3):289-94.
15. Alexiades-Armenakas MR, Bernstein LJ, Friedman PM, Geronemus RG. The safety and efficacy of the 308-nm excimer laser for pigment correction of hypopigmented scars and striae alba. Arch Dermatol. 2004;140(8):955-60.
16. Viennet C, Bride J, Cohen-Letessier A, Humbert P. Mechanical behavior of fibroblasts included in collagen lattices. J Soc Biol. 2001;195:427-30.
17. Burrows NP, Lovell CR. Disorders of connective tissue. In: Burns T, Breathnach S, Cox N, Griffith C, editors. Rook's Textbook of Dermatology. 7th ed. Oxford: Blackwcll Sciencc; 2004. pp. 46-7.
18. Hidalgo GL. Dermatological complications of obesity. Am J Clin Dermatol. 2002;3:497-506.
19. Watson RE, Parry EJ, Humphries JD, Jones CJ, Polson DW, Kielty CM, et al. Fibrillin microfibrils are reduced in skin exhibiting striae distensae. Br J Dermatol. 1998;138:931-7.
20. Dhepe N. Complications of fractional laser. In: Pai G, editor. Complications in Cosmetic Dermatology. New Delhi: Jaypee Medical Publisher (P) Ltd.; 2015.

CHAPTER 25

Nonablative Laser for Scar Reduction

Malavika Kohli, Banani Choudhury

INTRODUCTION

Since the invention of carbon dioxide lasers, two and half decades ago, which is a major breakthrough and gold standard for skin rejuvenation, there has been a laser swing to newer generations of lasers. Due to limitations of downtime and risks on Fitzpatrick type IV-VII skin, the pendulum has swung to nonablative lasers, which was considered as lunchtime procedures due to its minimal downtime. But because of their nonresurfacing properties and requierment of many sessions, the fractionated technology in 2004, came as a major breakthrough again, overcoming the scarring and postinflammatory changes from ablative lasers and acheiving increasing depth penetration in case of nonablative lasers.

History of Nonablative Lasers

During the early 1980s, Anderson and Parrish revolutionized dermatologic laser treatment by defining a concept known as selective photothermolysis.[1] This theory describes the use of laser energy to achieve localized photothermal injury of a targeted chromophore. From this idea, pulsed lasers were developed in which a short burst of photoenergy (photons) is delivered to a particular chromophore whose optimal wavelength of photoabsorption is distinct from its surrounding tissue.[1] This technique facilitates transfer of heat from photons, with the aim of keeping the converted thermal energy confined to a particular target, thereby diminishing widespread destructive or nonselective effects on normal surrounding tissue.[1]

In 1994, Alster[2] reported clinical and textural improvement in long-standing erythematous and hypertrophic scars, with 57% improvement following one pulsed dye laser (PDL) treatment and 83% improvement after two treatments. For a better result, Ebrahimi et al. recommended PDL within 2 weeks of surgery after sutures have been removed.[3]

Dierickx and colleagues[4] had similar findings the following year, in which they reported an average improvement of 77% after 1.8 laser treatments of erythematous or hypertrophic scars.

Later, Alster and Williams[5] compared the clinical, textural, histologic, and symptomatic responses in a split scar study involving hypertrophic and keloidal median sternotomy scars. Significant improvement in texture, erythema, scar height, and pruritus was observed at 6 months after the PDL treatment.[5] In addition, they histologically demonstrated increased numbers of mast cells at the lasered sites. Subsequent studies also showed improvement in keloid scars following PDL treatment. In 1996,[6] Alster and McMeekin also reported improvement in erythematous and hypertrophic facial acne scars following treatment with the 585 nm PDL.

McDaniel et al. demonstrated improvement in surface topography and increased dermal elastin in striae treated with the 585 nm PDL at low fluence.[7] Alster and colleagues[8] also found that low fluence PDL irradiation outperformed PDL fluences used for scars combined with pulsed carbon dioxide vaporization.

In the study by Bjerring et al.,[9] the biochemical analysis of interstitial fluid from forearm, performed before and 72 hours after laser administration of a single laser treatment at a subpurpura energy level, demonstrated that the 585 nm laser source induced an increase of 84% ($p < 0.05$) in the type III procollagen production rate compared with a nontreated control site.

Furthermore, in the study by Zelickson et al.,[10] histology showed accumulation of degenerated elastotic fibers in the dermis, the presence of activated fibroblasts 12 weeks after treatment, a thickening of the superficial collagen band, and an increase of the mucin in the superficial dermis, following treatment with the subpurpuric dose of 585 nm PDL.

BACKGROUND

The psychosocial impact of cutaneous scarring can be profound. The multifaceted causes of scaring, encountered by a dermatologist include traumatic, surgical procedures, and severe acne (grade III and IV).

TYPES OF SCARS

Hypertrophic and Keloid Scars

Hypertrophic scars are pink, raised, firm, erythematous scars. They occur approximately within a month following surgery or trauma and result from overzealous collagen synthesis coupled with limited collagen lysis during the remodeling phase of wound healing.[11] The result is the formation of thick collagen bundles consisting of fibroblasts and fibrocytes, arranged in nodules rather than in the normally smooth fashion.[12] Hypertrophic scars may be symptomatic, characterized by pruritus and/or dysesthesia,[1] and are more likely to arise in sites subjected to increased pressure or movement.[12]

Despite obvious tissue proliferation, hypertrophic scars remain within the confines of the original integumental injury, in distinction to keloid scars, which extend beyond the original cutaneous injury.[11] Unlike keloids, which tend to persist indefinitely, hypertrophic scars may regress spontaneously.[12]

Keloids are raised, reddish-purple, nodular scars that are firmer than hypertrophic scars,[11] and they may develop weeks or years after the initial insult, or even arise spontaneously.[12] Keloids develop during an extended proliferative phase of wound healing[12] and they demonstrate thick, hyalinized bundles of collagen arranged haphazardly in whorls, with increased hyaluronidase.[12] Unlike hypertrophic scars, keloids extend beyond wound margins and may even continue to grow over time.[12] Although they occur in all skin types, keloids are most common in patients with darker skin and like hypertrophic scars, may be associated with pruritus and/or dysesthesia.[12]

Striae Distensae

Striae distensae, or stretch marks, are linear bands of atrophic or wrinkled skin.[12] They result from excessive dermal stretching such as after rapid weight loss/gain, pregnancy, or pubertal growth spurts.[12] Dermal inflammation with mast cell degranulation, elastolysis, and dilated capillaries mark the initial presentation,[13] which results in an erythematous appearance of young striae distensae (striae rubra).[12] Later, striae appear hypopigmented and fibrotic owing to linear deposition of dermal bundles and thinning of the overlying epidermis (striae alba).[13] Their pathogenesis remains unclear, although estrogen and mast cell degranulation with elastolysis may be contributing factors.[12]

Atrophic Scars

Atrophic scars are dermal depressions that most commonly are the sequelae of an acute inflammatory process that has caused collagen destruction and dermal atrophy.[12] Examples of inciting events include cystic acne, varicella infection, surgery, and trauma.[12] On the skin, these pitted lesions form a surface resembling the dimples on a golf ball. This topographical irregularity tends to be difficult to treat, but therapy is generally aimed at resurfacing the distorted topography.[14]

Acne Scars

The acne scars should be properly evaluated and graded to determine the appropriate approach.

In 2007, Goodman and Baron proposed a global acne scarring classification of four grades.[15]

1. The first grade: consists of macular, hyper- or hypopigmented marks visible to an observer from any distance

2. The second grade: consists of mild atrophy or hypertrophy, but can be covered by makeup or a shaved beard
3. The third grade: moderate atrophic or hypertrophic scarring, not easily covered by makeup or a shaved beard in men that can be viewed at distances greater than 50 cm and can be flattened by stretching of the skin around the scar
4. The highest grade: severe atrophic or hypertrophic scaring that is visible at distances greater than 50 cm, and cannot be flattened by stretching the skin around the scar.

Goodman and Baron recommend that nonablative lasers are appropriate for patients in the second grade, and ablative lasers may be used for patients who fit criteria for the third grade.[15]

Acne scars may be categorized as hypertrophic or atrophic, the latter of which can be further characterized as ice pick, rolling, or boxcar scars.[14,16]

Ice pick scars are usually narrow (<2 mm), sharply demarcated tracts that can reach deep into the dermis or even the subcutaneous tissue.[16] They are typically wider at the epithelial surface and taper as they go deeper.[16] Rolling scars tend to be shallower, wider (4–5 mm), and produce an undulating appearance in otherwise normal appearing skin. This rise and fall of the skin surface is due to abnormal fibrous attachment of the dermis to the subcutis.[16] Boxcar scars are wider at the base than ice pick scars, but do not taper. These round to oval shaped skin dimples have sharp margins and can be either shallow (0.1–0.5 mm) or deep (>0.5 mm).[17]

Prescars

These are early wounds in scar prone skin. Prophylactic laser treatments immediately after injury helps to reduce or prevent scar formation in patients with high scarring tendency.

NONABLATIVE DEVICES AND LASERS

- 1,064 nm Q-switched neodymium doped yttrium-aluminium-garnet (Nd:YAG) laser/1,064 nm short-pulsed Nd:YAG laser
- 1,320 nm Nd:YAG laser
- 1,450 nm diode laser
- 1,540 nm erbium doped phosphate glass laser (Er:Glass)
- 585 nm PDL and intense pulsed light (IPL) system.

Infrared Lasers

Q-switched 1,064 nm Neodymium Doped Yttrium-aluminium-garnet Laser

The long-pulsed 1,064 nm Nd:YAG laser was primarily developed for the treatment of epidermal and dermal pigmentation and tattoos and became most popular for treating leg veins and hair removal, but some authors reported increased homogenization of the superficial collagen.[18]

Prieto et al. demonstrated that the 1,064 nm Nd:YAG laser can induce expression of heat shock protein 70 (HSP70) and type I procollagen by dermal dendritic cells, probably leading to collagen deposition in the papillary and reticular dermis resulting in improved appearance of scars.[19] It was also suggested that sufficient heat conducted from the heated blood vessels to the surrounding dermis may alter the fibrotic collagen in the scar. Furthermore, laser irradiation can cause microvasculature destruction via ischemia, causing collagenase production, which in turn can break down the collagen in the scar. These may be the possible mechanisms by which the 1,064 nm Nd:YAG laser can improve the cosmetic appearance of atrophic and mixed-pattern acne scars.

Neodymium Doped Yttrium-aluminium-garnet 1,320 nm Laser

A 1,320 nm Nd:YAG laser, the CoolTouch® laser was the first of the nonablative devices to be introduced for resurfacing, and utilizes a cryogen dynamic cooling spray for epidermal protection. It works on a similar principle to other nonablative devices—that of dermal injury by laser irradiation resulting in collagen remodeling and scar improvement.[20-22]

Diode 1,450 nm Laser

The 1,450 nm diode laser has been demonstrated to work in both acne and acne scars through its thermal action on the dermis and sebaceous glands.[23] This effect of the 1,450 nm laser on sebaceous glands was a coincidental finding when Ross et al. conducted a split face study on 16 patients, treating one half of the face with the 1,450 nm diode laser with four treatments at 3-week intervals, while the other half of the face was treated with cryogen cooling alone.[24] Mild-to-moderate improvement was observed in 12 out of 16 patients on the treated side. Besides these, sebaceous gland shrinkage was noted on histology. The same group treated some test areas on the back of 20 patients with the same laser, and 100% clearance of acne was noted after four treatments.

The first commercial fractional nonablative laser was Fraxel (1,550 nm), cleared by FDA for periorbital rhytides, pigmented lesions, melasma, skin resurfacing, acne scars, and surgical scars.

The next nonablative fractional thermolysis device to enter the market was known as Affirm (1,440 nm). Through original work by Weiss et al. and other investigation, Affirm was shown to be effective in the treatment of various skin conditions, wrinkles, scars, and pigmentary concerns.

Mode of Action

Nonablative devices deliver concomitant epidermal surface cooling with deeply penetrating infrared wavelengths that target tissue water and stimulate collagen production via controlled dermal heating with epidermal disruption. Also, absorption of the 1,064 nm wavelength by the blood vessels in the scar may lead to either conduction to surrounding dermis to alter fibrotic collagen within the scar or significant ischemia within laser treated tissue to affect collagen or to release collagenase.

No consensus exists regarding the mechanism by which the PDL achieves clinical improvement in scars. Purported mechanisms include:

- Laser induced microvasculature damage leading to tissue hypoxia with subsequent collagen degradation via release of collagenase[25,26]
- Thermal damage to collagen fibers dissipated from adjacent vessels with dissociation of disulfide bonds and collagen realignment[25]
- Increased regional mast cells, which may serve to stimulate collagen remodeling.[26]

In an experimental study investigating a diode laser in wound healing on hairless rats, Capon and colleagues demonstrated a phenomenon of scarless healing.[27,28] In this study, the laser irradiation led to a moderate increase in tissue temperature, insufficient to cause thermal damage, but high enough to stimulate HSP70. Heat shock protein 70 are chaperone proteins that are known to be involved in an inflammatory reaction and the wound healing process, playing a key role with coordinate expression of other growth factors, such as transforming growth factor-β (TGF-β), which in turn participates in inflammatory response and fibrogenic process.[29] It has been reported by some authors that TGF-β3 has a more dominant role in scarless healing than TGF-β1 or TGF-β2.[30,31]

This could suggest a possible relationship between laser irradiation, HSP70 upregulation, fibroblast activation, and scarless healing like phenomena. This could lead to improved outcomes in acne scarring when using the nonablative lasers.

FRACTIONAL NONABLATIVE LASER

This technology has been invented to overcome the disadvantage of conventional ablative and nonablative lasers. The concept behind fractional lasers "fractional photothermolysis" was described by Manstein D et al. (2004).[32] It produces small vertical zones of full thickness thermal damage by mid-infrared laser and the microscopic treatment zones snaps the tethered fibrotic bands.

Conceptually, it may be laser equivalent of skin micro-needling and can give benefit of ablative resurfacing.

Principle

- Nonablative mode of tissue coagulation with stratum corneum intact and the tissue not being vaporized
- Creation of multiple microthermal zones surrounded by islands of viable tissue
- Resurfacing with extrusion and replacement of damaged tissue with reepithelialization within 24 hours.

Devices

- 1,320 nm Nd:YAG
- 1,410 nm system
- 1,440 nm Nd:YAG laser
- 1,450 nm diode laser
- 1,540 nm Er:Glass
- 1,550 nm erbium laser.

Approach to Treatment

Scars can be treated depending on the type, stage, duration, color, and patient characteristics. Nonablative laser is effective for mild-to-moderate scars, particularly in skin type IV to VI, acne scars (grade I), and on patients who do not want downtime.

Fractional nonablative laser is particularly for patients who can afford a few days of downtime and for rolling and shallow boxcar scar.

Initially, authors approach the deep boxcar scar with subcision either with an 18 G needle or a blunt cannula and break the adhesions to the skin, and then we either go for microneedling radiofrequency or nonablative fractionated lasers.

Clinical Experience

The author has experience of 1,064 nm short-pulsed Nd:YAG for scar reduction in the clinic. The author recommends and counsels to the patients of acne with scarring tendency in the initial visit. Patients with resistant acne, cyclical isotretinoin (10 days a month) can be given with laser treatments placed in the remaining off days.

Authors' Experience (Figs 1 to 4)

According to authors' experience, IPL on erythematous acne scars bring good result after 4–6 sessions. We can combine fractionated skin resurfacing using radiofrequency energy, either in between IPL sessions or at the end for the resurfacing benefits. Nd:YAG 1,440 nm (affirm) for skin tightening and acne scar, has additional cooling system, allowing high power and deeper penetration.

Erbium glass 1,540 nm glass (palomer starlux), has additional cooling system allowing patient comfort and treating deeper scar. 1,410 nm (fraxel) is good for scars of superficial depth, but minimal downtime and versatile for broad spectrum of patients.

Combination modalities, like microneedling, microneedling radiofrequency, and skin reurfacing using radiofrequency, when combined with nonablative laser technologies, gives better result with reduction of number of sittings and high satisfactory result. Authors have experience of using combination modalities for most of the scar indications with high satisfactory score and great end result.

STUDIES AND RESULTS

In 1996, Alster and McMeekin demonstrated that the 585 nm PDL could improve erythematous and hypertrophic acne scars.[6] In 22 patients, significant improvements in texture and redness were seen after one or two treatments (6–7 J/cm^2; 7 mm spot size). Six weeks following only one laser treatment, the mean improvement was 67.5%. Eight of the patients received an additional laser treatment and showed an average improvement of 72.5% 6 weeks later.

Atrophic acne scarring has been treated with a 1,064 nm Q-switched Nd:YAG laser.[33] Eleven patients with mild-to-moderate atrophic scarring were treated with 5 laser sessions at 3-week intervals. The laser was set at an average fluence of 3.4 J/cm^2, 4–6 nanosecond pulse duration, and a 6 mm spot size. Skin roughness was significantly better (23.3%) 1 month after the fifth laser session. Further improvements continued with time. At the 6 month, follow-up, patients demonstrated a statistically significant 39.2% improvement from baseline measurements. Its efficacy has been seen in multiple studies. Friedman et al. assessed this laser for mild-to-moderate atrophic acne scarring by performing 5 treatment sessions at 3-week intervals. A total of 11 patients were treated in this study with the 1,064 nm

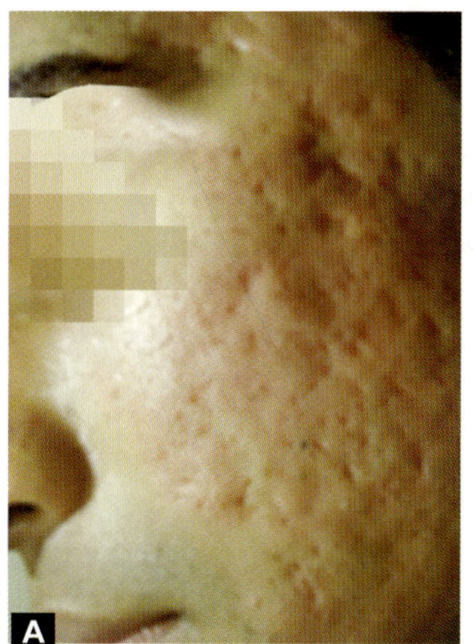

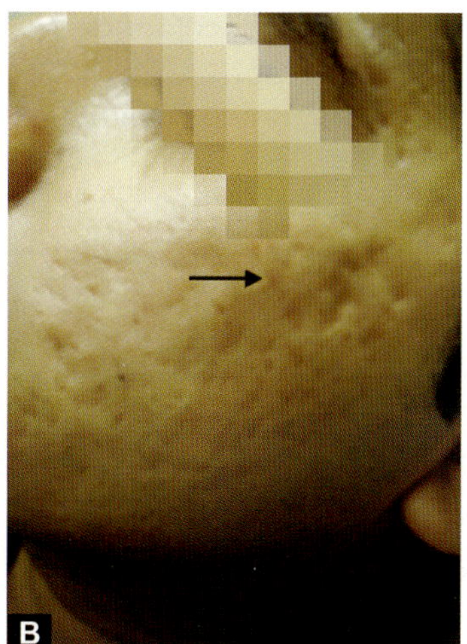

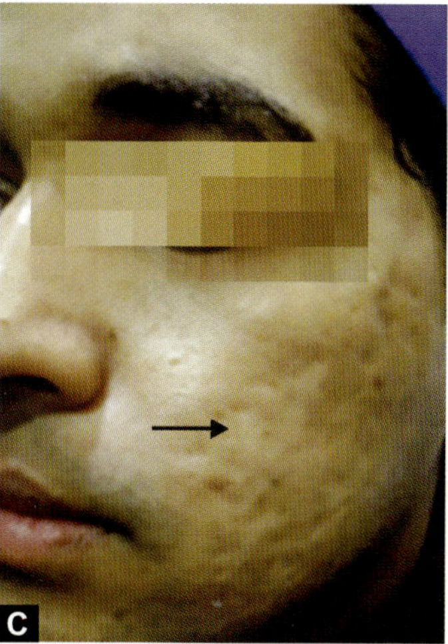

FIG. 1: Response of acne scar to combination of microneedling and 1,064 nm Nd:YAG laser; **A,** before treatment; **B,** 3 weeks post first session; **C,** 3 weeks post second session.

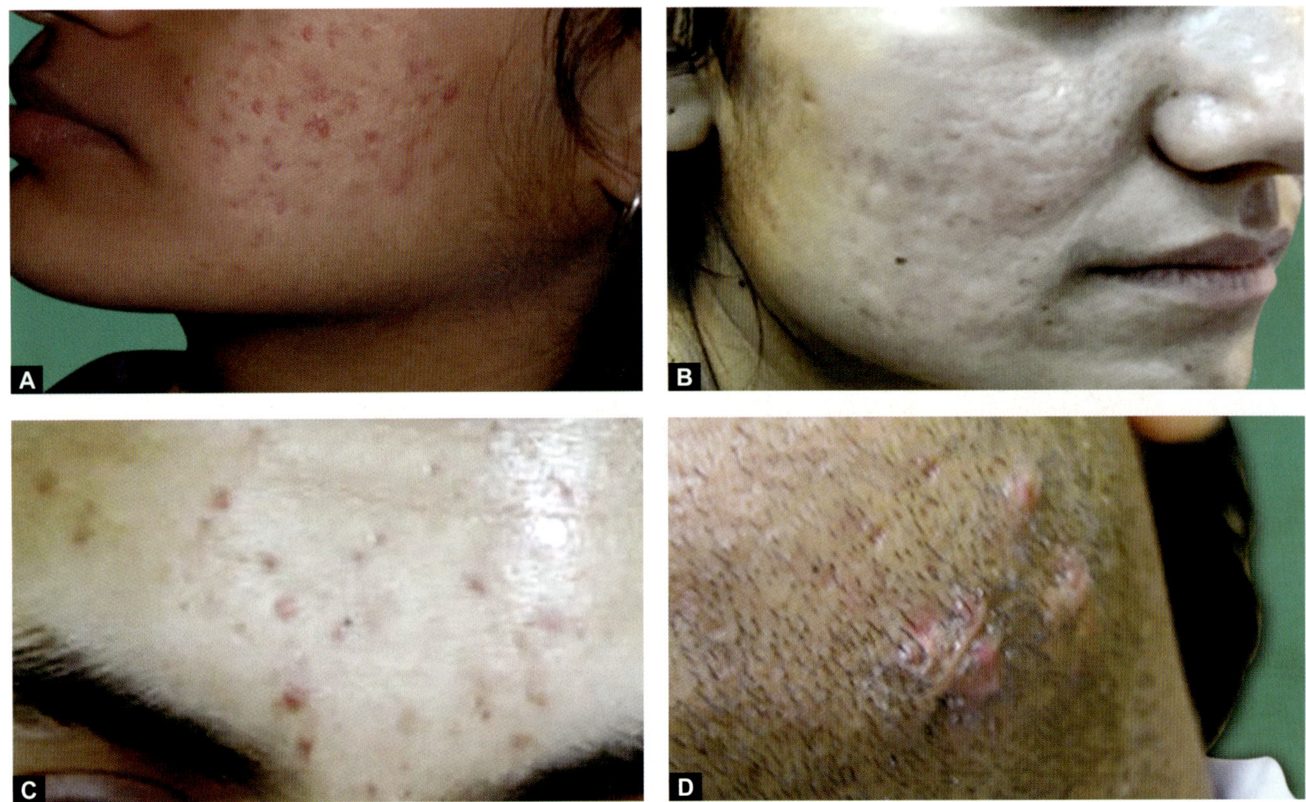

FIG. 2: Varied presentation of acne scars in Indian population; **A,** erythematous; **B,** undulating rolling; **C,** hyperpigmented; **D,** hypertrophic

Q-switched Nd:YAG laser. A month after the third treatment, an 8.9% improvement was observed in the roughness, and this improvement increased to 23.3, 31.6, and 39.2% at 1, 3, and 6 months after the fifth treatment, respectively. Transient erythema and mild pinpoint petechiae were the only adverse effects noted.

Keller et al. used a 1,064 nm Nd:YAG laser and studied its efficacy on 12 patients with mild-to-moderate atrophic acne scars who received five treatments. Three passes were performed and a water based cooling gel was used to provide epidermal protection.[34] Moderate improvement was noted in at least 50% of the patients. A significant increase in the quantity of dermal collagen fibers per unit area was observed by means of morphometry.

Lipper and Perez investigated the efficacy and safety of the short-pulsed 1,064 nm Nd:YAG laser on 10 patients with moderate-to-severe acne scarring.[35] They used a series of eight laser treatments (14 J/cm^2, 0.3 ms, 5 mm spot size, 7 Hz pulse rate, and 2,000 pulses per side of face). Acne scarring improved in 100% of the nine patients completing the study. Scar severity scores improved by a mean of 29.36%, with no adverse events reported. It was also concluded that at the settings used, the laser was most effective at reducing scar depth and softening scar contours.

The 1,320 nm Nd:YAG laser with a built-in cryogen cooling spray has been used for acne scarring. In 2004, Sadick and Schecter[37] treated eight patients with 6-monthly irradiations of three passes each and found a modest improvement. Ice pick scars without fibrosis responded more favorably than those with fibrous tracts. Statistically significant improvements were noted in seven of eight patients 5 months and 1 year after their final treatments. When only three treatments were used, another study found that atrophic scars improved the most. In Asian patients, there may be only a mild response. Of 27 patients treated, eight had no objective improvement and nine were only mildly better than at baseline. This modality may produce better results if combined with another modality, such as surgery or an IPL source.

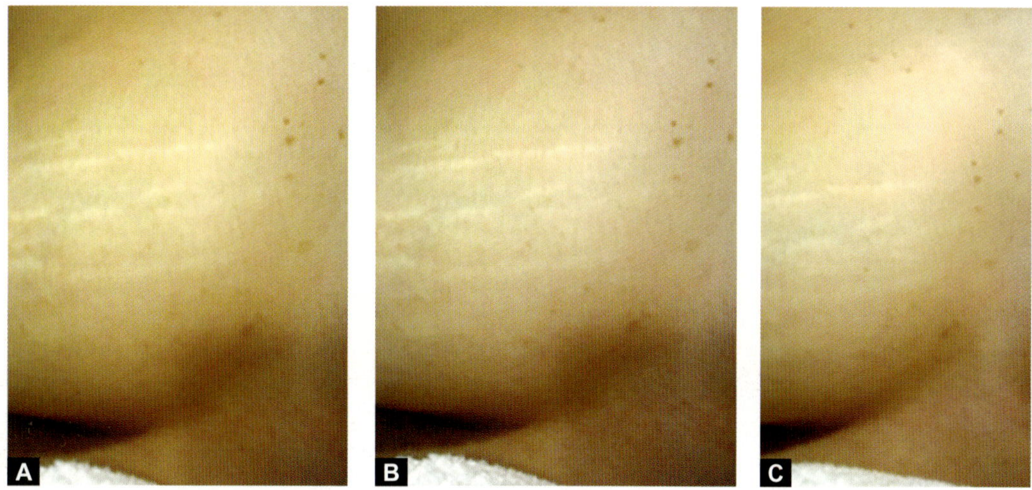

FIG. 3: Striae responds well to combination technologies(combination of 1064 Nd:YAG and fractionated skin resurfacing using radiofrequency) either on same sitting or at interval of 2 weeks; **A,** before treatment; **B,** 3 weeks post first session; **C,** 3 weeks post second session

A 2004 comparison by Tanzi and Alster[36] evaluated the efficacy of a 1,450 nm diode laser versus a 1,320 nm Nd:YAG for atrophic facial scars. Twenty patients with mild-to-moderate scarring each received 3-monthly treatments. Each half of the patient's face was randomized to one of the two lasers. After completing the treatments, the greatest clinical effect was seen at 6 months, which was consistent with the observed histologic increase in collagen production. Only modest improvements were seen with both lasers, but the 1,450 nm diode laser resulted in greater improvements.

Both lasers are safe, noninvasive options to improve the appearance of mild-to-moderate facial atrophic scars.

In a 2009 study, the efficacy and safety of the nonablative, 1,540 nm Er:Glass fractional laser in the treatment of surgical and post-traumatic scars was evaluated.[37] A histological study was conducted on a postsurgical scar to follow the time course of healing post-treatment and the impact of the fractional treatment on normalization of scar tissue, as compared with baseline histologic findings of the scar.

Histologic findings demonstrated rapid reepithelialization of the epidermis within 72 hours of treatment. Remodeling of scar tissue with renewal and reorganization of collagen fibers in the dermis was noted 2 weeks post-treatment. Relative to baseline, 73% of treated scars improved 50% or more and 43% improved 75% or more.[37]

Rogachefsky et al. investigated the treatment of atrophic or a mixed pattern (combination of atrophic and pitted, sclerotic or boxcar scars) acne scarring with 1,320 nm Nd:YAG laser.[20] They treated 12 individuals with these scars using three laser treatments 1 month apart with 13–22 J/cm^2 and 10 mm spot size. The scars were evaluated via a comparison of photographs taken at baseline and at the end of 6 months after last treatment by means of a 10 point severity scale (1:most imperceptible acne scars and 10:most severe acne scars) by both physicians and patients. The mean acne scar improvement was 1.5 points and 2.2 points on physician and patient assessments, respectively, demonstrating significant improvement in acne scars. It was also noted that atrophic acne scars improved more than mixed type acne scars.

Sadick and Schecter studied the efficacy of this laser and demonstrated significant acne scar improvement at 5 months (3.9 points) and 1 year (4.3 points).[22] The laser was studied in Asians for wrinkle reduction and treatment of atrophic acne scarring in 27 patients by Chan et al., and overall degree of patients' satisfaction was rated as 4.9 for wrinkle reduction and 4 for the treatment of acne scarring.[38]

In 2006, another study by Bhatia et al. with 34 patients assessed patient satisfaction with the 1,320 nm laser who had completed a series of 6-monthly nonablative treatments for photoaging or acne scarring.[39] Structured interviews were conducted at least 3 months (3–12 months range) after the cessation of the last treatment by researchers not involved in direct patient care. The patients reported a mean improvement of 4.5 (on a scale of 0–10; 10 being maximum improvement).

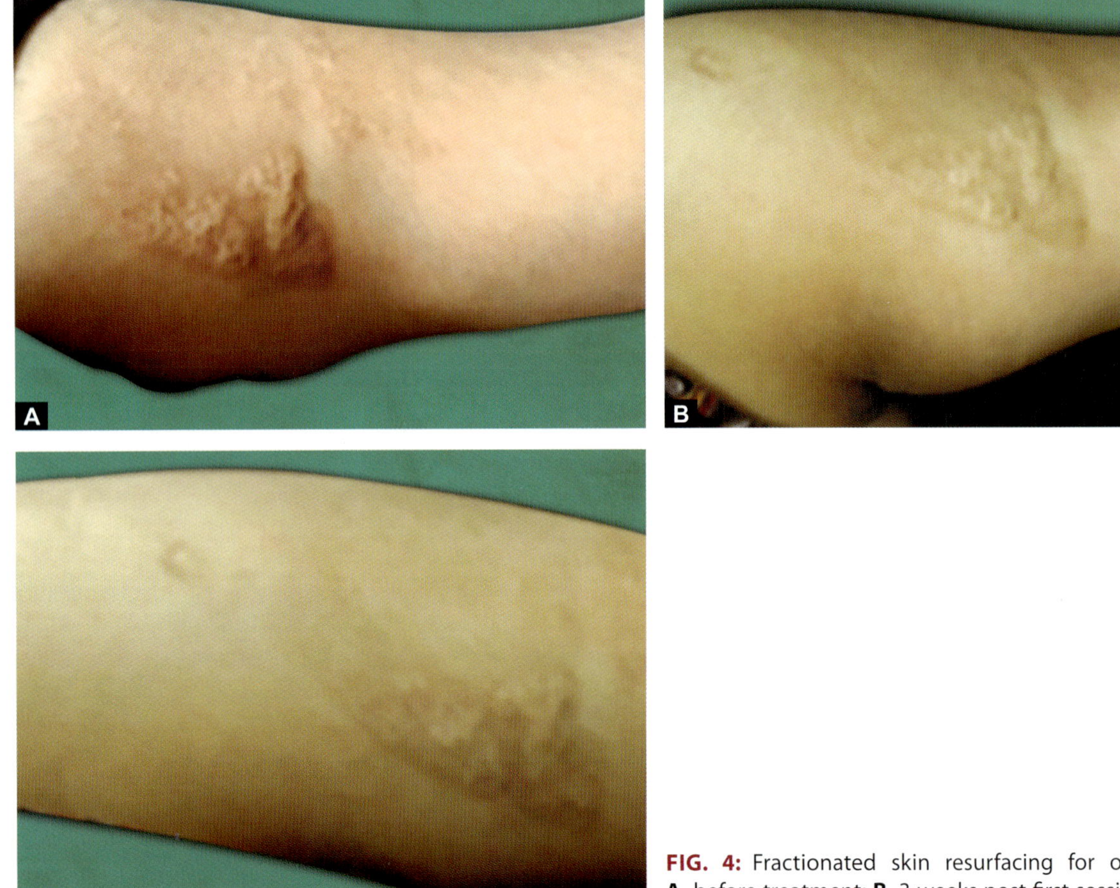

FIG. 4: Fractionated skin resurfacing for old Traumatic Scar; **A,** before treatment; **B,** 3 weeks post first session; **C,** 3 weeks post second session

Cho et al. studied the efficacy and safety of single session treatments of 1,550 nm erbium doped fractional photothermolysis systems and 10,600 nm carbon dioxide fractional laser systems for acne scars through a randomized, split face, evaluator blinded study with eight patients with acne scars.[40] Half of each subject's face was treated with a fractional photothermolysis system and the other half was treated with a carbon dioxide fractional laser system. At 3 months after treatment, the mean grade of improvement based on clinical assessment was 2 ± 0.5 for the fractional photothermolysis system and 2.5 ± 0.8 for the carbon dioxide fractional laser systems.

Tanzi and Alster compared the 1,320 and the 1,450 nm lasers in the treatment of atrophic facial scarring on 20 patients with mild-to-moderate acne scarring.[21]

Patients received three successive monthly treatments, with a long-pulsed 1,320 nm Nd:YAG laser on one facial half and a long-pulsed 1,450 nm diode laser on the contralateral facial half. Participants were evaluated using digital photography, three-dimensional *in vivo* microtopography measurements at each treatment visit and biopsy for histological evaluations after the first treatment and at 1, 3, 6, and 12 months postoperatively. Both of the lasers demonstrated clinical improvement without significant side effects or complications with better response seen with the 1,450 nm diode laser.

Carniol et al. evaluated the efficacy of treatment of acne scars with sequential combination of treatment using a 1,450 nm, mid-infrared, nonablative diode laser with cooling spray and trichloroacetic acid peels. In this prospective study, nine patients with atrophic rolling, boxcar, or both types of scars received 4-monthly treatments with the combination.[41] All types of scars showed improvement with a mean of 6.4 on a scale of 0–10. They concluded that the percentage improvement noted in this study was greater than that reported in any other studies with nonablative lasers. The improvement achieved by the laser treatments was enhanced by the chemical peels. No significant complications were noted.

Chua and coworkers aimed to determine the clinical efficacy and safety of a 1,450 nm laser in the treatment of atrophic facial acne scars in skin types IV–V, i.e., the darker skin types—in 57 patients.[42] In this prospective noncomparative open study, 4–6 laser treatment sessions were performed for each patient and final clinical assessment was performed 6 months after the last treatment.

A 2010 pilot clinical study demonstrated that lasers could also be used immediately after surgery to reduce the appearance of scars. The laser assisted skin healing (LASH) technique induces a temperature elevation in the skin, which modifies the wound healing process. Capon et al. demonstrated that 810 nm diode laser treatment, performed immediately after surgery, can improve the appearance of a surgical scar.[43] The dose plays a significant role in scar improvement and must be well-controlled. The authors additionally suggested that LASH could be used for hypertrophic scar revision.

Wada and colleagues performed an open study on 24 Japanese patients (17 female and 7 male, aged 15–44 years) with acne scars on the face treated with 5 sessions of low energy, double-pass, 1,450 nm diode laser at 4-week intervals.[44] The mean duration of the acne scars prior to receiving laser therapy was 4.8 years (range 1–9 years).

Clinical evaluation by physicians and with photographs was conducted at baseline, 1 month after the final treatment, and at a 3 month follow-up visit. Topical therapies for acne vulgaris were permitted during the follow-up period. All patients completed the 5 treatment sessions. Seventy-five percent of the subjects showed at least 30% improvement of acne scars. At the 3 month follow-up evaluation, 92.9% of the subjects with greater than 30% improvement maintained the effectiveness.[44]

Yoo et al. evaluated the efficacy and safety of 1,540 nm fractional photothermolysis (Starlux™ 1,540 nm) on 16 volunteers with Asian skin (Fitzpatrick III–IV) by treating them with 3 treatment sessions 4 weeks apart.[45] They demonstrated a mild-to-moderate clinical improvement in most patients, great improvement in the quality of life of all patients and significant collagen and elastic fiber increase. Minimal side effects, such as erythema and edema, were noted in 50% of patients. Hu et al. also demonstrated significant improvement in atrophic acne scars and texture after one treatment of nonablative 1,550 nm erbium doped fiber laser fractional photothermolysis in their study of 45 Asian patients (skin types III–IV). Similarly, significant improvement was observed by Mahmoud et al. with the same laser, while treating subjects with skin types IV–VI.

Specific Features of Nonablative Devices

Potassium titanyl phosphate or Frequency-doubled Neodymium Doped Yttrium-aluminium-garnet (532 nm)

Good for red, brown, and texture: the potassium titanyl phosphate (KTP) laser has traditionally been used for the treatment of small caliber focal facial telangiectasia and lentigines. Combined treatment with 532 nm KTP and 1,064 nm Nd:YAG lasers has been shown to provide synergistic benefits. When used with newer large spot sizes and scanner heads, the 532 nm laser can be used to nonablatively resurface the entire face rather than just fine vessels.

Pulsed Dye Laser (585 and 595 nm)

Good for red and texture: the pulsed dye laser, a workhorse in the treatment of facial telangiectasia, diffuse erythema, and other superficial vascular lesions, has also been used with intralesional steroids for the treatment of keloids and hypertrophic scars.

Intense Pulsed Light Device (500–1,200 nm)

Good for red, brown, and texture: intense pulsed light devices have been used for the treatment of telangiectasia and erythema, reduction of lentigines, and softening of facial lines and creases. The multiple skin improving functions of intense pulsed light have made it a favorite modality for nonablative therapy. While the degree of improvement of fine lines may be less remarkable, significant simultaneous improvement in brown spots and redness is conducive to overall patient satisfaction.

Neodymium Doped Yttrium-aluminium-garnet Laser (1,064 nm)

Good for brown and texture: the Q-switched Nd:YAG laser was developed for the treatment of skin pigments, including those present in lentigines and tattoos, but using low fluence has increasingly been used for nonablative rejuvenation, which is now popularly called "laser toning".

Mid-infrared Lasers (1,320 nm Neodymium Doped Yttrium-aluminium-garnet, 1,450 nm Diode, 1,540 nm erbium doped phosphate glass laser)

Best for texture, wrinkles, and texture. Do not help color: this class of lasers has been used to treat periocular and perioral fine rhytides, with the former tending to respond better. They are less effective at treating pigmentation and vascular lesions. The 1,450 nm laser has also been used for the nonablative treatment of acne via partial necrosis of sebaceous glands. Mid-infrared devices, like the 1,064 nm Nd:YAG, can induce serious eye damage in patients and operators if adequate eye protection is not used. Pain during treatment is common, and can be somewhat mitigated with topical anesthesia.

Nonablative lasers are one of the safest modalities with minimum downtime for all types of reduction, mostly atrophic acne scars.

Amongst acne scars, shallow boxcar scars and rolling scars show maximum benefit with nonablative lasers followed by deep boxcar scars with minimal improvement in ice pick scars.

Deeper scars need combination modalities of treatments like subscission, chemical reconstruction of skin scars using trichloroacetic acid (TCA CROSS), microneedling radiofrequency, and other ablative lasers like carbon dioxide lasers and erbium doped yttrium-aluminium-garnet lasers.

The results of scar reduction with nonablative lasers show only after a duration of 8–12 weeks. Also, multiple treatments of 4–6 sessions, 6–8 weeks apart are needed.

CONCLUSION

After reviewing all the laser technologies, definitely a clear trend arises. Nonablative lasers offer modrate results with fewer side effect and downtime and easier recovery. Fractionated technology has combined some of the best aspects of each category with shorter recovery time but results approaching those of ablative technology with a series of treatment. Nonablative laser is an excellent technology for scar reduction,safe for darker skin tone. Scars of varied etiologies can be targeted. Most commonly encounterd acne scar respond best followed by striae and traumatic scars.

Where We Stand Today?

In this decade, fractionated technology is preferred either in ablative or nonablative lasers for scar reduction because of increased efficacy and safety profile. The advantage of nonablative lasers are patient friendly, socially acceptable downtime, quicker recovery, and higher safety. However, one has to be prepared for more number of sessions in treating the scars. For more complete scar revision, combining results with fractionated ablative lasers and radiofrequency energy, depending on the case. Finally, the patients profile, selection, and physicians, judgement and expertize in operating laser and counseling the patient will help to ensure the satisfying result and meeting patients satisfaction.

REFERENCES

1. Anderson RR, Parrish JA. Selective photothermolysis: precise microsurgery by selective absorption of pulsed radiation. Science. 1983;220(4596):524-7.
2. Alster TS. Improvement of erythematous and hypertrophic scars by the 585-nm flashlamp-pumped pulsed dye laser. Ann Plast Surg. 1994;32(2):186-90.
3. Ebrahimi A, Kazemi HM, Nejadsarvari N. Experience with esthetic reconstruction of complex facial soft tissue trauma: application of the pulsed dye laser. Trauma Mon. 2014;19(3):e16220.
4. Dierickx C, Goldman MP, Fitzpatrick RE. Laser treatment of erythematous/hypertrophic and pigmented scars in 26 patients. Plast Reconstr Surg. 1995;95(1):84-90; discussion 91-2.
5. Alster TS, Williams CM. Treatment of keloid sternotomy scars with 585 nm flashlamp-pumped pulsed-dye laser. Lancet. 1995;345(8959):1198-200.
6. Alster TS, McMeekin TO. Improvement of facial acne scars by the 585 nm flashlamp-pumped pulsed dye laser. J Am Acad Dermatol. 1996;35(1):79-81.
7. McDaniel DH, Ash K, Zukowski M. Treatment of stretch marks with the 585-nm flashlamp-pumped pulsed dye laser. Dermatol Surg. 1996;22(4):332-7.
8. Alster TS, Lewis AB, Rosenbach A. Laser scar revision: comparison of CO2 laser vaporization with and without simultaneous pulsed dye laser treatment. Dermatol Surg. 1998;24(12):1299-302.
9. Bjerring P, Clement M, Heickendorff L, Egevist H, Kiernan M. Selective non--ablative wrinkle reduction by laser. J Cutan Laser Ther. 2000;2(1):9-15.
10. Zelickson BD, Kilmer SL, Bernstein E, Chotzen VA, Dock J, Mehregan D, et al. Pulsed dye laser therapy for sun damaged skin. Lasers Surg Med. 1999;25(3):229-36.
11. Alster TS, Handrick C. Laser treatment of hypertrophic scars, keloids, and striae. Semin Cutan Med Surg. 2000;19(4):287-92.
12. Lupton JR, Alster TS. Laser scar revision. Dermatol Clin. 2002;20(1):55-65.
13. Bak H, Kim BJ, Lee WJ, Bang JS, Lee SY, Choi JH. Treatment of striae distensae with fractional photothermolysis. Dermatol Surg. 2009;35(8):1215-20.
14. Omi T, Kawana S, Sato S, Bonan P, Naito Z. Fractional CO2 laser for the treatment of acne scars. J Cosmet Dermatol. 2011;10(4):294-300.
15. Goodman GJ, Baron JA. The management of postacne scarring. Dermatol Surg. 2007;33:1175-88.
16. Fabbrocini G, Annunziata MC, D'Arco V, De Vita V, Lodi G, Mauriello MC, et al. Acne scars: pathogenesis, classification and treatment. Dermatol Res Pract. 2010;2010:893080.

17. Rivera AE. Acne scarring: a review and current treatment modalities. J Am Acad Dermatol. 2008;59(4):659-76.
18. Menaker GM, Wrone DA, Williams RM, Moy RL. Treatment of facial rhytides with a nonablative laser: a clinical and histologic study. Dermatol Surg. 1999;25(6):440-4.
19. Prieto VG, Diwan AH, Shea CR, Zhang P, Sadick NS. Effects of intense pulsed light and the 1,064 nm Nd:YAG laser on sun - damaged human skin: histologic and immunohistochemical analysis. Dermatol Surg. 2005;31(5):522-5.
20. Rogachefsky AS, Hussain M, Goldberg DJ. Atrophic and a mixed pattern of acne scars improved with a 1320-nm Nd:YAG laser. Dermatol Surg. 2003;29(9):904-8.
21. Tanzi EL, Alster TS. Comparison of a 1450-nm diode laser with a 1320-nm Nd:YAG laser in the treatment of atrophic facial scars: a prospective clinical and histologic study. Dermatol Surg. 2004;30(2 Pt 1):152-7.
22. Sadick NS, Schecter AK. A preliminary study of utilization of the 1320-nm Nd:YAG laser for the treatment of acne scarring. Dermatol Surg. 2004;30(7):995-1000.
23. Alam M, Dover JS. Non ablative laser and light therapy: an approach to patient and device selection. Skin Therapy Lett. 2003;8(4):4-7.
24. Ross EV, Sajben FP, Hsia J, Barnette D, Miller CH, McKinlay JR. Nonablative skin remodeling: selective dermal heating with a mid-infrared laser and contact cooling combination. Lasers Surg Med. 2000;26(2): 186-95.
25. Tsao SS, Dover JS, Arndt KA, Kaminer MS. Scar management: keloid, hypertrophic, atrophic, and acne scars. Semin Cutan Med Surg. 2002;21(1):46-75.
26. Alster TS, Handrick C. Laser treatment of hypertrophic scars, keloids, and striae. Semin Cutan Med Surg. 2000;19(4):287-92.
27. Capon A, Mitchell VA, Sumian C, et al. Laser assisted skin closure (LASC) using a 815 nm diode laser system: determination of an optimal dose to accelerate wound healing. In: Brown S (Ed). Thermal Therapy, Laser Welding, and Tissue Interaction. SPIE, WA: USA; 1998. pp. 1-12.
28. Capon A, Souil E, Gauthier B, Sumian C, Bachelet M, Buys B, et al. Laser assisted skin closure (LASC) using a 815-nm diode-laser system accelerates and improves wound healing. Lasers Surg Med. 2001;28(2):168-75.
29. Souil E, Capon A, Mordon S, Dinh-Xuan AT, Polla BS, Bachelet M, et al. Treatment with 815-nm diode laser induces long-lasting expression of 72-kDa heat shock protein in normal rat skin. Br J Dermatol. 2001;144(2):260-6.
30. Shah M, Foreman DM, Ferguson MW. Neutralising antibody to TGF-β1, 2 reduces cutaneous scarring in adult rodents. J Cell Sci. 1994;107 (Pt 5):1137-57.
31. Shah M, Foreman DM, Ferguson MW. Neutralisation of TGF-β1 and TGF-β2 or exogenous addition of TGF-β3 to cutaneous rat wounds reduces scarring. J Cell Sci. 1995;108(Pt 3):985-1002.
32. Manstein D, Herron GS, Sink RK, Tanner H, Anderson RR. Fractional photothermolysis: a new concept for cutaneous remodeling using microscopic patterns of thermal injury. Laser Surg Med. 2004;34(5):426-38.
33. Friedman PM, Jih MH, Skover GR, Payonk GS, Kimyai-Asadi A, Geronemus RG. Treatment of atrophic facial acne scars with the 1064-nm Q - switched Nd:YAG laser: six-month follow-up study. Arch Dermatol. 2004;140(11):1337-41.
34. Keller R, Júnior J, Valente NY, Rodrigues CJ. Nonablative 1,064-nm Nd:YAG laser for treating atrophic facial acne scars : histologic and clinical analysis. Dermatol Surg. 2007;33(12):1470-6.
35. Lipper GM, Perez M. Nonablative acne scar reduction after a series of treatments with a short - pulsed 1,064-nm neodymium:YAG laser. Dermatol Surg. 2006;32(8):998-1006.
36. Sadick NS. Update on non – ablative light therapy for rejuvenation: a review. Lasers Surg Med. 2003;32(2):120-8.
37. Alster TS, Tanzi EL, Lazarus M. The use of fractional laser photothermolysis for the treatment of atrophic scars. Dermatol Surg. 2007;33(3):295-9.
38. Chan HH, Lam LK, Wong DS, Kono T, Trendell-Smith N. Use of the 1,320 nm Nd:YAG laser for wrinkle reduction and the treatment of atrophic acne scarring in Asians. Lasers Surg Med. 2004;34(2):98-103.
39. Bhatia AC, Dover JS, Arndt KA, Stewart B, Alam M. Patient satisfaction and reported long - term therapeutic efficacy associated with 1320 nm Nd:YAG laser treatment of acne scarring and photoaging. Dermatol Surg. 2006;32(3):346-52.
40. Cho SB, Lee SJ, Cho S, Oh SH, Chung WS, Kang JM. Non-ablative 1550-nm erbium - glass and ablative 10 600-nm carbon dioxide fractional lasers for acne scars: a randomized split - face study with blinded response evaluation. J Eur Acad Dermatol Venereol. 2010;24(8):921-5.
41. Carniol PJ, Vynatheya J, Carniol E. Evaluation of acne scar treatment with a 1450-nm midinfrared laser and 30% trichloroacetic acid peels. Arch Facial Plast Surg. 2005;7(4):251-5.
42. Chua SH, Ang P, Khoo LS, Goh CL. Nonablative 1450-nm diode laser in the treatment of facial atrophic acne scars in type IV to type V Asian skin: a prospective clinical study. Dermatol Surg. 2004;30(10): 1287-91.
43. Capon A, Iarmarcovai G, Gonnelli D, Degardin N, Magalon G, Mordon S. Scar prevention using Laser - Assisted Skin Healing (LASH) in plastic surgery. Aesthetic Plast Surg. 2010;34(4):438-46.
44. Wada T, Kawada A, Hirao A, Sasaya H, Oiso N. Efficacy and safety of a low-energy double-pass 1450-nm diode laser for the treatment of acne scars. Photomed Laser Surg. 2012;30(2):107-11.
45. Yoo KH, Ahn JY, Kim JY, Li K, Seo SJ, Hong CK. The use of the 1540 nm fractional photothermolysis for the treatment of acne scars in Asian skin: a pilot study. Photodermatol Photoimmunol Photomed. 2009;25(3): 138-42.

CHAPTER 26

Fractional Carbon Dioxide Lasers for Scar Reduction

Koushik Lahiri, Ishad Aggarwal

INTRODUCTION

Injury to skin initiates a cascade of organized sequential events of inflammation, granulation, and remodeling, which lead to wound healing. Any deviation in this process leads to formation of scars. In the world that constantly becomes centered upon appearance, scars could lead to significant psychological distress and loss of self-esteem. Consequently, cutaneous surgeons all across the globe, find themselves attending to an ever increasing desire amongst people for scar reduction. The field of laser scar reduction has seen a sea of change over the past few decades. The purpose of this chapter is to review the principles of fractional carbon dioxide (CO_2) laser for reduction of various kinds of scars, with special focus on Indian skin.

CONCEPT OF SELECTIVE PHOTOTHERMOLYSIS IN FRACTIONAL CARBON DIOXIDE LASERS: A HISTORICAL OVERVIEW AND BASIC PRINCIPLE

The earliest laser devices pioneered in 1970s were continuous wave lasers which had the ability to coagulate, cut, or ablate tissues nonspecifically, thereby leading to larger number of complications, mostly due to bulk tissue damage. Renaissance into the field of cutaneous laser medicine was heralded by the landmark theory of selective photothermolysis by Anderson and Parrish in the year 1983.[1] The theory describes localized photothermal injury to a specific chromophore. The idea is to selectively target the major chromophores such as water, melanin, and hemoglobin and contain the thermal damage into the target tissue without nonspecific destruction of the surrounding tissue. This is achieved by emitting photons of a specific wavelength which was specific to the target chromophore and differed from that of surrounding tissue, keeping the energy fluence sufficiently high to damage the target tissue and pulse duration less than or equal to thermal relaxation time (TRT) of the target chromophore.

Carbon dioxide laser became available for treatment in 1964 and since then it has been a popular ablative laser in dermatological practice. Carbon dioxide laser emits photons in the invisible infrared spectrum at 10,600 nm. The chromophore for this laser is water presenting both intracellularly and extracellularly. Water is abundantly present in epidermis and dermis which absorbs the incident light, causing vaporization of skin and coagulative necrosis of the dermis. The earlier CO_2 lasers were continuous wave lasers, which leave behind a thick zone of thermal necrosis measuring about 0.2–1 mm in thickness. The consequent risk of complications is higher and there runs a longer downtime of recovery.[2]

Laser resurfacing using CO_2 lasers saw a paradigm shift, when Manstein and colleagues came up with a novel concept of fractional photothermolysis in 2004.[3]

Although an extension of the principle of selective photothermolysis, fractional photothermolysis involved creation of pixelated patterns of full thickness columns of skin coagulation, which were termed as microthermal zones (MTZ).[3,4] By utilizing the principles of selective photothermolysis and creating short pulses of energy, the concept of fractional photothermolysis fosters the remodeling of collagen in these MTZs with aid of surrounding normal tissue. Fractional photothermolysis has become the industry standard of lasers which are involved in resurfacing and scar reduction, and, hence, the genesis of fractional CO_2 lasers.

HISTOGENESIS AND LASER TISSUE INTERACTIONS

In an ideal scenario, MTZ are cylindrical microscopic zones in dermis. The reparative capacity and resultant collagen remodeling is dependent upon the surrounding normal tissue. The diameter and depth of these zones is dependent upon a host of factors like fluence, wavelength, machine used, and number of stacking applied. Ablative fractional CO_2 lasers cause disruption of both epidermal and dermal tissue. Studies have shown that by 48 hours, invaginating epidermal keratinocytes replace the MTZ and there is extrusion of necrotic debris by 1 week also known as microscopic epidermal necrotic debris (MEND),[4] with complete replacement of stratum corneum by 1 month. Remodeling of collagen takes place by 3 months which is indicated by increased expression of heat shock protein 47 (Hsp47)[4] in this tissue, which is a marker of collagen synthesis. The depths of these MTZ vary between 100 and 160 μm and constitute 15–25% skin surface area under treatment per session. Carbon dioxide lasers vaporizes both epidermis and dermis to a depth of 20–60 μm while the thermal damage zone extends to another 20–50 μm. Approximately, 90% of CO_2 laser energy is absorbed in the initial 20–30 μm of skin. Theory of selective photothermolysis states that selective heating of the target chromophore can be achieved when using laser pulses shorter than the TRT of the chromophore (time required for chromophore to lose 50% of its heat to surrounding tissue). Thermal relaxation time for 20–30 μm of skin tissue is approximately 1 millisecond. Using the theory of selective photothermolysis, CO_2 lasers with pulse duration of less than 1 millisecond are capable of selectively vaporizing tissue with only very thin zone of residual thermal necrosis measuring approximately 100 μm. To have a clinical effect in the skin, laser energy must be absorbed by the target chromophore. Energy fluence (density) necessary to vaporize tissue is approximately 5 J/cm^2 (ablation threshold). Overall, delivering 1 millisecond CO_2 laser pulse with an energy fluence of approximately 5 J/cm^2, leads to tissue vaporization measuring 20–30 μm and residual thermal injury measuring 40–120 μm.[5] This zone of thermal necrosis is sufficient to seal small dermal blood vessels and lymphatics, yet narrow enough to reduce incidence of scarring.[5]

FRACTIONAL CARBON DIOXIDE LASERS FOR SCAR REDUCTION

Although ablative CO_2 lasers have been in use for skin resurfacing and scar reduction since 1960s, however, they came heavily upon the downtime and rate of complications. Nonablative lasers which selectively destroyed dermis, give lesser downtime and complications, but inferior results. Fractional lasers bridge the gap between these two modalities.

Two main types of fractional CO_2 lasers are currently being used by laser surgeons. They are:

- The scanning CO_2 laser
- The pulsed CO_2 laser.

The scanning CO_2 lasers use an optomechanical flash scanner connected to a continuous wave CO_2 laser, which efficiently distributes laser energy into train of pulses with dwell time shorter than TRT of the tissue, hence, mimicking a pulsed CO_2 laser.

Most conventional continuous wave CO_2 lasers can be converted into pulsed lasers by a pulsing technique. These pulsed lasers can produce a train of relatively high power, short duration pulses which work on the principle of selective photothermolysis. Some of these machines have computerized pattern generators which place individual laser beams into a specific pattern.

Pulsed Wave Carbon Dioxide Lasers

When the pulse length of the laser beam is shorter than the TRT of target tissue, it results in quick ablation of tissue with minimal thermal damage:

- Superpulsed lasers
- Ultrapulsed lasers.

Superpulsed CO_2 lasers were lasers with pulse duration of 10–100 milliseconds which have now been replaced by the ultrapulsed lasers which have pulse durations of submicroseconds.

INDICATIONS

Scars Amenable to Fractional Carbon Dioxide Lasers[6]

Of the wide variety of clinical scars a dermatosurgeon is confronted with, following types are the ones that shows significant improvement with fractional CO_2 lasers:

- Atrophic scars due to acne
- Atrophic scars due to nonacne etiologies such as trauma, post-varicella infection, or surgical scars
- Burn scars
- Striae distensae.

Patient Selection

When considering a patient for scar reduction using fractional CO_2 lasers, the caveats hold true as for different lasers otherwise and, especially, for ablative ones, the following points can generally be helpful to avoid complications and select patients for the procedure.

INDIAN SKIN TYPES

Color of Skin

The Indian skin type is predominantly Fitzpatrick types IV to V, although rarely skin types III and VI may also be seen in isolated cases. It is important to understand that the Indian skin may be more predisposed to develop keloids and hypertrophic scars after an ablative procedure, hence, appropriate history should be sought before performing the procedure. While discussing laser treatment outcomes with the patient, it is important that the treating physician be apprised with the possibility of developing transient postinflammatory hyperpigmentation.[7]

Concurrent Infections[8]

It is important to see that any infections seen on the cutaneous surface being treated, be free of any viral or bacterial infection which may otherwise flare up after treatment.

Coexistent Inflammatory Skin Conditions[8]

It is important that laser surgeon identify any inflammatory process, such as active acne, psoriasis, or contact dermatitis, and then treat prior to performing the procedure and treat them.

Medication[8,9]

Patients seeking treatment for atrophic scarring due to acne may have concurrent or recent history of isotretinoin intake. It has been shown that this could lead to development of hypertrophic scars due to isotretinoin effects on collagenase. There is much debate over the isotretinoin drug free interval and contrary to prevalent notion , many dermatologists treat patients on isotretinoin with fractional CO_2 lasers, the current consensus is to have a 6-month drug free interval before performing scar revision with these lasers.

Allergy to Systemic or Local Anesthetics

It is important to rule out history of developing any reaction to local or systemic anesthetics which are used during the procedure.[8]

Realistic Expectations

It is important to identify unrealistic expectations, psychological instability, and patients who will neither tolerate nor be compliant of postprocedure care.[8]

PRINCIPLES OF USING FRACTIONAL CARBON DIOXIDE LASER

The settings depend upon the types of scars being used and the machine that a treating laser surgeon has at his disposal. However, a few basic principles must be kept in mind before using a fractional CO_2 lasers:[10]

- Depth of skin vaporization and degree of thermal necrosis is directly proportional to pulse energy and number of passes performed
- The relationship between number of passes and depth of thermal damage is not linear. The first laser pass significantly ablates more tissue than the second or subsequent passes; an ablation plateau is reached in 3–4 passes, limiting ablation depth to approximately 250 μm. The effect of such passes is cumulative
- The goal of scar reduction using any CO_2 lasers system are to achieve a soft transition between atrophic indentation and surrounding normal skin; to stimulate collagen in the indented area. To get a desirable result, entire cosmetic unit should be treated together. To avoid sharp demarcation lines between treated and untreated skin, it is important to perform a technique called feathering, in which the surrounding normal skin is treated with lower energy

- In case multiple passes are required, the partially desiccated tissue should be removed with saline soaked gauze to prevent charring
- Another important parameter in fractional CO_2 devices is the density of the MTZ that are active in the beam of light. The higher the density, higher is the vaporisation of the tissue.

SCARS CHARACTERISTICS AND PARAMETERS

Scar characteristics, such as size, color, morphology, and history of previous treatments are essential to be determined because such differences could require modifications of treatment protocols.

Atrophic Scars

Atrophic scars are depressions seen on the surface of skin which is the result of inflammatory processes such as acne, varicella infection, or trauma.

Atrophic Acne Scars[11,12]

Atrophic acne scars are classified and have traditionally been classified as ice picks, rolling, or boxcar scars. Ice pick scars are typically narrow (<2 mm), sharp tracts that extend into the dermis or may even go as deep as the subcutis. These scars taper down and are wider at the surface. Rolling scars are wide and produce undulations over the surface of the skin. Boxcar scars are round to oval depressions over the surface of skin and show no tapering. It is, however, prudent to state, that due to the complexity of the nature of acne scars, fractional CO_2 lasers although represents a major advancement in treatment modality for acne scars, it does, however, come with certain limitations and hence, a combination of scar revision techniques are advocated for best results. Most studies have reported good outcomes in superficial and medium depth scars, thereby making it a good treatment modality for superficial boxcar scars. In ice pick scars and depressed boxcar scars, the aim is to soften the abrupt transition between the scar edge and normal skin and to stimulate collagen in the dermis. However, in rolling scars, the treatment outcome depends upon the severity to which the scar is tethered to underlying dermis and subcutis. Such scars present an ideal opportunity for a dermatosurgeon to perform subcision before attempting ablation with fractional CO_2 lasers.

Laser parameters for atrophic acne scars vary with different machines with different settings.[13] Many manufacturers provide different handpieces which differ in amount of energy released and depth of penetration. With a CO_2 laser, a fluence of 300 μJ with 60 watt power is typically used in a single pass to achieve ablation of epidermis with variable sized and shaped parameters.[14] Depending upon the scar severity, 2–3 passes may be required, with depth of ablation increasing at each successive pass. It is advisable to avoid overlapping in lasers with computer generated pattern and clean debris with saline soaked gauze in between passes.[15] The second pass after the first pass may also be given in a direction perpendicular to the initial pass. Cosmetic end point in a session is ablation of the tissue, however, safety end point is considered to be attained when the treated skin color appears yellowish even after it is washed with saline.

Outcomes in Atrophic Acne Scar Reduction with Fractional Carbon Dioxide Lasers

In a study conducted in India by Majid et al., 43.3% of the patients showed excellent response to fractional CO_2 lasers as monotherapy for atrophic acne scars.[16] They used fluence of 15–20 J/cm^2 with a density of 100–150 MTZ/cm^2 with single or double pass and repeated sessions every 6 weeks for 3–4 sessions. They found good results in rolling scars and boxcar scars. Wang YS et al. conducted a study on type IV Asian skin, and found similar results.[17] Their parameters were fluence of 28 J/cm^2 and 20% coverage in single pass.

Suffice to say that fractional CO_2 lasers can bring good outcomes in acne scars; however, the laser parameters need to be picked carefully to prevent complications, especially, in Asian skin types. Results shown by Yuan XH et al. shows that lower fluence of 10 J/cm^2 shows comparable results and fewer complications in Asian skin(Figs 1 to 3).[18]

COMBINATION OF FRACTIONAL CARBON DIOXIDE LASER WITH OTHER TREATMENT MODALITIES

Due to versatility of acne scars, most treating dermatologists find it more rewarding to combine different therapeutic modalities to achieve the most optimum results. The most commonly used modalities are non-ablative lasers, microneedling techniques, and chemical peels.[13]

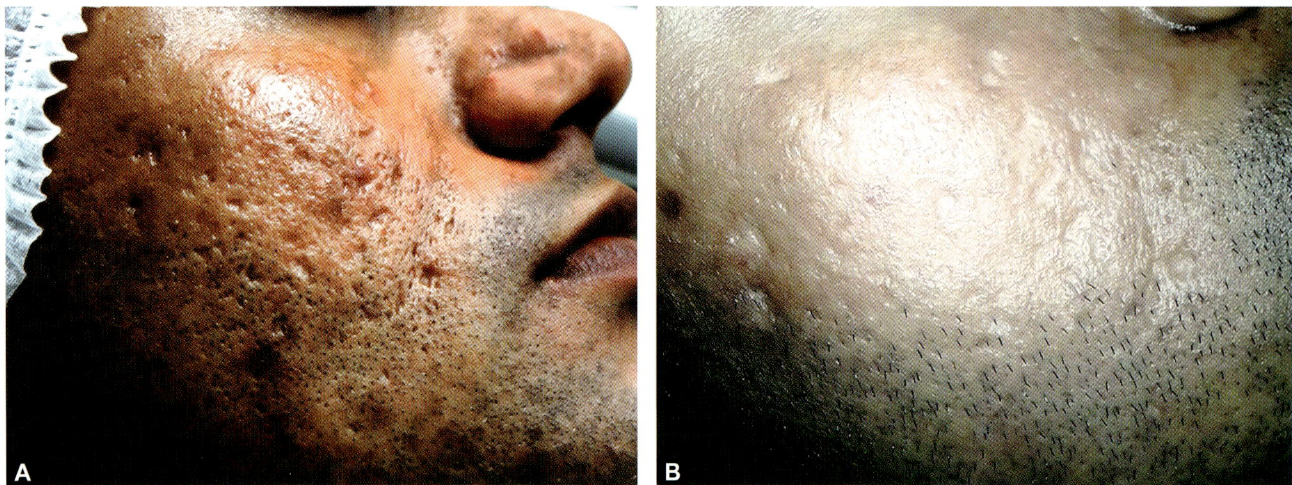

FIG. 1: A, Box and ice pick types of post acne scars; **B,** improvement after four sessions of fractional carbon dioxide laser treatment

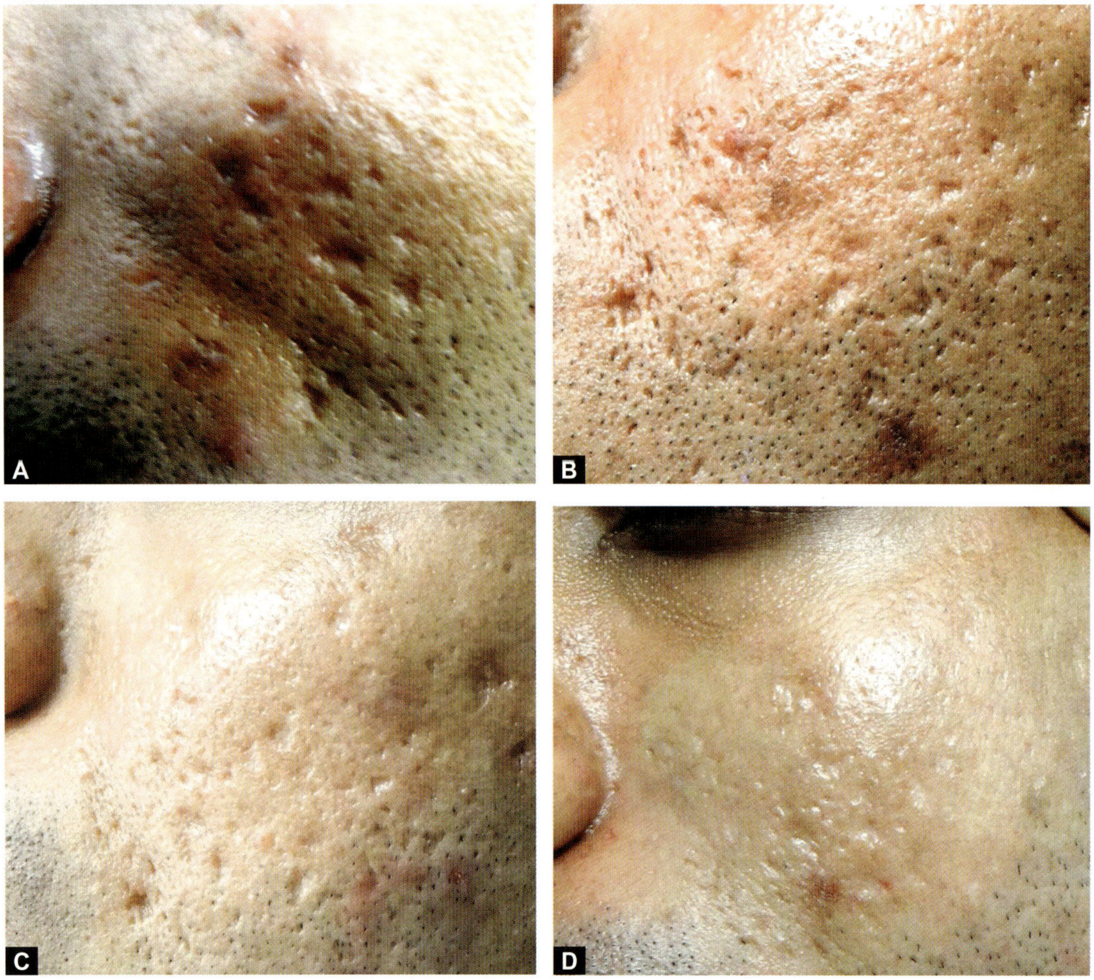

FIG. 2: A, Atrophic acne scars before treatment; **B,** improvement after three sessions of fractional carbon dioxide laser treatment; **C,** improvement after four sessions of fractional carbon dioxide laser treatment; **D,** improvement after five sessions of fractional carbon dioxide laser treatment

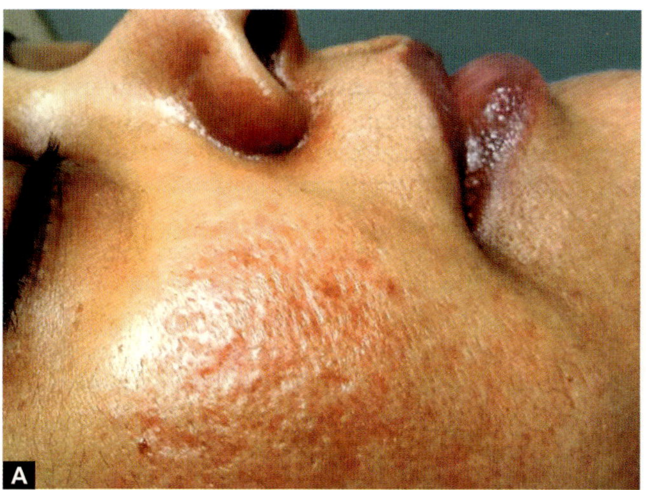

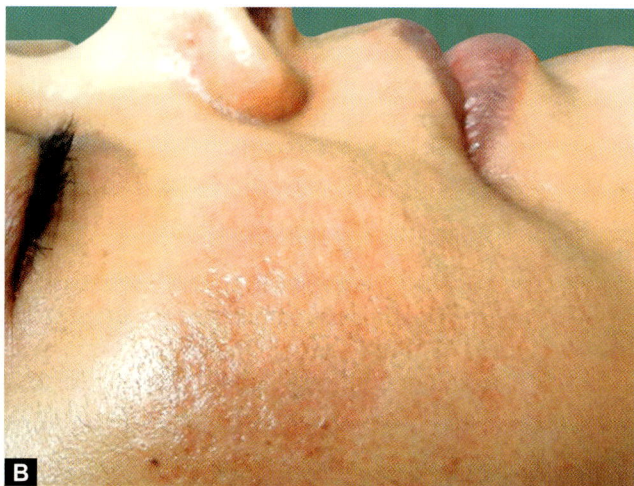

FIG. 3: A, Post acne scars before therapy of fractional carbon dioxide laser; **B,** improvement seen after two sessions of fractional carbon dioxide laser treatment

WHAT IS NEW FOR FRACTIONAL CARBON DIOXIDE LASER

- Focal acne scar treatment technique, a recently introduced concept, challenges the common know-how and envisages the usage of higher fluence focused beam of laser only over the scar area, thus, sparing the normal skin. It has been used with comparable results in ice pick scars which hitherto have been lesser responsive to fractional CO_2 lasers[19]
- Radiofrequency microplasma technique has been introduced for scar correction. In combination with fractional CO_2 laser, it has been shown to reduce complications and give better results[20]
- Fractional CO_2 laser may also be used to inject substances like poly L-lactic acid inside scars to give better cosmetic outcome.[21]

FRACTIONAL CARBON DIOXIDE LASER IN NONACNE SCARS

Nonacne Atrophic Scars

Fractional CO_2 lasers are currently commonly used in practice for treatment of scars caused by varicella, although studies for this indication are largely lacking. However, extrapolating from data obtained for acne scars, it could be good treatment modality for correction of post-varicella scars. Fractional CO_2 laser has been used to treat atrophic scars due to leishmaniasis in 11 subjects by Alghamadi and Khurram and they showed more than 50% improvement in all patients at 3 months follow-up.[22]

Scars due to Trauma and Surgery

Scar reconstruction after trauma and surgery could be a challenge. Fractional CO_2 lasers have been found to reduce the scar size and volume in post-traumatic and surgical scars and are more effective for atrophic scars than hypertrophic scars. A study conducted by Wiess et al. demonstrates a 38.0% mean reduction of volume and 35.6% mean reduction of maximum scar depth in nonacne atrophic scars due to trauma and surgery. In another Korean study on 23 post-thyroidectomy scars treated with fractional CO_2 laser, 12 out of 23 patients showed more than 51% improvement at 3 weeks after surgery.[23] The parameters used were single session of two passes of a CO_2 fractional laser system with a pulse energy setting of 50 µJ and a density of 100 spots/cm^2, 2–3 weeks after surgery.[24] Both fractional CO_2 laser and pulsed dye laser (PDL) have been used for scar revision, but it has been seen that fractional CO_2 laser give better scar contour and PDL gives better color improvements.

Postburn Mature Scars[25]

Histological and biochemical analyses have been performed over mature burn scars treated with fractional CO_2 laser and it was found that there is increase in collagen remodeling and expression of growth factors and ribonucleic acid with statistically significant clinical improvement. However, given the nature of scars, multiple sessions may be required and other lasers like PDL may be used in combination to give better cosmetic improvement, more so in the color of scars, especially, in keloidal and hypertrophic burns scar (Fig. 4).

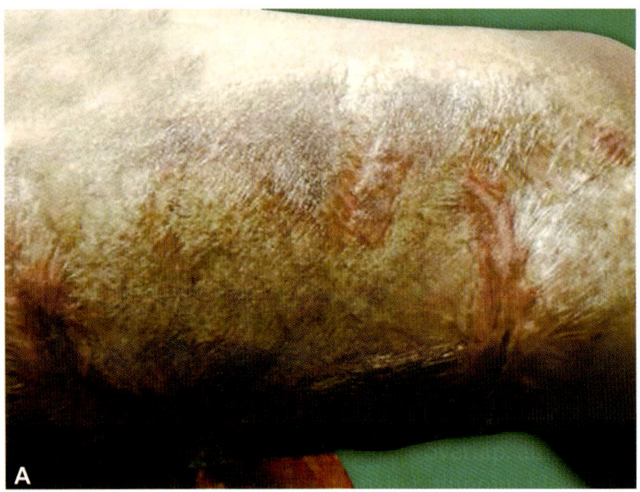

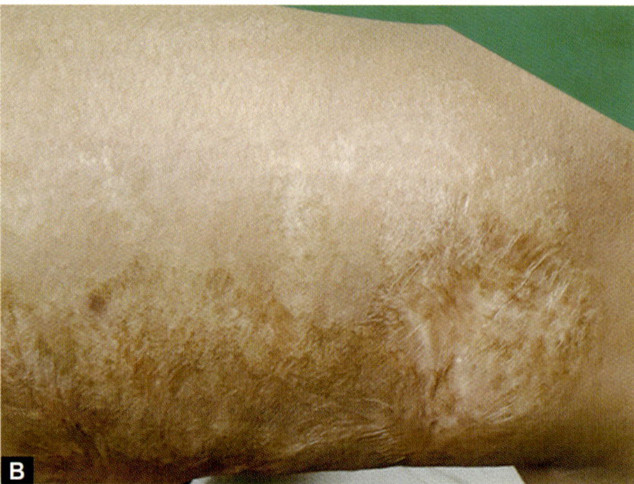

FIG. 4: A, Postburn scar before treatment; **B,** improvement noted after treatment with fractional carbon dioxide laser

Striae Distensae

Traditional PDL has been used to treat striae distensae, but there is growing evidence of fractional CO_2 laser's efficacy in this condition. Combination of PDL with fractional CO_2 laser has been shown to be more efficacious than either modality alone.[26] In a Korean study, energy of 10 μJ and area coverage of 10% were used to treat striae in single session and good outcomes were reported.[27]

COMPLICATIONS AFTER FRACTIONAL CARBON DIOXIDE LASER TREATMENT[28,29] AND MANAGEMENT

Since fractional CO_2 laser ablates the skin and imparts thermal energy to skin, some effects are expected, therefore, these side effects must be differentiated from complications.

Some of these immediate effects include post-procedure pain, edema, pruritus, and scab formation.[12] Application of ice, postprocedure analgesics, efficacious sun protection, and emollients help to alleviate these effects and must be given to all the patients.[30]

Mild complications sometimes occur and usually are of minimal consequence. Minor complications include milia formation, perioral dermatitis, acne and/or rosacea exacerbation, contact dermatitis, and postinflammatory hyperpigmentation. Transient postinflammatory hyperpigmentation is very commonly seen in the Indian skin types and generally resolves within a few days.

The first postoperative week is critical. It is important to closely monitor patients for appropriate healing responses and complications such as dermatitis and infection. Carbon dioxide laser reepithelialization requires 7–10 days.

Moderate complications include localized viral, bacterial, and candidal infection, delayed hypopigmentation, persistent erythema, and prolonged healing. The most severe complications are hypertrophic scarring, disseminated infection, and ectropion. Early detection of complications and rapid institution of appropriate therapy are extremely important. Delay in treatment can have severe deleterious consequences, including permanent scarring and dyspigmentation.

Erythema

Erythema may persist for 12 weeks or more. Mild corticosteroids twice a day for 3–4 weeks can be used for persistent focal areas of erythema. Diffuse erythema may be secondary to contact dermatitis. This may occur with excessive intraoperative use of wet gauze or early postoperative use of topical tretinoin.

Dyspigmentation

A significant adverse effect that may occur with fractional CO_2 laser is transient hyperpigmentation. Although hyperpigmentation is more common in patients with darker skin tones, it may occur in any skin type. Transient hyperpigmentation is observed early in the postoperative course, occurring approximately 1–2 months after treatment.[28,29] While the process is usually self-limited, resolution may be hastened with depigmenting creams (e.g., hydroquinone, arbutin) or acid preparations (e.g., glycolic, retinoic, azelaic, kojic, ascorbic).[8] Hypopigmentation is a relatively late sequel of treatment (typically observed ≥6 months postoperatively) and appears to be permanent.

Infection[8]

Significant pain that occurs at day 2 after procedure may indicate a bacterial, fungal, or viral infection. A high degree of vigilance and suspicion is necessary because signs may be subclinical, and the patient may be dismissed as having a low pain threshold. They should be identified early and treated accordingly. Incidence can be reduced with appropriate use of prophylactic antibiotics and, more importantly, aggressive postoperative wound care.

Scarring[28]

Postprocedure scarring may occur with excessive thermal damage or infection. Treatment should be instituted as early as signs of scarring are evident. Treatment with potent topical steroids, intralesional steroids, and silicone gel may be given.

CONCLUSION

In a world where technology has made us fickle and even impatient, where everyone wants everything now, where micro is becoming nano, fractional CO_2 lasers find themselves comfortably placed. With ever increasing demand, lesser downtime and better results, they have become a reliable tool for the ambitious cosmetic surgeons. With careful watch, thoughtful mind, and sound knowledge of the principles, we could offer more with this technology.

REFERENCES

1. Anderson RR, Parrish JA. Selective photothermolysis: precise microsurgery by selective absorption of pulsed radiation. Science. 1983;220(4596):524-7.
2. Ross EV, Domankevitz Y, Skrobal M, Anderson RR. Effects of CO_2 laser pulse duration in ablation and residual thermal damage: implications for skin resurfacing. Lasers Surg Med. 1996;19(2):123-9.
3. Manstein D, Herron GS, Sink RK, Tanner H, Anderson RR. Fractional photothermolysis: a new concept for cutaneous remodeling using microscopic patterns of thermal injury. Lasers Surg Med. 2004;34(5):426-38.
4. Laubach HJ, Tannous Z, Anderson RR, Manstein D. Skin responses to fractional photothermolysis. Lasers Surg Med. 2006;38(2):142-9.
5. Janik JP, Markus JL, Al-Dujaili Z, Markus RF. Laser resurfacing. Semin Plast Surg. 2007;21(3):139-46.
6. Alster TS, West TB. Resurfacing of atrophic facial acne scars with a high-energy, pulsed carbon dioxide laser. Dermatol Surg. 1996;22(2):151-4.
7. Alster T, Zaulyanov L, Zaulyanov-Scanlon L. Laser scar revision: a review. Dermatol Surg. 2007;33(2):131-40.
8. Alster TS. Cutaneous resurfacing with CO_2 and erbium: YAG lasers: preoperative, intraoperative, and postoperative considerations. Plast Reconstr Surg. 1999;103(2):619-32; discussion 633-4.
9. Zachariae H. Delayed wound healing and keloid formation following argon laser treatment or dermabrasion during isotretinoin treatment. Br J Dermatol. 1988;118(5):703-6.
10. Fitzpatrick RE, Tope WD, Goldman MP, Satur NM. Pulsed carbon dioxide laser, trichloroacetic acid, Baker-Gordon phenol, and dermabrasion: a comparative clinical and histologic study of cutaneous resurfacing in a porcine model. Arch Dermatol. 1996;132(4):469-71.
11. Goodman GJ, Baron JA. The management of postacne scarring. Dermatol Surg. 2007;33:1175-88.
12. Thiboutot D, Gollnick H, Bettoli V, Dréno B, Kang S, Leyden JJ, et al; Global Alliance to Improve Outcomes in Acne. New insights into the management of acne: an update from the Global Alliance to Improve Outcomes in Acne Group. J Am Acad Dermatol. 2009;60(5):S1-S50.
13. Omi T, Kawana S, Sato S, Bonan P, Naito Z. Fractional CO_2 laser for the treatment of acne scars. J Cosmet Dermatol. 2011;10(4):294-300.
14. Groover IJ, Alster TS. Laser revision of scars and striae. Dermatol Ther. 2000;13(1):50-9.
15. Kang WH, Kim YJ, Pyo WS, Park SJ, Kim JH. Atrophic acne scar treatment using triple combination therapy: dot peeling, subcision and fractional laser. J Cosmet Laser Ther. 2009;11(4):212-5.
16. Majid I, Imran S. Fractional CO_2 laser resurfacing as monotherapy in the treatment of atrophic facial acne scars. J Cutan Aesthet Surg. 2014;7(2):87-92.
17. Wang YS, Tay YK, Kwok C. Fractional ablative carbon dioxide laser in the treatment of atrophic acne scarring in Asian patients: a pilot study. J Cosmet Laser Ther. 2010;12(2):61-4.
18. Yuan XH, Zhong SX, Li SS. Comparison study of fractional carbon dioxide laser resurfacing using different fluences and densities for acne scars in Asians: a randomized split-face trial. Dermatol Surg. 2014;40(5):545-52.
19. Schweiger ES, Sundick L. Focal Acne Scar Treatment (FAST), a new approach to atrophic acne scars: a case series. J Drugs Dermatol. 2013; 12(10):1163-7.
20. Tenna S, Cogliandro A, Piombino L, Filoni A, Persichetti P. Combined use of fractional CO_2 laser and radiofrequency waves to treat acne scars: a pilot study on 15 patients. J Cosmet Laser Ther. 2012;14(4):166-71.
21. Sadove R. Injectable poly-L-lactic acid: a novel sculpting agent for the treatment of dermal fat atrophy after severe acne. Aesthetic Plast Surg. 2009;33(1):113-6.
22. AlGhamdi K, Khurrum H. Successful treatment of atrophic facial leishmaniasis scars by CO_2 fractional laser. J Cutan Med Surg. 2014;18(6):379-84.
23. Weiss ET, Chapas A, Brightman L, Hunzeker C, Hale EK, Karen JK, et al. Successful treatment of atrophic postoperative and traumatic scarring with carbon dioxide ablative fractional resurfacing. Quantitative volumetric scar improvement. Arch Dermatol. 2010;146(2):133.
24. Jung JY, Jeong JJ, Roh HJ, Cho SH, Chung KY, Lee WJ, et al. Early postoperative treatment of thyroidectomy scars using a fractional carbon dioxide laser. Dermatol Surg. 2011;37(2):217-23.
25. Cho SB, Lee SJ, Chung WS, Kang JM, Kim YK. Treatment of burn scar using a carbon dioxide fractional laser. J Drugs Dermatol. 2010;9(2): 173-5.
26. Naein FF, Soghrati M. Fractional CO_2 laser as an effective modality in treatment of striae alba in skin types III and IV. J Res Med Sci. 2012;17(10): 928-33.
27. Cho SB, Lee SJ, Lee JE, Kang JM, Kim YK, Oh SH. Treatment of striae alba using the 10,600-nm carbon dioxide fractional laser. J Cosmet Laser Ther. 2010;12(3):118-9.
28. Nanni CA, Alster TS. Complications of carbon dioxide laser resurfacing. An evaluation of 500 patients. Dermatol Surg. 1998;24(3):315-20.
29. Bernstein LJ, Kauvar AN, Grossman MC, Geronemus RG. The short- and long-term side effects of carbon dioxide laser resurfacing. Dermatol Surg. 1997;23(7):519-25.
30. Alexiades-Armenakas MR, Dover JS, Arndt KA. The spectrum of laser skin resurfacing: nonablative, fractional, and ablative laser resurfacing. J Am Acad Dermatol. 2008;58(5):719-37; quiz 738-40

CHAPTER 27

Erbium Doped Yttrium-aluminium-garnet Laser Treatment for Scars

Rajetha Damisetty

INTRODUCTION

Erbium doped yttrium-aluminium-garnet (Er:YAG) laser is an ablative laser with a wavelength of 2,940 nm. Its only chromophore in the human body is water. It is very avidly absorbed by water; as water is present abundantly in all layers of the skin, Er:YAG laser ablates all the layers of skin that it reaches, leaving very little collateral thermal damage.[1]

In its conventional and fractionated forms, it has been used for a myriad of indications in dermatology ranging from preparing the recipient site in vitiligo surgery to enhancing the elimination of tattoo pigment after Q-switched laser treatments. It has been used extensively in the treatment of atrophic postacne scars and various other kinds of scars.

MECHANISM OF ACTION

Improvement in scars occurs due to collagen induction, which ensues when water in the dermis absorbs the light waves and gets heated up. This leads to stimulation of neocollagenesis[2] by the dermal fibroblasts.

Resurfacing also adds to the effect, resulting in an improvement in skin texture.

Conventional Erbium Doped Yttrium-aluminium-garnet Resurfacing versus Fractional Resurfacing (Fig. 2)

Ablative resurfacing in the late 1990s was the first paradigm in laser treatment of acne scars, following the use of dermabrasion in 1980s. Mechanical and chemical ablative techniques have largely been overtaken by ablative or nonablative laser techniques for resurfacing, which are technically easier to perform and tend to produce less variable results.[2]

Use of the erbium laser in the treatment of acne scars began to be reported in the literature in 1999, when Weinstein[2] studied its effects on 63 out of 78 patients. The other 15 patients were treated with a combined erbium/carbon dioxide laser. It was noted that 55 out of 78 or 71% of the patients showed 70–90% improvement, and 23 out of 78 or 29% had 50–70% improvement. Weinstein reported that there were no excellent or poor results.

Average of 51–75% improvement was reported by a few other workers using slightly different protocols.[3,4] Asian patients with skin phototypes III, IV, and V were treated too,[5] using extra-long pulse widths up to 1,500 ms in some cases.[6]

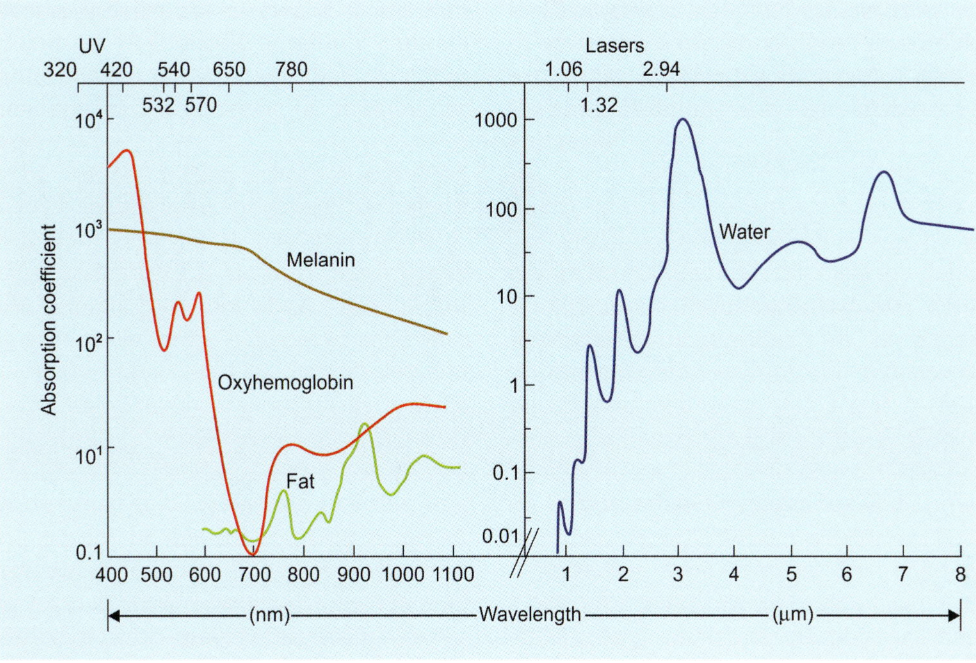

UV, ultraviolet.

FIG 1: Various chromophores in human skin and their absorption spectra

In conventional ablative laser resurfacing, skin is treated with long-wave lasers (carbon dioxide or Er:YAG) and is heated to above 100°C, resulting in vaporization of a portion of the treated area. The tissue ablation results in removal of abnormal pigmentation and reduction of wrinkles.[7] This method of rejuvenation is widely considered to be the most effective, but also the riskiest. It had to be performed in the operation theatre, required general anesthesia, hospitalization for a week or so, and resulted in morbidity due to viral, bacterial, and fungal infections to which the completely denuded skin was susceptible to.

Religious sun protection was mandatory for up to 6 months. Yet those with colored skin could not undergo this treatment as the chances of prolonged or permanent pigment anomalies (both hyper- and hypopigmentation) and keloidal or hypertrophic scars was too high.

As the entire epidermis and upper dermis had to be removed, healing was dependent on pilosebaceous units. So this procedure's utility was limited to the face where the density of pilosebaceous units was sufficiently high to allow healing by primary intention. Any other area of the body, such as neck and hands, would develop scarring when subjected to conventional laser resurfacing.

Nonablative laser resurfacing, using neodymium doped yttrium-aluminium-garnet (Nd:YAG) 1,064 nm heats skin to lower temperatures, resulting in thermal injury without vaporization of skin.[8] This method, though much safer, suffered from significantly reduced efficacy.[9]

In 2004, Manstein et al[10] introduced the concept of fractional photothermolysis (FPT). This new paradigm completely transformed laser resurfacing and the way acne scars were treated. Their concept was to heat only columns of skin and not the entire skin to high enough temperatures to induce injury, which would result in wound healing with subsequent dermal remodelling and improved appearance. These zones of injury are microscopic in nature and separated from each other by areas of undamaged skin, allowing for rapid healing.

Splitting of the laser beam allowed healing to happen from the intentionally untreated islands of skin within the treatment area. Pilosebaceous units were not required for healing. Hence, any part of the body could be safely treated. The process was much simpler and could be performed with topical anesthesia as an outpatient procedure. Healing would be complete after a minimal downtime of 5–7 days and morbidity due to infections became exceedingly rare. Even skin of color could be

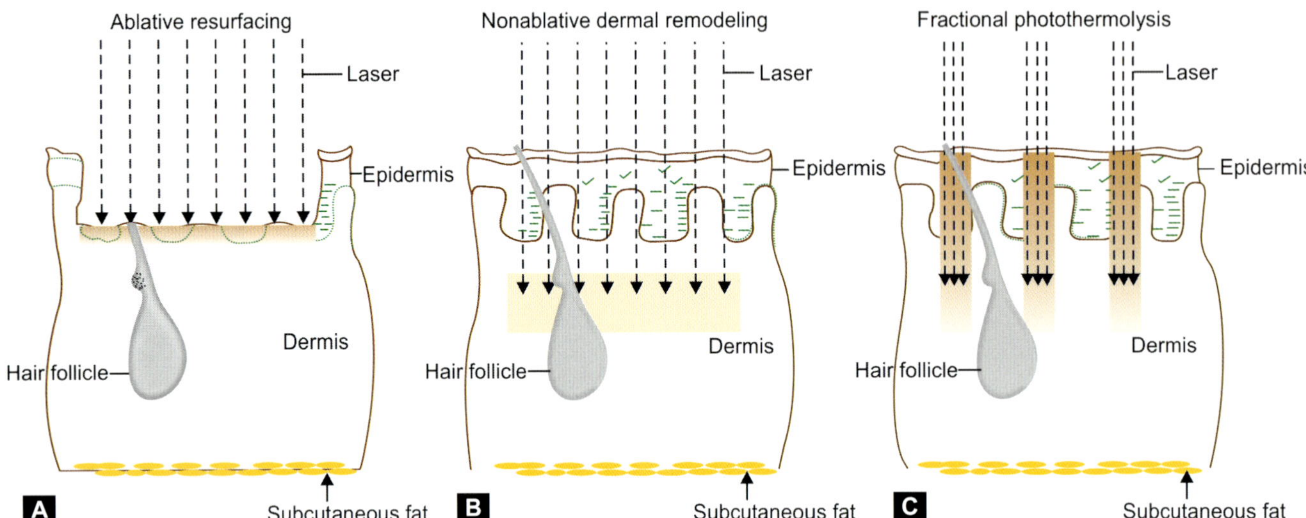

FIG. 2: Conceptual comparison of ablative skin resurfacing, nonablative dermal remodeling, and fractional photothermolysis. **A,** Ablative skin resurfacing removes the epidermis and causes residual thermal damage within the dermis. Reepithelialization is delayed because of relative long migratory path lengths for keratinocytes that repopulate from skin appendages. **B,** Nonablative dermal remodeling creates a layer of thermal damage below the surface without causing epidermal removal or damage. **C,** Fractional photothermolysis is the distribution of microscopically small volumes of thermal damage, microthermal treatment zones, within the skin. Epidermal repair is fast due to small wounds and short migratory paths for keratinocytes.

treated with remarkable safety and cost of treatment reduced drastically.

Fractionated resurfacing attempted to bridge the divide between high risk efficacious procedures and low risk poorly efficacious ones. Unlike both ablative and nonablative resurfacing devices, which attempt to uniformly damage skin at varying depths, FPT induces pixelated microscopic columns of thermal injury. It leaves normal undamaged intervening tissue around the treated area. However, the trade off is reduced efficacy and requirement for increasing number of treatments.

Multiple sessions (four in number) of fractional Er:YAG laser have comparable effects to a single session of ablative Er:YAG laser on dermal collagen type I, III, and VII, but pure ablative laser has more effect on elastic tissue and epidermal thickness.[1]

Ten years after the introduction of the concept of FPT, pure ablative laser resurfacing was re-explored.[11] While good (51–75%) to excellent (75–100%) improvement was noted, 45.5% of the 22 patients developed postinflammatory hyperpigmentation including one patient who had the pigmentation persisting for more than 3 months. Complete wound healing occurred between 6 and 9 days. Erythema occurred in all patients and lasted longer than 3 months in two patients (9.1%). Mild-to-moderate acne flare-up occurred in five patients (22.7%).

In a study of 25 patients with Fitzpatrick's phototypes IV and V in South India,[12] 96% showed at least fair (26–50% or more) improvement. Rolling and superficial box scars showed higher significant improvement when compared with ice pick and deep box scars. Patient's satisfaction of improvement was higher when compared to physician's observations. The difference in agreement was noticed when observing the number of patients reporting more than 50% improvement (good to excellent) compared with the observers' rating. Forty percent of the subjects noticed good to excellent improvement as opposed to 20–24% in the observers. Patients felt better probably because of the additional benefits of fractional laser in decreasing pigmentation and fine lines, skin tightening, and pore reduction. This is the reason why though the patients had only a fair improvement after pixel laser (Alma Lasers' fractionated Er:YAG), they felt the laser's efficacy to be good or excellent. Twelve percent of the patients reported excellent improvement with the highest being 85% improvement. Downtime was also acceptable in the study with mean value less than 7 days in all four sittings. No serious adverse effects were noted with exacerbation of acne lesions forming the majority. It was concluded that ablative FPT using Er:YAG laser is both effective and safe treatment for atrophic acne scars in Indian skin.

TYPES OF ACNE SCARS IMPROVED BY ERBIUM DOPED YTTRIUM-ALUMINIUM-GARNET

Evaluation of scar type and its severity is a very important step to select the most appropriate therapeutic option among the currently available ones. There have been several approaches to classify acne scars in order to evaluate objectively type and severity.

Jacob et al.[13] proposed a descriptive, simple, universally applicable acne scar classification system that includes three scar types: ice pick, rolling, and boxcar. They also developed an effective treatment algorithm for reconstructing and improving the appearance of acne scars including punch excision, punch elevation, subcutaneous incision (subcision), and laser skin resurfacing. Papular acne scars,[14] also known as perifollicular elastolysis or "postacne anetoderma-like scars" have been described on the upper trunk but are commonly encountered on the face, especially on the nose and chin (author's personal experience). Both elastic and collagen fibers were found to be attenuated in comparison with those in normal adjacent dermis.

The ice pick scars, which represent almost the 60–70% of atrophic scars, are usually punctiform, sharp and deep, and have a "V" shape in longitudinal section. The boxcar ones are round or oval shaped, from 1.5 through 4.0 mm in diameter, wide at the surface and the base, showing ''U'' shape and representing 20–30% of total atrophic scars. Finally, the rolling scars have ''M'' shape and, therefore, give a rolling appearance to the skin; they usually have a diameter of 4–5 mm and represent from 15 through 25% of atrophic scars.[13]

Frequently, all these types of atrophic scars coexist in the same patient. For this reason, several classifications and evaluation scales have been proposed by other authors. Goodman and Baron proposed a qualitative scale[15] and then presented a quantitative scale (Table 1).[16] Dreno et al. introduced the ECCA scale[17] (Echelle d'Evaluation Clinique des Cicatrices d'Acné) which is the only validated scoring scale.

While rolling scars respond best to subcision followed by collagen induction using fractionated Er:YAG or other modalities, boxcar scars need "shouldering"[15] with a pure ablative laser to attenuate the sharp margin and convert it into a gently sloping one which is esthetically more acceptable.

Ice pick scars respond poorly to fractional lasers[18] or other methods of collagen induction but show excellent results with the chemical reconstruction of skin scars (CROSS)[19] technique using 50–100% trichloroacetic acid (TCA).[19,20] Chemical reconstruction of skin scars is a technique comprising of focal application of higher TCA concentrations by pressing hard on the entire depressed area of depressed acne scars using a sharpened wooden applicator. Ice pick scars have been reported to respond to laser "punch-out"[21] using 3–7 continuous passes of carbon dioxide laser only on the affected area.

Focal acne scar treatment (FAST),[22] a new approach to atrophic acne scars was described in 2013 in which only the

TABLE 1: Goodman and Baron acne scarring grading system[15]

Grade	Level of disease	Characteristics	Examples of scars
1	Macular disease	Erythematous, hyper- or hypopigmented flat marks visible to patient or observer irrespective of distance	Erythematous, hyper- or hypopigmented flat marks
2	Mild disease	Mild atrophy or hypertrophy that may not be obvious at social distances of 50 cm or greater and may be covered adequately by makeup or the normal shadow of shaved beard hair in males or normal body hair if extrafacial	Mild rolling, small soft papular
3	Moderate disease	Moderate atrophic or hypertrophic scarring that is obvious at social distances of 50 cm or greater and is not covered easily by makeup or the normal shadow of shaved beard hair in males or body hair if extrafacial, but is still able to be flattened by manual stretching of the skin	More significant rolling, shallow boxcar, mild-to-moderate hypertrophic or papular scars
4	Severe disease	Severe atrophic or hypertrophic scarring that is obvious at social distances of 50 cm or greater and is not covered easily by makeup or the normal shadow of shaved beard hair in males or body hair (if extrafacial) and is not able to be flattened by manual stretching of the skin	Punched out atrophic (deep boxcar), ice pick, bridges and tunnels, gross atrophy, dystrophic scars, significant hypertrophy or keloid

scarred areas were treated with fractional carbon dioxide laser, resulting in 40–70% improvement. Higher energy and density levels can be used when utilizing this technique, resulting in improved outcomes when compared with whole face fractional carbon dioxide laser resurfacing. Healing is improved and faster with this technique and no increased incidence of permanent adverse events were found. Only temporary postinflammatory hyperpigmentation was encountered in a few patients. Presumably, similar effects could be obtained with the use of Er:YAG, in pure ablative and fractionated modes for laser punch-out and FAST, respectively.

Hence, the way forward for the use of Er:YAG laser for extensive resurfacing would be in its fractional mode, judiciously combining the use of pure ablative Er:YAG for shouldering of boxcar scars, flattening of excess skin of papular scars, and laser punch-out of ice pick scars. Trichloroacetic acid CROSS is an option for laser punch-out while subcision prior to fractional resurfacing helps in optimizing the results of the latter.

ERBIUM DOPED YTTRIUM-ALUMINIUM-GARNET VERSUS CARBON DIOXIDE LASER

The two most commonly used ablative lasers for acne scars are the carbon dioxide and Er:YAG lasers. The carbon dioxide laser emits light at the 10,600 nm wavelength. It vaporizes both the epidermis and papillary dermis to 20–60 µm in depth, while the thermal necrosis zone extends another 20–50 µm.[23]

The Er:YAG laser[24] emits a 2,940 nm light and ablates 10–20 µm of tissue with each pass using a fluence of 5 J/cm^2. The Er:YAG laser's residual zone of thermal damage does not extend beyond 15 µm, in comparison with the 20–60 µm thermal damage zone that occurs with the carbon dioxide laser.[25]

Ablative lasers have previously been noted to be successful in the treatment of atrophic scars. Traditionally, the carbon dioxide ablative laser has been thought of as a more effective laser, albeit with more side effects in comparison to the erbium laser, which is a less effective laser, with less risk of side effects. Edema, oozing, crusting, and burning discomfort during the first week following treatment and prolonged erythema are common. In addition, patients may experience long-lasting pigmentary changes, scarring, and infection. These side effects are unacceptable for many patients. The Er:YAG laser is associated with milder side effects compared with the carbon dioxide laser, including transient postinflammatory hyperpigmentation,[26] acneiform eruptions,[27] and post-treatment erythema, peeling, and crusting.[28,29]

Ablative skin resurfacing with the Er:YAG laser was introduced as a gentler alternative to the carbon dioxide laser.[25] The Er:YAG laser has a shallower absorption depth, which leads to less residual thermal damage and faster healing, but the Er:YAG is less effective for dermal collagen remodeling because the laser does not affect the dermis as significantly as the carbon dioxide laser. The most effective Er:YAG lasers for the treatment of rhytides use longer pulse durations to increase the residual thermal damage depth.[25] To enhance wound healing without sacrificing efficacy, a combined approach has become popular for ablative skin resurfacing.[30]

Skin resurfacing with conventional single pass carbon dioxide or conventional multiple pass long-pulsed Er:YAG laser techniques yielded comparable postoperative healing times and complication profiles.[31]

A split side comparison of fractional carbon dioxide and Er:YAG revealed comparable outcomes of scar treatment, but fractional carbon dioxide laser was associated with greater treatment discomfort.[26] However, another study showed that compared with a fractionated Er:YAG laser, better skin smoothening was achieved by fractional carbon dioxide laser treatment.[32]

COMBINING ERBIUM DOPED YTTRIUM-ALUMINIUM-GARNET LASER RESURFACING WITH OTHER MODALITIES OF SCAR TREATMENT TO OPTIMIZE RESULTS

Treatment of acne scars can be optimized only when each of the scars is treated in an appropriate manner.[33] As discussed earlier, every individual with acne scars has different types of scars. The treatment plan should address each type of scar; hence, combining more than one modality is required.

Subcision, also called as subcutaneous incisionless surgery, a term coined by Orentreich and Orentreich in 1995[34] to describe the minor surgical procedure for treating depressed scars and wrinkles using a tri-beveled hypodermic needle inserted through a puncture in the skin surface (hence, “incisionless” surgery), and its sharp edges maneuvered under the defect to make subcuticular cuts or -cisions. The principle of this procedure is to break the fibrotic strands, which tether the scar to the underlying subcutaneous tissue. The sunken skin is lifted

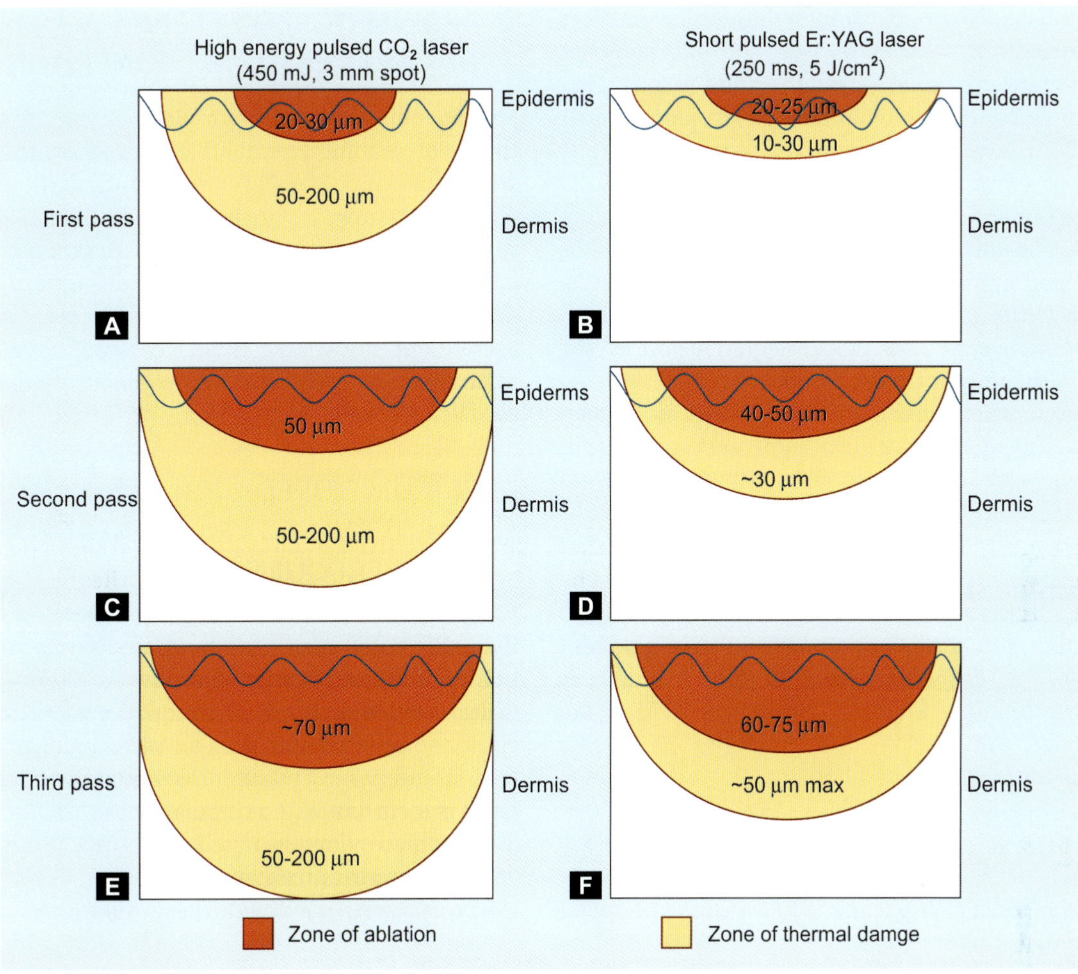

CO_2, carbon dioxide; Er:YAG, erbium doped yttrium-aluminium-garnet.

FIG. 3: Depth of ablation and thermal injury produced by the high energy pulsed carbon dioxide and the short-pulsed erbium doped yttrium-aluminium-garnet laser

by the releasing action of the procedure, as well as from connective tissue that forms during the course of normal wound healing.

Number 18 or 20 G needle or a Nokor needle (1.5 inch, 18 G is inserted adjacent to the scar with the bevel upwards parallel to the skin surface, into the deep dermis and moved back and forth in a fan-like motion under the scar to release fibrous bands at dermal or deep dermal subcutaneous plane. A snapping sound is heard as the fibrous bands are broken. "Stabbing" motion and to and fro movement in a linear fashion helps in cutting the stubborn bands makes the process of "fanning" easier (author's experience). The needle is removed and squeezed circumferentially around exit point to evacuate excess blood and prevent large hematoma formation. A small hematoma is allowed to be formed, which supports the released scar. Bleeding and nodule formation are the main side effects. Nodule formation can be improved with low dose intralesional steroid injections, but often resolves without treatment in 2–3 months. Ideally, subcision should be performed before any other acne scar treatment. One session would suffice if all or most scars are treated in that session, using adequate anesthesia. Other treatments may be initiated once the hematoma resolves completely, after 10–30 days.

Punch Excision, Punch Elevation, and Punch Grafting Techniques

Punch excision is mainly indicated for ice pick or boxcar scars. According to diameter, depth, and shape of scar, a biopsy punch of appropriate size is used to excise the scar and, then, closure or elevation or grafting is possible options to perform. Scar is excised and sutured after undermining, in a parallel direction to the relaxed skin tension lines. The goal is to trade a larger, deeper scar for a smaller, linear closure that will hopefully be less noticeable.

If the depressed scar has a normal surface texture, it is incised up to the subcutaneous tissue and its base is elevated and, then, sutured to the level of the surrounding skin. Scar is excised and replaced with an autologous, full thickness punch graft. The postauricular region or the buttocks are the most used donor sites.

Scars larger than 4 mm have to be excised in a staged manner. It is ideal to perform these procedures prior to laser resurfacing,[35] so that the smaller scars that ensue are further improved by the laser treatment.

Tissue Augmenting Agents

Augmentation is a further alternative for management of acne scarring, especially when the time available is short, e.g., prior to a wedding. Hyaluronic acid is the recommended one. Results are temporary as it gets degraded within 6–12 months.[36]

Platelet Rich Plasma

Autologous platelet rich plasma (PRP) has been applied after fractional Er:YAG resurfacing and was found to be effective and safe; it enhanced the recovery of laser damaged skin.[37] Combining PRP with fractional carbon dioxide laser led to enhanced improvement, more safety, and lesser downtime.[38]

Table 2 enumerates the various modes of treatment needed for different types of acne scars.

TABLE 2: Various modes of treatment needed for different types of acne scars

Type of scar	Modality of treatment
Rolling scars	Subcision + fractional laser resurfacing/ bipolar microneedling radiofrequency
Boxcar scars	Subcision, punch elevation/excision/ grafting, "shouldering", laser resurfacing/ bipolar microneedling radiofrequency
Ice pick scars	TCA CROSS, laser "punch-out", bipolar microneedling radiofrequency
Hypertrophic or keloidal scars	Intralesional triamcinolone with or without 5-fluorouracil

TCA, trichloroacetic acid; CROSS, chemical reconstruction of skin scars.

ERBIUM DOPED YTTRIUM-ALUMINIUM-GARNET VERSUS MICRONEEDLING

Microneedling with dermaroller is a simple and cheap means of treatment modality for acne scars remodulation with little downtime. It is also known as the poor man's "fractional laser". An improvement of 50–75% was reported in a majority of patients with skin types IV and V after five sittings of dermaroller under topical anesthesia at monthly intervals.[39] Pain during the procedure is a frequent drawback. Head to head comparisons of microneedling with fractional lasers do not exist, but it is believed to be inferior to them.

ERBIUM DOPED YTTRIUM-ALUMINIUM-GARNET VERSUS MICRONEEDLING RADIOFREQUENCY

Fractional radiofrequency uses an array of electrodes that allows for zones of thermal wounds to be made between areas of unaffected zones, thus stimulating dermal remodeling and allowing for a supply of reservoir cells to promote healing.[40] Variations of fractional radiofrequency exist that employ microneedles to deliver electrical current to a particular depth within the dermis that decreases damage to the epidermis. Improvement in cosmetic appearance in between 25 and 75% of affected skin can be expected with these treatments. It takes an average of three to four treatment sessions with 1–2 passes and 3 months post-treatment for these results to be fully appreciated.

This is most likely due to the required time for adequate activation of fibroblasts and the upregulation of the collagen production needed to replace the dermal matrix. Side effects that can be expected from radiofrequency treatments include transient pain, erythema, and scabbing that resolve within 3–5 days; albeit, the pain is significantly less with radiofrequency compared to fractional laser treatment. Fine lines and wrinkles, brightness, tightness, acne scar texture, pigmentation, and pore size were all improved significantly.[40]

Patients with ice pick type of scars reported the maximum improvement, while those with predominant box type scars had poor improvement. Rolling type scars had variable results with patients reporting both excellent to poor response to therapy. Performing subcision prior to radiofrequency in box type scars resulted in better improvement.[41] Microneedling fractional radiofrequency was found to be efficacious for the treatment of moderate and severe acne scars in south Indian patients with type

IV and V Fitzpatrick's phototypes, with 80% showing improvement by two grades and 20% improvement by one grade in the Goodman-Baron qualitative assessment. About 58% of the patients had moderate, 29% had minimal, 9% had good, and 3% showed very good improvement. Adverse effects were limited to transient pain, erythema, edema, and hyperpigmentation.[42] Fractional bipolar radiofrequency and fractional erbium doped glass have similar effectiveness for the treatment of atrophic acne scars, but the former had a higher safety profile.[43]

Comparison of a fractional microplasma radiofrequency technology and carbon dioxide fractional laser for the treatment of atrophic acne scars in a randomized split-face clinical study revealed that both modalities have good effects on treating atrophic scars.[44] Postinflammatory hyperpigmentation was encountered in 30.3% of treatment sessions using fractional carbon dioxide but was not seen with the fractional microplasma radiofrequency, which might make it a better choice for patients with darker skin.

ADVERSE EVENTS

Most common side effect seen after 100 sittings (25 patients × 4 sittings each) of Er:YAG 2,940 nm fractional laser resurfacing was exacerbation of acne lesions (13%) which was treated with oral antibiotics.[12] Post-treatment pigmentation was seen only in 2% and was effectively treated with demelanizing creams. Prolonged crusting (more than 7 days) was seen after 3% of the sittings. None of the patients had prolonged erythema (more than 4 days) after undergoing treatment sessions. The mean erythema duration was less than 2 days and mean crusting was around 5 days in all sittings (Table 3).

TABLE 3: Robert's hyperpigmentation (H) scale[45] (Measures propensity for pigmentation)[46]

Type H0	Hypo-pigmentation
Type HI	Minimal and transient (<1 year) hyperpigmentation
Type HII	Minimal and permanent (>1 year) hyperpigmentation
Type HIII	Moderate and transient (<1 year) hyperpigmentation
Type HIV	Moderate and permanent (>1 year) hyperpigmentation
Type HV	Severe and transient (<1 year) hyperpigmentation
Type HVI	Severe and permanent (>1 year) hyperpigmentation

USING ERBIUM DOPED YTTRIUM-ALUMINIUM-GARNET LASER CONCOMITANTLY WITH ORAL ISOTRETINOIN TREATMENT

Unlike earlier days, it is now proven that acne scar treatments using varied modalities can be done while the patient is concomitantly taking isotretinoin. Studies proving the safety of this approach on Asian skin have been published.[47,48]

Treatment Protocol for the Use of Erbium Doped Yttrium-aluminium-garnet Laser for Acne Scars on Colored Skin

Fractionated Er:YAG is a safe and effective modality of treatment for acne scars in coloured individuals[1], provided prudent clinical judgment is used. Pure ablative Er:YAG is used for shouldering[15] the edges of boxcar scars and flattening papular scars.

Client Selection

Patients with atrophic acne scars with sound mental health are ideal candidates for fractional Er:YAG treatment. Those with body dysmorphic disorder[45] and picking tendency should not be treated. Those with predominant ice pick scars should be first treated with TCA CROSS[19] as fractionated Er:YAG alone would not yield satisfactory results.

Contraindications[12] are mentioned below:

1. Active infection at the site of treatment
2. Active keloidal tendency
3. Active vitiligo, psoriasis, or other disorders which may koebnerize
4. Pregnancy
5. Impaired immune system.

Concomitant use of oral isotretinoin is no longer considered a contraindication, as elaborated later in this chapter. Caution should be exercised while treating those with diabetes mellitus and autoimmune diathesis, especially those associated with photosensitivity.

Prerequisites

Assessment of the skin type (Fitzpatrick's phototype, predilection to hyperpigmentation as described by Roberts[46] and scarring tendency should be done while formulating the treatment plan and determining the fluence and the density of microthermal treatment zones.

Those with poor Robert's skin types whose post-inflammatory hyperpigmentation (PIH) tends to persist should be treated with lower fluences and lower treatment densities.

Priming with a topical retinoid for at least two weeks followed by a gap of 5–7 days helps in prevention of PIH. About 2–4% hydroquinone may be added to the primimg regimen for those with Robert's H2, H3, H4, and H5. It is risky to treat those with Robert's H6 skin type with this modality.

A laser patch test on the side of the neck would help from a medico-legal perspective, to give the patient an idea of what kind of downtime to expect and to identify poor Robert's skin types. It is prudent to use less fluence than that planned for the first session as this area is not primed.

Prelaser Documentation

High resolution photographs of cleansed face in frontal and profile view, with standardized distance and lighting avoiding direct flash should be taken at every session.[12]

Informed consent mentioning downtime to be expected, degree of anticipated improvement, and possibility of new scars appearing if acne recurs should be taken.

The grade of acne scars should be clearly documented. Qualitative Goodman and Baron grading of acne scars is a simple and reproducible way of documentation.

Topical anesthetic cream (eutectic mixture of local anesthetics) applied under occlusion for 60–90 minutes makes the pain of laser resurfacing tolerable in most patients.

Performing Erbium Laser Resurfacing

It is advisable to start with the use of pure ablative erbium for shouldering before using the fractionated hand-piece. Care should be taken to shoulder only the edges of the boxcar scars to prevent widening of the scars. Very extensive use of pure ablative erbium YAG should be avoided.

The number of stacks should be decided based on the depth of the scars and the manufacturers recommendation. Typically 4–6 stacks are needed for moderate to deep scars.

While using the fractionated tip, number of passes should not exceed four lest the advantage of fractionated technology be lost.

Postlaser Resurfacing Steps

Cold compress may be given and a soothing cream with sucralfate or antibiotic cream like mupirocin may be used. Use of mild steroid cream in combination with antibiotic is advocated by some but is best avoided as it increases re-epithelisation time.

Postcare consists of a gentle non-foaming cleanser, moisturizing sunscreen and emollient applied to the treated area at least 5–8 times a day. Twice a day usage of antibiotic is advocated.

Anti-herpes prophylaxis is initiated 24 hours prior to the procedure and continued for seven days, till complete re- epithelisation.

Patient is called for a review after one week and the procedure repeated after 4 weeks.

For moderate to severe scars, 4–8 sessions are recommended. The percentage of improvement expected varies from 50 to 80%.

Aligning Patients about Results to be Expected

It should be clearly explained that the effects of collagen induction become obvious only after 2–3 months and continue for up to six months after the last session. The effects of shouldering become obvious by day seven. Also obvious is the improved skin texture and lightening of skin, which is very pleasing to patients,[12] though it imay be temporary(Figs 4 and 5).

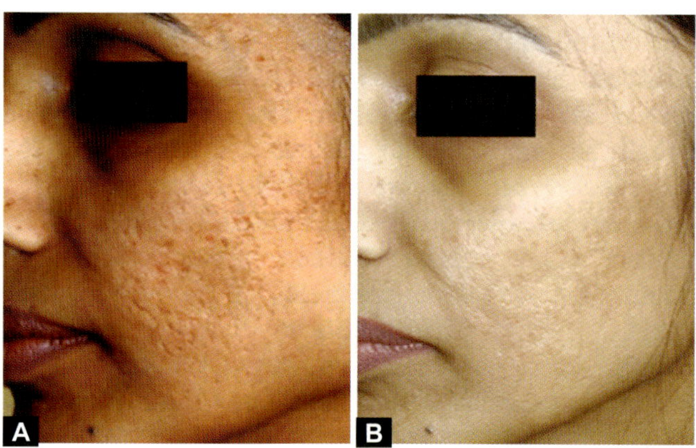

FIG. 4: Improvement in acne scars and skin color after 4 sessions of erbium laser resurfacing

Photo courtesy: Alma lasers.

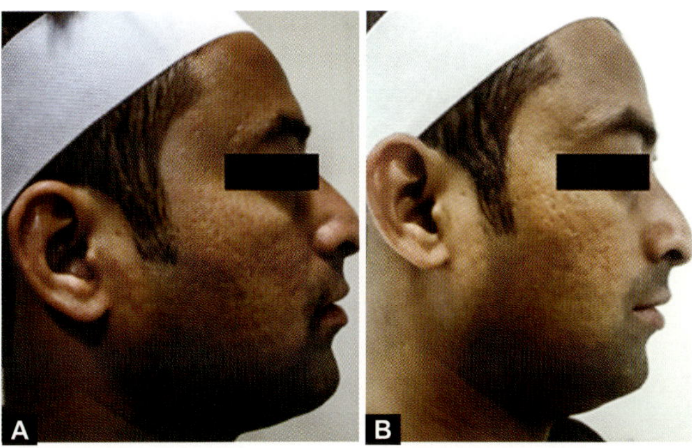

FIG. 5: Improvement in acne scars and skin color after subcision and 3 sessions of erbium laser resurfacing. Patient was on 0.4mg/kg of isotretinoin three months prior and throughout the duration of laser treatment

OPTIMIZING THE RESULTS OF ERBIUM DOPED YTTRIUM-ALUMINIUM-GARNET FOR SCAR TREATMENT

Erbium doped yttrium-aluminium-garnet resurfacing is an effective and safe modality in the treatment of acne scars. In depth knowledge of the patient's skin type, propensity to scarring and hyperpigmentation, and the morphology of scars is essential in preparing an effective treatment strategy and combining various modalities to achieve optimal results.

CONCLUSION

Erbium doped yttrium-aluminium-garnet laser resurfacing is a time tested, safe, and effective modality of treatment of acne scars. It has advantages over carbon dioxide laser in terms of less risk of PIH while treating coloured skin. Its role in future has to be watched in view of the introduction of color blind technologies with higher safety margin and minimal downtime like microneedling radiofrequency.

Treating colored skin with ablative lasers is similar to a tight rope walk. A competent laser surgeon judiciously combines selective use of pure ablative Er:YAG and fractionated Er:YAG with other modalities of acne scar treatment, such as subcision and TCA CROSS, to balance safety and efficacy.

REFERENCES

1. El-Domyati M, Abd-El-Raheem T, Abdel-Wahab H, Medhat W, Hosam W, El-Fakahany H, et al. Fractional versus ablative erbium:yttrium-aluminum-garnet laser resurfacing for facial rejuvenation: an objective evaluation. J Am Acad Dermatol. 2013;68(1):103-12.
2. Weinstein C. Modulated dual mode erbium/CO_2 lasers for the treatment of acne scars. J Cutan Laser Ther. 1999;1(4):203-8.
3. Jeong JT, Park JH, Kye TC. Resurfacing of pitted facial acne scars using Er:YAG laser with ablation and coagulation mode. Aesthetic Plast Surg. 2003;27(2):130-4.
4. Tanzi EL, Alster TS. Treatment of atrophic facial acne scars with a dual-mode Er:YAG laser. Dermatol Surg. 2002;28(7):551-5.
5. Tay YK, Kwok C. Minimally ablative erbium:YAG laser resurfacing of facial atrophic acne scars in Asian skin: a pilot study. Dermatol Surg. 2008;34(5):681-5.
6. Wanitphakdeedecha R, Manuskiatti W, Siriphukpong S, Chen TM. Treatment of punched-out atrophic and rolling acne scars in skin phototypes III, IV, and V with variable square pulse erbium:YAG laser resurfacing. Dermatol Surg. 2009;35(9):1376-83.
7. Hruza GJ, Dover JS. Laser skin resurfacing. Arch Dermatol. 1996;132(4):451-5.
8. Herne KB, Zachary CB. New facial rejuvenation techniques. Semin Cutan Med Surg. 2000;19(4):221-31.
9. Grema H, Greve B, Raulin C. Facial rhytides—subsurfacing or resurfacing? A review. Lasers Surg Med. 2003;32(5):405-12.
10. Manstein D, Herron GS, Sink RK, Tanner H, Anderson RR. Fractional photothermolysis: a new concept for cutaneous remodeling using microscopic patterns of thermal injury. Lasers Surg Med. 2004;34:426.
11. Lee SJ, Kang JM, Chung WS, Kim YK, Kim HS. Ablative non-fractional lasers for atrophic facial acne scars: a new modality of erbium:YAG laser resurfacing in Asians. Lasers Med Sci. 2014;29(2):615-9.
12. Nirmal B, Pai SB, Sripathi H, Rao R, Prabhu S, Kudur MH, et al. Efficacy and safety of erbium-doped yttrium aluminium garnet fractional resurfacing laser for treatment of facial acne scars. Indian J Dermatol Venereol Leprol. 2013;79:193-8.
13. Jacob CI, Dover JS, Kaminer MS. Acne scarring: a classification system and review of treatment options. J Am Acad Dermatol. 2001;45(1):109-17.
14. Wilson BB, Dent CH, Cooper PH. Papular acne scars. a common cutaneous finding. Arch Dermatol. 1990;126:797-800.
15. Goodman GJ, Baron JA. Postacne scarring: a qualitative global scarring grading system. Dermatol Surg. 2006;32:1458-66.
16. Goodman GJ, Baron JA. Postacne scarring: a quantitative global scarring grading system. J Cosmet Dermatol. 2006;5:48-52.
17. Dreno B, Khammari A, Orain N, Noray C, Mérial-Kieny C, Méry S, et al. ECCA grading scale: an original validated acne scar grading scale for clinical practice in dermatology. Dermatology. 2007;214: 46-51.
18. Sardana K, Manjhi M, Garg VK, Sagar V. Which type of atrophic acne scar (ice-pick, boxcar, or rolling) responds to nonablative fractional laser therapy? Dermatol Surg. 2014;40(3):288-300.
19. Lee JB, Chung WG, Kwahck H, Lee KH. Focal treatment of acne scars with trichloroacetic acid: chemical reconstruction of skin scars method. Dermatol Surg. 2002;28(11):1017-21.
20. Khunger N, Bhardwaj D, Khunger M. Evaluation of CROSS technique with 100% TCA in the management of ice pick acne scars in darker skin types. J Cosmet Dermatol. 2011;10(1):51-7.

21. Koo SH, Yoon ES, Ahn DS, Park SH. Laser punch-out for acne scars. Aesthetic Plast Surg. 2001;25(1):46-51.
22. Schweiger ES, Sundick L. Focal Acne Scar Treatment (FAST), a new approach to atrophic acne scars: a case series. J Drugs Dermatol. 2013; 12(10):1163-7.
23. Tanzi EL, Alster TS. Laser treatment of scars. Skin Therapy Lett. 2004; 9:4-7.
24. Ross EV, McKinlay JR, Sajben FP, Miller CH, Barnette DJ, Meehan KJ, et al. Use of a novel erbium laser in a Yucatan minipig: a study of residual thermal damage, ablation, and wound healing as a function of pulse duration. Lasers Surg Med. 2002;30(2):93-100.
25. Khatri KA, Ross V, Grevelink JM, Magro CM, Anderson RR. Comparison of erbium:YAG and carbon dioxide lasers in resurfacing of facial rhytides. Arch Dermatol. 1999; 135(4): 391-7.
26. Manuskiatti W, Lamphonrat T, Wanitphakdeedecha R, Eimpunth S. Comparison of fractional erbium-doped yttrium aluminium garnet and carbon dioxide lasers in resurfacing of atrophic acne scars in Asians. Dermatol Surg. 2013; 39(1 Pt 1): 111-20.
27. Tanzi EL, Alster TS. Treatment of atrophic facial acne scars with a dual-mode Er:YAG laser. Dermatol Surg. 2002; 28(7);551-5.
28. Wanitphakdeedecha R, Manuskiatti W, Siriphukpong S, Chen TM. Treatment of punched-out atrophic and rolling acne scars in skin phototypes III, IV, and V with variable square pulse erbium:YAG laser resurfacing. Dermatol Surg. 2009;35(9):1376-83.
29. Tay YK, Kwok C. Minimally ablative erbium:YAG laser resurfacing of facial atrophic acne scars in Asian skin: a pilot study. Dermatol Surg. 2008; 34(5): 681-5.
30. Millman AL, Mannor GE. Combined erbium:YAG and carbon dioxide laser skin resurfacing. Arch Facial Plast Surg. 1999; 1(2): 112-6.
31. Tanzi EL, Alster TS. Single-pass carbon dioxide versus multiple-pass Er:YAG laser skin resurfacing: a comparison of postoperative wound healing and side-effect rates. Dermatol Surg. 2003; 29(1):80-4.
32. Reinholz M, Schwaiger H, Heppt MV, Poetschke J, Tietze J, Epple A, et al. Comparison of two kinds of lasers in the treatment of acne scars. Facial Plast Surg. 2015; 31(5): 523-31.
33. Goodman G. Post acne scarring: a review. J Cosmet Laser Ther. 2003; 5: 77-95.
34. Orentreich DS, Orentreich N. Subcutaneous incisionless (subcision) surgery for the correction of depressed scars and wrinkles. Dermatol Surg. 1995;21:543-9.
35. Grevelink JM, White VR. Concurrent use of laser skin resurfacing and punch excision in the treatment of facial acne scarring. Dermatol Surg. 1998; 24: 527-30.
36. Cooper JS, Lee BT. Treatment of facial scarring: lasers, filler, and nonoperative techniques. Facial Plast Surg. 2009; 25: 311-5.
37. Zhu JT, Xuan M, Zhang YN, Liu HW, Cai JH, Wu YH, et al. The efficacy of autologous platelet-rich plasma combined with erbium fractional laser therapy for facial acne scars or acne. Mol Med Rep. 2013;8(1): 233-7.
38. Gawdat HI, Hegazy RA, Fawzy MM, Fathy M. Autologous platelet rich plasma: topical versus intradermal after fractional ablative carbon dioxide laser treatment of atrophic acne scars. Dermatol Surg. 2014; 40(2):152-61.
39. Dogra S, Yadav S, Sarangal R. Microneedling for acne scars in Asian skin type: an effective low cost treatment modality. J Cosmet Dermatol. 2014; 13(3): 180-7.
40. Gold MH, Biron JA. Treatment of acne scars by fractional bipolar radiofrequency energy. J Cosmet Laser Ther. 2012; 14(4): 172-8.
41. Ramesh M, Gopal M, Kumar S, Talwar A. Novel technology in treatment of acne scars: the matrix tunable radiofrequency technology. J Cutan Aesthet Surg. 2010; 214:46-51.
42. Chandrashekar BS, Sriram R, Mysore R, Bhaskar S, Shetty A. Evaluation of microneedling fractional radiofrequency device for treatment of acne scars. J Cutan Aesthet Surg. 2014; 7: 93-7.
43. Rongsaard N, Rummaneethorn P. Comparison of a fractional bipolar radiofrequency device and a fractional erbium-doped glass 1,550-nm device for the treatment of atrophic acne scars: a randomized split-face clinical study. Dermatol Surg. 2014; 40(1): 14-21.
44. Zhang Z, Fei Y, Chen X, Lu W, Chen J. Comparison of a fractional microplasma radio frequency technology and carbon dioxide fractional laser for the treatment of atrophic acne scars: a randomized split-face clinical study. Dermatol Surg. 2013; 39(4): 559-66.
45. Crerand CE, Franklin ME, Sarwer DB. Body dysmorphic disorder and cosmetic surgery. Plast Reconstr Surg. 2006; 118(7): 167e-80e.
46. Roberts WE. The Roberts skin type classification system. J Drugs Dermatol 2008; 7(5): 452-6.
48. Chandrashekar BS, Varsha DV, Vasanth V, Jagadish P, Madura C, Rajashekar ML. Safety of performing invasive acne scar treatment and laser hair removal in patients on oral isotretinoin: a retrospective study of 110 patients. Int J Dermatol. 2014; 53(10): 1281-5.
47. Khatri KA, Iqbal N, Bhawan J. Laser skin resurfacing during isotretinoin therapy. Dermatol Surg. 2015; 41(6): 758-9.

CHAPTER 28

Evidence Based Approach to Laser Scar Reduction

Vijay P Zawar, Madhuri H Agarwal

INTRODUCTION

The definition of scar is a mark left on the skin or body tissue after a burn, injury, or wound which does not heal completely and there is development of fibrous connective tissue.

Cutaneous scars can be manifested due to various reasons such as acne, accidental or trauma injuries, surgical procedures, etc. These scars have an immense psychological, physical, and cosmetic impact on the person's quality of life. Cutaneous scars can lead to negative perception of body image, social stigmata, and disconnect from peers and dissatisfaction in all aspects of life.

There have been various treatments performed over the last few decades for minimizing or reducing the scars. Treatments range from surgical excision, topical lightening agents containing retinoid and hydrocortisone, chemical peels, dermabrasion, injectable soft tissue filler, and autologous fat transfer. All these treatments have been employed in different kinds of scars with varying degree of results and successes. The adverse effects and downtime associated with the above procedures had created the requirement of treatment devices which are completely noninvasive or minimally invasive, superior efficacy in couple of sessions, and zero-to-negligible adverse effects.

In the last decade, lasers have gained popularity at a rapid acceleration for treatment of scars. There is a plethora of laser devices that fit the above criteria and have changed the face of scar treatments.

We will discuss and review the different types of scars with their practical aspects and treatment recommendations in our chapter.

TYPES OF SCARS

Cutaneous scars can be of various types due to different etiology.

- Hypertrophic scars
- Keloids
- Atrophic scars
- Acne scars
- Prescars.

Hypertrophic Scars

Hypertrophic scars are red or pink, firm, nodular raised scars due to increased proliferation of collagen. The common sites of hypertrophic scars are areas that have a slow or low wound healing time and areas of friction or movement. The scars typically start developing within a month of injury and then resolve subsequently over time. They generally do not exceed the margins of original wound. Hypertrophic scars are formed at the time of wound healing due to excessive collagen synthesis along with reduced collagen lysis in the matrix remodeling phase.[1-6] Histologically, they contain collagen type III parallel to the epidermis containing abundant fibroblasts and large extracellular collagen filaments. There are two types of hypertrophic scars: (1) linear and (2) widespread hypertrophic scars. Linear hypertrophic scars are red, elevated scars limited to the boundary of the original wound and commonly seen in surgical incision. They usually mature to have a raised, increased girth with rope-like appearance. Widespread hypertrophic scars are seen after burns and are red, raised, and occasionally, itchy scars.[6]

Keloids

Keloids are firm, pink to purple colored, nodular scars that are well demarcated and irregular in outline. They develop spontaneously for up to years after minor injuries or at times spontaneously on the midchest, shoulders, neck, and presternum. Keloids are not self-limiting, persist for many years, and extend beyond the margins of the original wound. They exhibit more pain and itching as compared to hypertrophic scars. There is generally a history of genetic predisposition in keloids and it is more common in darker skin type individuals. Keloid can be stimulated by hormonal changes such as puberty and pregnancy. Histologically, keloids comprise of haphazardly arranged collagen type I and III with excessive fibroblasts.[1-5,7] There are two types of keloids: (1) minor and (2) major keloids. Minor keloids are itchy, elevated scars that form up to 1 year after injury and do not resolve with time.[6] Major keloids are large, raised scars which extend beyond the original wound. They persistently extend over long period of time.[6]

Atrophic Scars

In inflammatory skin disorders, such as varicella or cystic acne or post-trauma and surgery, the collagen destruction caused by the disease process leads to dermal depression and atrophy. The resulting scars are called atrophic scars. Initially, the atrophic scars are red but with time settle down to fibrotic, hypopigmented scars.[1-5]

Acne Scars

Acne vulgaris is a common skin concern seen in ages of 11–30 years and it is prevalent in in 80% of the population. The active acne generally results in fulminant scars of different variety that have severe psychological and social negative impact. The treatment of these acne scars are often challenging for both patients and physicians.

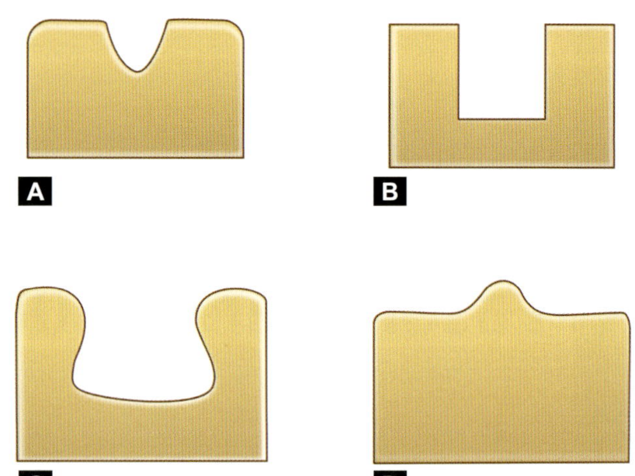

FIG. 1: Illustrations of different types of acne scars. **A,** Ice pick scar; **B,** box scar; **C,** rolling scar; **D,** hypertrophic scar

Courtesy: Sketches drawn by Himanish M Agarwal.

The classification of acne scars is macular, ice pick, rolling, and box scar (Fig. 1).[8-10] Macular scars result from early inflammatory acne. The macular scars can be erythematous, hyper- or hypopigmented flat scars. Hyperpigmented scars are commonly seen in dark skinned individuals.[9,10] Ice pick scars or pitted scars are circular, deep pit-like scars that extend deep into the subcutaneous tissues and are very narrow. Rolling scars are broader than ice pick scars. They are distensible scars that have shallow depression with sloping edges. The rolling scars are caused by dermal tethering to underlying subcuticular tissues.[5] Box scars are punched out scars that have a wide surface and base. The box scars can extend from mid-dermis to reticular dermis.[9,10] The acne scars are of different variety and physical characteristics and hence, require customized treatments.

HISTORY OF LASERS IN SCAR REVISION

The treatment of scars started with use of pressure for keloids in 1835 and slowly gained popularity till 1970.[3] The treatment of scars has involved various techniques such as surgical excision and grafting, pressure therapy, intralesional steroids, topical retinoids, and cryosurgery. Most of these procedures have poor outcomes and undesirable adverse effects such as worsening of scars, atrophy, and pain. The recurrence of scars post these treatments is also faster.[1] In the past three decades, laser surgery has evolved and developed as minimally invasive and successful treatment option for scars. Anderson and Parrish's theory of selective photothermolysis is the backbone of laser treatment and has revolutionized the use of lasers in dermatology.[11] Their theory is founded on the principle of thermal relaxation time and based on it, lasers were developed to generate light pulses of the duration that corresponds to the thermal relaxation time of the target tissue. This theory of selective photothermolysis has led to the productions of lasers which are highly efficacious and safe.[12] The theory by Anderson and Parrish paved the way for invention of pulsed lasers which were highly selective and target-specific. Continuous wave argon, neodymium doped yttrium-aluminium-garnet (Nd:YAG), 1,064 nm and carbon dioxide (CO_2) lasers were the initial lasers used in the treatment of keloids and hypertrophic scars.[2,13] In the early 1990s, the widely used laser for vascular lesions such as port wine stains and telangiectasias was the 585 nm pulsed dye laser (PDL). In 1994, Alster reported the use of PDL lasers in erythematous and hypertrophic scars. Alster observed 57–83% clinical and textural improvement in these scars after one to two sessions of PDL lasers.[14] Dierickx et al. reported similar results of scar improvement by 77% after 1.8 PDL laser treatments.[15] A combination of lasers such as CO_2 and PDL lasers were also been studied for the nonerythematous, minimally hypertrophic scars. In 1998, Alster et al. utilized CO_2 laser followed by PDL laser for treatment of scars.[16] In 1990s, Kaufmann and his colleagues researched and demonstrated the potential of the erbium doped yttrium-aluminium-garnet (Er:YAG) laser as it had tremendous decrease in the residual thermal dermal damage.[12,17,18] The reduced postprocedure erythema and rapid healing time were strong evidence for the efficacy and safety of the Er:YAG laser. However, a section of laser surgeons were of the opinion that CO_2 laser was more efficacious than Er:YAG.[18] The concern with CO_2 lasers, was the high adverse effect profile of hyperpigmentation and hypopigmentation especially in a darker skin type and worsening of the scars.[5]

In the past decade, fractional photothermolysis is the newest technology in the cutaneous laser surgery portfolio. The principle of fractional photothermolysis is to thermally ablate fractions of skin, leaving untouched the intervening areas of skin. These intact areas quickly repopulate the ablated areas of skin tissue.[19] The fractional resurfacing lasers have lesser side effects and faster healing time as compared to the conventional ablative lasers. The fractional technology is of two types: (1) nonablative and (2) ablative fractional lasers. The ablative fractional technology has been reported to show successful outcomes in moderate-to-severe scars and photoaging.[5]

LASER TREATMENT OF HYPERTROPHIC AND KELOID SCARS

In the past few years, multiple lasers have been researched for the treatment of hypertrophic and keloid scars. The common ones are PDL, CO_2, Er:YAG, and fractional lasers. Pulsed dye laser laser with spectrum of 585–595 nm is the most preferred laser used in comparison to other lasers. In 1994, Alster et al. studied and presented evidence of the effective parameters in hypertrophic scars and keloids with PDL 585 nm.[14] The recommended protocols for PDL lasers in these scars are to start with low energy densities and gradually increase the energy levels only when the previous readings deliver inadequate results. The entire scar area must be treated with nonoverlapping laser shots. The PDL parameters used for these scars range from 6.0 to 7.5 J/cm^2 with a spot size of 5 or 7 mm and 4.5–5.5 J/cm^2 with a spot size of 10 mm.[12,14,20] The energy densities must be decreased by 10% in cases of patients with darker skin type or patients with scars in thin skinned areas such as anterior chest.[4,20-22] The sessions are generally done at an interval of 6–8 week but it is advisable to increase the time interval in darker skin types and patients with scars in sensitive areas. In cases of poor scar response to PDL treatment, a concomitant use of intralesional corticosteroids or 5-fluorouracil has demonstrated a superior result.[23,24] Postprocedure purpura is the most common side effect seen with the PDL and it is persistent for several days to a week.

The other lasers used with some degree of success in hypertrophic scars and keloids is ablative CO_2 and Er:YAG lasers. Early intervention with these lasers in form of resurfacing wound edges prior to suturing or immediately after surgery decreases the intensity of scars.[19] In cases where the ablative resurfacing is done within 6–10 weeks after trauma or surgery, the scars show a drastic healing and response rate. The common adverse effects with ablative resurfacing lasers are erythema that lasts for 1–4 months after laser sessions, acneiform eruptions, and dyspigmentation. Dyspigmentation is usually encountered in darker skin types (Fitzpatrick skin type III–VI).[19]

Since last decade, the nonablative fractional lasers have shown considerable promise in the treatment of scars. These lasers have shown successful outcomes in the treatment of hypertrophic, hypopigmented, and atrophic scars by delivering dramatic improvement in the thickness and pigmentation of surgical scars.[25] Tierney et al. conducted a comparative study of PDL and nonablative fractional laser for the treatment of surgical scars to study the improvement in scar thickness, texture, pigmentation, and overall cosmetic results.[25] The study showed that 83.3% patients found the half area of scar treated with the nonablative fractional laser showed better results. The pain sensation was higher with the nonablative laser as compared to the PDL, hence, it is advisable to perform the nonablative lasers under the cover of topical anesthetic.[25] Niwa et al. so studied the safety and efficacy of nonablative fractional 1,550 nm erbium doped fiber laser in eight patients of hypertrophic scars.[13] Niwa reported a mean improvement ranging from 26 to 75% at the end of 4 weeks after last treatment. Transient edema and erythema were the only side effects seen in this study.[13] Thus, nonablative fractional laser has emerged as a safe and effective treatment option for hypertrophic scars with minimal adverse effects and negligible downtime.

LASER TREATMENT FOR ATROPHIC SCARS

The objective of atrophic scar treatment with lasers is to trigger the neocollagenesis in the depressed scar and improve the texture of scar, so, it blends with the normal skin. Atrophic scars have been treated with dermabrasion and soft tissue fillers for many years; however, the limitation of these treatments is the short longevity of efficacy, side effects, and operator-dependent results. Carbon dioxide and Er:YAG lasers have been preferred in the correction of atrophic scars over the last few years. This is due to the fact that these lasers show reproducible results, are not totally operator-dependent and have longer-lasting efficacy.[2,5,20] The protocol followed is to ablate the entire epidermis in the vicinity of the scar in a single session instead of just treating the solitary scar. This will induce a larger neocollagenesis stimulation and overall collagen tightening of the surface area, thus yielding superior results in the atrophic scars. In CO_2 laser, a single pass at 250–350 mJ and 60 watts is sufficient to achieve a good ablation of epidermis. Erbium doped yttrium-aluminium-garnet laser requires several passes at 5–15 J/cm^2 with a 5 mm spot size for similar results.[2,20] The process of reepithelialization takes about 7–10 days in CO_2 laser and 4–7 days in Er:YAG laser so it is essential to counsel the patients on the downtime before starting the procedure. The treated skin appears erythematous and edematous immediately post the laser procedure and there is usually worsening of the skin 24–48 hours after procedure. The other adverse effect is transient hyperpigmentation, but it is more common in darker skin types.

Nonablative laser systems have been studied and employed in atrophic scars in the recent years, as the prolonged downtime and side effects of ablative CO_2 and Er:YAG laser does not make it an attractive option. The most widely used nonablative lasers are 1,450 nm diode and the 1,320 nm Nd:YAG.[26-28] The laser systems are developed to achieve stimulation of collagen production by targeting the tissue water and dermal heating without impacting the epidermis as the systems parallel deliver epidermal surface cooling.[29] The recommended protocol is three to five treatments consecutively on a monthly basis and the desired clinical results are achieved after 3–6 months of the last laser session. The results are long-lasting and around 40–45% results are achieved in the atrophic scars with these laser systems.[4] The quantum of clinical results are significantly less than ablative systems. However, the negligible side effect profile of postinflammatory hyperpigmentation makes it a preferred option for atrophic scars especially in the darker skin types.

In recent times, the fractional ablative and nonablative systems are popularly utilized in the treatment of scars. Fractional technology is shown to yield better efficacy in atrophic and pigmented scars as opposed to hypertrophic scars and keloids.[30] There is an overall improvement in the scar color, texture, and quality of atrophic scars after multiple sessions with fractional lasers.[30] Behroozan et al. used 1,550 nm Fraxel SR on chin surgical scar and in a single treatment reported 75% improvement.[31] In a study by Glaich et al., drastic improvement was reported in atrophic scars after 3 months of completion of five sessions of fractional laser.[32] The side effects noted with fractional laser systems are minimal and transient in form of edema and erythema. The side effects have higher incidence in case aggressive doses or higher stackings are delivered to achieve results.[30,33] Fractional lasers have great promise for the treatment of atrophic scars.

LASER TREATMENT OF ACNE SCARS

Despite various treatment modalities available for acne scars, laser resurfacing has yielded the best results in post-acne scarring. Carbon dioxide lasers are effective in treating mild-to-moderate acne scars. Both CO_2 and Er:YAG are considered the gold standard for treating acne scars and shown clinical efficacy ranging from 25 to 90% depending on the scar age, depth, texture, and patient skin type.[34] There have also been some studies conducted for comparison of CO_2 and Er:YAG laser efficacy. These studies have revealed that while CO_2 is more clinically efficacious than Er:YAG, due to the lesser downtime Er:YAG is better tolerated than CO_2.[19]

Nonablative lasers such as 585 nm PDL, 1,064 and 1,320 nm Nd:YAG, and 1,450 nm diode lasers have delivered dramatic improvements in post-acne scarring by inducing neocollagenesis and scar remodeling while preserving the epidermal surface.[34] The advantages of these lasers are low side effect profile and negligible downtime. Tanzi et al. conducted a comparative study between 1,320 nm Nd:YAG and 1,450 nm diode laser. The study showed both lasers delivered an improvement in the range of 25–50% at the end of 6 months. The study also noted that by stacking three passes of 1,450 nm Nd:YAG, the acne scar results were on par with the 1,450 nm diode laser resurfacing.[26] Another laser which can be utilized in acne scars is PDL. Pulsed dye lasers lasers are effective in hypertrophic and hyperpigmented acne scars and result in improvement of scar color and texture.[19]

There have been number of studies on fractional lasers as it is safe and effective modality for treatment of acne scarring. The fractional lasers yield excellent results in superficial to medium depth scars.[30,35-44] A study was done by Chapas et al. with ablative fractionated CO_2 laser in moderate-to-severe acne scarring. They noted 26–50% improvement in atrophy and texture and overall improvement of acne scars with the fractional CO_2 laser.[43] Nonablative fractional lasers have also delivered clinical efficacy in post-acne scarring. Alster et al. conducted a study with 1,550 nm erbium doped fiber laser for atrophic acne scars. The study demonstrated 91% patients had an improvement of 25–50% after a single treatment of the laser and 51–75% improvement in 87% patients after minimum three laser sessions.[36] Nirmal and his colleagues studied the safety and efficacy of ablative fractional 2,940 nm Er:YAG laser in Indian skin. They found that 96% patients showed fair improvement. Superficial box and rolling scars had a higher degree of improvement in comparison to deep box and ice pick scars. They also noted that the patient's satisfaction on efficacy was more than the physician observations.[45] Most of the studies found that while superficial and medium depth scars respond well to the laser treatments, ice pick and deep scars have poor response.

It is recommended that in these poor to non-responsive acne scars, laser treatments must be combined with other modalities of treatment such as subcision, dermabrasion, and chemical peels for optimum clinical efficacy.[19,30]

RADIOFREQUENCY FOR SCARS

With evolving technologies, there are now unconventional and newer modalities in treatment of scars. Radiofrequency (RF) is rapidly developing as an alternative or is combined with other laser treatments in scar treatments. There are three major types of RF systems available: (1) unipolar, (2) bipolar, and (3) fractional. Unipolar or monopolar RF is the most basic RF device and delivers deeper penetration in the dermis using a single electrode and a grounding pad on the skin. The second RF is bipolar which offers more focused RF energy to the dermis and is less painful than monopolar as it utilizes lesser amounts of energy to achieve the same thermal effects as monopolar. The third type, i.e., fractional RF stimulates dermal remodeling by using a series of electrodes that creates areas of thermal wounds with intervening intact areas of normal skin.[46,47] There are also variations in the RF systems that combine microneedles with RF system. The principle in this variation is to protect the epidermis and employ the microneedles to deliver electrical current to the desired dermal depth. There are also systems which combine the nonablative lasers and RF in the same system. The thought process in this again is to lower the tissue impedance with the pretreatment of nonablative laser and thus ensure deeper penetration of the RF energy to achieve optimum clinical results with less discomfort to the patient.[48] Various studies have shown that fractional bipolar RF and microneedle fractional bipolar RF have so far superior clinical efficacy in acne scars. Approximately 25–75% clinical improvement is seen in the scars with these RF technologies. The protocol is to perform three to four RF sessions delivering one to two passes. The desirable clinical results are usually seen 3 months after the last RF session. The common adverse effects with RF treatments are transient erythema, crusting, and pain that settle down in 4–7 days.[49]

CONCLUSION

Laser technology is a convenient, easy, and efficacious tool in treating patients of different types of scars. It can be safely adopted and performed in darker skin types without the concern of long-lasting, undesirable adverse effects. Lasers can be used in all types of scars such as keloids, hypertrophic, traumatic, surgical, and acne scars. It is vital to remember pertinent points of ideal patient selection, customization of lasers according to skin color and scar characteristics, the recommended pre- and postprocedure care and focused patient counseling and result expectation setting.

REFERENCES

1. Groover IJ, Alster TS. Laser revision of scars and striae. Dermatol Ther. 2000;13:50-9.
2. Nouri K, Alster TS, Ballard CJ, Vejjabhinanta V. Laser revision of scars. [online] Available from http://emedicine.medscape.com/article/1120673-overview. [Accessed February, 2016].
3. Wolfram D, Tzankov A, Pülzl P, Piza-Katzer H. Hypertrophic scars and keloids—a review of their pathophysiology, risk factors, and therapeutic management. Dermatol Surg. 2009;35:171-81.
4. Tanzi EL, Alster TS. (2015). Laser treatment of scars. [online] Available from http://www.skintherapyletter.com/2004/9.1/2.html. [Accessed February, 2016].
5. Khatri KA, Mahoney DL, McCartney MJ. Laser scar revision: a review. J Cosmet Laser Ther. 2011;13:54-62.
6. Mustoe TA, Cooter RD, Gold MH, Hobbs FD, Ramelet AA, Shakespeare PG, et al. International clinical recommendations on scar management. Plast Reconstr Surg. 2002;110(2):560-71.
7. Gauglitz GG, Korting HC, Pavicic T, Ruzicka T, Jeschke MG. Hypertrophic scarring and keloids: pathomechanisms and current and emerging treatment strategies. Mol Med. 2011;17(1-2):113-25.
8. Jacob CI, Dover JS, Kaminer MS. Acne scarring: a classification system and review of treatment options. J Am Acad Dermatol. 2001;45(1):109-17.
9. Goodman GJ. Treatment of acne scarring. Int J Dermatol. 2011;50:1179-94.
10. Khunger N; IADVL Task Force. Standard guidelines of care for acne surgery. Indian J Dermatol Venereol Leprol. 2008;74:S28-36.
11. Anderson RR, Parrish JA. Selective photothermolysis: precise microsurgery by selective absorption of pulsed radiation. Science. 1983;220(4596):524-7.
12. Kauvar AN, Hruza GJ. Principles and Practices in Cutaneous Laser Surgery. Boca Raton, FL: Taylor and Francis Group; 2005. pp. 12-29.
13. Niwa AB, Mello AP, Torezan LA, Osorio N. Fractional photothermolysis for the treatment of hypertrophic scars: clinical experience of eight cases. Dermatol Surg. 2009;35:773-8.
14. Alster TS. Improvement of erythematous and hypertrophic scars by 585-nm flashlamp-pumped pulsed dye laser. Ann Plast Surg. 1994;32(2):186-90.
15. Dierickx C, Goldman MP, Fitzpatrick RE. Laser treatment of erythematous/hypertrophic and pigmented scars in 26 patients. Plast Reconstr Surg. 1995;95(1):84-90; discussion 91-2.
16. Alster TS, Lewis AB, Rosenbach A. Laser scar revision: comparison of CO2 laser vaporization with and without simultaneous pulsed dye laser treatment. Dermatol Surg. 1998;24(12):1299-302.
17. Kaufman R, Hibst R. Pulsed Erbium:YAG laser ablation in cutaneous surgery. Lasers Surg Med. 1996;19:324-30.
18. Khatri KA, Ross V, Grevelink JP, Magro CM, Anderson RR. Comparison of erbium:YAG and carbon dioxide lasers in resurfacing of facial rhytides. Arch Dermatol. 1999;135:391-7.
19. Alexiades-Armenakas MR, Dover JS, Arndt KA. The spectrum of laser skin resurfacing: nonablative fractional, and ablative laser resurfacing. J Am Acad Dermatol. 2008;58(5):719-37.
20. Alster TS, Zaulyanov L. Laser scar revision: a review. Dermatol Surg. 2007;33:131-40.
21. Alster TS. Laser treatment of scars and striae. In: Alster TS (Ed). Manual of Cutaneous Laser Techniques. Philadelphia: Lippincott-Raven; 2000. pp. 89-107.
22. Macedo O, Alster TS. Laser treatment of darker skin tones: a practical approach. Dermatol Ther. 2000;13:114-26.
23. Alster TS. Laser scar revision: comparison study of 585-nm pulsed dye laser with and without intralesional corticosteroids. Dermatol Surg. 2003;29:25-9.
24. Manuskiatti W, Fitzpatrick RE. Treatment response of keloidal and hypertrophic sternotomy scars: comparison among intralesional corticosteroid, 5-fluorouracil, and 585-nm flashlamp-pumped pulsed-dye laser treatments. Arch Dermatol. 2002;138:1149-55.
25. Tierney E, Mahmoud BH, Srivastava D, Ozog D, Kouba DJ. Treatment of surgical scars with nonablative fractional laser versus pulsed dye laser: a randomized controlled trial. Dermatol Surg. 2009;35:1172-80.
26. Tanzi EL, Alster TS. Comparison of a 1450-nm diode laser and a 1320-nm Nd:YAG laser in the treatment of atrophic facial scars: a prospective clinical and histologic study. Dermatol Surg. 2004;30:152-7.
27. Rogachefsky AS, Hussain M, Goldberg DJ. Atrophic and a mixed pattern of acne scars improved with a 1320-nm Nd:YAG laser. Dermatol Surg. 2003;29:904-8.
28. Friedman PM, Jih MH, Skover GR, Payonk GS, Kimyai-Asadi A, Geronemus RG. Treatment of atrophic facial acne scars with the 1064-nm Q-switched Nd:YAG laser: six-month follow-up study.. Arch Dermatol. 2004;140:1337-41.
29. Friedman PM, Skover GR, Payonk G, Kauvar AN, Geronemus RG. 3D in-vivo optical skin imaging for topographical quantitative assessment of non-ablative laser technology. Dermatol Surg. 2002;28:199-204.
30. Goel A, Krupashankar DS, Aurangabadkar S, Nischal KC, Omprakash HM, Mysore V. Fractional lasers in dermatology—current status and recommendations. Indian J Dermatol Venereol Leprol. 2011;77:369-79.
31. Behroozan DS, Goldberg LH, Dai T, Geronemus RG, Friedman PM. Fractional photothermolysis for the treatment of surgical scars: a case report. J Cosmet Laser Ther. 2006;8:35-8.
32. Glaich AS, Goldberg LH, Friedman RH, Friedman PM. Fractional photothermolysis for the treatment of postinflammatory erythema resulting from acne vulgaris. Dermatol Surg. 2007;33:842-6.
33. Metelitsa AI, Alster TS. Fractionated laser skin resurfacing treatment complications: a review. Dermatol Surg. 2010;36:299-306.
34. Asilian A, Salimi E, Faghihi, Dehghani F, Tajmirriahi N, Hosseini SM. Comparison of Q-Switched 1064-nm Nd: YAG laser and fractional CO2 laser efficacies on improvement of atrophic facial acne scar. J Res Med Sci. 2011;16(9):1189-95.
35. Hasegawa T, Matsukura T, Mizuno Y, Suga Y, Ogawa H, Ikeda S. Clinical trial of a laser device called fractional photothermolysis system for acne scars. J Dermatol. 2006;33:623-7.
36. Alster TS, Tanzi EL, Lazarus M. The use of fractional laser photothermolysis for the treatment of atrophic scars. Dermatol Surg. 2007;33:295-9.
37. Gold MH, Heath AD, Biron JA. Clinical evaluation of the SmartSkin fractional laser for the treatment of photodamage and acne scars. J Drugs Dermatol. 2009;8:s4-8.
38. Hu S, Chen MC, Lee MC, Yang LC, Keoprasom N. Fractional resurfacing for the treatment of atrophic facial acne scars in Asian skin. Dermatol Surg. 2009;35:826-32.
39. Rahman Z, Tanner H, Jiang K. Treatment of atrophic scars with the 1550-nm erbium-fiber fractional laser. Lasers Surg Med. 2006;38:24.
40. Geronemus RG. Fractional photothermolysis: current and future applications. Lasers Surg Med. 2006;38:169-76.
41. Lee HS, Lee JH, Ahn GY, Lee DH, Shin JW, Kim DH, et al. Fractional photothermolysis for the treatment of acne scars: a report of 27 Korean patients. J Dermatolog Treat. 2008;19:45-9.
42. Ong MW, Bashir SJ. Fractional laser resurfacing for acne scars: a review. Br J Dermatol. 2012;166:1160-9.
43. Chapas AM, Brightman L, Sukal S, Hale E, Daniel D, Bernstein LJ, et al. Successful treatment of acneiform scarring with CO2 ablative fractional resurfacing. Lasers Surg Med. 2008;40:381-6.

44. Kim S. Clinical trial of a pinpoint irradiation technique with the CO2 laser for the treatment of atrophic acne scars. J Cosmet Laser Ther. 2008;10(3):177-80.
45. Nirmal B, Pai SB, Sripathi H, Rao R, Prabhu S, Kudur MH, et al. Efficacy and safety of erbium-doped yttrium-aluminium garnet fractional resurfacing laser for treatment of facial acne scars. Indian J Dermatol Venereol Leprol. 2013;79:193-8.
46. Simmons BJ, Griffith RD, Falto-Aizpurua LA, Nouri K. Use of radiofrequency in cosmetic dermatology: focus on nonablative treatment of acne scars. Clin Cosmet Investig Dermatol. 2014;7:335-9.
47. Lolis MS, Goldberg DJ. Radiofrequency in cosmetic dermatology: a review. Dermatol Surg. 2012;38(11):1765-76.
48. Hruza G, Taub AF, Collier SL, Mulholland SR. Skin rejuvenation and wrinkle reduction using a fractional radiofrequency system. J Drugs Dermatol. 2009;8(3):259-65.
49. Rongsaard N, Rummaneethorn P. Comparison of a fractional bipolar radiofrequency device and a fractional erbium-doped glass 1,550-nm device for the treatment of atrophic acne scars: a randomized split-face clinical study. Dermatol Surg. 2014;40(1):14-21.

CHAPTER 29

Excimer Lasers

Atul Taneja, Tolongkhomba Potsangbam

INTRODUCTION

Excimer lasers are ultraviolet lasers which use a combination of a noble gas (argon, krypton, or xenon), which are very inert and normally do not combine with other elements; and a reactive gas (fluorine or chlorine). With electrical stimulation and high pressure inside a discharge tube, a pseudomolecule called an excimer ("ex"cited di"mer") is created, which exists in an energized state very transiently and rapidly goes back to unbound ground state and emits usually in the ultraviolet (UV) spectrum between 157 and 351 nm.[1]

Excimers have several attractive properties of immense help in engineering and in medicine. Excimers have the property to cause "cold ablation" by breaking interatomic bonds, without heating peripheral material or causing bulk heating. They also have a very low pulse duration of around 10 nanoseconds, which again prevents bulk heating. The short wavelengths allows for less diffraction and more precision. The high repetition rate of 100 kHz allows for rapid work. All these properties allow excimers to create or work rapidly on tiny materials with no thermal damage and are indispensible for creating dense, tiny microchips for computers creating flat panel displays or for creating fine nozzles for printers. In medicine, they are useful for removing precise layers of skin or cornea (193 nm), surface modification of dental tissue (248 nm), and removal of plaques from blood vessels (308 nm).[2-4] The xenon chloride laser at 308 nm is used in dermatology but its mechanism of action is probably different as discussed below.

BACKGROUND

The 308 nm excimer laser has a wavelength which is very close to the wavelength of narrow-band ultraviolet B (NB-UVB) light at 311 nm (Fig. 1). In a landmark experiment in 1981 at Massachusetts General Hospital, Harvard Medical School, Parrish had determined that out of the several wavelengths from 254–313 nm, a very "narrow" band from 311–318 nm was most effective in flattening lesions of psoriasis.[5] Since then, many studies have established NB-UVB phototherapy as useful in the treatment of a variety of skin conditions like psoriasis, vitiligo, alopecia areata, atopic dermatitis, cutaneous lymphomas, and lichen planus.[6] It was presumed that the 308 nm excimer laser would work in a similar fashion to the 311 nm NB-UVB phototherapy and a series of experiments were conducted in the same and other institutes to assess its activity in a variety of skin disorders. The obvious advantage of a laser over conventional phototherapy is to allow higher doses of UV light to be delivered only to affected areas, while leaving unaffected normal skin unexposed to radiation. This results in faster clearing of lesions at a much lower cumulative dose. Lamps emitting noncoherent light at 308 nm, monochromatic excimer light (MEL) have recently been introduced to be used for the same indications as the 308 nm excimer laser (Fig. 2).[7]

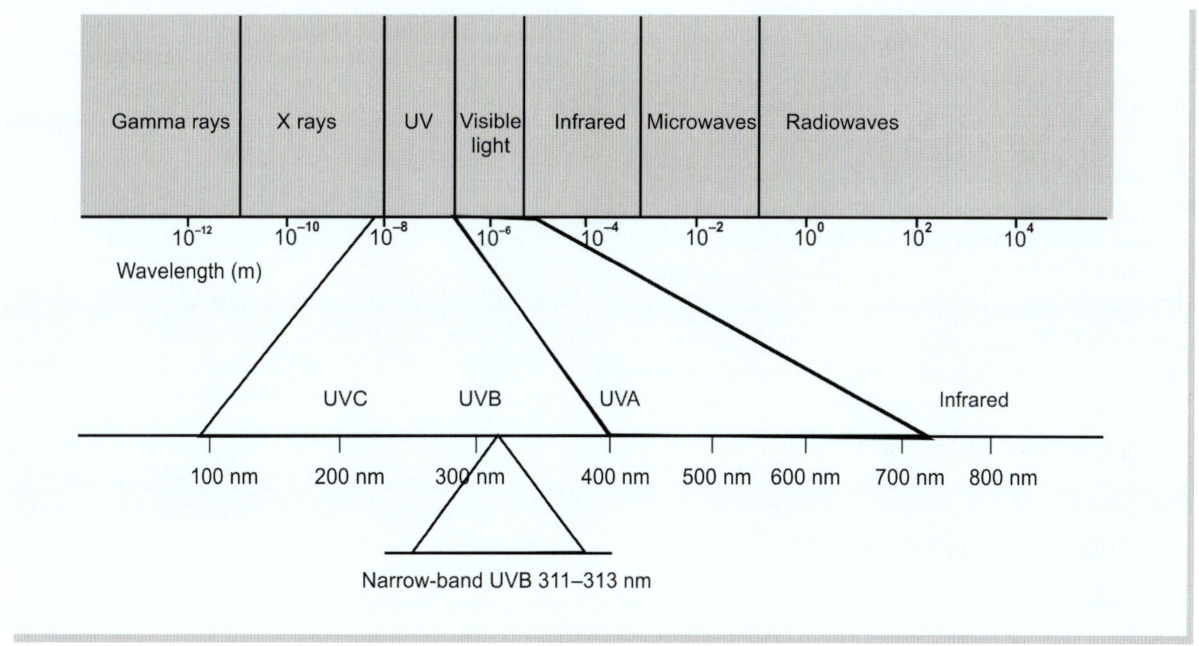

UV, ultraviolet.

FIG. 1: Electromagnetic spectrum showing excimer laser 308 nm—super narrow-band ultraviolet B

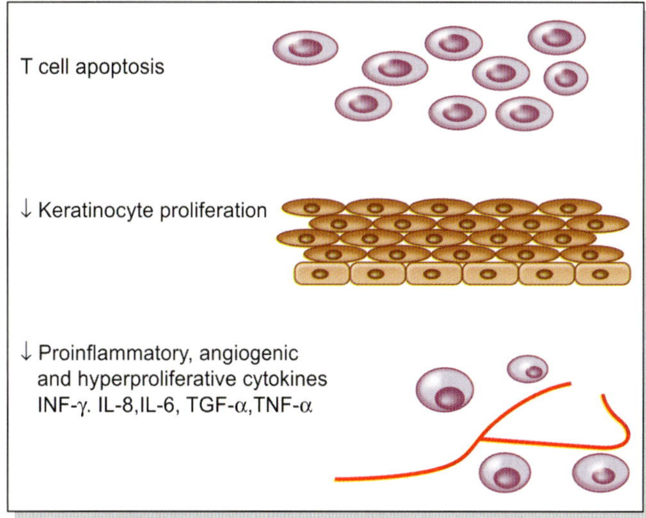

INF-γ, interferon-γ; IL, interleukin; TGF-α, transforming growth factor-α; TNF-α, tumor necrosis factor-α.

FIG. 2: Possible mechanisms of action of excimer laser: (i) depletion of T cell by causing apoptosis; (ii) decreased keratinocyte proliferation; (iii) depletion of proinflammatory, angiogenic, and hyperproliferative cytokines; (iv) upregulation of endothelin-1 release from keratinocytes may play a role in ultraviolet B-related melanocyte migration from the outer root sheath of hair follicles

MECHANISMS OF ACTION

There are only a few studies examining the mechanisms by which the 308 nm excimer laser works in different skin conditions, leaving exact mechanisms still open to debate. Based on the current studies, it seems likely that this laser works on the cellular level and has immunosuppressive properties.[8] Ultraviolet B exposure leads to deoxyribonucleic acid (DNA) damage in the form of photoproduct formation (like pyrimidine dimers), which leads to suppression of DNA synthesis in the hyperplastic psoriatic epidermis. In addition, it induces apoptosis of T cells, which are important in initiating inflammatory skin diseases. In psoriasis, there is hyperproliferation of keratinocytes, infiltration of the epidermis with activated T cells, secretion of proinflamatory cytokines and increased expression of leukocyte trafficking adhesion molecules. With 308 nm radiation on psoriatic lesions, it was demonstrated that the number of CD3+ T cells started depleting within two treatment sessions and this was progressive with continuation of treatment.[9] Immunochemistry, flow cytometery, and cell morphology studies demonstrated progressive increase in apoptotic cells with continued radiation. There was change of molecular targets with upregulation of p53 antigen and decreased expression of B-cell lymphoma 2. Proinflammatory, angiogenic and hyperproliferative cytokines like interferon-γ, interleukin 8 (IL-8), IL-6, transforming growth factor-α, and tumor necrosis factor-α (TNF-α) were drastically decreased in psoriatic lesions treated with MEL 308.[10] The quantitative induction of T cell apoptosis is greater with excimer laser (MEL) than with conventional broadband (BB), or NB-UVB phototherapies.[11] It is thought that the capability to induce T cell apoptosis is an indicator of clinical efficacy. In vitiligo, NB-UVB light and the 308 nm excimer were both found to upregulate endothelin-1 (ET-1) release from keratinocytes. This may play a role in UVB-related melanocyte migration from the outer root sheath of hair follicles.[12]

EXCIMER LASER IN PSORIASIS

The excimer laser is indicated for localized psoriasis and is especially useful for treating localized, thick, stubborn plaques. Psoriatic lesions that occur in the groin and axilla (inverse psoriasis), where light from conventional UV machines reaches with difficulty, respond well to the excimer laser.[13] The excimer laser also works well for recalcitrant psoriatic lesions in areas such as the palms, soles, and scalp.[14] It may also be used in combination with other systemic and topical treatments.[15] The only contraindication for this treatment is a photosensitive psoriatic patient. Most studies demonstrate that the excimer is able to flatten out psoriatic lesions much faster (about a third number of treatments) compared with conventional NB-UVB phototherapy and at a much lower cumulative dose.

TREATMENT PROTOCOLS IN PSORIASIS

Initial evaluation of patients should include extent, distribution, and past treatments. The skin should be free of any topical agents. Eye protection should be worn by all persons in the treatment room. Application of a small amount of mineral oil to thick scaly plaques helps reduce light scatter and allows better penetration of light.

There is as yet still no standard protocol for treatment. In the initial study by Bónis,[16] patients were treated on alternate days, starting with dose increments of about 20% every treatment and compared with NB-UVB treatments. Patients required a mean of 8.33 treatments and received a mean cumulative dose of 4.81 J/cm^2 of irradiation, while patients treated with NUVB required a mean of 30.1 treatments and a mean cumulative dose of 31.1 J/cm^2.

Box 1: Induration based dosimetry for treatment of individual psoriatic plaques

- Determine induration of the psoriatic plaque
- Apply oil before treatment to allow easy penetration of laser light
- Use initial doses based solely on induration component of modified PASI score. For a score of 1, the first dose can be 400 mJ/cm^2, for a score of 2; 600 mJ/cm^2 and for a score of 3; 900 mJ/cm^2
- Subsequent doses are based solely on change in induration. In the first few weeks, the increments in the dose are higher; about 40–50% increment, if there is no change in the induration; 20–25% increment if there is some improvement but no change in the induration score; no increment if there is decrease in the score by 1. As plaques become thinner later on in treatments the increments in doses are lesser
- Four consolidation doses are given after 90% clearing of the plaque. For thick skin like knees and elbows the dose is up to 1.5 J/cm^2 and 1 J/cm^2 for other places

PASI, Psoriasis Area Severity Index.

Subsequently, Taylor et al. at Harvard Medical School conducted the largest series of studies with the excimer in psoriasis and a variety of other conditions.[17] Initial protocols were based on minimal erythema dose (MED). The MED is determined by using incremental doses of radiation (in this case the excimer) on distinct areas of nonphotoexposed part of the body like the lower back or gluteal skin and then examined for erythema after 24 hours. The lowest dose that produces mild, distinct, well-marginated erythema is chosen as the MED for that patient. Induration based dosimetry is another easier way to use the excimer laser and may be more appropriate and practical for day-to-day clinical practice. A convenient protocol for the excimer in psoriasis is mentioned in box 1.

Protocols Based on Minimal Erythema Doses

Dose Response Study

Asawanonda et al. used a variety of doses for stable plaque-type psoriasis.[18] Selected areas in single psoriatic plaques were treated twice weekly with: low dose (0.5, 1 MED multiples), medium dose (2, 3, 4, and 6 MED multiples) and high dose (8 and 16 MED). At 4 months follow-up, all sites that received low or medium fluences had recurrences, whereas those that underwent even a single treatment at 8 and 16 MED multiples remained in remission. It was noted that psoriatic plaques can tolerate several times the MED of normal skin without burning. Lesions exposed to three to four times the MED demonstrated early clearance and longer remissions. Doses greater than six times the MED, however, were shown to be complicated by blistering, pain, and reduced compliance.

Medium dose protocols

Trehan and Taylor used standard phototherapy schedules of thrice weekly treatments with escalations from 0–30%, every week in 15 patients.[19] More than 95% clearance was seen in a mean number of 10.6 treatments with a cumulative dose per plaque of 6.1 J/cm^2.

In 2002, Feldman performed a multicentric study on 80 patients.[20] The initial UV dose administered was based on the MED and the physical characteristics (location, size, and thickness) of the plaque. An initial dose of 1 to 3 MED was generally used and the initial dose was maintained twice weekly until plaques thinned or flattened considerably or pigment appeared. About 75% or greater clearance was achieved in 72% of subjects in an average of 6.2 treatments.

Gerber et al. treated 120 patients with plaque psoriasis.[21] The initial dose was 3 MED, treatments twice weekly with increments of 1 MED per session. About 85.3% of patients showed more than 90% improvement in Psoriasis Area and Severity Index (PASI) after 13 sessions with a cumulative UVB dose of 11.25 $\pm$ 4.21 J cm^2 and average treatment time of 7.2 weeks. Another 43 patients were treated with 1 MED with subsequent doses based on PASI scores and showed nearly identical rates of clearance (83.7%).

Kollner et al. compared UVB treatments with the 308 nm excimer and with the 308 nm excimer lamp.[22] A stepwise regimen and an accelerated dosage schedule were used thrice weekly. The excimer was able to clear psoriasis faster only with the accelerated regimen but side effects of crusting and blistering were also more.

High dose protocol

A single dose of 8 MED was given to one plaque and another single dose of 16 MED was given to another plaque in 16 patients.[23] Half of each plaque was left untreated as control. Bullae developed on treated areas within 6–12 hours and healed over 1–2 weeks. Eleven patients showed significant response, while five patients with very thick acrally located thick lesions with PASI of more than 7 showed minimal response. Out of the 11 patients who responded, 5 had complete clearance of the lesion even at 4 months follow-up.

A recent study used a sub-blistering protocol to treat a single patient with Fitzpatrick type 1V skin type with psoriasis resistant to topical and NB-UVB treatment.[24] The minimum blistering dose was determined to be 1,500 mJ/cm^2, therefore an initial dose of 1,300 mJ/cm^2 was administered. Topical clobetasol propionate was used and after 12 days another dose of 800 mJ/cm^2 was administered to clear the plaque by 79% in just two treatments. Biopsies taken before and after treatment reveal a dramatic decrease in CD4+T cells as well as TNF-α and IL-2 producing T cells.

Protocol Based on Induration of Individual Plaques

Treatments based on MED's have several disadvantages. For determination of MED, one has to wait for at least 24 hours before actual treatments can begin. It is not easy to read an MED on darker skin types. Different plaques have different thicknesses and different amounts of scale and giving the same dose to each and every plaque would give variable results. Exposure to even a single dose alters the optical properties of the plaque and the subsequent optimal dosage for that plaque needs to be adjusted upwards to compensate for acclimatization and downwards after flattening of that plaque. To overcome these problems, Taneja, et al. introduced a new, convenient, induration-based dosage schedule for treatment of plaque psoriasis to be used independent of Fitzpatrick skin types.[25] Plaques were treated twice weekly with an initial dose based solely on the most important induration component, while ignoring the scaling and erythema component of the modified PASI score for each individual lesion and also completely ignoring the MED. Subsequent treatments were twice a week with aggressive dosage increments of up to 50%, based on change in induration. Unlike in conventional phototherapy and other protocols, where doses are sometimes escalated in a fixed pattern, a gradually tapering dosage schedule was used. As plaques become thinner with each treatment, they also become prone to blistering reactions and a flexible, tapering escalation allows lowering of doses without burning the skin. Forty four plaques were treated in 14 patients. The mean modified PASI scores of the treated plaques improved steadily as treatment progressed: from 6.2 (control, 6.4) before treatment; to 2.6 (control, 6.2) after treatment number 5; to 1.2 (control, 6.9) after treatment number 10; to 1.0 (control, 7.0) after treatment number 13 (Fig. 3). At follow-up, the mean modified PASI scores of all treated lesions gradually regressed from 1.0 at the time of the last treatment; to 2.0 by the end of the 3rd month; to 3.1 at the 6 months follow-

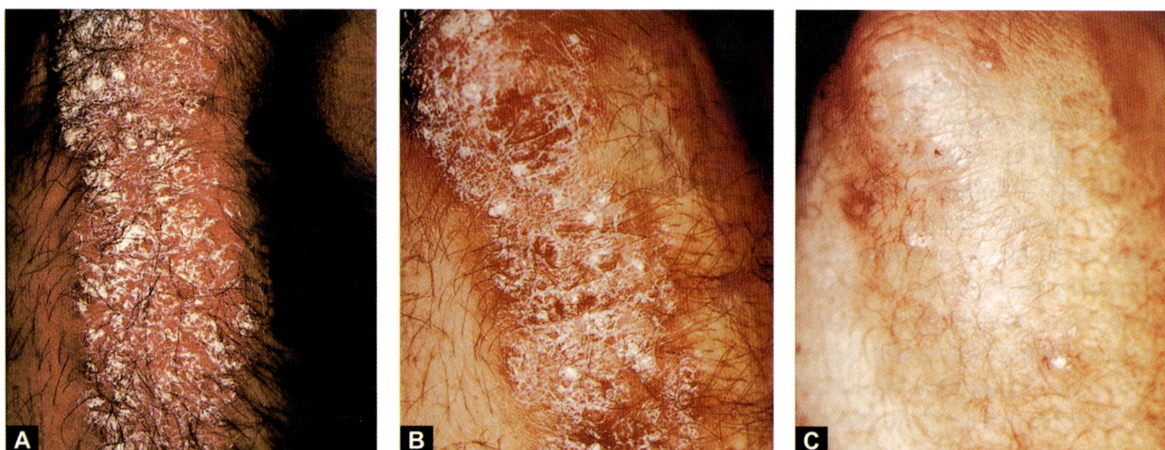

FIG. 3: **A,** Typical plaque psoriasis on the elbow resistant to other treatments; **B,** after five treatments, the lesion has flattened significantly with reduced induration and scaling and small areas of normal skin; **C,** after 12 treatments there is almost complete clearing with only few persistent points of scaling

Source: Taneja A, Trehan M, Taylor CR. 308-nm excimer laser for the treatment of psoriasis. Induration-based dosimetry. Arch Dermatol. 2003;139(6):759-64, with permission..

up. The relapse was mild in all cases and mostly focal in 20 of 44 cases. This protocol may have special significance in the darker skin types, not only because of practical convenience but also because MED determinations are often not performed and not easy to read on darker skin.

SCALP, PALMOPLANTAR, CHILDHOOD, AND NAIL PSORIASIS, AND COMBINATIONS

It is not easy to treat scalp psoriasis with phototherapy simply because hair comes in the way of radiation targeted for scalp skin. Attachments to conventional phototherapy devices are often cumbersome. A fiberoptic comb device was first used by Taneja and Taylor to administer UVB radiation for scalp psoriasis.[26] The same group performed simultaneous studies using the 308 nm excimer laser to target scalp psoriasis.[27] A scalp delivery device fashioned by Anderson was used to blow hair out of the way of excimer radiation for targeting psoriatic plaques on the scalp.[28] An initial dose of 1 MED followed by conservative phototherapy protocols allowed reduction of 4 in PASI scores in 13 patients after a mean of 29 treatments.

Palmoplantar psoriasis is also amenable to treatment with the excimer laser and compares well with cream psoralen + UVA (PUVA) treatments and with lesser side effects.[29] Nail psoriasis does not respond well to the laser.[30]

Regarding combination therapies, Trott et al. administered 4 doses of 308 nm excimer radiations on selected lesions of psoriasis which were already being treated with PUVA therapy.[31] Compared to controls, these lesions went into remission in half the time and with half the cumulative dose. Other studies have used topical corticosteroids, calcipotriene, and tacrolimus in combination with the excimer and found improved long-term efficacy, reduced cumulative doses and lesser adverse events.[32-34]

EXCIMER LASER IN VITILIGO

Several different forms of light therapy have been used effectively for the treatment of vitiligo, including PUVA, BB (290–320 nm) light sources, and NB-UVB (311–313 nm) light sources. Since NB-UVB at 311 nm is an effective and standard mode of the therapy for vitiligo, a very proximal wavelength of the excimer at 308 nm was used for targeting only the affected areas of skin. Unlike in other forms of phototherapy which exposes unaffected normal skin to radiation or requires psoralens, side effects of erythema, blisters, carcinogenesis, and cataracts can be avoided by targeted therapy of the excimer. The 308 nm excimer shows better and faster repigmentation compared with NB-UVB.[35] It should be the preferred modality in children and patients with sun-damaged skin and patients with a history of long-term UVB treatment.

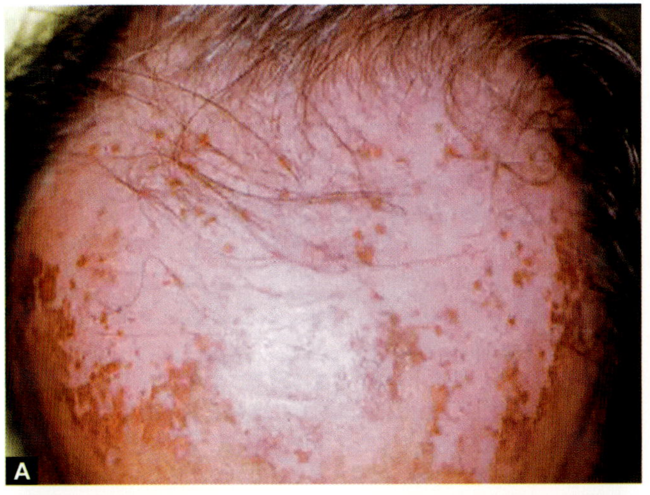

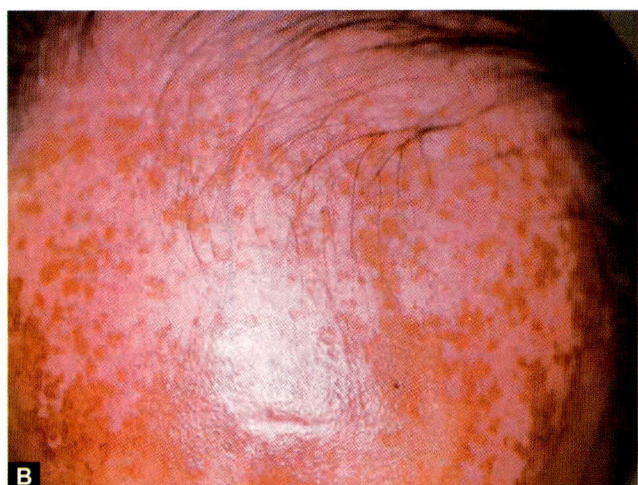

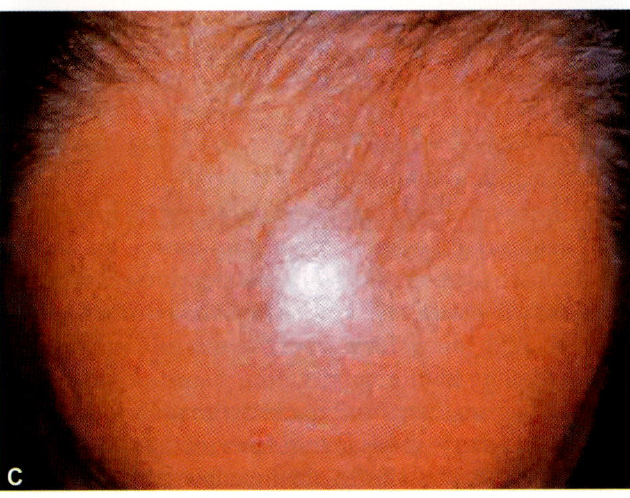

FIG. 4: **A,** Vitiligo lesion on scalp before treatment; **B,** after 15 treatments there is definite perifollicular repigmentation; **C,** after 22 treatments there is complete repigmentation. Interestingly, this patient also noticed slight improvement in hair density after use of the excimer in this area

Source: Taneja A, Trehan M, Taylor CR. 308-nm excimer laser for the treatment of localized vitiligo. Int J Dermatol. 2003;42(8):658-62, with permission.

Baltás et al. reported the initial patient whose vitiligo lesion responded to the 308 nm excimer.[36] Spencer et al. performed a short, 4 weeks study, treating 18 patients thrice weekly. Twelve patients received at least six treatments and showed some repigmentation in 57% of the patches. Six patients received all 12 treatments and showed some repigmentation in 82% of the patches.[37] Taneja et al. initiated a more involved 30 weeks study and treated recalcitrant lesions twice weekly with dose increments of 10–25%, till erythema for 60 treatments (Fig. 4, Box 2).[38] They determined that the excimer was effective in treating vitiligo lesions, with the best improvement seen on the face followed by the axillae and the least improvement in acral areas. This study also made an interesting observation that compared with lighter skin types, lesions in darker individuals required higher fluences to achieve erythema, suggesting that there are factors other than melanin which are important for photoprotection. Since then, many studies using different regimes have been conducted confirming the efficacy of this laser for vitiligo treatments.[39]

Box 2: Recommended 308 nm excimer laser treatment for vitiligo

- Determination of MED is not necessary for vitiligo patients because the calculated MED of the normal skin will not be indicative of the skin affected by vitiligo
- For thinner areas like face or for fair skin, initial doses of 100–150 mJ/cm^2 are appropriate. Darker skin and thicker skin areas like hands and feet can be given higher initial doses of 400–600 mJ/cm^2
- Subsequent doses are gradually increased by fixed increments or by using standard phototherapy increments of 20/10/0, meaning a 20% increase if there is no erythema, 10% increase if there is transient erythema lasting for less than 8 hours, no increase if there is erythema lasting for 8 hours or more
- The dose is held at a given level once asymptomatic pink erythema persisting for more than 8 hours is seen
- If a severe burn occurs, the dose is reduced by half, or the next treatment is skipped
- Treatments can be two to three times per week with a gap of at least 48 hours between two consecutive treatments
- If treatments are missed for more than 2 weeks, fresh treatments are begun using initial starting doses.

TECHNIQUES IN VITILIGO

Initial evaluation of potential candidates with vitiligo should include extent, distribution, and past treatments. A Wood's light may be used for better visualization of vitiligo lesions in patients with pale skin. Risks and benefits should be discussed including the frequent and potentially long duration of therapy. The skin should be free of any topical agents. Eye protection should be worn by all persons in the treatment room. The patient should be protected from natural sunlight between treatments. Determination of MED is not necessary for vitiligo patients as the calculated MED for the surrounding normal skin is not indicative for the skin affected by vitiligo. The starting dose for Fitzpatrick type 1 and 2 skin is normally conservative at 100–150 mJ/cm^2 given the presumed sensitivity of amelanotic lesions.[40] As discussed above, darker skin types seem to tolerate higher doses as also thicker skin areas, like hands and feet and allowing higher initial doses of 400–600 mJ/cm^2. Subsequent doses are gradually increased by fixed increments or by using standard phototherapy increments of 20/10/0; meaning a 20% increment if there is no erythema, 10% increment if there is transient erythema lasting for less than 8 hour, and no increment if there is erythema lasting for 8 hours or more. The dose is held at a given level, once asymptomatic pink erythema persisting for more than 8 hours is achieved. If a severe burn occurs, the dose is reduced by half or the following treatment is skipped. Consecutive day treatments should not be done. Different dosage schedules varying from one to three sessions per week and with low fluences have been tried successfully. Although repigmentation occurs fastest with thrice weekly treatment, the ultimate repigmentation initiation seems to depend entirely on the total number of treatments, not their frequency.[41] Anatomic location is a major predictor of response rate with the best improvement seen on "UV sensitive" areas of face, neck, and trunk and lesser improvement in "UV resistant" areas like the extremities and bony prominences.[42] No relationship could be established between efficacy and age, sex, skin type, MED, and duration of evolution of vitiligo. Hair follicles are also probably important for repigmentation.[43] The pathway of repigmentation with the excimer may be different than of 311 NB-UVB and may account for faster appearance of pigmentation with the laser.[44] The laser has also been used in combination with topical corticosteroids, calcineurin inhibitors and vitamin D analogs, and surgical procedures, thus further expanding treatment options for patients with vitiligo.[45-48] The only contraindication is a photosensitive patient. High cost of therapy is a matter of concern.

OTHER HYPOPIGMENTARY DISORDERS

Using similar techniques as in the treatment of vitiligo, other hypopigmented disorders also show improvement with the use of the 308 nm excimer laser. Armenekas et al. used low-dose biweekly treatments with the laser to achieve 61% improvement in scars and 69% in striae alba. However, hypopigmentation reappeared on 6 months follow-up and maintenance treatment ever 1–4 months is recommended.[49] Pityriasis alba in 12 patients with Fitzpatrick skin types III-V was treated with the excimer and showed near complete resolution of hypopigmentation with 12 weeks of biweekly treatment.[50] Postsurgical hypopigmentation sometimes seen after laser resurfacing or punctuate leukoderma sometimes seen after the use of low-dose Q-switched 1,064 nm lasers or after tattoo removals is also amenable to treatment with the excimer.[51,52]

LICHEN PLANUS

Oral lichen planus is an autoimmune condition which is often difficult to manage and can be refractory to treatment. Kollner et al. treated eight patients with the excimer for 9 to 32 treatments; six patients showed clinical improvement with two showing complete remission with relapse after 4 weeks in one patient.[53] Subsequently, Passeron et al. treated four patients with erosive lichen planus with disappointing results.[54] Trehan and Taylor treated nine patients with refractory oral lichen planus with once weekly low doses of the excimer with five patients showing excellent improvement after seven treatments.[55] The study used a reusable handpiece for easy delivery of light to the oral mucosa and the authors speculate about the interesting possibility of using similar fiberoptic UV devices to treat other inflammatory conditions beyond dermatology, such as in dentistry, oncology, rheumatology, gastroenterology, urology, and gynecology. An improvement in allergic rhinitis with the use of this laser has been reported.[56]

ALOPECIA AREATA

Using the immunosuppressive properties of the excimer laser, two patients showed successful and stable regrowth of hair with 11 and 12 sessions over a period of 9 and 11 weeks.[57] The doses varied from 300–2,300 mJ/cm^2.

No relapse was observed on follow-up at 5 months and 18 months. Childhood alopecia areata is also responsive to the excimer and in a study on nine patients the laser was used twice weekly for 12 weeks. Regrowth of hair was seen in 60% of scalp patches while control patches and patches on extremities showed no change.[58]

ATOPIC DERMATITIS

Based on the knowledge that NB-UVB at 311 nm is an effective and safe treatment for the treatment of atopic dermatitis, Baltas et al. tried the proximal wavelength of 308 nm excimer in 15 atopic patients who had less than 20% body surface involvement. Twice weekly treatments were performed and severity was assessed on clinical scores, quality of life scores, and a Visual Analogue Scale. All scores improved after 1 month of therapy.[59] Prurigo lesions in atopic dermatitis also respond to the excimer and a prospective randomized within patient controlled study was performed on 13 patients comparing the laser with topical clobetasol propionate for 10 weeks.[60] Both treatments showed significant improvement with the excimer laser treated lesions showing better improvement on follow-up.

CUTANEOUS LYMPHOMAS

Primary cutaneous lymphomas are heterogeneous, clonal lymphoproliferative disorders, and are often amenable to treatment with phototherapy. Nistico et al. treated 10 lesions of early mycosis fungoides in five patients with the eximer, using initial doses of 2 MED with increments of 150–500 mJ/cm^2 in subsequent sessions for a maximum of 10 sessions and cumulative doses of 6–12 J/cm^2.[61] All lesions remained in remission at 1 year follow-up. Passerson et al. treated five patients with patch and plaque stage primary cutaneous lymphoma with doses 50 mJ/cm^2 below the MED.[62] Treatments were twice weekly with dose increments of 100 mJ/cm^2 every two sessions till remission or more than 90% improvement. Clinical healing was achieved in an average of 15 sessions with no relapse at 3 months.

REFERENCES

1. Basting D, Marowsky G. Excimer Laser Technology. 1st ed. Heidelberg: Springer-Verlag; 2005. p. 42.
2. Flammer J, Mozaffarieh M, Bebie H. Interventions with Laser Light. In: Flammer J, Mozaffarieh M, Bebie H, editors. Basic Sciences in Ophthalmology. Heidelberg: Springer-Verlag; 2013. pp. 105-15.
3. Moss JP, Patel BC, Pearson GJ, Arthur G, Lawes RA. Krypton fluoride excimer laser ablation of tooth tissues: precision tissue machining. Biomaterials. 1994;15(12):1013-8.
4. Ambrosini V, Sorropago G, Laurenzano E, Golino L, Casafina A, Schiano V, et al. Early outcome of high energy Laser (Excimer) facilitated coronary angioplasty ON hARD and complex calcified and balloOn-resistant coronary lesions: LEONARDO Study. Cardiovasc Revasc Med. 2015;16(3):141-6.
5. Parrish JA, Jaenicke KF. Action spectrum for phototherapy of psoriasis. J Invest Dermatol. 1981;76(5):359-62.
6. Farkas A, Kemeny L. Applications of the 308-nm Excimer Laser in Dermatology. Laser Physics. 2006;16:876-83.
7. Mavilia L, Mori M, Rossi R, Campolmi P, Puglisi Guerra A, Lotti T. 308 nm monochromatic excimer light in dermatology: personal experience and review of the literature. G Ital Dermatol Venereol. 2008;143(5): 329-37.
8. Bianchi B, Campolmi P, Mavilia L, Danesi A, Rossi R, Cappugi P. Monochromatic excimer light (308 nm): an immunohistochemical study of cutaneous T cells and apoptosis-related molecules in psoriasis. J Eur Acad Dermatol Venereol. 2003;17(4):408-13.
9. Hassan, NFM, Soleiman AN. 308 nm excimer laser induces apoptosis of T cells within psoriatic lesions. J Egypt Wom Dermatol Soc. 2006;3:19-25.
10. Cappugi P, Mavilia L, Mavilia C, Brazzini B, Rossi R, Hercogova J, et al. 308 nm monochromatic excimer light in psoriasis: clinical evaluation and study of cytokine levels in the skin. Int J Imm Pharm. 2002;13(Suppl 1):14-19.
11. Ozawa M, Ferenczi K, Kikuchi T, Cardinale I, Austin LM, Coven TR, et al. 312-nanometer Ultraviolet B Light (Narrow-Band UVB) Induces Apoptosis of T Cells Within Psoriatic Lesions. J Exp Med. 1999;189(4):711-8.
12. Noborio R, Morita A. Preferential induction of endothelin-1 in a human epidermal equivalent model by narrow-band ultraviolet B light sources. Photodermatol Photoimmunol Photomed. 2010:26(3):159-61.
13. Mafong EA, Friedman PM, Kauvar AN, Bernstein LJ, Alexiades-Armenakas M, Geronemus RG. Treatment of inverse psoriasis with the 308 nm excimer laser. Dermatol Surg. 2000;28(6):530-2.
14. Al-Mutairi N, Al-Haddad A. Targeted phototherapy using 308 nm Xecl monochromatic excimer laser for psoriasis at difficult to treat sites. Lasers Med Sci. 2013;28(4):1119-24.
15. Passeron T, Ortonne JP. Use of the 308-nm excimer laser for psoriasis and vitiligo. Clin Dermatol. 2006;24(1):33-42.
16. Bónis B, Kemény L, Dobozy A, Bor Z, Szabó G, Ignácz F. 308 nm UVB excimer laser for psoriasis. Lancet. 1997;350(9090):1522.
17. Taylor CR, Taneja A, Gupta S, Racette A, Asawanonda P, Trehan M. 022 308 excimer laser treatment of psoriasis. Photodermatol Photoimmunol Photomed. 2002;18(2):107.
18. Asawanonda P, Anderson RR, Chang Y, Taylor CR. 308-nm excimer laser for the treatment of psoriasis: a dose-response study. Arch Dermatol. 2000;136(5): 619-24.
19. Trehan M, Taylor CR. Medium-dose 308-nm excimer laser for the treatment of psoriasis. J Am Acad Dermatol. 2002;47(5):701-8.
20. Feldman SR, Mellen BG, Housman TS, Fitzpatrick RE, Geronemus RG, Friedman PM, et al. Efficacy of the 308-nm excimer laser for treatment of psoriasis: results of a multicenter study. J Am Acad Dermatol. 2002;46(6):900-6.
21. Gerber W, Arheilger B, Ha TA, Hermann J, Ockenfels HM. Ultraviolet B 308-nm excimer laser treatment of psoriasis: a new phototherapeutic approach. Br J Dermatol. 2003;149(6):1250-8.
22. Köllner K, Wimmershoff MB, Hintz C, Landthaler M, Hohenleutner U. Comparison of the 308-nm excimer laser and a 308-nm excimer lamp with 311-nm narrowband ultraviolet B in the treatment of psoriasis. Br J Dermatol. 2005;152(4):750-4.
23. Trehan M, Taylor CR. High-dose 308-nm excimer laser for the treatment of psoriasis. J Am Acad Dermatol. 2002;46(5):732-7.
24. Debbaneh MG, Levin E, Sanchez Rodriguez R, Leon A, Koo J, Rosenblum MD. Plaque-based sub-blistering dosimetry: Reaching PASI-75 after two treatments with 308-nm excimer laser in a generalized psoriasis patient. J Dermatolog Treat. 2015;26(1):45-8.

25. Taneja A, Trehan M, Taylor CR. 308-nm excimer laser for the treatment of psoriasis: induration-based dosimetry. Arch Dermatol. 2003;139(6):759-64.
26. Taneja A, Racette A, Gourgouliatos Z, Taylor CR. Broad-band UVB fiber-optic comb for the treatment of scalp psoriasis: a pilot study. Int J Dermatol. 2004;43(6):462-7.
27. Taylor CR, Racette AL. A 308-nm excimer laser for the treatment of scalp psoriasis. Lasers Surg Med. 2004;34(2):136-40.
28. Gupta SN, Taylor CR. 308-nm excimer laser for the treatment of scalp psoriasis. Arch Dermatol. 2004;140(5):518-20.
29. Neumann NJ, Mahnke N, Korpusik D, Stege H, Ruzicka T. Treatment of palmoplantar psoriasis with monochromatic excimer light (308-nm) versus cream PUVA. Acta Derm Venereol. 2006;86(1):22-4.
30. Aubin F, Vigan M, Puzenat E, Blanc D, Drobacheff C, Deprez P, et al. Evaluation of a novel 308 nm monochromatic excimer light delivery system in dermatology: a pilot study in different chronic localized dermatoses. Br J Dermatol. 2005;152(1):99-103.
31. Trott J, Gerber W, Hammes S, Ockenfels HM. The effectiveness of PUVA treatment in severe psoriasis is significantly increased by additional UV 308-nm excimer laser sessions. Eur J Dermatol. 2008;18(1):55-60.
32. Tang YJ, Xu WW, Liu XM, Zhang RZ, Xu CX, Xu B, et al. Self-control study of combination treatment of 308 nm excimer laser and calcipotriene ointment on stable psoriasis vulgaris. Int J Clin Exp Med. 2014;7(9):2844-50.
33. Carrascosa JM, Soria X, Domingo H, Ferrándiz C. Treatment of inverse psoriasis with excimer therapy and tacrolimus ointment. Dermatol Surg. 2007;33(3):361-3.
34. Levin E, Debbaneh M, Malakouti M, Brown G, Wang E, Gupta R, et al. Supraerythemogenic excimer laser in combination with clobetasol spray and calcitriol ointment for the treatment of generalized plaque psoriasis: Interim results of an open label pilot study. J Dermatolog Treat. 2014;26(1):16-8.
35. Alhowaish AK, Dietrich N, Onder M, Fritz K. Effectiveness of a 308-nm excimer laser in treatment of vitiligo: a review. Lasers Med Sci. 2013;28(3):1035-41.
36. Baltás E, Nagy P, Bónis B, Novák Z, Ignácz F, Szabó G, et al. Repigmentation of localized vitiligo with the xenon chloride laser. Br J Dermatol. 2001;144(6):1266-7.
37. Spencer JM, Nossa R, Ajmeri J. Treatment of vitiligo with the 308-nm excimer laser: a pilot study. J Am Acad Dermatol, 2002;46(5):727-31.
38. Taneja A, Trehan M, Taylor CR. 308-nm excimer laser for the treatment of localized vitiligo. Int J Dermatol. 2003;42(8):658-62.
39. Sun Y, Wu Y, Xiao B, Li L, Li L, Chen HD, et al. Treatment of 308-nm excimer laser on vitiligo: A systemic review of randomized controlled trials. J Dermatolog Treat. 2015;26(4):347-53.
40. Alhowaish AK, Dietrich N, Onder M, Fritz K. Effectiveness of a 308-nm excimer laser in treatment of vitiligo: a review. Lasers Med Sci. 2013;28(3):1035-41.
41. Hofer A, Hassan AS, Legat AS, Kerl H, Wolf P. Optimal weekly frequency of 308-nm excimer laser treatment in vitiligo patients. Br J Dermatol. 2005;152(5):981-5.
42. Ostovari N, Passeron T, Zakaria W, Fontas E, Larouy JC, Blot JF, et al. Treatment of vitiligo by 308-nm excimer laser: an evaluation of variables affecting treatment response. Lasers Surg Med. 2004;35(2):152-6.
43. Goldstein NB, Koster MI, Hoaglin LG, Spoelstra NS, Kechris KJ, Robinson SE, et al. Narrow Band Ultraviolet B Treatment for Human Vitiligo Is Associated with Proliferation, Migration, and Differentiation of Melanocyte Precursors. J Invest Dermatol. 2015;135(8):2068-76.
44. Yu H, Lan CE. Differential effects of excimer light (308nm) and narrow-band UVB (311nm) on pigment cell development: Novel insights for better phototherapeutic strategy. J Invest Dermatol. 2012;132:S120.
45. Sassi F, Cazzaniga S, Tessari G, Chatenoud L, Reseghetti A, Marchesi L, et al. Randomized controlled trial comparing the effectiveness of 308-nm excimer laser alone or in combination with topical hydrocortisone 17-butyrate cream in the treatment of vitiligo of the face and neck. Br J Dermatol. 2008;159(5):1186-91.
46. Bae JM, Yoo HJ, Kim H, Lee JH, Kim GM. Combination therapy with 308-nm excimer laser, topical tacrolimus, and short-term systemic corticosteroids for segmental vitiligo: A retrospective study of 159 patients. J Am Acad Dermatol. 2015;73(1):76-82.
47. Oh SH, Kim T, Jee H, Do JE, Lee JH. Combination treatment of non-segmental vitiligo with a 308-nm xenon chloride excimer laser and topical high-concentration tacalcitol: a prospective, single-blinded, paired, comparative study. J Am Acad Dermatol. 2011;65(2):428-30.
48. Ebadi A, Rad MM, Nazari S, Fesharaki RJ, Ghalamkarpour F, Younespour S. The additive effect of excimer laser on non-cultured melanocyte-keratinocyte transplantation for the treatment of vitiligo: a clinical trial in an Iranian population. J Eur Acad Dermatol Venereol. 2015;29(4):745-51.
49. Alexiades-Armenakas MR, Bernstein LJ, Friedman PM, Geronemus RG. The safety and efficacy of the 308-nm excimer laser for pigment correction of hypopigmented scars and striae alba. Arch Dermatol. 2004;140(8):955-60.
50. Al-Mutairi N, Hadad AA. Efficacy of 308-nm xenon chloride excimer laser in pityriasis alba. Dermatol Surg. 2012;38(4):604-9.
51. Friedman PM, Geronemus RG. Use of the 308-nm excimer laser for postresurfacing leukoderma. Arch Dermatol. 2001;137(6):824-5.
52. Kim HS, Jung HD, Kim HO, Lee JY, Park YM. Punctate leucoderma after low-fluence 1,064-nm quality-switched neodymium-doped yttrium aluminum garnet laser therapy successfully managed using a 308-nm excimer laser. Dermatol Surg. 2012;38(5):821-3.
53. Köllner K, Wimmershoff M, Landthaler M, Hohenleutner U. Treatment of oral lichen planus with the 308-nm UVB excimer laser—early preliminary results in eight patients. Lasers Surg Med. 2003;33(3):158-60.
54. Passeron T, Zakaria W, Ostovari N, Mantoux F, Lacour JP, Ortonne JP. Treatment of erosive oral lichen planus by the 308 nm excimer laser. Lasers Surg Med. 2004;34(3):205.
55. Trehan M, Taylor CR. Low-dose excimer 308-nm laser for the treatment of oral lichen planus. Arch Dermatol. 2004;140(4):415-20.
56. Csoma Z, Ignacz F, Bor Z, Szabo G, Bodai L, Dobozy A, et al. Intranasal irradiation with the xenon chloride ultraviolet B laser improves allergic rhinitis. J Photochem Photobiol B. 2004;75(3):137-44.
57. Gundogan C, Greve B, Raulin C. Treatment of alopecia areata with the 308-nm xenon chloride excimer laser: case report of two successful treatments with the excimer laser. Lasers Surg Med. 2004;34(2):86-90.
58. Al-Mutairi N. 308-nm excimer laser for the treatment of alopecia areata in children. Pediatr Dermatol. 2009;26(5):547-50.
59. Baltás E, Csoma Z, Bodai L, Ignácz F, Dobozy A, Kemény L. Treatment of atopic dermatitis with the xenon chloride excimer laser. J Eur Acad Dermatol Venereol. 2006;20(6):657-60.
60. Brenninkmeijer EE, Spuls PI, Lindeboom R, van der Wal AC, Bos JD, Wolkerstorfer A. Excimer laser vs. clobetasol propionate 0·05% ointment in prurigo form of atopic dermatitis: a randomized controlled trial, a pilot. Br J Dermatol. 2010;163(4):823-31.
61. Nisticò S, Costanzo A, Saraceno R, Chimenti S. Efficacy of monochromatic excimer laser radiation (308 nm) in the treatment of early stage mycosis fungoides. Br J Dermatol. 2004;151(4):877-9.
62. Passeron T, Zakaria W, Ostovari N, Perrin C, Larrouy JC, Lacour JP, et al. Efficacy of the 308-nm excimer laser in the treatment of mycosis fungoides. Arch Dermatol. 2004;140(10):1291-3.

CHAPTER 30

Endovenous Laser Ablation in the Treatment of Varicose Veins

Ankur Talwar, Kshama Talwar

INTRODUCTION

Saphenous vein reflux is the underlying primary abnormality in the majority of cases of superficial venous insufficiency. Thus, approaches to dealing with saphenofemoral junction and saphenous truncal incompetence have dominated the thinking of phlebologists (Fig. 1). Although conservative management with compression therapy may improve the symptoms of chronic venous insufficiency, it does not cure it.

The standard treatment for varicose veins associated with small saphenous reflux is ligation of the saphenopopliteal junction (SPJ) with or without stripping of the small saphenous vein (SSV) under general anesthesia. However, recurrence rate following surgery may be as high as 50%[1] at 3 years. In many instances, this is the result of inaccurate ligation of the SPJ. In addition, neovascularization, which is the most common cause for recurrence following saphenofemoral ligation and stripping,[2] may have a role.

Over the years, the ligation and stripping technique has largely been replaced by percutaneous endovenous thermal ablation. Two types of thermal ablation procedures exist: endovenous laser ablation (EVLA) and radiofrequency ablation. Both procedures are associated with high success and low complication rates. The procedures are generally performed on an ambulatory basis with local anesthetic and typically require no sedation.

INDICATIONS

The common indications in patients with varicose veins in which EVLA is performed are:

- Symptoms associated with chronic venous hypertension, e.g., throbbing pain, cramps, heaviness, spontaneous hemorrhage, etc.
- Cutaneous changes associated with chronic venous hypertension, e.g., stasis eczema, lipodermatosclerosis, atrophie blanche, etc.
- Stasis ulcer
- Cosmetic concerns due to unsightly appearance of the dilated veins.

CONTRAINDICATIONS

The contraindications to endovenous treatment are:

- Hypercoagulable states
- Nonambulatory patient
- Obstruction of the deep venous system
- Excessive tortuosity of the superficial veins making passage of an endovenous device impossible
- Allergy to the local anesthetics
- Pregnancy or patient with poor general health.

MECHANISM OF ACTION

The underlying goal for all thermal ablation procedures is to deliver sufficient thermal energy to the wall of

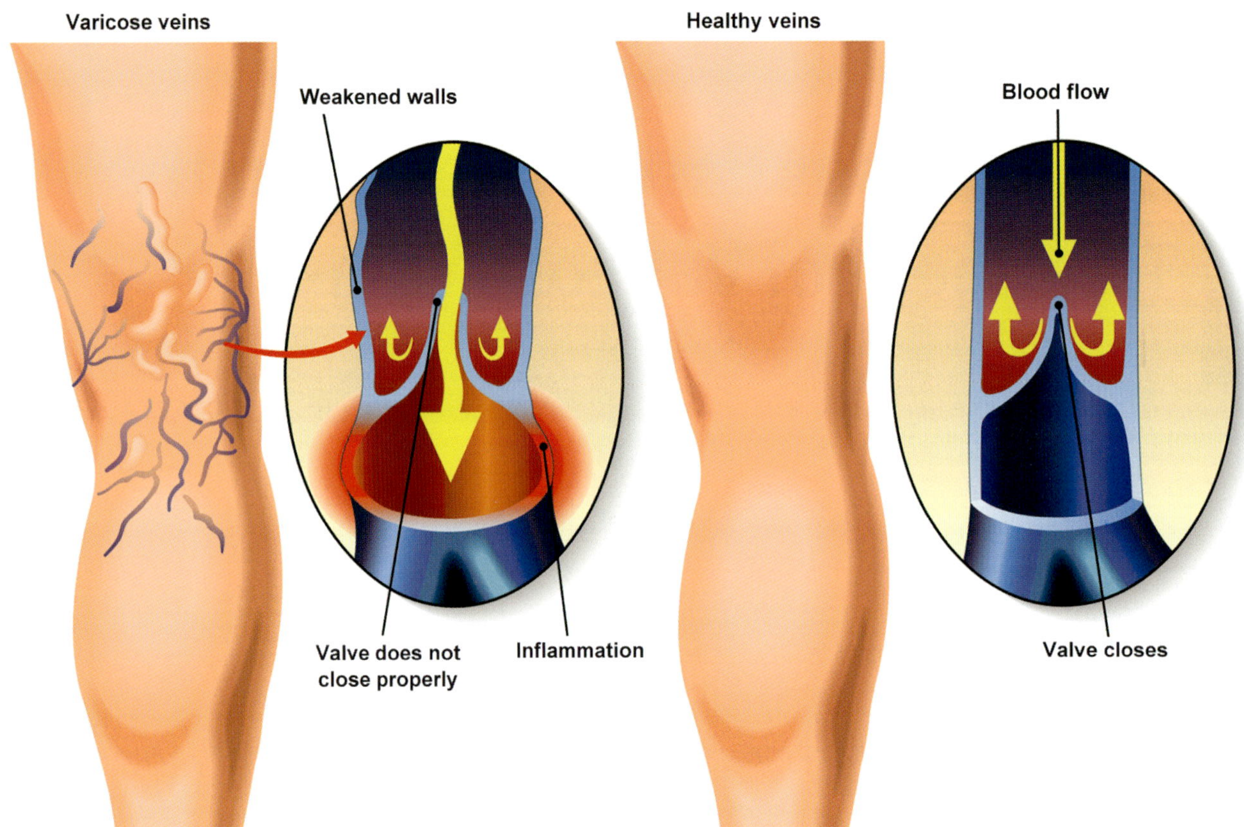

FIG. 1: Pathophysiology behind the development of varicose veins

an incompetent vein segment to produce irreversible occlusion, fibrosis, and ultimately, disappearance of the vein. It has been postulated that vein wall injury is mediated both by direct effect of the laser on the vessel wall and indirectly via laser induced steam generated by heating of small amounts of blood within the vein (Fig. 2).[3] Some heating may occur by direct absorption of photon energy by the vein wall as well as by convection from steam bubbles and conduction from heated blood.

The following wavelengths are in current use for EVLA: 810, 940, 980, 1,064, 1,320, and 2,068 nm. The main chromophore of 1,320 and 2,068 nm lasers, at least initially, is water, while other wavelengths used for EVLA primarily target hemoglobin. Although, it is still not definitively established in the literature, some authors suggest that the higher wavelength lasers produce similar efficacy at lower power settings with less postprocedure symptoms.[4]

Mean peak intravascular temperatures during EVLA measured flush with the laser tip, averaged 729°C, while those 4 mm distal to the tip averaged 93°C.[5] There appears to be a very rapid fall-off in temperature over short distances during EVLA. The risk of collateral thermal injury to surrounding structures depends on perivenous tissue heating, not intravascular temperature. These findings seem to explain the very low reported incidence of nerve injury and skin burns following EVLA.

LASER USED

Historically, laser ablation has been primarily performed with 810 nm diode lasers. The laser beam is delivered through extremely fine bare tipped fibers which are capable of entering the dilated vein (Fig. 3).

There are now many different forms of endovenous laser, i.e., 810, 940, 941, 1,064, and 1,320, and other wavelengths, different sized sheaths, end-firing lasers fibers and side-firing laser fibers, etc. However, all of them are forms of EVLA—as they all ablate veins from within using laser. Limited data are available that compare the different configurations, but anecdotally, it is thought that higher, water specific wavelengths produce less postprocedure pain with equivalent outcomes.

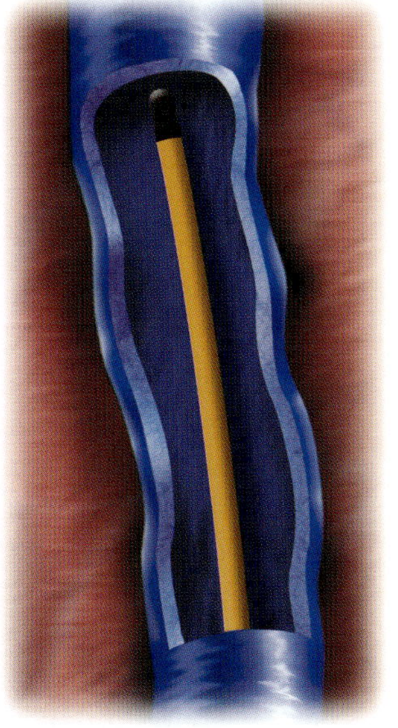

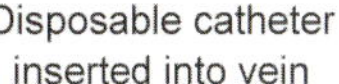

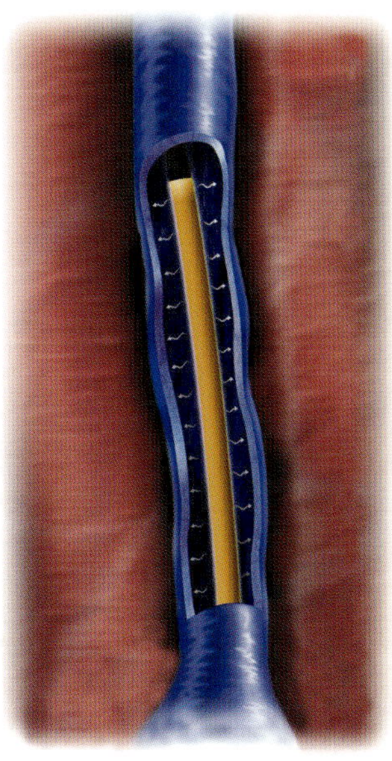

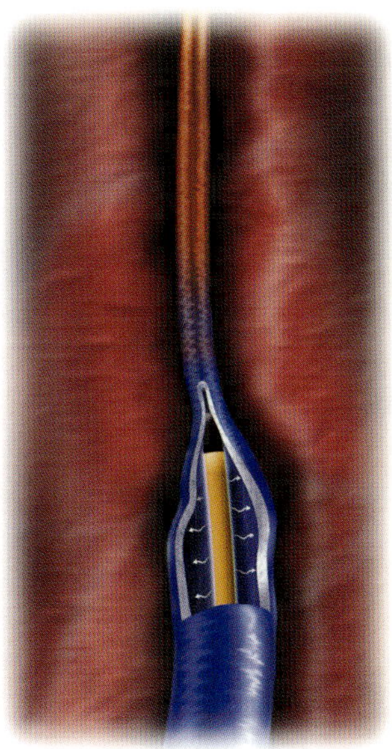

FIG. 2: Principle of endovenous laser ablation treatment
Photo courtesy: Vascular Surgery Associates, LLC.

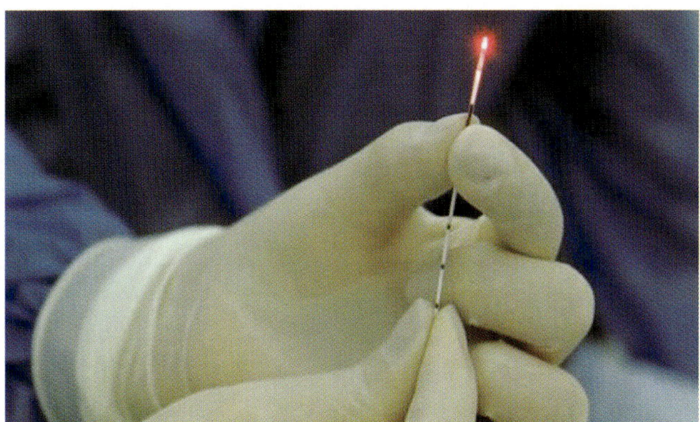

FIG. 3: The fine bare tipped laser probe

PROCEDURE

A preprocedure marking of the veins is done using a Doppler ultrasound. The course of the vein and important anatomical landmarks are mapped out.

Endovenous laser ablation should be performed under local tumescent anesthesia using large volumes of a dilute solution of lidocaine and epinephrine (average volume of 200–400 mL of 0.1% lidocaine with 1:1,000,000 epinephrine) that is buffered with sodium bicarbonate. This solution should be delivered either manually or with an infusion pump under ultrasound guidance, so the vein is surrounded with an anesthetic fluid along the entire length of the segment to be treated. In addition to the anesthetic effect, the use of large volume tumescent anesthesia for EVLA allows for separation of the vein to be treated from the surrounding structures along with its ability to empty the vein due to compression, which maximizes the effect of treatment on the vein wall. Further, an anesthetic solution provides a protective heat sink around the treated vein which reduces peak temperatures in the surrounding tissues.

Under ultrasound guidance, a needle is introduced into the great saphenous vein at or slightly above the level of knee using a Seldinger technique. A guidewire is passed through this needle up into the vein. The intravenous placement of the guidewire is then confirmed with Doppler. The needle is subsequently removed and a catheter is passed over the guidewire.

Once the catheter is inside the vein, the guidewire is taken out and the laser fiber is passed up the catheter so its tip lies at the highest point to be heated. Once the placement has been confirmed, the laser source is switched on and the laser fiber is gradually withdrawn slowly so that 5–6 pulses of laser energy are delivered per cm vein.

Early data on treatment of the great saphenous vein with 810 and 940 nm devices suggest treatment failure is uncommon in patients treated with more than 70 J/cm.[6] A withdrawal rate of 2 mm/s at 14 watts delivers 70 J/cm.

The treatment takes about 20–30 minutes per leg. Following treatment, a nonstretch compression bandage is applied to the limb for 1 week followed by a class 2 support stocking for a further week.

POSTOPERATIVE CARE

Immediately postoperatively, some form of compression is recommended. The most common recommendation is for class 2 compression stockings (30–40 mmHg) applied immediately after the procedure and worn for 1–2 weeks. Further, patients are encouraged to ambulate for at least 30–60 minutes after leaving the procedure room and at least 1–2 hours daily for 1–2 weeks. Nonsteroidal anti-inflammatory drugs may be given for 3 days to reduce inflammatory "phlebitis" of the treated veins.

PROTOCOL

The success of EVLA is correlated to the amount of thermal energy delivered. With laser, energy deposition has been described as that deposited per centimeter of vein length (J/cm). Most studies have made it clear that an energy density more than or equal to 60 J/cm is central to achieving complete saphenous vein occlusion.[7] This equates to 5 pulses/cm vein when using 12 watts power, 1 second pulses, and 1 second intervals for laser fiber withdrawal, i.e., 2 mm pullback during each 1 second interval.

Further, some data support the notion that complications and adverse effects are not increased with energies up to 140 J/cm.

Newer data suggests that the energy delivery required to achieve reliable vein ablation and low recanalization rates is dependent not only on the quantity of energy delivered but also on vein diameter.[8] Although a protocol delivering more than or equal to 60 J/cm would be straightforward, it should be used with caution if the vein for ablation is particularly superficial (within <1 cm of skin surface).

RESULTS

Short-term and mid-term studies of EVLA, regardless of wavelength used, seem remarkably consistent, typically reporting ablation of refluxing saphenous veins in 90% or more of cases.[9,10] Outcomes seem equal to or better than those of stripping, with better quality of life scores in the postoperative period compared to stripping.

Further, reports suggest, that in contrast to ligation and stripping, endovenous ablation techniques are associated with a very low incidence of neovascularization.[11] It may be that the development of neovascularization is largely prevented by avoiding groin dissection and by preserving venous drainage in normal junctional tributaries.

ADVERSE EVENTS

Adverse events following EVLA are generally common but minor. Ecchymosis over the treated segment frequently occurs and normally lasts for 7–14 days. Short-term pain following the procedure is also commonly reported. In a short-term review, intermittent-pulsed laser fiber pullback has been reported to cause significantly greater levels of post operative pain and bruising, compared with a continuous pullback protocol.[12] Use of a short-stretch bandage for 3 days following intermittent mode EVLA has been found to substantially reduce patient reported bruising and pain.

Superficial thrombophlebitis is another uncommon side effect of EVLA, being reported in about 5% of treatments.

More significant adverse events reported following EVLA include neurologic injuries, skin burns, and deep vein thrombosis (DVT). Skin burns following EVLA have been reported but are fortunately relatively rare and seem to be avoidable with adequate tumescent anesthesia. As nerves can lie alongside the veins, these may also become damaged by the heat and a few patients notice small patches of numbness on their skin. Tumescent anesthesia has been demonstrated to reduce perivenous temperatures with laser ablation and leads to reduced incidence of cutaneous and neurologic thermal injuries.

Deep vein thrombosis following EVLA is unusual. Deep vein thrombosis can occur as an extension of thrombus from the treated superficial vein across the junctional connection into the femoral or popliteal veins. Various large scale studies have found the risk of DVT following EVLA to be less than 1%.[11,13] The protocol to immediately ambulate the patient following the procedure further reduces any such risk.

CONCLUSION

Endovenous laser ablation, like radiofrequency ablation and foam sclerotherapy, is a less invasive alternative to vein stripping. Endovenous laser ablation is indicated in an ambulatory patient with great, small, or accessory saphenous vein reflux with surface varices and/or symptoms or complications related to superficial venous insufficiency. Endovenous laser ablation is routinely performed using dilute local anesthesia, with or without supplemental oral anxiolytics, in an office setting. Generally, taking 30-60 minutes to perform, procedure times are dependent on the length of segment treated, experience of the operator, and whether ancillary procedures, such as ambulatory phlebectomy, are done.

REFERENCES

1. van Rij AM, Jiang P, Solomon C, Christie RA, Hill GB. Recurrence after varicose vein surgery: a prospective long-term clinical study with duplex ultrasound scanning and air plethysmography. J Vasc Surg. 2003;38(5):935-43.
2. Jones L, Braithwaite BD, Selwyn D, Cooke S, Earnshaw JJ. Neovascularisation is the principal cause for varicose vein recurrence: results of a randomised trial of stripping the long saphenous vein. Eur J Vasc Endovasc Surg.1996;12(4):442-5.
3. Proebstle TM, Sandhofer M, Kargl A, Gül D, Rother W, Knop J, et al. Thermal damage of the inner vein wall during endovenous laser treatment: key role of energy absorption by intravascular blood. Dermatol Surg. 2002;28:596-600.
4. Sadek M, Kabnick LS, Berland T, Cayne NS, Mussa F, Maldonado T, et al. Update on endovenous laser ablation: 2011. Perspect Vasc Surg Endovasc Ther. 2011;23(4):233-7.
5. Weiss RA. Comparison of endovenous radiofrequency versus 810 nm diode laser occlusion of large veins in an animal model. Dermatol Surg. 2002;28(1):56-61.
6. Timperman PE, Sichlau M, Ryu RK. Greater energy delivery improves treatment success of endovenous laser treatment of incompetent saphenous veins. J Vasc Interv Radiol. 2004;15:1061-3.
7. Theivacumar NS, Dellagrammaticas D, Beale RJ, Mavor AI, Gough MJ. Factors influencing the effectiveness of endovenous laser ablation (EVLA) in the treatment of great saphenous vein reflux. Eur J Vasc Endovasc Surg. 2008;35(1):119-23.
8. Proebstle TM, Moehler T, Herdemann S. Reduced recanalization rates of the great saphenous vein after endovenous laser treatment with increased energy dosing: definition of a threshold for the endovenous fluence equivalent. J Vasc Surg. 2006;44:834-9.
9. Min RJ, Khilnani N, Zimmet SE. Endovenous laser treatment of saphenous vein reflux: long-term results. J Vasc Interv Radiol. 2003;14:991-6.
10. Kabnick LS. Outcome of different endovenous laser wavelengths for great saphenous vein ablation. J Vasc Surg. 2006;43:88-93.
11. Ravi R, Rodriguez-Lopez JA, Trayler EA, Barrett DA, Ramaiah V, Diethrich EB. Endovenous ablation of incompetent saphenous veins: a large single-center experience. J Endovasc Ther. 2006;13:244-8.
12. Zimmet SE. Pain, bruising and short-term efficacy after endovenous laser treatment of the greater saphenous vein: the effect of operative technique and postoperative care. Paper presented at the 16th Annual Congress of the American College of Phlebology. Florida: Fort Lauderdale; 2002.
13. Agus GB, Mancini S, Magi G. The first 1000 cases of Italian Endovenous-laser Working Group (IEWG). Rationale, and long-term outcomes for the 1999-2003 period. Int Angiol. 2006;25:209-15.

CHAPTER 31

Laser Lipolysis

Jayashree Venkataram, Venkataram Mysore, Aniketh Venkataram

INTRODUCTION

Suction lipoplasty or liposuction has been the gold standard for removing fat over the last four decades.[1] Several efforts have been made with technology of different energy sources such as lasers, and ultrasound to enhance the efficacy of this procedure. Recent devices have shown gradually increasing efficacy, but a perfect device is yet not available. Hence, while tumescent liposuction continues to be the gold standard, these alternatives are being accepted as at least additional procedures, if not as replacement.[2] This chapter reviews laser lipolysis (LAL), which is also known as laser lipoplasty or laser-assisted liposuction.

HISTORY

The technology has had a chequered history. The first documented use of LAL was by Dressel in1990.[3] Apfelberg et al. later reported efficacy of a 1,064 nm light source.[4] These initial efforts did not show much promise and the field lagged behind as tumescent liposuction (both manual and powered) established its dominance. Recent advances in laser technology, such as introduction of a laser beam via a liposuction cannula,[5] have stimulated interest again in this field and LAL is beginning to find its place in the sun.

Laser is being used currently in two ways:

1. Laser-assisted liposuction which means destruction of fat by laser followed by suction aspiration as in any liposuction for all large areas
2. Laser lipolysis which means only destruction without aspiration useful, in small fat deposits.

INDICATIONS

In the current scenario, LAL is useful for the following scenarios:

- Like liposculpture, the main indication for LAL is for body contouring[6]
- Laser cannulae are smaller and hence, more easily maneuverable in fibrous tight areas, such as upper chest, male breast, and flanks in abdomen, which do not allow sufficient tumescent fluid infiltration and where larger aspiration cannulae cause pain[7]
- Small areas, such as double chin, neck, arms, periumbilical areas, i.e., liposuction regions where destroyed fat can be left behind without aspiration; here also smaller laser cannulae lead to smaller adits and hence, more acceptable scars[8]
- As an additional technique in large areas wherein limitations of upper limit of tumescent anesthesia does not allow adequate anesthesia and aspiration[9]

- Areas with loose skin where the purported benefits of laser induced collagenogenesis and remodeling can lead to skin tightening, e.g., neck, abdomen.
- Additional revision or touch-up liposuctions for small areas after an initial liposuction.[9,10]

ADVANTAGES

Several advantages have been advocated by laser manufacturers. These include:

Lesser Downtime

The most commonly mentioned advantages of LAL relate to the ease of patient recovery.[6,7,11,12] Compared to traditional liposuction, LAL may diminish postoperative pain, and decrease the extent of edema and bruising following the procedure.[6,7,9,12-14] Laser operated liposuction reduces trauma to the tissue during fat removal, resulting in improved wound healing.[15] As a result, patients may have a more rapid return to daily activities.[5,15]

Lesser Bleeding

Laser induced thrombosis of blood vessels and closure of lymphatic channels may explain the reduction in severity of bruising and swelling after LAL.[11] Operator as well as patient safety is increased with the procedure.

Ease of Procedure

The process of laser induced fat emulsification allows more efficient fat extraction with less surgeon fatigue.[4,10,11] The need for repeat procedures may also be decreased by use of laser.[8]

Skin Tightening

Laser induced photobiological changes can induce some skin tightening when treating areas of skin laxity by inducing collagen production and subsequent skin contraction.[6,10-12]

Location of LAL is shown in figures 1 and 2.

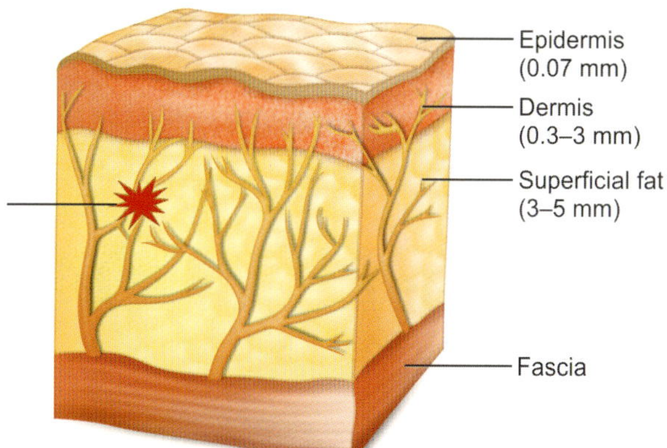

FIG. 1: Superficial lipolysis for skin tightening

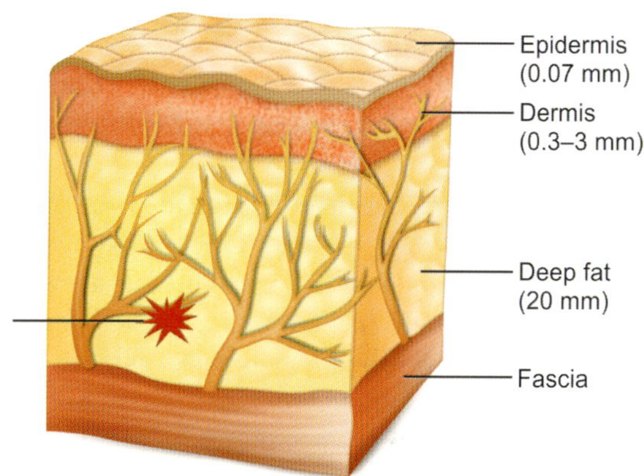

FIG. 2: Deep laser lipolysis for lipolysis

DISADVANTAGES

Several disadvantages exist, some of which are as follows:

- As explained above, in most situations, it is an adjuvant procedure and not a replacement for traditional liposuction[9]
- Cost of laser machine is high
- Efficacy of LAL as a solo procedure is yet to be established and some studies have not demonstrated any definitive benefit of using the laser[11,12]
- Since aspiration is essential even after using laser, duration of surgery is increased in an already lengthy procedure. Simultaneous aspiration with laser using dual functioning cannulae allowing laser delivery and aspiration has been attempted in recent machines,[16] but are yet to find uniform acceptance
- As with any laser, burns are a possibility
- There is a learning curve with the machine.[9]

LASER PHYSICS AND MECHANISM OF ACTION

The basic principle of LAL as in all laser indications is the principle of selective photothermolysis with fat and water, and possibly hemoglobin as chromophores (Fig. 3). According to the theory of selective photothermolysis,

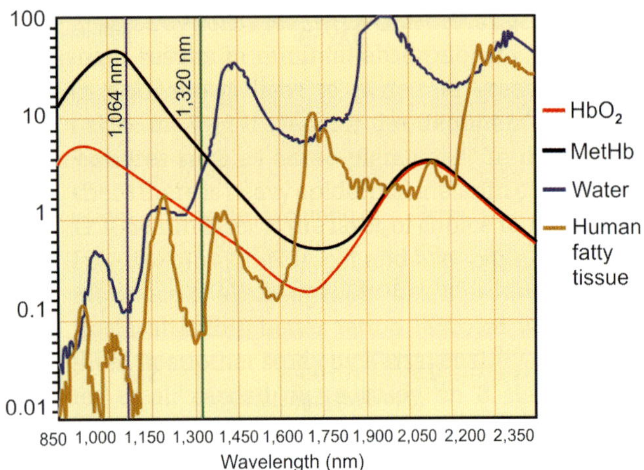

HbO_2, oxyhemoglobin; MetHb, methemoglobin.

FIG. 3: Absorption coefficients of water and fatty tissue

these chromophores will preferentially absorb laser energy on the basis of their absorption coefficients at specific wavelengths.[6] Several wavelengths have been found to be absorbed by fat—924, 968, 980, 1,064, 1,319, 1,320, and 1,344 nm. Some wavelengths have unique advantages. The 924 nm wavelength has the highest selectivity for fat melting,[12] while 1,064 nm targets oxyhemoglobin leading to coagulation of blood vessels and therefore, lesser bleeding.[14] The 1,320 nm wavelength penetrates deeper and hence, causes lesser tissue damage in dermis.[12]

Mechanism of Action

Different mechanisms such as photoacoustic,[10] photomechanical, photostimulatory, and photothermal effects have been proposed for destruction of fat.[6,17] But the most important mechanism is perhaps a pure thermal effect, referred to as photohyperthermia.[10] Heat produces coagulation of collagen, vessel thrombosis, and damage to fat cells by degradation of cell membrane and protein denaturation.[10,15] It is also proposed that the tumescent fluid acts as a heat sink and aids in dissipation of fat to lower dermis where it leads to neocollagenogenesis as happens in any laser rejuvenation. This effect is thought to explain the skin tightening benefit of LAL.[18]

It is said that temperatures of 48–50°C must be reached within the dermis to induce collagen contraction and resultant skin tightening.[12,18,19] A dermal temperature between approximately 50 and 70°C translates to a skin surface temperature of approximately 40–41°C.[12,18] Amount of damage depends on total energy delivered and hence, determination of optimum levels is important.[2,14]

Thermal damage promotes collagen remodeling, leading to increases in skin tone and texture. These effects continue to improve for 3–6 months after the procedure.[9,16]

Laser Lipolysis Technology

Devices of three wavelengths have been approved by the Food and Drug Administration for use in the United States for LAL: diode 924–980 nm (continuous wave), neodymium doped yttrium-aluminium-garnet (Nd:YAG) 1,064 nm, and 1,320 nm.[6]

- Diode laser: 924 nm wavelength has a high specificity for fat, while the 970 nm targets collagen to promote tissue tightening. A 980 mm device is also available.[12] Dual technology devices are available but have not demonstrated any additional benefit
- Neodymium doped yttrium-aluminium-garnet laser devices: Nd:YAG laser at 1,064 nm is one of the earliest lasers to be used to destroy fat. It is absorbed by collagen and fat bound water, though less efficiently than 1,320 nm diode, but it has the advantage of being absorbed by oxyhemoglobin (thus producing hemostasis)
- 1,320 nm: 1,320 nm is one of the longest wavelength available and targets water in adipocytes and bound to collagen, and hence is thought to produce greater skin tightening
- Multiplex devices using different wavelengths (1,064 and 1,320 nm) have been introduced. The scientific premise for combining the 1,064 and 1,320 nm wavelengths is to exploit their individual properties and allow for them to act synergistically, particularly with regards to hemostasis. The 1,320 nm wavelength converts hemoglobin to methemoglobin. The 1,064 nm not only targets oxygenated hemoglobin, but has a great affinity to methemoglobin, thereby enhancing the effects of the 1,320 nm firing.[12]

The authors use Fotona (Slovenia) machine which uses a quasicontinuous pulsed Nd:YAG device with maximum power of 35 watt, pulse energy of 50 watt, repetition rate of 100 Hz (Figs 4 and 5). The machine has been used by us for nearly 2 years since 2013 in 252 patients. The machine is bulky, but easy to use. Our experience shows that machine is useful in the following ways:

- Initial laser damage to fat to facilitate aspiration—this is done at 25 watt fluence of 3000–5000 J over 100 cm^2
- The laser cannulae are 1.5 mm in size while aspiration cannulae are 3–4 mm in size. This facilitates its use in tight areas such as upper chest, around umbilicus and flanks

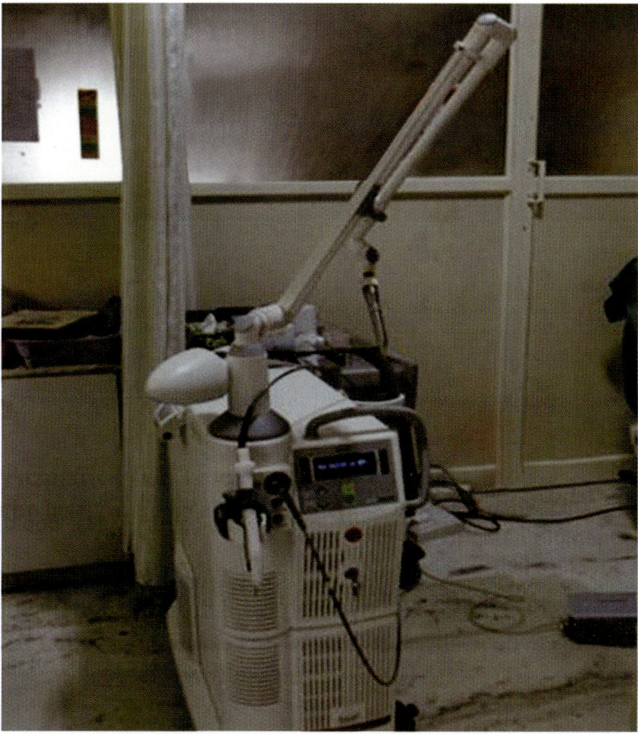
FIG. 4: Neodymium doped yttrium-aluminium-garnet laser machine

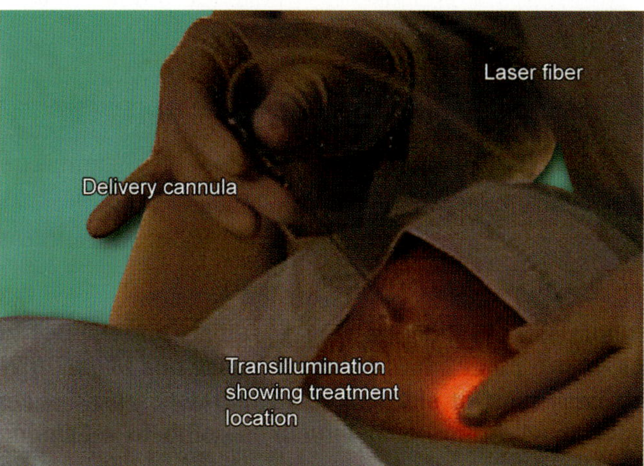

FIG. 5: Laser beam

- At the end of the liposuction, laser is used to create a heat sink in residual tumescent fluid for diffusion into lower dermis, and possible skin tightening
- While performing large areas, it is somewhat difficult to give adequate anesthesia as upper safety limits are approached. In such areas, we use laser as a lipolytic device without aspiration.

A practical advantage of having the machine that the authors have noticed is that it can impress a patient who might be seeking a "high tech" device, as compared to regular liposuction. However, the machine is expensive if bought for use in liposuction only. This machine, however, is a platform with several applications such as skin tightening, acne, post-acne scarring, hair removal, pigmented lesions, etc. This fact is of use in a dermatological setup for other indications.

Technique of Laser Lipolysis

Patient Counseling

Patient counseling is in general similar to those undergoing liposuction. Patients often have a high expectation from a high tech device and it should be properly explained as to what can be reasonably expected.

Preparation

Preparation is similar to the preparation of liposuction patient. Procedure is performed under tumescent anesthesia. The authors do not advocate the use of intramuscular, spinal, or general anesthesia.

Initial phase of infiltration is also entirely similar to that in liposuction and the reader is referred to appropriate books on liposuction for this purpose. If only LAL is planned as in cases of small areas such as chin, small adits of 2 mm are adequate. If suction is needed after lipolysis as is the case with most procedures, adits of size 3–3.5 mm are needed as in any case of liposuction. The laser is applied in two ways:

1. Initial lipolysis soon after tumescence at fluence levels 25 watt and 5000 J over 100 cm^2. The laser movement can be made out by the red beam guide. The movements have to be smooth and below upwards in layers. The same area should not be targeted more than once for fear of burning and a fan shaped movement is advocated. Protective eye glasses should be used by all the staff in the theater. Adequacy of lipolysis is judged by crackling sound (popcorn effect) and the feeling of heat felt by the nonoperating hand. While fluence levels needed may vary depending on the machine, 3000–5000 J is what we usually use for 100 cm^2 area. Once adequate soft feeling is felt, aspiration by conventional cannulae is performed
2. A second use of the laser is at the end of the surgery; at reduced fluences 10 watt to produce skin tightening.

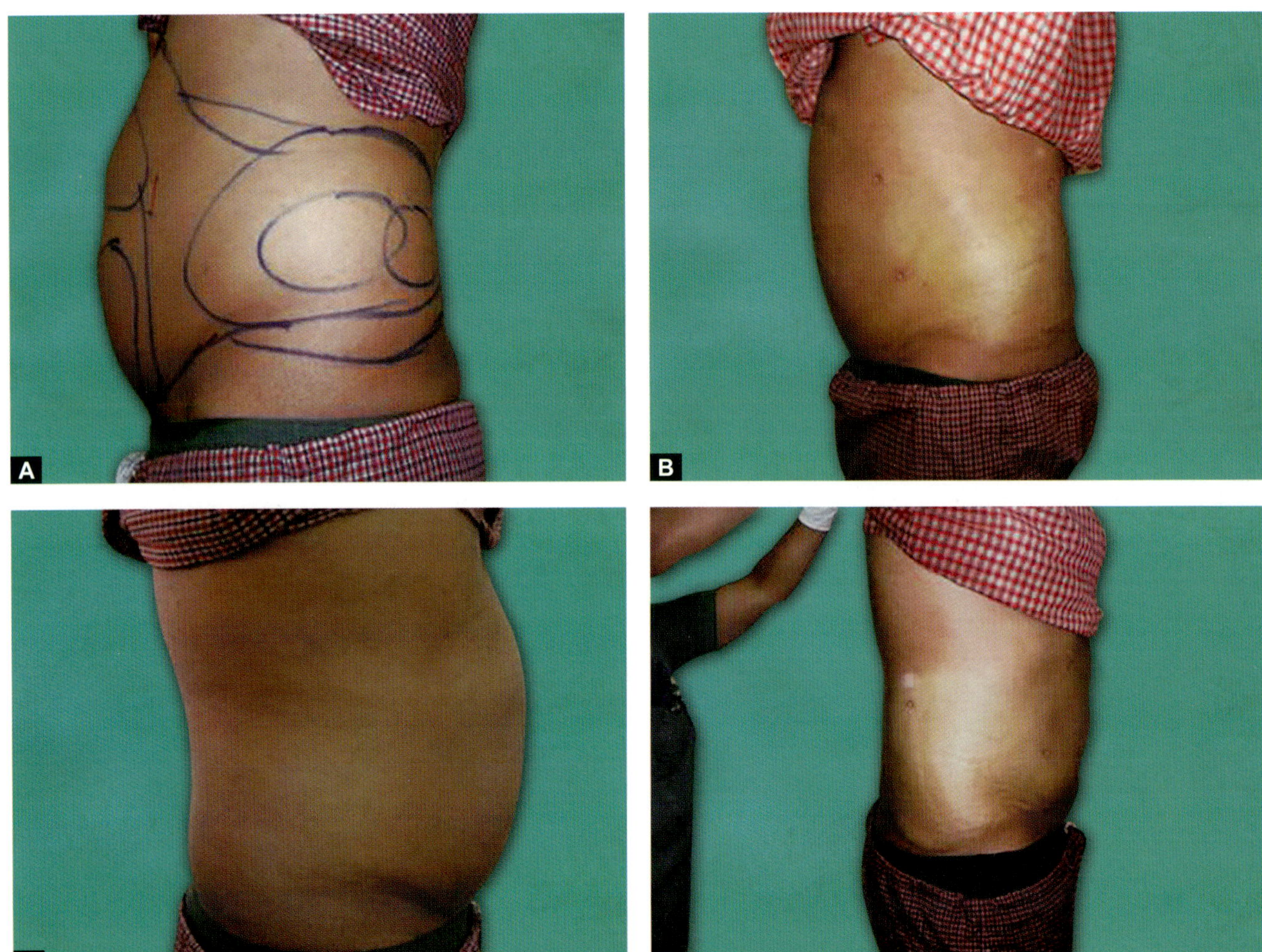

FIG. 6: Results after combination of liposuction and lipolysis

Since the amount of fat left is small, laser has to be used carefully to avoid burning.

After LAL is complete, the emulsified fat may be removed by aspiration with traditional liposuction. This part is again similar to that is done in liposuction and hence, will not be elaborated. Adit sites are left open for drainage and wound dressings applied in a manner similar to traditional tumescent liposuction. Patients wear compression bandages or garments for 2–3 weeks. Patients may resume daily activities as tolerated, usually within 24 hours. Pain management usually requires only acetaminophen, and occasionally, a codeine-containing medication. Patients can usually resume vigorous physical activity within days. Postoperative physiotherapeutic treatments or lymphatic drainage massage are used by some to accelerate patient recovery and enhance the clinical result (Fig. 6).

COMPLICATIONS/ADVERSE EFFECTS/PRECAUTIONS

The complication rate after LAL is extremely low in well-trained hands, estimated at 0.93% according to a prospective trial in 537 patients.[8]

- Ecchymoses, edema, and pain are common but minor and self-limiting, similar to those expected after liposuction[10,17,20]
- Laser burns are rare;[17,20] we have not witnessed this complication in any patient thus far
- Paresthesias and hyperpigmentation have also been reported[6,20]
- Rare side effects similar to liposuction related complications are also possible, including seroma, infection, neuropathy, and minor contour irregularities. The presence of tumescent fluid may provide some

epidermal protection. According to Mordon et al.,[18] cooled tumescent fluid infiltration decreases skin surface temperature greatly

- A theoretic concern of LAL is its effects on serum lipid levels. Laser induced adipocyte rupture causes the release of intracellular lipid contents, and how this is metabolized by the body is unclear. Studies on lipid levels after LAL indicate no change in serum lipid levels after the procedure.[18,20]

Mordon et al.[18] followed serial lipid panels in four patients for 30 days after LAL and found no deviation from baseline levels. Goldman et al.[21] conducted LAL with a 1,064 nm and observed no increase in cholesterol or triglyceride levels after the procedure. Woodhall et al.[16] also found no change in triglycerides in 39 patients undergoing LAL with the 1,064 nm, 1,320 nm, or multiplex (1,064–1,320 nm) device. Given the lack of serum lipid level elevation, there seems to be no lipid related renal or hepatotoxicity risk. Lipid metabolism after LAL has not been specifically studied although mechanisms of action have been postulated. Lipid metabolism may occur slowly, avoiding changes in serum lipid levels or alternatively, lipids may be cleared through a phagocytic route via macrophage digestion.[18]

CONCLUSION

Despite laser technology being available for a number of years, the laser is yet to find a prime place in routine liposuction. This reflects both the outstanding efficacy and safety of tumescent liposuction and also the evolving phase of laser. While recent machines have established safety profile, improved efficacy and additional benefit for skin tightening, the scenario is changing and laser lipolysis has emerged as a useful procedure for small areas and as an adjuvant procedure for liposuction. With further advances, such as use of simultaneous aspiration and suction, and dual wavelength technologies, this field may emerge as an alternative to liposuction.

ACKNOLWEDGEMENT

The authors gratefully acknolwedge the assistance of Dr Gayatri Khatri MD DNB FRUGHS in proof correction of this chapter.

REFERENCES

1. Venkataram J. Tumescent liposuction: a review. J Cutan Aesthet Surg. 2008;1(2):49-57.
2. Mordon S, Eymard-Maurin AF, Wassmer B, Ringot J, et al. Histologic evaluation of laser lipolysis: pulsed 1064-nm Nd:YAG laser versus cw 980-nm diode laser. Aesthet Surg J. 2007;27(3):263-8.
3. Apfelberg DB. Results of multicenter study of laser-assisted liposuction. Clin Plast Surg. 1996;23(4):713-9.
4. Apfelberg DB, Rosenthal S, Hunstad JP, Achauer B, Fodor PB. Progress report on multicenter study of laser-assisted liposuction. Aesthet Plast Surg. 1994;18(3):259-64.
5. Uebelhoer NS, Ross EV. Introduction. Update on lasers. Semin Cutan Med Surg. 2008;27(4):221-6.
6. Goldman A, Gotkin RH. Laser-assisted liposuction. Clin Plast Surg. 2009;36(2):241-53.
7. Katz B, McBean J Cheung JS. The new laser liposuction for men. Dermatol Ther. 2007;20(6):448-51.
8. Katz B, McBean J. Laser-assisted lipolysis: a report on complications. J Cosmet Laser Ther. 2008;10(4):231-3.
9. Badin AZ, Moraes LM, Gondek L, Chiaratti MG, Canta L. Laser lipolysis: flaccidity under control. Aesthet Plast Surg. 2002;26(5):335-9.
10. Goldman A. Submental Nd: Yag laser-assisted liposuction. Lasers Surg Med. 2006;38(3):181-184.
11. Reynaud JP, Skibinski M, Wassmer B, Rochon P, Mordon S, et al. Lipolysis using a 980-nm diode laser: a retrospective analysis of 534 procedures. Aesthet Plast Surg. 2009;33(1):28-36.
12. Parlette EC, Kaminer ME. Laser-assisted liposuction: here's the skinny. Semin Cutan Med Surg. 2008;27(4):259-63.
13. Mordon SR, Wassmer B, Reynaud JP, Zemmouri J. Mathematical modeling of laser lipolysis. Biomed Eng Online. 2008;7:10.
14. Sun Y, Wu SF, Yan S, Shi HY, Chen D, Chen Y. Laser lipolysis used to treat localized adiposis: a preliminary report on experience with Asian patients. Aesthet Plast Surg. 2009;33(5):701-5.
15. Badin AZ, Gondek LB, Garcia MJ, Valle LC, Flizikowski FB, de Noronha L. Analysis of laser lipolysis effects on human tissue samples obtained from liposuction. Aesthet Plast Surg. 2005;29(4):281-6.
16. Woodhall KE, Saluja R, Khoury J, Goldman MP. A comparison of three separate clinical studies evaluating the safety and efficacy of laser-assisted lipolysis using 1064 nm, 1320 nm, and a combined 1064/1320 nm multiplex device. Dermatol Surg Med. 2009;41(10:774-8.
17. Goldman A, Gotkin RH, Sarnoff DS, Prati C, Rossato F. Cellulite: a new treatment approach combining subdermal Nd:YAG laser lipolysis and autologous fat transplantation. Aesthet Surg J. 2008;28(6):656-62.
18. Mordon S, Wassmer B, Rochon P, Desmyttere J, Grard C, Stalnikiewicz G, et al. Serum lipid changes following laser lipolysis. J Cosmet Laser Ther. 2009;11(2):74-7.
19. DiBernardo BE, Reyes J, Chen B. Evaluation of tissue thermal effects from 1064/1320-nm laser-assisted lipolysis and its clinical implications. J Cosmet Laser Ther. 2009;11(2):62-9.
20. Kim KH, Geronemus RG. Laser lipolysis using a novel 1,064 nm Nd:YAG laser. Dermatol Surg. 2006;32(2):241-8.
21. Goldman AG, Schavelzon D, Blugerman GS, et al. Liposuction using Nd: YAG laser. Rev Soc Bras Cir Plast. 2002;17:17-26.

CHAPTER 32

Cryolipolysis: Hype or Hope

Ankur Talwar, Kshama Talwar

INTRODUCTION

Body contouring remains among the most common cosmetic surgical procedures performed worldwide. In fact, liposuction was found to be the most common surgical procedure performed in the United States in the year 2013 followed by breast augmentation. Despite its popularity, there remain rare but significant risks regarding liposuction, including complications from anesthesia, infections, and even death.[1] Although liposuction is an effective therapeutic option for the removal of excess adipose tissue, it remains an invasive procedure and carries the inherent risks associated with surgery. In recent years, a number of modalities have become available for the noninvasive reduction of adipose tissue, including cryolipolysis, radiofrequency, low level laser, and high intensity focused ultrasound. Each technology employs a different mechanism of action to cause apoptosis or necrosis of the targeted adipocytes. These modalities primarily target the physical properties of fat that differentiate it from the overlying epidermis and dermis, thus resulting in selective destruction of fat.

Cryolipolysis is defined as noninvasive cooling of adipose tissue to induce lipolysis—the breaking down of fat cells—to reduce body fat without damage to other tissues.

HISTORY

The scientific principles of cryolipolysis were discovered by Manstein and Anderson, at Massachusetts General Hospital in Boston.[2] The development behind cryolipolysis stems from the clinical observation of cold-induced panniculitis which leads to transient fat necrosis. These observations led to the concept that lipid-rich tissues are more susceptible to cold injury than the surrounding water-rich tissue.

MECHANISM OF ACTION

The principle behind this technology exploits the premise that adipocytes are more susceptible to cooling than other skin cells. Precise application of cold temperatures triggers the death of adipocytes that are subsequently engulfed and digested by macrophages.[3] Immediately following the treatment, an inflammatory process is triggered by the apoptosis of adipocytes, as reflected by an influx of inflammatory cells, which can be seen within 3 days after treatment and peaks at approximately 14 days as the adipocytes become surrounded by histiocytes, neutrophils, lymphocytes, and other mononuclear cells. At 14–30 days after treatment, macrophages and other phagocytes surround, envelope, and digest the lipid cells as part of the body's natural response to injury. Four weeks after treatment, the inflammation lessens and the adipocyte volume is decreased.

No changes in subcutaneous fat are seen immediately after treatment. The loss in volume of adipose tissue occurs gradually over time as the adipocytes are removed through an inflammatory clearing process that peaks within 2–3 months after cold exposure.[3] By this time, the fat volume in the treated area is apparently decreased and the septae account for the majority of the tissue volume.[4]

CONTROVERSIES

With the removal of the adipocytes internally, there has been concern that cryolipolysis may cause rising blood lipid levels and elevations in liver enzymes that may put the patient at additional risk, particularly for cardiovascular parameters. However, multiple studies have demonstrated that cholesterol, triglycerides, low density lipoprotein, high density lipoprotein, aspartate transaminase/alanine transaminase, total bilirubin, albumin, and glucose remained within normal limits during and after cryolipolysis.[5,6] It is not surprising that cryolipolysis has no effect on lipid levels since the resorption of fat after cryolipolysis occurs at a very slow rate.

EFFICACY

Preliminary human studies have evaluated efficacy of the cryolipolysis procedure using several measures: visible change in the surface contour, photographic assessment of baseline untreated area versus the same area post-treatment, and reduction in the fat layer thickness as measured with ultrasound. Data for six subjects treated on a single flank with the Zeltiq clinical prototype device at cooling intensity factor (CIF) 33 for 60 minutes showed a reduction in the size of the treated love handle in comparison to an untreated contralateral control.[7] Ultrasound at 2 months demonstrated an average fat layer reduction of 20.4% across the treated area. These findings were also supported by efficacy data from a larger study of 32 subjects treated with above parameters for 60 minutes that resulted in an average fat layer reduction of 22.4% at 4 months post-treatment.[8] A third study demonstrated similar efficacy using a range of treatment parameters (CIF 37–42, for 30 or 45 minutes) with evidence of fat layer reduction at 6 months.[9]

Another study used a three-dimensional camera to evaluate the amount of fat loss after cryolipolysis.[10] Mean fat loss between baseline and the 2-month follow-up visit was 56.2 ± 25.6 mL on the treated side and 16.6 ± 17.6 mL on the control side ($p < 0.0001$). Two months post-treatment, the mean difference in fat loss between the treated and untreated sides was 39.6 mL.[10]

The long-term duration of effect of cryolipolysis has not been evaluated as yet. Although little is known about the durability of fat loss induced by selective cryolipolysis, there is no evidence that the fat lost after cold exposure could regenerate. A small study of two cases who were followed up for a period of 5 years post procedure found the fat reduction to be durable despite fluctuations in the body temperature. [11]

SIDE EFFECTS

A low profile of adverse effects is one of the main advantages with cryolipolysis, especially when compared with more invasive measures. Only mild, short-term side effects, such as erythema, bruising, changes in sensation, and pain, were reported in the studies reviewed. The most common complaint is late-onset pain, occurring 2 weeks postprocedure that resolves without intervention. Erythema was noted in multiple studies immediately after the treatment and subsided within a week.[12] Swelling and bruising of the area were shown to a slightly lesser extent than erythema. Hyper- and hyposensitivity were shown in studies but were never debilitating nor persisted beyond 1 month. Coleman et al. demonstrated that patients exhibiting reduction in sensation recovered normal sensation in 3.6 weeks.[7] This study also showed that a nerve biopsy taken at 3 months after treatment showed no long-term changes to nerve fibers concluding that temperature and duration of cryolipolysis have no permanent effect on nervous tissue.[7]

A rare side effect of this technique is paradoxical adipose hyperplasia with an estimated incidence of 0.0051%, or approximately one in 20,000.[13] Affected patients exhibit fat loss after therapy and then develop a large, demarcated, tender fat mass at the site 2–3 months later. The hypothesized pathogenesis includes recruitment of stem cells and hypertrophy of existing fat cells in the area.[13]

AVAILABLE DEVICES AND THE PROCEDURE

In 2010, the Food and Drug Administration (FDA) cleared a cryolipolytic device (CoolSculpting®) for reduction of flank and abdominal fat. In April 2014, the FDA also cleared this system for the treatment of subcutaneous fat in the thighs (Fig. 1). One part of the device is a cup-shaped applicator with two cooling panels that is applied to the treatment area (Fig. 2). The tissue is drawn into the handpiece under moderate vacuum and the selected temperature is modulated by thermoelectric elements and controlled by sensors that monitor the heat flux out of the tissue (Fig. 3). Each area is treated for approximately 45–60 minutes.

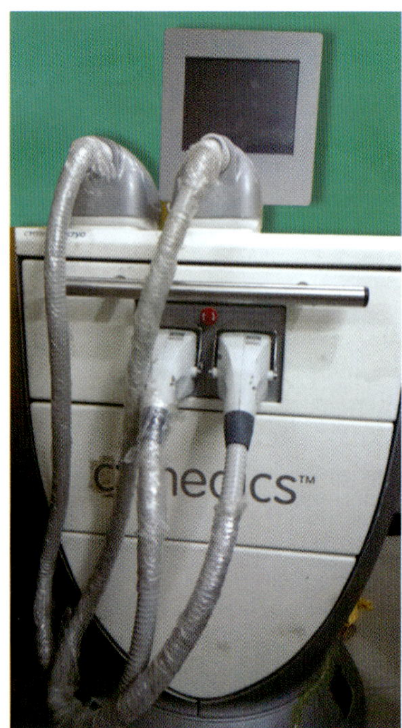

FIG. 1: Cryolipolysis machine with the display monitor and two cup-shaped applicators
Courtesy: Cymedics Cryolipolysis Ltd.

There has been a study which concluded that addition of a 2 minutes massage to the treated area immediately after the procedure enhanced the efficacy of a single cryolipolysis treatment.[14] The procedure described consists of 1 minute of vigorous kneading of the treated tissue between the thumb and fingers followed by 1 minute of circular massage of the treated tissue against the patient's body. Another study described cryolipolysis with 5 minutes of post-treatment integrated preset mechanical massage using the device applicator with excellent outcomes.

The patient is then discharged home and is free to resume normal activities immediately after treatment.

The number of treatment cycles needed depends on the treatment area. While good results at the flanks can usually be achieved with only one treatment, the back and the inner and outer thighs often require more than two treatments. Repeated treatment sessions should be spaced 8 weeks apart to allow the inflammatory process to resolve.[15] The body sites at which cryolipolysis was most effective were the abdomen, back, and flank.[16]

Because cryolipolysis is still a relatively new procedure, treatment protocols have yet to be optimized to maximize results. Many studies assessed the theoretical enhanced efficacy with multiple treatments in the same anatomic area and demonstrated that a second successive course of cryolipolysis treatment led to further fat reduction.[17] It is

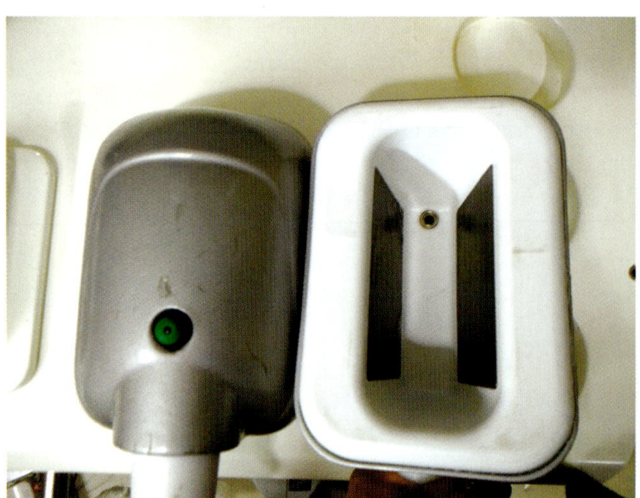

FIG. 2: Cryolipolysis applicator showing the two cooling panels on the inner surface

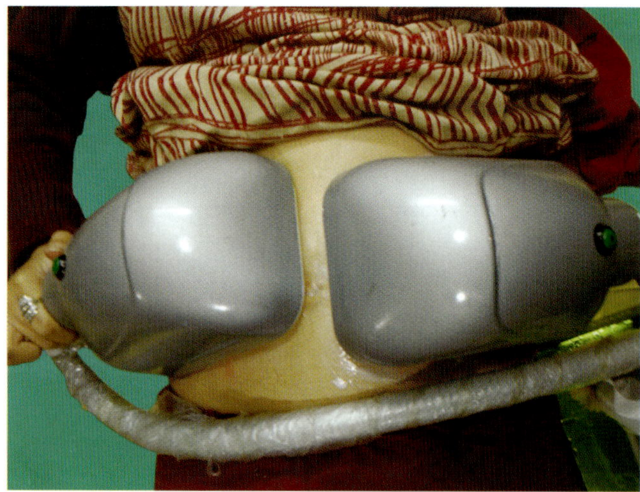

FIG. 3: Applicators attached on both sides of abdomen to reducer "belly" fat

important to note that although a subsequent treatment leads to further fat reduction, the extent of improvement was not as dramatic as the first treatment. Interestingly, one study demonstrated that a second treatment enhanced fat layer reduction in the abdomen area but not the love handles.[18]

LIMITATIONS

Although cryolipolysis is a promising new technology, it is important to bear in mind a few potential limitations. In the human clinical studies, results were most visible in patients with discrete, localized fat bulges. Cryolipolysis does not appear to be as effective in obese patients or patients with excess skin laxity. It is unclear whether the device itself is less effective in these patients or whether the potential improvement associated with cryolipolysis treatment is harder to observe in these patients. Thus, patients seeking large scale fat removal, which can be achieved with liposuction, may not achieve their desired outcomes with cryolipolysis. It is, therefore, important for physicians to carefully select potential cryolipolysis treatment patients, as well as educate them regarding their expected outcomes and potential limitations.

Additionally, the improvement following cryolipolysis is not immediate but rather occurs slowly over the course of 2–3 months.

CONCLUSION

Body contouring remains among the most common cosmetic surgical procedures performed. Although liposuction is an effective therapeutic option for the removal of excess adipose tissue, it remains an invasive procedure and carries the inherent risks associated with surgery. In recent years, new modalities have been developed to address body contouring from a less invasive perspective. These modalities primarily target the physical properties of fat that differentiate it from the overlying epidermis and dermis, thus resulting in selective destruction of fat.

Cryolipolysis is a novel procedure, which uses controlled cold exposure, known as energy extraction, to produce noninvasive, effective, and selective damage to adipocytes. In animal and human clinical studies, cryolipolysis has been shown to result in significant improvement in the clinical appearance of fat. Additionally, reductions in the thickness of the subcutaneous fat layer of up to 50% can occur following a single cryolipolysis treatment. Clinical studies have shown potential efficacy in the treatment of excess back fat, flank fat, and abdominal fat; the potential efficacy of cryolipolysis in other treatment areas and for the treatment of cellulite remains to be determined. In these initial studies, cryolipolysis treatments have been well-tolerated by patients with transient, mild adverse events, such as erythema and bruising, occurring in treated patients (Fig. 4). No cases of ulceration, scarring, or significant changes in lipid profiles and liver function tests have been reported following cryolipolysis. Cryolipolysis, therefore, appears to be a safe and effective treatment option for reduction of excess adipose tissue. The device is particularly appealing given that it is noninvasive, requires not much or no downtime for patients following treatment, and does not require local or regional anesthesia. Ongoing clinical studies will help to determine the full potential and efficacy of this device. Cryolipolysis appears to be a promising new technology for safe, effective, and noninvasive treatment of fat.

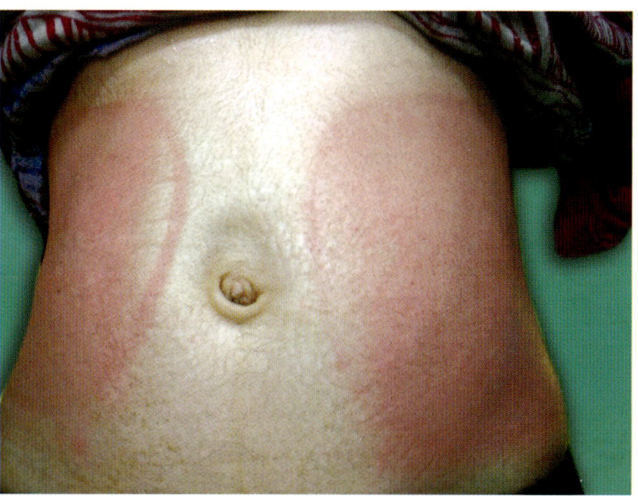

FIG. 4: Erythema and edema seen immediately following the removal of handpiece post procedure

REFERENCES

1. Rao RB, Ely SF, Hoffman RS. Deaths related to liposuction. N Engl J Med. 1999;340(19):1471-5.
2. Manstein D, Laubach H, Watanabe K, Farinelli W, Zurakowski D, Anderson RR. Selective cryolysis: a novel method of non-invasive fat removal. Lasers Surg Med. 2008;40(9):595-4.
3. Zelickson B, Egbert BM, Preciado J, Allison J, Springer K, Rhoades RW, et al. Cryolipolysis for noninvasive fat cell destruction: initial results from a pig model. Dermatol Surg. 2009;35(10):1462-70.
4. Nelson AA, Wasserman D, Avram MM. Cryolipolysis for reduction of excess adipose tissue. Semin Cutan Med Surg. 2009;28(4):244-9.
5. Ferraro GA, De Francesco F, Cataldo C, Rossano F, Nicoletti G, D'Andrea F. Synergistic effects of cryolipolysis and shock waves for noninvasive body contouring. Aesthetic Plast Surg. 2012;36(3):666-79.

6. Riopelle JT, Kovach B. Lipid and liver function effects of the cryolipolysis procedure in a study of male love handle reduction. Lasers Surg Med. 2009;82.
7. Coleman SR, Sachdeva K, Egbert BM, Preciado J, Allison J. Clinical efficacy of noninvasive cryolipolysis and its effects on peripheral nerves. Aesthetic Plast Surg. 2009;33:482-8.
8. Dover J, Burns J, Coleman S, Fitzpatrick R, Garden J, Goldberg D, et al. A prospective clinical study of noninvasive cryolipolysis for subcutaneous fat layer reduction—Interim report of available subject data. Lasers Surg Med. 2009;41(S21):43.
9. Riopelle J, Tsai M, Kovach B. Lipid and liver function effects of the cryolipolysisTM procedure in a study of male love handle reduction. ASLMS e-Poster, 2009.
10. Bernstein EF. Longitudinal evaluation of cryolipolysis efficacy: two case studies. J Cosmet Dermatol.2013;12(2):149-52.
11. Dierickx CC, Mazer JM, Sand M, Koenig S, Arigon V. Safety, tolerance, and patient satisfaction with noninvasive cryolipolysis. Dermatol Surg. 2013;39(8):1209-16.
12. Jalian HR, Avram MM, Garibyan L, Mihm MC, Anderson RR. Paradoxical adipose hyperplasia after cryolipolysis. JAMA Dermatol. 2014;150(3):317-9.
13. Boey GE, Wasilenchuk JL. Enhanced clinical outcome with manual massage following cryolipolysis treatment: a 4-month study of safety and efficacy. Lasers Surg Med. 2014;46(1):20-6.
14. Sasaki GH, Abelev N, Tevez-Ortiz A. Noninvasive selective cryolipolysis and reperfusion recovery for localized natural fat reduction and contouring. Aesthet Surg J. 2014;34(3):420-31.
15. Avram MM, Harry RS. Cryolipolysis for subcutaneous fat layer reduction. Lasers Surg Med. 2009;41(10):703-8.
16. Dierickx CC, Mazer JM, Sand M, Koenig S, Arigon V. Safety, tolerance, and patient satisfaction with noninvasive cryolipolysis. Dermatol Surg. 2013;39(8):1209-16.
17. Pinto HR, Garcia-Cruz E, Melamed GE. A study to evaluate the action of lipocryolysis. Cryo Letters. 2012;33(3):177-81.
18. Shek SY, Chan NP, Chan HH. Non-invasive cryolipolysis for body contouring in Chinese—A first commercial experience. Lasers Surg Med. 2012;44(2):125-30.

CHAPTER 33

Lasers in Onychomycosis

Aarti Sarda, Nidhi Sharma

INTRODUCTION

Onychomycosis is undoubtedly the most common disease affecting the nails, representing up to 50% of all ungual pathologies.[1,2] More than just a cosmetic concern, onychomycosis has no tendency for spontaneous remission and is an extremely difficult condition to treat. High prevalence of the disease together with limited efficacy of conventional therapies, has stimulated the development of new and more effective approaches in treating the disease.[3]

Many device based therapies have been used recently in the treatment of onychomycosis. Lasers that have been used for this indication include the carbon dioxide, neodymium doped yttrium-aluminium-garnet (Nd:YAG), 870/930 nm combinations, and femtosecond infrared 800 nm lasers.[4] The 2,940 nm erbium doped yttrium aluminium garnet (Er:YAG) laser has been used to ablate the nail plate to enhance topical drug delivery.[3]

MECHANISM OF ACTION

Lasers emit narrow spectra light to achieve photo-effect in the targeted tissue. The effects can induce photochemical, photomechanical and photothermal changes in the target. The primary mechanism of action of most lasers is photothermal, wherein light energy is converted to heat, which in turn damages the target tissue.[5]

To treat onychomycosis by thermal means, the laser must have the ability to penetrate under the nail plate in order to reach the fungal colonies of the nail bed and nail matrix. When it gets to that point, it should be able to induce high temperatures in the fungal matter under the nail plate for long enough periods to cause fungal thermolysis, while keeping the surrounding temperature below the threshold for pain and necrosis.[6,7] Though laser energy has been shown to eliminate dermatophytes *in vitro*, direct laser elimination of onychomycosis is not successful due to difficulties in delivering laser energy to deeper levels of the nail plate without collateral damage.[8]

Selective photothermolysis is a mechanism by which there is specific targeting of certain tissue or foreign matter, causing locally confined heating and minimal effects in the surrounding tissues.[9] The wavelength of light is a primary laser parameter required for selective photothermolysis. The choice of wavelength depends on the choice and distribution of chromophobe and the required penetration depth of light. To target the chromophobe, distribution and density of the chromophobe has to be kept in mind. The targeted chromophobe should be abundant in fungal hyphae and conidia and less prevalent in the nail plate, nail bed and surrounding skin. Possible chromophobes include chitin, melanin, and other common fungal pigments. Density of chromophobe should be much higher in the target than the surrounding tissue so more heat is imparted into the target.[5]

It is suspected that due to its longer wavelength, the 1,064 nm Nd:YAG is able to more deeply penetrate tissue and efficiently target fungal overgrowth in the nail bed.[10] The 532 nm wavelength is well absorbed by red pigment, xanthomegnin in *T. rubrum*, which has peak absorption between 406 and 555 nm.[11] This, thereby generates mechanical damage in the irradiated fungal colony. The 1,064 nm setting is beyond the absorption spectrum of xanthomelanin, but its effectiveness is due to another chromophobe, perhaps melanin, which is present in the fungal cell wall.[12]

Besides the wavelength to target a certain chromophobe, there are several laser parameters that must be calibarated to selectively target fungal matter. These parameters include the spatial and temporal pulse format, peak and average power, pulse energy, and spot size of the laser beam.[5] The setting should be able to destroy the target chromophobe without damaging the surrounding nail tissue.

The temporal pulse format of the laser is the way in which the pulse energy is distributed in time, including pulse duration, substructure, and pulse repetition rate. For photothermal interactions to be selective, the duration of pulse should be shorter than the thermal relaxation time of the target.

Fungal hyphae are cylindrical structures with a thin chitin wall, which is a better insulator than the dermal cell membrane. Conidia are spherical and have a thicker wall than hyphae. Since heat loss occurs through surface, cylindrical hyphae would have a thermal relaxation time roughly three-fourths of the conidia of similar composition and dimension but the relaxation time for long cylindrical mycelia would be only two-thirds of that of conidia. To confine heat in both the fungal structures, the pulse duration should be of a few microseconds or shorter.[5]

Proper spacing of the pulses helps in dissipation of heat in the healthy tissue. Dermal cells have a highly conducive membrane and high water content than fungi and hence have higher thermal conductivity than fungal cells. Circulatory system and lymphatics, as well as convective airflow and radiation, act to dissipate heat from the lasered tissue.

The pulse structure should be designed so as to target fungal elements, inducing a progressive and absorption, high water content tissues, and vascular flow will help in rapid dissemination of laser energy, thus antitargeting the nail bed and other dermal tissues.

The effective penetration depth and irradiated tissue volume depends on the spot size and beam shape. The fluence that falls off with the penetration depth can be reduced by using a large spot size, however, large high energy beams heat large tissue volumes and can thus lead to side effects. It is best to select a spot size that provides a fluence needed to treat the fungus. The peak power should be kept below the ablation threshold of the nail plate and healthy dermal tissues.[5]

LASER USED FOR ONYCHOMYCOSIS

In vitro studies of commercial laser models have yielded poor to mixed results. Long pulse systems cause bulk heating of fungal colonies in the nail bed with associated discomfort which necessitates multiple treatments and a high treatment failure.[13] Clinical trials have largely been open label trials with mixed results ranging from 0 to 100% mycological cure rates[14-22] (Table 1).

CONCLUSION

Due to their minimally invasive nature and potential to restore clear nail growth with relatively few sessions, lasers potentially represent a bright future as regards to onychomycosis treatment. Lasers have the advantage of having few contraindications and minimal side effects. The fungal elements are believed to be forming a biofilm, making them refractory to therapy. Laser therapy seems not to be affected by this biofilm formation.

Available data on the use of lasers in onychomycosis is still incipient. Primary research on fungal chromophobes, the thermal properties of the fungal hyphae, and a clear understanding on laser penetrance through an infected nail plate are essential to achieve selective photothermolysis. The results of early in vitro and *in vivo* studies have yielded poor results. This is most likely attributable to the use of nonoptimal preexisting laser systems without reoptimization for the fungal target. Randomized control trials are needed to determine the efficacy of lasers in onychomycosis. Further efforts toward the establishment of standard treatment schedules as well as the best pulse characteristics with regards to fluence, length and format, are still required.

TABLE 1: Clinical trials of laser therapy for onychomycosis

Study	Laser	No. of patients	Diagnosis	Pulse duration	Frequency	Spot size	Energy	Sessions	Follow-up	Cure rate	Adverse effect
Morais et al.	Er:YAG Etherea 2,940 nm	–	–	2 ms	1 Hz	–	50 ms/mtz (microthermal zone)	–	–	–	Mild discomfort, pain, overheating sensation, bleeding
Myres et al.	Q-switch eye-safe Er:YAG 1,534 nm	12	–	6 ns–3 ms	Single shot, 3 Hz, 5 Hz	2 mm	15–100 mJ	1–2	<6 months	–	–
Bornstein et al.	Dual wavelength, 870/930 nm	–	Culture	–	–	–	–	4	2 months	4/7 pts	Heat, tingling
Landsman et al.	Dual wavelength near infrared diode laser (Noveon)	26	Culture	–	–	15 mm	204–424	4	6 months	85%	–
Afpelberg et al.	CO_2	8	–	–	–	–	–	1	–	6/8	–
Bovoroy et al.	CO_2	200	–	–	–	–	–	–	3 years	75	–
Harris et al.	PinPointe Footlaser	14	–	–	–	2.5 mm	–	1	6 months	80%	–
Kozarev et al., 2011	Long pulsed VSP Nd:YAG Dualis,SP,Fotona	14	Microscopy/ culture	25 ms	1	4 mm	35–40 J/cm^2	4	3 months	93	Pain
Kozarev et al., 2010	Long pulsed VSP Nd:YAG Dualis, SP, Fotona	162	Microscopy/ culture	35 ms	1	4 mm	35–40 J/cm^2	4	12–30 months	95.8%	–
Weiss et al.	Long pulsed VSP Nd:YAG Cutera Genesis plus	7	Not specified	300 µs	2	5 mm	16	2	12 months	70%	–
Hochman	1,064 nm Nd:YAG Light Pod Neo	8	Culture/ microscopy	0.65 ms	–	2 mm	223 J/cm^2	2–3	6 months	87.5%	–
Kimura	1,064 nm Nd:YAG	13	Microscopy	0.30 ms	–	5 mm	14 J/cm^2	1–3	4 months	51%	–
Waibel et al.	Nd:YAG Clearsense	7	Culture/PAS	300 µs	6	-	13	4	6 months	100%	–
Carney et al.	Nd:YAG Laser Genesis	14	Culture	0.3 ms	2	5	16	5	6 months	33%	–
Hollmig et al.	Nd:YAG Joule Clearsense	17	Culture/PAS	300 µs	6	6	5	2	3 months	33%	–
Noguchi et al.	Nd:YAG Gentle Yag Candela	12	Culture	500 µs	2	6	10	3	6 months	0%	–
Moon et al.	Nd:YAG Clearsense	13	Culture/KOH	300 µs	5	6	5	5	6 months	70%	–

Continued

Continued

Study	Laser	No. of patients	Diagnosis	Pulse duration	Frequency	Spot size	Energy	Sessions	Follow-up	Cure rate	Adverse effect
Hees	Short pulsed Nd:YAG	10	Culture/HPE	40 µs		3	50	2	9 months	20	–
Kalokasidis et al.	Q-switchd Q clear Lightage 532/1064	131	Microscopy/ culture	ns, µs	5 Hz	2.5 mm	14 J/cm2	2	3 months	95.4	Mild pain
Garcia et al.	Q-clear Lightage	62	KOH	ns, µs	3	3	19	1	9 months	100%	–
Ortiz et al.	Nd:YAG 1,320 nm CT3Plus Coolbreze	10	–			5	3	4	3 months	50%	–
Zhang et al.	Long pulsed Nd:YAG 1,064 nm	33patients (154 nails)	–	–	–	–	–	4–8	6 months	51–68%	–
Gupta et al.	Nd:YAG JOULE Clearsense	21	Microscopy/ culture	0.3 ms	6	–	13	4	3 months	95%	–
Gupta et al.	Nd:YAG Q Clear	100	Microscopy/ culture	3-10 ns	–	2.5–6 mm	2–14	1	4 months	95%	–
Nouri et al.	Nd:YAG	1	–	–	–	–	–	4	3 months	–	–

Nd:YAG, neodymium doped yttrium-aluminum-garnet; Er:YAG, erbium doped yttrium-aluminum-garnet; PAS, periodic acid–Schiff; KOH, potassium hydroxide; HPE, histopathological examination; mtz, microthermal zone.

REFERENCES

1. Araújo AJG, Bastos OMP, Souza MAJ, Oliveira JC. Occurrence of onychomycosis among patients attended in dermatology offices in the city of Rio de Janeiro, Brazil. An Bras Dermatol. 2003;78:299-308.
2. Gupta AK, Simpson FC. New therapeutic options for onychomycosis. Expert Opin Pharmacother. 2012;13:1131-42.
3. Morais O, Costa I, Gomes C, Shinzato D, Ayres G, Cardoso RM. The use of the Er-YAG 2940nm laser associated with amorolfine lacquer in the treatment of onychomycosis. An Bras Dermatol. 2013;88(5):847-9.
4. Ledon J, Savas J, Franca K, Nouri K. Laser and light therapy for onychomycosis: a systematic review. Lasers Med Sci. 2014;29(2):823-9.
5. Gupta A, Simpson FC, Heller DF. The future of lasers in onychomycosis. J Dermatolog Treat. 2016;27(2):167-72.
6. Essien JP, Umoh AA, Akpan EJ, Eduok DI, Umoiyoho A. Growth, keratinolytic proteinase activity and thermotolerance of dermatophytes associated with apolecia in Uyo, Nigeria. Acta Microbiol Immunol Hung. 2009;56(1):61-9.
7. Essien JP, Umoh AA, Akpan EJ, Eduok DI, Umoiyoho A. Heat resistance of dermatophyte's conidiospores from athletes kits stored in Nigerian University Sport's centre. Acta Microbiol Immunol Hung. 2009;56(1):71-9.
8. Manevich Z, Lev D, Hochberg M, Palhan M, Lewis A, Enk CD. Direct antifungal effect of femtosecond laser on Trichophyton rubrum onychomycosis. Photochem Photobiol. 2010;86:476-9.
9. Anderson RR, Pariiish JA. Selective photothermolysis: precise microgurgery by selective absorption of pulsed radiation. Science. 1983;220:524-7.
10. Yang MU, Yaroslavsky AN, Farinelli Wa, Flotte TJ, Rius-Diaz F, Tsao SS, et al. Long pulsed neodymium-aluminium-garnet laser treatment for port wine stains. J Am Acad Dermatol. 2005;52(3 Pt 1):480-90.
11. Gupta AK, Ahmad I, Borst I, Summerbell RC. Detection of xanthomegnin in epidermal materials infected with Trichophyton rubrum. J Invest Dermatol. 2000;115(5):901-5.
12. Vural E, Winfield HL, Shingleton AW, Horn TD, Shafirstein G. The effects of laser irradiation on Trichophyton rubrum growth. Lasers Med Sci. 2008;23:349-53.
13. Kostas K, Onder M, Traketelli M, Richard B, Fritz K. The Effect of Q-Switched Nd:YAG 1064 nm/532 nm Laser in the Treatment of Onychomycosis In Vivo. Dermatol Res Pract. 2013;2013:379725.
14. Myres MJ, Myres JA, Roth F, Guo B, Hardy CR, Myres S, et al. Treatment of toe nail fungus infection using an AO Q-switched eye-safe erbium glass laser at 1534 nm. Photonic Therapeutics and Diagnostics, Paper No. 8565-31.
15. Carney C, Cantrell W, Warner J, Elewski B. Treatment of onychomycosis using a submillisecond 287 1064 nm neodymium:yttrium-aluminum-garnet laser. J Am Acad Dermatol. 2013;69(4):578-82.
16. Hochman LG. Laser treatment of onychomychosis using a novel 0,65-milisecond pulsed Nd:YAG-nm laser. J Cosmet Laser Ther. 2011;13(1): 2-5.
17. Landsman AS, Robbins AH, Angelini PF, Wu CC, Cook J, Oster M, et al. Treatment of mild, moderate, severe onychomycosis using 870 and 930 nm light exposure. J Am Podiatr Med Assoc. 2010;100(3):166-77; Waibel J, Wulken AJ, Rudnick A. Prospective efficacy and safety evaluation of laser treatments with real-time temperature feedback for fungal onychomycosis. J Drugs Dermatol. 2013;12(11):1237-42.
18. Ledon JA, Savas J, Franca K, Chacon A, Nouri K. Laser and light therapy for onychomycosis: a systematic review. Lasers Med Sci. 2014;29(2):823-9.
19. Bornstein E. A review of current research in light-based technologies for treatment of podiatric infections disease states. J Am Pediatr Med Assoc. 2009;99(4):348-52.
20. Kimura U, Takeuchi K, Kinoshita A, Takamori K, Hiruma M, Suga Y. Treating onychomycosis of the toenail: clinical efficacy of the sub-millisecond 1,064 nm Nd:YAG laser using a 5 mm spot diameter. J Drugs Dermatol. 2012;11(4):496-504.
21. Naouri M, Mazer JM. Traitment d'une onychomycose digitale à Candida tropicalis par laser Nd:YAG short pulse. Ann Dermatol Venereol. 2013;140(10):610-3.
22. Carney C, Cantrell W, Warner J, Elewski B. Treatment of onychomycosis using a submillisecond 1064-nm neodymium:yttrium-aluminum-garnet laser. J Am Acad Dermatol. 2013;69(4):578-82.

CHAPTER 34

Laser Training in India and the World

Rashmi Sarkar, Bhawna Wadhwa

INTRODUCTION

Laser, as a part of dermatosurgery, is gaining a lot of momentum in dermatological practice these days. An appropriate set of guidelines for laser training are lacking in India. According to Indian Association of Dermatologists, Venereologists, and Leprologists (IADVL),[1] a physician performing laser should have the following qualifications:

- He/she should be a qualified dermatologist (MD or DVD)
- The physician should have basic knowledge and training about laser physics and laser tissue interaction
- The training may be obtained during postgraduation if the institute for postgraduation provides such training or later in dedicated workshops. Proper hands on training should be obtained from equipment supplier's medical experts or from a dermatologist or plastic surgeon experienced in performing the procedure
- The physician should be familiar with early recognition, prevention, and treatment of postlaser complications like hypopigmentation or hyperpigmentation, scarring, burns, etc.

There are several laser and dermatosurgery centers in India and abroad which offer training and fellowships in lasers. Information about these centers is patchy in the literature. Most of them are providing training for part time technicians. We will mention a few of them, mainly those run by dermatologists and plastic surgeons and that offer training to dermatologists.

INDIAN CENTERS

Indian Association of Dermatologists, Venereologists, and Leprologists Training Fellowships[2]

These are open to any life or provisional member of IADVL, who is not working in the same institution, who have completed their degree or diploma and whose age is less than 35 years at the time of commencement of fellowship. The duration of training is 4 weeks. The training is provided at one of the following places, as selected by the candidate:

- All India Institute of Medical Sciences, New Delhi
- Postgraduate Institute of Medical Education and Research, Chandigarh. It provides Maya Devi Fellowship in Dermatosurgery
- Rita Skin Foundation, Kolkata. It provides Fellowship in Dermatosurgery and Cosmetology under Dr Malakar
- Amala Institute of Medical Sciences, Kerala provides Fellowship in Dermatosurgery under Dr Criton
- In Thiruvananthapuram, Kerala—Fellowship in Lasers under Dr Nair
- AKJN Skin and Laser Center, Chennai holds Laser Dermatology Fellowship under Dr Selvam.

These may vary after every couple of years. The details are made available at the website www.iadvl.org.

Laser training at Derma-Care,[3] Mangalore, under Dr Pai: it trains skin specialists, general doctors, and aestheticians in laser and cosmetology. Dermatologists require 2 weeks while others need 4 weeks training, including hands-on training on lasers like erbium doped yttrium-aluminium-garnet, Pixel erbium, Q-switched neodymium doped yttrium-aluminium-garnet, intense pulsed light (IPL), diode, and Soprano diode.

Certificate training in lasers at SP Derma Center,[4] Madurai, Tamil Nadu, under Dr Prasad: it offers dermatosurgery and laser surgery training program as a certificate course for dermatologists and plastic surgeons. It is a one-to-one intensive training program for a compulsory period of 2–4 weeks, depending on the training module selected. First week is an observership week and second week is hands-on training. During observership, the doctor has to learn all preoperative, postoperative, dressings, and complication handling connected with the procedure.

Laser training at Cosmetic Dermatology India,[5] at Aayna, New Delhi, under Dr Soin: doctors are trained in lasers in batches of one or two only.

FOREIGN CENTERS

Gateway Aesthetic Institute and laser center,[6] Salt Lake City, Utah, headed by Dr taylor: it offers a 1-year preceptorship open to board certified dermatologists or plastic surgeons. The course is for 40 hours per week.

Stanford School of Medicine, Redwood City,[7] Los Angeles: it offers 1-year pediatric dermatology fellowship of which laser surgery is a part.

National Laser Institute[8], United States: it offers a 12-day professional training for doctors in medical aesthetics including latest cosmetic lasers and injectables.

Northern Virginia Laser Training[9] or Nova Laser Training at Virginia Premier School for Laser: it provides advanced laser specialist certification course of 40 hours in mainly laser hair removal and IPL.

Esthetic Advisor Laser Academy,[10] Scottsdale: it provides 40 hours basic laser operative course and 48 hours hands-on laser course.

School of Medicine, University of California[11], Irvine: it offers procedural dermatology fellowship program, which is a 1-year Accreditation Council for Graduate Medical Education (ACGME) approved program and gives extensive training in dermatosurgery including laser surgery. Monthly hands-on workshops are carried on. Lasers for tattoo, hair, pigment, and vessel removal, non-ablative and ablative laser resurfacing, fractional erbium and carbon dioxide lasers are taught.

SkinCare Physicians, Boston Dermatologist Training Center[12]: each year, skin care physicians train three board eligible dermatologists in its cosmetic surgery and laser fellowship program which is accredited by American Society for Dermatologic Surgery (ASDS). The program is under the direction of Kenneth A Arndt, Jeffrey S Dover, Michael S Kaminer and Thomas E Rohrer.

In addition, lasers can be learnt in IADVL hands-on workshops and workshops held in conferences of Association of Cutaneous Surgeons of India (ACSI) and Cosmetic Dermatology Society of India (CDSI). Fellowships are also offered by ACSI and internationally under international mentorship program of International Society of Dermatology and ASDS.

CONCLUSION

So, with so many Indian and foreign laser training centres available at our disposal, dermatologists should make an effort to get basic laser training before starting a laser treatment centre to avoid any patient related issues in their practice.

REFERENCES

1. Dhepe N. Minimum standard guidelines of care on requirements for setting up a laser room. Indian J Dermatol Venereol Leprol. 2009;75:S101-10.
2. Indian Association of Dermatologists, Venereologists, and Leprologists. [online] Available from www.iadvl.org [Accessed February, 2016].
3. Derma-Care, Mangalore. [online] Available from www.derma-care.in [Accessed February, 2016].
4. SP Derma Center, Madurai. [online Available from www.spdermacenter.com [Accessed February, 2016].
5. Cosmetic Dermatology India, New Delhi. [online] Available from www.cosmeticdermatologyindia.com/doctortrainingcourse.php [Accessed February, 2016].
6. Gateway Aesthetic Institute and Laser Center, Salt lake City. [online] Available from gatewaylasercenter.com [Accessed February, 2016].
7. Stanford School of Medicine, Los Angeles. [online Available from http://dermatology.stanford.edu/fellowships/pedsfellowship.html [Accessed February, 2016].
8. National Laser Institute, United States. [online] Available from nationallaserinstitute.com [Accessed February, 2016].
9. Northern Virginia Laser Training or Nova Laser Training at Virginia Premier School for Laser. [online Avaliable from www.northernvirginialasertraining.com [Accessed February, 2016].
10. Esthetic Advisor laser academy, Scottsdale. [online] Available from www.aestheticlaseracademy.com [Accessed February, 2016].
11. School of Medicine, University of California, Irvine. [online] Available from www.dermatology.uci.edu/fellowships.asp [Accessed February, 2016].
12. SkinCare Physicians. [online] Available from www.skincarephysicians.net [Accessed February, 2016].

CHAPTER 35

When Lasers Go Wrong!

Chakravarthi R Srinivas, Muthuvel Kumaresan

INTRODUCTION

Laser procedures are commonly used in dermatology due to their low invasiveness, good results, and rapid recovery time. Laser devices offer high levels of safety, however, they can cause serious complications if used improperly. Adverse effects can still occur even with the best technology and physician care.

GENERAL SAFETY CONSIDERATIONS

- Lasers come under the category of class IV medical devices. These devices are dangerous to view either directly or when diffusely scattered, may cause significant skin damage and are a potential fire hazard
- Laser room should have a sign indicating when the laser is in use
- All the windows and doorways should be covered to prevent the escape of laser beam
- The laser machine should have an emergency shutdown option in case of any emergency
- Accidental fire during the laser procedure can be prevented by minimizing exposure to anesthetic gases, supplemental oxygen, and alcohol based products during the procedure
- Lasers should be kept in the standby mode when not in use to avoid inadvertent firing
- Persons unnecessary to the laser operation should be kept away from the laser operating area
- Appropriate eye safety wear should be provided according to the wavelength of the laser used to all the personnel in the treatment room.

OCULAR SAFETY FOR LASERS[1]

Eye protection is of prime importance during the laser procedure. Nature of the ocular injury depends on the wavelength of the laser. The target chromophores in the eye are melanin within the retinal pigmented epithelium, the iris, sclera, and choroid, hemoglobin within the retinal vasculature and water within the cornea and lens. Wavelength specific eye protection is recommended for the patient and the operator. Metal eye shields are recommended for the periocular area treatment and the metal eye shields for the treatment of facial lesions.

Exposure to lasers in the wavelength range of 400–1,400 nm may lead to partial or complete visual loss depending on the extent of injury and proximity of injury to the fovea, due to absorption by melanin within the retinal pigment epithelium. Direct foveal injury may lead to focal scotoma as well as complete blindness, while parafoveal injury may be limited to local inflammation and edema associated with transient visual loss. Exposure to ultraviolet and far-infrared wavelengths (1,400–10,600 nm) absorbed by water may lead to thermal injury to the cornea and lens.

COMPLICATIONS ASSOCIATED WITH ABLATIVE FRACTIONAL LASERS

Fractional carbon dioxide (CO_2) and erbium doped yttrium-aluminium-garnet (Er:YAG) lasers are increasingly used now for resurfacing. Adverse effects are commonly encountered with these devices irrespective of the precautions followed.

Erythema and Edema

Erythema and edema are commonly encountered following ablative laser resurfacing, usually subsides within few days. But rarely, these may persist for weeks or months. Supportive treatment with ice compressions and topical steroids reduces the erythema and edema over the treated areas.

Infections

The risk for bacterial, fungal, and viral infection is high following resurfacing lasers until skin has reepithelialized. Infection should be promptly recognized and treated to prevent delayed wound healing and scarring. Herpes simplex virus is the most common infection following ablative lasers.[2] Postablation herpes infection can occur despite antiviral prophylaxis and in those who report no prior herpes infection. The common bacterial infections following the laser treatment are usually due to staphylococcus, pseudomonas, klebsiella, and enterobacter. Candidiasis may present as prolonged erythema and pruritus.[3]

Scarring

Scarring could be secondary to infection or operator error like high fluence/density and pulse stacking. Neck, eyelids, and chest are more prone to scarring.[4]

Dyschromia

Postinflammatory Hypo- or Hyperpigmentation

Transient hyperpigmentation is the most common complication seen following cutaneous laser resurfacing. Hyperpigmentation secondary to Er:YAG is not as persistent as that of CO_2 laser. Darker skin has a high risk for hyperpigmentation.

Milia and Acne

Milia and acne are usually due to the occlusive dressing used after the ablative procedure. Flare-up of acne in predisposed individual is commonly observed. Mild flares of acne and milia resolve spontaneously.

LASER TATTOO REMOVAL

Q-switched neodymium doped yttrium-aluminium-garnet (Nd:YAG) laser is commonly used for tattoo removal. Although this laser is considered very safe to use, still complications occur.

Immediate Complications

Pain, crusting, blistering, and pinpoint hemorrhage are the most common complications following the laser tattoo removal. The reasons are excess fluence, smaller spot size, dark skin, dense tattoo, and multiple passes.[5] Acute urticarial reactions has been documented following laser tattoo removal.[6] Urticarial reaction usually subsides in few hours. Treatment of these complications includes supportive measures and sunscreens.

Late Complications

Purpura and bruising are the late complication, and are usually due to higher fluence and may persist for 1–2 weeks.[5]

Delayed Complications

The most common delayed complication are hypo-/hyperpigmentation. Pigmentary changes following laser are usually transient. In darker skin, long-lasting pigmentary alteration can occur.[7] Increasing the treatment interval reduces the chances of dyspigmentation in high risk individuals.

Allergic Reactions

Allergic reactions are reported in red or yellow ink tattoo removal. These reactions may be early or delayed after several weeks.[8] Allergic reactions should be treated with topical and intralesional corticosteroids. Laser tattoo removal in the presence of hypersensitivity reactions should be avoided due to risks of inducing systemic hypersensitivity reactions and anaphylaxis. Ablative methods of removal, such as CO_2 or Er:YAG lasers, or dermabrasion may be used.

Paradoxical Tattoo Darkening

Tattoos that contain ferric oxide or titanium oxide become oxidized and turn black following Q-switched lasers.[9] Additional procedures, such as surgical excision or CO_2 laser ablation, may be necessary for elimination of these types of tattoos.

Incomplete Removal

Some tattoos may not be removed entirely, particularly the multicolored professional tattoos and residual pigment can remain or there may be a ghost image. Textural changes can occur and these may be transient or permanent.

Scarring

Atrophic and hypertrophic scarring can occur with excessive fluences relative to the amount of chromophore present.

Tips for Laser Tattoo Removal

- Laser tattoo removal is usually well-tolerated, but usually requires several treatment sessions for a good result
- Small spot size and greater densities are better avoided
- For a treatment resistant tattoo, switching to a different laser wavelength might be useful
- Patients with allergy to tattoo ink should not be subjected to laser
- For high risk individuals, a test spot is suggested.

COMPLICATIONS OF LASER FOR HAIR REMOVAL

Photoepilation is one of the most common laser procedure performed. There are various laser and light devices available for photoepilation. These devices work on the principle of selective photothermolysis by targeting the follicular melanocytes. Unwanted light absorption by melanin within epidermal melanocytes and keratinocytes may lead to thermal injury to the overlying skin leading to complications. The wide array of available laser and light sources used in photoepilation differ in their efficacy and complication rates, owing to differing characteristics of optical penetration and absorption.

Pain, Erythema, and Edema

Transient pain, edema, and erythema following the treatment is expected and indicates the efficacy of the laser treatment. Deeper erythema and persistent pain are associated with excessive thermal injury. Epidermal cooling reduces the erythema and thermal injury to the epidermis.

Laser Burns

Dark skin, excessive fluence, and lack of adequate cooling are the common reasons for the burns.

Ocular Complications[10,11]

The absence or improper use of eye shielding can result in serious and long-lasting ocular damage like corneal burns, uveitis, cataract formation, and retinal burns. Common patient symptoms are blurred vision, photophobia, pain, and conjunctival hyperemia. If patients complain of eye pain, then the procedure should be terminated immediately, and the patient should receive ophthalmic consultation.

Total body bromhidrosis and hyperhidrosis are potential complications of total body laser hair removal.[12] Possible mechanisms include the activation of dormant bacteria in the skin flora, sweat gland dysfunction, altered skin flora, sweat gland hormone receptor disturbances, and genetic factors.[12]

Paradoxical Hypertrichosis

Paradoxical hypertrichosis can occur within and adjacent to treated areas following photoepilation with several laser and intense pulsed light (IPL) devices.[13] The exact underlying mechanism is not known, has been hypothesized to result from aberrant follicular cycling following suboptimal thermal injury or the effects of local inflammation.[13]

Transient and Persistent Leukotrichia

Subtherapeutic injury to the melanocytes within the hair matrix leads to leukotrichia. This adverse effect is reported more with the IPL devices than the lasers.[14]

Persistent Local Erythema

Persistent reticulate erythema has also been described in patients following photoepilation with diode laser.[15]

An unknown laser-tissue interaction involving the local vasculature is likely to be responsible.

Urticarial-like Plaques

Pruritic, urticarial-like plaques have been described following laser photoepilation. Lesions may persist for several days to weeks and may involve significant edema. Symptomatic improvement may be achieved with the use of topical corticosteroids and antihistamines.

COMPLICATIONS OF LASERS FOR VASCULAR LESIONS

The pulsed dye laser (PDL) is commonly used to treat vascular lesions. It is generally safe and has low risk for complications. Long-pulsed Nd:YAG laser is also used for some vascular lesions and is associated with adverse effects.

Purpura

Transient purpura is the most common complication following PDL. This is due to vaporization of capillaries and extravasation of red blood cells. The use of purpuric fluences is required for treatment of various vascular lesions. The newer PDL with extended pulse duration allows the use of subpurpuric fluencies for the treatment. Treatment of purpura is supportive with the use of ice compressions, topical steroids, and sunscreens.

Erythema and Edema

Transient erythema and edema is common following the laser treatment. Excessive pulse stacking and multiple passes are associated with long-lasting edema.[16]

Superficial Crusting and Hyperpigmentation

Hyperpigmentation and superficial crusting are rare complications due to higher fluencies and in dark skin. Epidermal cooling prevents these complications.

Ulcerations and Scarring[17]

Marked erythema and graying of skin are signs of excessive thermal injury. Immediate tissue injury should be carefully observed with vessel coagulation and no change in the epidermis. Scarring and ulceration is more commonly seen in Nd:YAG laser than with PDL. Use of longer pulse width and Nd:YAG lasers should be reserved for experts with good experience in lasers.

Dermal Depressions

Dermal depressions are a rare complication following vascular lasers. This is due to the spatial defects in the dermis persisting after vessel dissolution or thermal injury to surrounding collagen diffusing from the target vessel. This complication usually resolves spontaneously over time.

CONCLUSION

Lasers are prone for complications due to human and technical error. A thorough knowledge about the laser and the safety precautions to the physician and the patient is necessary to avoid the adverse effects.

REFERENCES

1. Barkana Y, Belkin M. Laser eye injuries. Surv Ophthalmol. 2000;44(6):459-78.
2. Alster TS, Nanni CA. Famciclovir prophylaxis of herpes simplex virus reactivation after laser skin resurfacing. Dermatol Surg. 1999;25:242-6.
3. Alam M, Pantanowitz L, Harton AM, Arndt KA, Dover JS. A prospective trial of fungal colonization after laser resurfacing of the face: correlation between culture positivity and symptoms of pruritus. Dermatol Surg. 2003;29:255-60.
4. Avram MM, Tope WD, Yu T, Szachowicz E, Nelson JS. Hypertrophic scarring of the neck following ablative fractional carbon dioxide laser resurfacing. Lasers Surg Med. 2009;41:185-8.
5. Khunger N, Molpariya A, Khunger A. Complications of tattoos and tattoo removal: stop and think before you ink. J Cutan Aesthet Surg. 2015;8:30-6.
6. Kirby W, Koriakos A, Desai A, Desai T. Undesired pigmentary alterations associated with Q-switch laser tattoo removal. Skin Aging. 2010;18:38-40.
7. Liu XJ, Huo MH. Permanent leukotrichia after Q-switched 1064 nm laser tattoo removal. Indian J Dermatol Venereol Leprol. 2011;77:81-2.
8. Bernstein EF. Laser tattoo removal. Semin Plast Surg. 2007;21:175-92
9. Bencini PL, Cazzaniga S, Tourlaki A, Galimberti MG, Naldi L. Removal of tattoos by q-switched laser: variables influencing outcome and sequelae in a large cohort of treated patients. Arch Dermatol. 2012;148:1364-9.
10. Lapidoth M, Shafirstein G, Ben Amitai D. Reticulate erythema following diode laser-assisted hair removal: a new side effect of a common procedure. J Am Acad Dermatol. 2004;51:774-7.
11. Parver DL. Ocular phototoxicity. In: Huang D, Kaiser PK, Lowder CY, Traboulsi EI (Eds). Retinal Imaging. Philadelphia: Mosby Elsevier; 2006. pp. 421-6.
12. Helou J, Haber R, Kechichian E, Tomb R. A case of generalized bromhidrosis following whole-body depilatory laser. J Cosmet Laser Ther. 2015;19:1-3.
13. Alajlan A, Shapiro J, Rivers JK. Paradoxical hypertrichosis after laser epilation. J Am Acad Dermatol. 2005;53:85-8.
14. Radmanesh M, Mostaghimi M, Yousefi I, Mousavi ZB, Rasai S, Esmaili HR, et al. Leukotrichia developed following application of intense pulsed light for hair removal. Dermatol Surg. 2002;28:572-4.
15. Lapidoth M, Shafirstein G, Ben Amitai D, Hodak E, Waner M, David M. Reticulate erythema following diode laser-assisted hair removal: a new side effect of a common procedure. J Am Acad Dermatol. 2004;51:774-7.
16. Alam M, Omura NE, Dover JS. Clinically significant facial edema after extensive treatment with purpura-free pulsed-dye laser. Dermatol Surg. 2003;29:920-4.
17. Yang MU, Yaroslavsky AN, Farinelli WA. Long-pulsed neodymium:yttrium-aluminum-garnet laser treatment for port-wine stains. J Am Acad Dermatol. 2005;52:480-90.

CHAPTER 36

Purchasing a Laser: Tips and Tricks

Abhishek De, Aarti Sarda, Anupam Das

INTRODUCTION

The advent of lasers has revamped the prospects of a dermatology practice. With better understanding of laser-tissue interaction, lasers are now being used for various indications. Conditions which were untreatable can now be treated with lasers. With the beginning of new millennium, dermatology and plastic surgery practices are being more and more dependent on lasers. Though buying the right lasers and using them appropriately can generate big revenue for the doctors; purchasing lasers involve huge financial implications. Therefore, one should do meticulous planning regarding the type of machine, specifications, financial aspects, maintenance, and warranties. As laser is being used for more and more conditions, and more and more laser companies are coming with many options, all having some benefits over the others, buying a laser is no more an easy task. The authors here would like to emphasize that there can be no particular guideline for buying a laser. A particular laser of a particular make may suit the practice of a particular doctor but may not be suitable for others. Therefore, the present article would rather aim at discussing various pros and cons of different types of lasers; forming a check list for the reader before buying a machine and also try to answer various frequently asked questions that may cross the readers mind.[1]

The buck does not stop at just buying a laser system, ensuring regular maintenance and after-sales service for the machine is vital to having a smooth laser practice. There is considerable ambiguity with regards to the postsales maintenance policies including annual maintenance contracts (AMC) and annual service visit.[2] Majority of the doctors may be unaware of the technical aspects of these contracts and can land in considerable trouble during postsales maintenance.

FREQUENTLY ASKED QUESTIONS BEFORE BUYING A LASER

When Is the Right Time to Buy a Laser in a Mixed Dermatology-esthetic Practice for a Beginner?

Key to start a successful laser practice is to prepare for it. The doctor should understand that this is an entirely different field, and many amongst us, were not trained in lasers during our residency. The doctor needs to read and understand the basic physics of lasers thoroughly, then get himself trained under suitable mentor, either in some laser fellowship or in workshops. He should also understand the nature of his practice, demography of the locality where he practices before venturing into a laser practice. Patients' attitude, paying capacity, esthetic consciousness, and financial capacity are to be considered by the practicing doctor. For more established practitioners, financial implication may not be a deterrent, but even then the consultant should understand the demographics well before buying the laser technology.

What Is the First Laser to Buy in Laser Practice?

The common consensus on the first laser to buy in practice is a hair reduction laser. The high prevalence of hirsutism coupled with increased awareness and predictable result makes a hair reduction laser, the most viable.[3] However, the doctor may also consider buying a fractional ablative laser as the first one, as this gives the consultant an edge over mushrooming chains of beauty parlors, many of which possess a hair reduction device.[4] Next laser to buy is usually a pigment laser, and for Indian context, it is nearly always a Q-switched neodymium doped yttrium-aluminium-garnet laser.[5] Intense pulsed light (IPL) is often a cheaper device to buy in comparison with a laser, and offers great flexibility. Body shaping and tightening energy devices have much less evidence and should only be reserved as adjuvant for standard laser practice. Excimer lasers are important for the treatment of vitiligo and psoriasis, but its use and procurement are limited to a very few institutions. One must also remember that the laser parameters from publication from the West cannot be extrapolated on our patients due to differences in the skin type.

Should We Buy a Platform Laser or Go for Standalone Technologies?

There is nothing much to choose between a good quality platform laser and a good quality standalone technology. Both have some pros and cons. Platform technology gives the user benefit of choosing from multiple handpieces, which is expandable as the practice grows. It limits the initial costs, but also comes with problem of long waiting period in a particularly busy practice. The benefit of platform lasers is also in the fact that maintenance is less costly, and required less office space. However, if the platform breaks down, none of the handpieces can be used for any indication. Standalone technologies have the benefit of being employed simultaneously in different procedure rooms, and avoid long waiting period for the patients. In general, standalone systems are suitable for established practitioner with steady inflow of patients, while platforms are more suited for beginners and if different doctors wish to share the machine.[2,6]

If We Have a Budget Constrain, Should We Compromise on the Make of the Laser and Buy a Cheaper One than the Market Leaders?

The authors strongly believe the doctor should be absolutely sure about the authenticity of the manufacturer. It is of utmost importance that the laser machine delivers the requisite power consistently, to ensure desired effect with minimal side effect. An incompetent system may not only fail to deliver the clinical result but also may cause undesired complication. Money lost in a system may be recovered in due course of time, but the confidence lost by the doctor on laser and the patients on the doctor, in such cases, are invaluable losses.

What Is the Checklist Before We Buy a Laser from a Particular Company?

The doctor must cross check the following before buying a machine:[1,2,6]

- Full specification of the machine: power, wavelength—when introduced, when the next upgradation due, and what are various wavelength available, if it is a platform laser
- Model number, year of manufacture, time gap before delivery of the system or parts
- Accessories included in the purchase
- Purchase of contract to be read carefully
- Warranty or extended warranty
- Annual maintenance: charge and how much comprehensive
- Reliability/credibility of the vendor, whether the company has a direct distributor
- If the custom clearance and transportation charge will be provided by the dealer
- If the company or the distributor have a service engineer stationed in the city
- How many free visit does the AMC cover
- Insurance for the laser
- Cost of the consumable required
- Life of the laser: approximate of how many shots can be delivered from the system
- Provision of a standby system in case of a delay in repair
- If there is a chance of upgradation of the laser
- How many systems were sold in the city or the country: may ask for list of the existing users and cross check with one or two of the users. It is always advisable for the beginners not to be the first buyer of a particular

system as he runs the risk of buying a not-tested system and also to be the last buyer of a system where he may be sold an outdated technology
- If the company is providing with some training facilities.

LASERS TRAINING FOR BEGINNER[7]

Before starting the practice, the doctor may consider getting himself well-versed with the principles of laser physics and also can get some first-hand training. He/she may opt to a member of the society dedicated for laser practice, attend conferences and observational and hands-on workshops to refresh his knowledge. Short dedicated fellowship on lasers in some reputed institute also may help. Laser companies often arrange training for the buyer; ensure that before buying a system. Going through the materials and manuals provided by the companies on the particular device is also helpful to know how the particular technology works.

JUDGING THE SUITABILITY OF A LASER[1,2,6,8,9]

After completion of basic training, the suitability of a particular system may be analyzed in a step-by-step process.

1. Laser specification: the doctor needs to know the spot size, pulse duration, peak power, and customization options for the particular system. A large spot size is preferable for laser hair removal as it allows deeper penetration and faster treatments. The curve of the energy beam is also important. Top-hat beam profile is preferable for Q-switched lasers over the Gaussian beam as that can prevent "hot spots". The fractional laser should preferably have variable scan density, adjustable and variable scan patters, changeable spot size of each microbeam, and high power (e.g., minimum 30 watts for fractional carbon dioxide). Correct wavelength of filters, variable on time, and off time are essential for an IPL system. An inbuilt appropriate cooling system for IPL for hair reduction device is also very important
2. One should try to find out if there is any publication in peer-reviewed journals for a particular system. If published, the data should be analyzed to see if it suits the predominant skin types of his patients
3. Try to collect feedback from the other users and discuss in detail about their experience with system and also with postsales support by the vendor. It is prudent to ask the competitor companies for an opinion, to judge unbiased
4. Always insist upon demonstration session where the machine can be kept in the clinic for a few days and a few sessions may be done before buying the system
5. Check if the machine is generating correct output with the help of a power meter, which the service engineer should provide
6. Ask the company in detail the electrical connections and power backup required, and make suitable arrangement in the clinic
7. Go through the laser manual in details
8. Ensure that right quality of laser glasses is provided in sufficient quantity and perfect working condition both for the surgeon and for the supporting staff. Also ensure the provision of the ocular shields for the patient.

NEGOTIATION FOR THE BEST COST[2]

The key to negotiate the best cost is not to hurry in buying a laser. It is important to take quotations from multiple competitive brands, which often helps in getting the best deal. While calculating the cost-benefit ratio, one has to keep in mind the depreciation value of the machine. It is also not practical to buy and own every new laser that is launched in the market. It is prudent to evaluate each technology in depth and choose only that system which will benefit the practice maximum.

FUNDING[2]

A doctor may have to take a bank loan to purchase the laser. One should the interest rates in competing banks and required documents to procure the loan. The following is a rough checklist of the documents needed for procuring a loan for medical equipment:

- Quotation from the company
- Purchase contract
- Income tax returns
- Registration documents of the clinic
- Clinic building documents
- Medical council registration
- Personal documents such as identity, address proofs, taxation documents.

Laser Purchase Contract[2]

After finalizing what laser to buy, the doctor should get a detailed contract signed with vendor which should clearly mention amount paid in advance, clause of bank payment, warranty, clause of repair, etc. Checking the contract prepared by the vendor by a professional lawyer is a good option for further safety.

Annual Maintenance Contract[2]

The doctor should take either the labor maintenance contract which is generally 5–7% of the invoice value and valid only for servicing or AMC, which is generally 22% of the invoice value and includes all parts and maintenance, after the initial warranty period is over. Annual maintenance contract is also essential for insurance purpose.

Insurance[2]

Insurance coverage is a must following installation of the device. Insurance should cover all parts of the device and also cover for fire or burglary or damage incurred during shifting the machine.

CONCLUSION

In this rapidly evolving era of aesthetic consciousness, lasers have emerged as the most rewarding procedures, both for the patients and the treating physician. We have reviewed the basic whereabouts regarding the purchase of laser equipment. Most of the frequently asked questions have been dealt with. Buying lasers should be easier now. However, the reader should also keep in the mind the variation of local socioeconomic status, aesthetic requirements, and most importantly should understand his own practice.

REFERENCES

1. Mackety CJ. Purchasing lasers and related accessories. Hosp Purch Manage. 1985;10(11):7-10.
2. Aurangabadkar SJ, Mysore V, Ahmed ES. Buying a laser—tips and pearls. J Cutan Aesthet Surg. 2014;7(2):124-30.
3. Buddhadev RM. IADVL Dermatosurgery Task Force. Standard guidelines of care: laser and IPL hair reduction. Indian J Dermatol Venereol Leprol. 2008;74:68-74.
4. Goel A, Krupashankar DS, Aurangabadkar S, Nischal KC, Omprakash HM, Mysore V. Fractional lasers in dermatology—current status and recommendations. Indian J Dermatol Venereol Leprol. 2011;77(3):369-79.
5. Aurangabadkar S, Mysore V. Standard guidelines of care: lasers for tattoos and pigmented lesions. Indian J Dermatol Venereol Leprol. 2009;75(Suppl 2):111-26.
6. Dhepe N. Minimum standard guidelines of care on requirements for setting up a laser theatre. Indian J Dermatol Venereol Leprol. 2009;75:101-10.
7. Plee J, Barbe C, Richard MA, Dreno B, Bernard P. Survey of post-graduate training for Dermatology and Venereology residents in France (2005-2010). Ann Dermatol Venereol. 2013;140(4):259-65.
8. Kerr DR, Malhotra IV. Electrical design and safety in the operating room and intensive care unit. Int Anesthesiol Clin. 1981;19:27-48.
9. Alster TS. Getting started: setting up a laser practice. In: Alster TS, editor. Manual of Cutaneous Laser Techniques, 2nd ed. Philadelphia: Lippincott Williams and Wilkins; 2000. pp. 2-4.

CHAPTER 37

Ethical Promotion on Social Media of Laser Facilities Offered by a Dermatologist

Emily M Altman

INTRODUCTION

The practice of medicine is rooted in a covenant of trust among patients, physicians, and society. The ethics of medicine must seek to balance the physician's responsibility to each patient and the professional, collective obligation to all who need medical care. This statement articulates core values and principles that are shared by all physicians, in a range of settings and circumstances, including the use of new technologies of communication, regardless of specialty.[1]

HISTORICAL AND PRESENT SCENARIO

Throughout history, people have been seeking ways to enhance their appearance. In ancient Egypt, ingredients such as sour milk were used for masks. Ancient Greeks are rumored to have used snail mucus, a natural source of glycolic acid for its skin softening properties.[2] Makeup in the ancient world was the sign of wealth and status. Rosy cheeks, red lips, and smooth skin tone have always been recognized as signs of youth and beauty.

The second half of the 20th century brought a number of new powerful cosmetic treatments and devices. Neuromodulators, dermal fillers, and lasers made cosmetic treatments accessible to the general public. Cutaneous laser surgery, in particular, began to be seen as "state-of-the-art" treatment for a number of conditions, many of them cosmetic in nature.[3]

Although the theoretical foundation for lasers was laid early in the 20th century, the first laser was invented in 1960. By 1961, Goldman, a dermatologist whom the American Society for Laser Medicine and Surgery honors as the "father of lasers in medicine in the United States," founded the first biomedical laser laboratory at the University of Cincinnati.[4] In the early 1980s, Anderson and Parrish from the department of dermatology at the Harvard Medical School revolutionized the practice of cutaneous laser surgery by developing the theory of selective photothermolysis. Several years later, the first lasers were approved by the Food and Drug Administration for cosmetic procedures such as the ruby laser for the permanent removal of pigmented hair and the Q-switched neodymium doped yttrium-aluminium-garnet (Nd:YAG) for the treatment of tattoos. Today, many medical and surgical specialties use lasers for diagnosis and treatment of a wide variety of diseases.[5] Often described as painless and exaggerated as producing perfect results,[3] lasers are often seen by the public as the proverbial magic bullet for enhancement of beauty and perhaps, even for recapture of lost youth. Stylianou and Talias[6] call this the myth of the "magic light," the belief that laser light is harmless and has magical powers.

In their discussion of the modern concepts of beauty, Adamson and Galli[7] argue that beauty and youth are hardwired into our brains and have survival value for us as individuals and as a species. They further argue that the increasing numbers of cosmetic surgery procedures done today are due to our drive for a youthful appearance that results in an enhanced self-esteem, loss of anxiety about certain body parts, increased vitality, enjoyment of life, and also improves the chances for reproductive success. One might say that the use and advertisement of these new technological tools for "circumventing evolution" does and should place the physicians practicing cosmetic surgery in situation after situation where ethics and business success may come into conflict.

This is just one of the numbers of such ethical conflicts that cosmetic surgeons face. As De Sousa states in his scathing article, even the nature of nontherapeutic cosmetic surgery and the justification for altering the body for purposes other than to cure disease raises ethical questions.[8] He goes further to question whether cosmetic surgery even constitutes healthcare. A number of authors have placed the practice of cosmetic surgery as outside traditional medicine.[9]

As Baumann states in her examination of ethics in cosmetic dermatology, a number of functions that cosmetic dermatologists must perform, such as advertising and hiring public relations specialists, are also outside traditional scope of the medical field.[10] Baumann goes on to note that the goal of improving patients' appearance and skin health places the practice of cosmetic dermatology firmly in the arena of traditional medicine, however, she questions whether financial motivations can cloud the cosmetic dermatologists' judgment.

According to Baumann, a successful cosmetic dermatologist must be a scientist, a marketer, an artist, and a business person. Because cosmetic dermatology is a direct-to-consumer cash based business, marketing and advertising are essential for the dermatologist to be noticed and chosen over the competition.[11] And, there is plenty of competition from multiple sources outside the core cosmetic specialties. Numerous family practitioners, internists, obstetricians, dentists, and nurse practitioners perform cosmetic procedures in their practices. How does one stand out from the competition both within and outside the core cosmetic specialties? The internet offers numerous avenues of interaction with existing and potential patients via social media, such as Facebook, Twitter, Pinterest, and multiple other sites that can bring potential patients to your website and into your office. The conundrum is how to use these valuable interactive platforms while keeping to the high ethical and moral standards that are integral to being a physician.

To consider the ethical implications of advertising laser dermatology services on social media, such as Facebook and Twitter among others, one must look at the ethics of advertising, social media, and medicine, and determine if there is a unifying principle that would allow cosmetic and laser dermatologists to advertise to their potential patients in an educational and ethical way.

ADVERTISING

Advertising is "a public notice meant to convey information and invite patronage or some other response". Its purpose is to inform and persuade ("stimulate demand"). It is a paid form of nonpersonal communication about an organization and/or its products that is transmitted to a target audience through a mass medium."[12] By itself, advertising is morally neutral, neither good nor bad. Good advertising can appeal on many levels from creativity to humor to esthetics. However, advertising can also be deceptive. It may exploit emotions and sidestep logical thought processes, therefore, undermining personal autonomy and freedom of choice.

Advertising in medicine is a relatively recent phenomenon. In some countries, it is still not allowed. In its original 1847 Code of Ethics, the American Medical Association (AMA) banned medical advertising as "highly reprehensible in a regular physician" and "derogatory to the dignity of the profession." In 1980, these prohibitions were reversed when a second circuit appellate court ordered the AMA to stop restraints on advertising, ruling that such restraints violated fair trade laws.[13] Soon to follow, in 1986, the British General Medical Council signaled its acceptance of the distribution of information material about general practitioners and their services to persons who are not their patients. Since that time, medical advertising has been growing by leaps and bounds and so has the criticism that advertising solicits patients and differentiates the physician from his peers and not just disseminates information but blurs the distinction between the physician and the "itinerant merchant of nostrums" by emphasizing the commercial aspects of the practice.[14] Similar sentiments exist in the Indian Medical Council (professional conduct, etiquette, and ethics) Regulations 2002, Section 6.1 which states that "soliciting of patients directly or indirectly by a physician or a group of physicians or an organization, by advertisement or publicity through any mode so as to invite attention to his professional qualifications, skills, achievements, appointments or honors is unethical."[15] Roman Gaehwiler of Oxford University's philosophy department blog "Practical Ethics" compares plastic surgeons who practice cosmetic surgery individual enhancement "Dr Salesmen," and bluntly states that they are no better than "Bentley car-salesmen."[16]

SOCIAL MEDIA

Putting the "physician versus salesman" argument aside, let's look at the ethics of social media and the ethics that are desperately trying to catch up with the meteoric rise of the use of social media throughout the world. Although it seems like it has been around for decades, social media was truly born in the 21st century.

The first message was sent over the internet (or Advanced Research Projects Agency Network, as it was known then) almost exactly 45 years ago, on October 29, 1969, as a communication between two computer science laboratories at the University of California, Los Angeles and Stanford Research Institute. It was not until the late 1980s that the internet as we know it today came into being.

It was not until 2002 that social networking hit its stride with the creation of Friendster, which promoted an online community for people with common bonds.[17] The most popular social network, Facebook, did not launch until 2004 at Harvard University and remained a campus-only social site for 2 years.

However, as with any new and, especially, revolutionary technology, there has to be new ethics developed. Moor describes a policy vacuum that occurs when new technologies allow us to perform activities in new ways and we do not have adequate policies in place to guide us. We need to formulate and justify new policies for acting in these new situations.[18] According to Moor, formulating and justifying new policies for new technologies is made far more complex by our limitations as how to understand the new matter at hand, something he calls a conceptual muddle. Moor's Law states, "As technological revolutions increase their social impact, ethical problems increase."

With the advent of social media, advertising can now reach staggering numbers of people. It is no longer a stack of pamphlets one hands out on the street or even a newspaper that reaches a larger audience. Facebook alone has over 1.44 billion monthly active users as of the first quarter of 2015. The concerns about the ethics of marketing on social media are heard loud and clear. Because social media can track personal preferences, shopping habits, interests, and multiple other variables of its users, even brand marketers themselves share concerns about using such information for advertising.

The Social Content Marketing author, Barry, explores some ethical dilemmas faced by brand marketers and advertisers on social media:[19]

- Invasion of privacy of social networking participants, which includes behavioral targeting
- Spamming overpromoting unsolicited messages
- Public bashing or disparaging others, such as your competition
- Dishonesty and distortions of information about the product or brand
- Distorted endorsements and misrepresentations of one's credentials, affiliations, and expertize.

The Australian Advertising Standards Bureau published a list of key issues regarding the use of advertising on social media.[20] The bureau prohibits the following:

- Advertising directly to children, requiring social media advertisers to limit the age of their audience to over 18 years
- Discrimination and vilification, particularly of competitors
- Objectification, such as employing sexual appeal in a manner which is exploitative and degrading of any individual or group of people
- Sex, sexuality, and nudity issues must be targeted at the relevant audience, particularly limitation of that audience by age
- Use of strong or obscene language.

Interestingly, most of these ethically questionable practices are frowned upon not only by the Internet marketing experts, but are also seen in the advertising and internet ethics guidelines of a number of medical societies, particularly, the core specialties for cosmetic procedures.

THE ETHICS OF MEDICINE

Dyer[14] notes that the medical profession is increasing identified with technical expertize, but technical expertize is not sufficient to characterize a profession without an ethical dimension. So, then, how do medical ethics relate to physician advertising for cosmetic procedures?

Ethics is considered to be the summation of morals, values, and codified laws of professional behavior.[21] For any physician, no matter which hat he must wear in the course of his day (doctor, business owner, etc.), medicine as a profession and a calling must come first. Although the original formulation of medical ethics is ascribed to Hippocrates, the foundation of modern medical ethics came from the work of Childress and Beauchamp who based medical ethics on the following four principles:[22]

1. Autonomy
2. Beneficence
3. Nonmaleficence
4. Justice.

Autonomy

The patient must have autonomy of thought, intention and action when making decisions regarding healthcare procedures. Such decision-making process must be free of coercion or coaxing. To make such a decision, the patient must understand all the risks and benefits of the procedure and the likelihood of success.

Autonomy is self-governance, the presence of understanding and decision-making capacity, the right to choose or refuse treatment. The competent adult patient has the right to choose or refuse his/her treatment. The patients' autonomous decisions should be free from external constraint, coercion, or coaxing. The patient must give informed consent to a treatment with understanding of all the risks and benefits, the likelihood of success, and alternative treatments.

Of interest, out of a total library search of 1,00,000 plastic surgery oriented articles, Chung et al. found that only 110 clearly focused on ethical principles.[23] Of the four principles of medical ethics, autonomy was most commonly addressed (53%). This finding was not surprising given that the issues addressed by autonomy, such as informed consent, photography, and advertising, are particularly pertinent to plastic surgery.

Crisp's discussion of persuasive advertising and its effect on autonomy argues that persuasive advertising overrides the autonomy of consumers in that it manipulates them without their knowledge.[24] Crisp points out that such advertising causes desire in such a way that a necessary condition of autonomy—the possibility of decision—is removed, since autonomous action depends on autonomous desire, rational desire, free choice, and control of manipulation.

Beneficence

Requirement that medical professionals act in the patients' best interests.[25] More specifically, medical practitioners should prevent harm, remove harm, and promote good for the patient.[26]

The procedure must be provided with the intent of doing well for the patient. Demands that the healthcare provider develop and maintain skills and knowledge, continually update training, consider individual circumstances of all patients, and strive for net benefit.

Nonmaleficence

The procedure should not harm the patient or others in society.

Justice

Fair distribution of scarce resources, competing needs, rights and obligations, and potential conflicts with established legislation. In the case of cosmetic dermatology, justice considers the limited number of doctors that deliver medical care in a particular specialty and the decrease in that number, should the doctor decide to perform primarily cosmetic procedures.

In this sea of new technologies, new procedures, and new access to previously unreachable audiences, how do we strike the right balance between educating our patients and the public at large about the procedures we do and new developments in the field and yet steer clear of crossing any ethical lines? The four core cosmetic specialties (dermatology, ophthalmology, otolaryngology, and plastic surgery) have all addressed ethical advertising with prohibition against use of deceiving, or misleading credentials, photographs, statements or testimonials.[27]

One of the well-thought out documents regarding adherence to the ethical standards in advertising for cosmetic physician services comes from the American Society of Plastic Surgeons (ASPS) advertisers guidelines for compliance with ASPS Code of Ethics.[28] The society drafted a document, which it suggests, should be signed by the advertising entity and the physician, which clearly delineates the rules and conditions of advertising by their member physicians.

As a member of the medical profession and the ASPS (the "society"), the member has a duty, when communicating with the public, through professional announcements, telephone and medical directories, computer bulletin boards, internet webpages, and broadcast and electronic media, to do so truthfully, honestly, and accurately. The society's Code of Ethics contains specific requirements and prohibitions about the member's actions and statements as well as statements made on the member's behalf. These are summarized below with examples. At the request of the company, the member will provide a copy of the complete Code of Ethics to the company.

The member is prohibited from:

- Including misrepresentations of facts or omissions which make a statement deceptive or misleading
- Using exaggerated claims intended to or likely to attract patients
- Including statements or claims which are intended or likely to create false or unjustified expectations of favorable results
- Making representations or statements of opinion as to the superior quality of professional services which are not susceptible to verification by the public nor include statements representing that the member possess skills or provides services superior to those of other physicians with similar training unless such representation can be factually substantiated
- Appealing to the layperson's fears, anxieties, or emotional vulnerabilities. Either failing to include reasonable warnings and disclosures or making representations of fact or implications regarding matters material to a person's decision to utilize the member's services that are likely to cause an ordinary, prudent person to misunderstand or be deceived; including predictions of future success or guarantees that satisfaction or a cure will result from the performance of the member's services
- Compensating, directly or indirectly, in cash or in-kind, a representative of the press, radio, television, or other communication medium in anticipation of or return for recommending the member's services or for professional publicity, except for payment of the cost of advertising or promotional services; the company will disclose that an advertisement or solicitation is paid for where it is not apparent from the context alone.

Photographs or images will not:

- Falsely or deceptively portray a physical or medical condition, injury, disease, including obesity, or recovery or relief therefrom
- Portray persons who have received the services advertised, but who experienced results that are not typical of the results obtained by the average patient without clearly and noticeably disclosing this fact
- Portray persons before and after receiving services, which use different light, poses, or photographic techniques that misrepresent the actual results achieved
- Use photographs of models who have not received the advertised services in any manner suggesting that the model received the advertised services; such photographs must clearly and noticeably disclose the fact that the model did not receive the advertised services.

Testimonials will not:

- Include statements pertaining to the efficacy or quality of medical care if the experience of the endorser does not represent the typical experience of other patients or if, due to the infrequency and/or complexity of such care, the results in other cases cannot be predicted with any degree of accuracy.
- Include statements or endorsements pertaining to the quality of the member's medical care or qualifications if the endorser has been compensated by the member or the company for making such testimonial or endorsement.

CONCLUSION

The ethics of cosmetic or laser dermatology or ethics or advertising of the developing ethics of social media, they all call for the same ethical principles: guard your patients' privacy, be truthful, do not overpromise what the device can deliver, disclose your connections with the company that makes the device you advertise, disclose any compensation to the persons giving their testimonials in support of your work, do not take advantage of your audience's fears, lack of education, weaknesses, or low self-esteem. Deliver excellent care by undergoing extensive and continuing training in your area of practice; teach present and prospective patients about new technologies, good and bad. Ethics, in addition to technical expertize, is what defines a profession, particularly medicine. Doctors, no matter what the specialty, are honor and duty-bound to help patients. The education that the audience derives from a doctor's advertising can and should be part of the same. As Anderson said, "In short, the patients are ours, and we should make better patient care the only real bottom line.[29,30]

REFERENCES

1. Charles SC, Lazarus JA. Reframing the professional ethic: the Council of Medical Specialty Societies consensus statement on the ethic of medicine. West J Med. 2000;173(3):198-201.
2. Perdis N. Back to the future: ancient beauty secrets. New York: Huffington Post; 2013.
3. Low DW. Lasers in Plastic Surgery. In: Charles HT (Ed). Grabb and Smith's Plastic Surgery, 6th ed. Philadelphia: Lippincott Williams & Wilkins; 2007. pp. 169-76.
4. Geiges ML. History of Lasers in Dermatology. Current Problems in Dermatology. In: Bogdan AI, Goldberg DJ (Eds). Basics in Dermatological Laser Applications. Switzerland: S. Karger; 2011.

5. Wheeland RG, McBurney E, Geronemus RG. The role of dermatologists in the evolution of laser surgery. Dermatol Surg. 2000;26(9):815-22.
6. Stylianou A, Talias MA. The 'Magic Light': A Discussion on Laser Ethics. Sci Eng Ethics. 2015;21(4):979-98.
7. Adamson PA, Doud Galli SK. Modern concepts of beauty. Curr Opin Otolaryngol Head and Neck Surg. 2003;11:295-300.
8. De Sousa A. Concerns about cosmetic surgery. Indian J Med Ethics. 2007;4(4):171-3.
9. Sullivan DA. Cosmetic surgery–the cutting edge of commercial medicine in America. New Brunswick: Rutgers University Press; 2001.
10. Baumann L. Ethics in cosmetic dermatology. Clin Dermatol. 2012;30(5): 522-7.
11. Advertising and Marketing for Cosmetic Surgery Practices. Healthcare Success Strategies. [online] Available from: http://www.healthcaresuccess.com/medical/cosmetic-surgery [Accessed February 2016].
12. Ethics of Advertising. Carroll College. [online] Available from: https://www.carroll.edu/msmillie/busethics/ethadvertising.htm [Accessed February 2016].
13. Schenker Y, Arnold RM, London AJ. Response to open peer commentaries on "The ethics of advertising for health care services". Am J Bioeth. 2014; 14(4):W3-4.
14. Dyer AR. Ethics, advertising and the definition of a profession. J Med Ethics. 1985;11(2):72-8.
15. Kumar H. The Ethics of Advertising in Medicine. Amrita Journal of Medicine. 2012;8(1):2.
16. Gaehwiler R. 2010. Cosmetic Surgery–What is the Matter with Dr Salesman? Practical Ethics. [online] Available from: http://blog.practicalethics.ox.ac.uk/2010/08/cosmetic-surgery-what-is-the-matter-with-dr-salesman/. [Accessed February 2016].
17. Staff, Digital Trends. 2014. The History of Social Networking. Digital Trends. [online] Available from: http://www.digitaltrends.com/features/the-history-of-social-networking/. [Accessed February 2016].
18. Moor, James H. Why we need better ethics for emerging technologies. Ethics and Information Technology. 2005;7:111-9.
19. Barry J. (2014). 7 Ethical Dilemmas Faced in Content Marketing. Social Content Marketing. [online] Available from: http://blog.socialcontentmarketing.com/7-ethical-dilemmas-faced-in-social-media-marketing/. [Accessed February 2016].
20. Ad Standards—Social media advertising. Ad Standards. 2013. [online] Advertising Standards Bureau. [online] Available from: http://www.adstandards.com.au/process/theprocesssteps/specificproductsandissues/socialmedia. [Accessed February 2016].
21. Meffert JJ. Ethics? Morals? Values? Clinics in Dermatology. 2009;(27):327-30.
22. Smith R, Chalmers I. In: Ashcroft RE, Dawson A, Draper H, McMillan JR (Eds). Principles of Health Care Ethics, 2nd ed. West Sussex: John Wiley & Sons; 2007.
23. Chung KC, Pushman AG, Bellfi LT. A systematic review of ethical principles in the plastic surgery literature. Plast Reconstr Surg. 2009;124(5):1711-8.
24. Crisp R. Persuasive Advertising, autonomy, and the creation of desire. Journal of Business Ethics. 1987;6(5):413-8.
25. Mousavi, SR. The ethics of aesthetic surgery. J Cutan Aesthet Surg. 2010;3(1):38-40.
26. Snyder JE, Gauthier CC. Chapter 2. The Underlying Principles of Ethical Patient Care. Evidence-Based Medical Ethics: Cases for Practice-Based Learning. New York: Humana Press; 2008.
27. Wong WW, Camp MC, Camp JS, Gupta SC. The quality of Internet advertising in aesthetic surgery: an in-depth analysis. Aesthet Surg J. 2010;30:735-43.
28. Advertisers Guidelines for Compliance with ASPS Code of Ethics. American Society of Plastic Surgeons. [online] Available from: http://www.plasticsurgery.org/Documents/medical-professionals/ASPS%20Ethics%20Advertiser%20Guidelines%20FINAL.pdf. [Accessed February, 2016].
29. Dryden, Jane. Autonomy. Internet Encyclopedia of Philosophy. [online] Available from: http://www.iep.utm.edu/autonomy/#SH4b. [Accessed February 2016].
30. Business Dictionary. [online] Available from: http://www.businessdictionary.com/definition/advertising.html. [Online] [Accessed March, 2016.]

CHAPTER 38

What is New in Lasers?

Vandana Mehta

INTRODUCTION

Laser technology and other energy sources are rapidly finding a place in dermatology armamentarium. In the field of skin rejuvenation by fractional photothermolysis, several new devices have emerged over the recent years which although appear less effective than ablative lasers, but are safer. This article provides an insight into the existing and available new laser technologies for the purpose of skin rejuvenation.

ADVANCES IN HAIR REMOVAL LASERS

Since its introduction in 1995, laser hair removal is one of the most sought after cosmetic procedures. The efficacy of various laser systems to destroy the hair follicles is based on the theory of selective photothermolysis.[1] The hair shaft is produced by rapidly dividing matrix stem cells located 2–7 mm deep. Thus technically, the matrix stem cells are the best target for hair removal. However, recent evidence states that the pleuripotent epithelial cells located in the bulge region about 1–1.5 mm deep should also be targeted. From personal experience, the author feels that in terms of safety and efficacy the alexandrite (GentleLase and GentleMax) and long-pulsed diode laser (Soprano XL, LightSheer, MedioStar) are the most popular systems suitable for skin types I to IV, however, for darker skin types V and VI, the neodymium doped yttrium-aluminium-garnet (Nd:YAG) laser (CoolGlide, MedLite IV, GentleMax) is preferred. In addition to the wavelength, a larger spot size is chosen in order to improve the efficacy of treatment by enhancing the depth of penetration and also reducing the time for treatment.[2]

Of late, scanners have been incorporated to the laser systems so that large areas of the body can be treated in a short period of time (Arion single spot scan alexandrite laser and LEDA EPI continuous scan diode laser. A recent advancement has been the simultaneous use of 755 nm alexandrite laser and 1,064 nm Nd:YAG laser in a single laser beam which has been made possible by the EV laser systems (StarDuo EVO Mix) giving us the freedom to choose the percentage of each laser required. For example, in case of phototype IV, 60% Nd:YAG and 40% alexandrite can be used during the treatment.

LASERS FOR ACNE

Acne is a chronic inflammatory disease of pilosebaceous units and the multiple factors are involved in its pathogenesis. Lasers and light based devices may be used as an adjunct to conventional acne modalities in selected patients. Many light sources may affect *Propionibacterium acnes* such as the blue, red, and ultraviolet light, intense pulsed light (IPL) devices (broadband light), potassium titanyl phosphate lasers (532 nm), pulsed dye lasers (PDLs) (585–595 nm), and infrared lasers (1,440 nm diode, 1,540 nm erbium glass).

There are several studies showing the efficacy of blue light as well as a combination of both blue and red light for the treatment of mild-to-moderate acne. The 585 nm PDL targets oxyhemoglobin and has been used to cause selective photothermolysis of the dilated vascular component in acne. At low nonpurpuric doses, this laser can reduce the inflammatory acne by reducing the *P. acnes*. Seaton et al. demonstrated a 49% reduction in inflammatory lesion counts versus 10% in controls 12 weeks after treatment using a 585 nm PDL.[3]

The infrared lasers cause selective thermal damage to the sebaceous glands by targeting the water which is the dominant chromophore in the sebaceous gland, thereby decreasing the overproduction of sebum and eliminating acne. The 1,450 nm diode laser (SmoothBeam) is Food and Drug Administration (FDA) approved for the treatment of mild-to-moderate inflammatory acne vulgaris on the face.[4] The authors have also noted excellent results with the SmoothBeam laser performed at weekly intervals for inflammatory acne of the face for 3–4 weeks at fluences of 14 J with a dynamic cooling device. The SmoothBeam laser has also been used by the authors for the residual atrophic acne scars with good result at monthly intervals. The 595 nm PDL has also been used in conjunction with the 1,450 nm diode laser to treat both acne vulgaris and postinflammatory erythema resulting from acne.[5] The 1,540 nm is a nonablative erbium glass laser and after four treatments at 4-week intervals, a 78% reduction in acne lesions and decreased skin oiliness was noted in 25 patients by Boineau et al.[6]

Chun et al. reported that application of a topical carbon lotion followed by the use of Q-switched frequency, doubled Nd:YAG laser in a quasi long-pulsed mode followed immediately by Q-switched mode using a 7 mm handpiece gave very good clearance for inflammatory acne with minimal patient downtime.[7]

LASERS FOR PIGMENTATION AND TATTOOS

The use of lasers in ethnic skin is challenging as it is prone to develop postinflammatory hyperpigmentation (PIH) due to thermal injury of the laser. Kim et al. demonstrated a significant improvement in PIH following the use of subthermogenic low fluence Q-switched Nd:YAG laser.[8] With regards to melasma though topical therapy remains the mainstay of management studies have shown synergistic benefits when topical therapy was combined with a PDL or a low fluence Q-switched Nd:YAG laser to target the vascular and pigmentary component of melasma.[9] The fractionated thulium laser 1,927 nm which is a relative newcomer has shown some benefit in the management of melasma.[10,11]

The nanosecond lasers (Q-switched) are the gold standard for tattoo removal. These systems can cause a mechanical rupture of the tattoo pigment through a photoacoustic effect where the traditional millisecond lasers can cause scarring. The Q-switched Nd:YAG can treat most colors, but green or blue responds to Q-switched alexandrite, purple to Q-switched ruby, and red to Q-switched 532 nm laser.

PicoSure is the first FDA approved picosecond 755 nm alexandrite laser introduced in 2013 which uses very short pulse duration for the treatment of tattoos. Saedi et al. reported the safety and efficacy of picosecond laser in professional and amateur tattoos with 100% patient satisfaction rate.[12] The smaller the target, the shorter will be the thermal relaxation time and hence, shorter pulse durations will be required. Recent studies have demonstrated that performing multiple treatments on a tattoo separated over a period of 20 minutes during a single office visit could improve the treatment outcome popularly known as the R20 method of tattoo removal.[13] Fractional lasers 2,940 nm are also starting to be used for resistant tattoos in combination with the Q-switched 1,064 nm laser, but this indication is still a subject of debate and more studies are needed to confirm the benefit.[14]

LASERS FOR VASCULAR LESIONS

The vascular lasers work on the principle of selective photothermolysis and the 585 nm PDL is the gold standard for the treatment of port wine stain (PWS) and capillary vascular malformations. Children under the age of 1 year tend to respond better. The author generally uses a 10 mm spot size, 1.5 millisecond pulse duration with fluence ranging from 6 to 9 J and intense epidermal cooling. The end result is darkening of the vascular lesion and treatments are carried at 3–4 weekly intervals. For darker and resistant PWS, studies have demonstrated the sequential use of a PDL and 1,064 nm Nd:YAG laser (Cynergy MultiPlex) to be useful. The improved results here could be attributed to the fact that the oxyhemoglobin coefficient peaks at 595 nm and the methemoglobin coefficient aligns well with 1,064 nm laser.[15]

Though gross purpura formation after a vascular laser is necessary, a recent concept that has been reported by Huang et al. states that purpura formation is an insufficient prognostic indicator of photocoagulation.

Treatment areas were found to harbor persistent pools of perfusion regardless of the presence of purpura.[16] Here, the addition of topical rapamycin which belongs to the class of macrocyclic immunosuppressives could play a beneficial role in view of its antiangiogenic properties. Hence, combined vascular laser and topical rapamycin might serve as a useful adjunct in the clearance of PWS.[17]

The newer generations of IPL such as the AcuTip 500 and Lux G (StarLux) have further improved vascular applications. Reddy et al. have reported the safety and efficacy of frequency-doubled 532 nm Nd:YAG laser with short pulse durations for the treatment of cutaneous vascular lesions resistant to PDL treatment.[18] The authors have also noted good improvement with a PDL for nonfacial viral warts. The effects could be explained due to photocoagulation of the feeding vessels of the wart.

LASERS FOR SKIN REJUVENATION

Fractional photothermolysis has revolutionized the use of lasers for skin resurfacing and photorejuvenation. Facial resurfacing with fractional carbon dioxide (CO_2) lasers is currently claimed to be one of the most effective treatment options for facial scars.[19] Fractional lasers treat only a fraction or a column of the affected skin causing microscopic thermal treatment zones leaving intervening areas of skin untreated. Thermal damage initiates a biological signaling cascade leading to increased expression of heat shock protein which causes upregulation of transforming growth factor-β, a facilitator of collagen synthesis. The untreated areas help in rapid reepithelialization of the skin, minimizing the chances of prolonged and serious adverse effects.[20]

Fractional lasers are divided into either nonablative or ablative fractional lasers. While, the ablative lasers (fractional CO_2 and fractional erbium 2,940 nm) are considered to be more effective, they still run the risk of developing side effects in dark skin. The nonablative ones were developed to combat the side effects of the ablative lasers and provide modest improvement in mild-to-moderate photodamage, acne scars, wrinkles, and textural imperfections.[21] The nonablative fractional lasers currently available on the market are Fraxel Restore 1,550 nm, 1,550 nm erbium glass, and 1,927 nm thulium fiber (Restore Dual), 1,540 nm Palomar Star, 1,440 nm Cynosure Affirm, 1,410 nm Solta Fraxel Refine. The popular ablative fractional ablative lasers are 10,600 nm $C0_2$ laser (Lumenis UltraPulse, Encore, Fraxel Repair), fractional 2,940 nm erbium doped yttrium-aluminium- garnet (Alma Lasers Harmony platform, Sciton ProFractional XC), 2,790 nm fractional erbium doped yttrium-scandium-gallium-garnet (Cutera Xeo Platform). Lumenis recently introduced the SCAAR FX™ (Synergistic Coagulation and Ablation for Advanced Resurfacing) mode to its UltraPulse CO_2 laser for the treatment of surgical and acne scars as well as hypertrophic scars. The nonablative nonfractional lasers produce controlled thermal injury in the dermis stimulating dermal collagen remodeling and are particularly popular with the darker skin tones as they do not produce any abnormal pigmentation. At present, the 1,320 nm Nd:YAG laser (CoolTouch, Alma Harmony XL) , SmoothBeam 1,450 nm, and the 1,319 nm pulsed energy (Sciton ThermaScan) are the nonablative nonfractionated lasers available.[22] Radiofrequency microneedling (Infini microneedling fractional radiofrequency) is currently classified under nonablative systems, but appears to be promising in the treatment of wrinkles and acne scars as it has the advantage of a higher penetration depth, while aiming for collagen shrinkage and skin tightening.[23]

RECENT ADVANCES IN FACE AND BODY CONTOURING

Noninvasive devices which entered the market only a few years ago have transformed approaches to body contouring which relied formerly only on liposuction. Velasmooth, Accent, Thermage, Sciton, Liposonix, and SmartLipo are some of the devices currently available. CoolSculpt is a relatively new device which works on the principle of cryolipolysis by inducing a localized cold panniculitis followed by selective fat reduction in the affected areas. Once the fat cells are destroyed, the body disposes out the liquefied fat through normal biological pathways. Dover et al. found a visible contour change for the flank and back fat pads by using cryolipolysis in 32 subjects.[24] Cellulaze (1,440 nm laser) is the first minimally invasive laser approved by the FDA in 2012. It involves the insertion of a tiny optic fiber beneath the skin to break the fibrotic bands responsible for creating cellulite.[25] Intense focused ultrasound is another noninvasive device that is FDA approved for lifting of skin of the eyebrows, chin, and neck. The clinician here has the added advantage of varying the depth of treatment depending of the degree of sagging. Effects of skin tightening are visible in 3–4 treatments.[26]

LOW LEVEL LASER THERAPY (COLD LASER) AND LIGHT EMITTING DIODES

Light emitting diodes (LED) are devices which emit light in the wavelength of 630–850 nm. They have a high penetrating power and are used currently for the purpose of photorejuvenation, acne treatment, and several types of dermatitis. Low level laser therapy works on the principle of photobiostimulation of the skin primarily by increasing the permeability of mitochondrial membranes and raising the pH, activating the cyclic adenosine monophosphate and increasing the deoxyribonucleic acid/ribonucleic acid synthesis. Low level laser therapy has more recently been used to promote hair growth in male and female pattern baldness. The HairMax LaserComb, Revage 670 which is a low level diode laser, and TOPHAT 655 are the devices which have been granted FDA clearance for the same.[27]

CONCLUSION

With rapid advancements in the field of laser technology and the preference of patients toward more of noninvasive treatments, new lasers continue to emerge. Hence, a sound clinical judgment on the part of the treating physician is very important to ensure that these new devices are used ethically and appropriately for patient care. It is of utmost importance that the need for repetitive treatments should be addressed beforehand in order to avoid an unhappy patient and to maintain satisfactory results.

REFERENCES

1. Manstein D, Herron GS, Sink RK, Tanner H, Anderson RR. Fractional photothermolysis: A new concept for cutaneous remodeling using microscopic patterns of thermal injury. Lasers Surg Med. 2004;34:426-38.
2. Gan SD, Graber EM. Laser hair removal: a review. Dermatol Surg. 2013;39:823-38.
3. Seaton ED, Charakida A, Mouser PE, Grace I, Clement RM, Chu AC. Pulsed-dye laser treatment for inflammatory acne vulgaris: Randomised controlled trial. Lancet. 2003;362:1347-52.
4. Laubach HJ, Astner S, Watanabe K, Clifford J, Rius-Diaz F, Zurakowski D, et al. Effects of a 1,450 nm diode laser on facial sebum excretion. Lasers Surg Med. 2009;41:110-5.
5. Glaich AS, Friedman PM, Jih MH, Goldberg LH. Treatment of inflammatory facial acne vulgaris with combination 595-nm pulsed-dye laser with dynamic-cooling-device and 1,450-nm diode laser. Lasers Surg Med. 2006;38:177-80.
6. Boineau D, Angel S, Auffret N, Dahan S, Mordon S. Treatment of active acne with an erbium glass (1.54 micron) laser. Lasers Surg Med. 2004;16:S55.
7. Chun SI. Carbon assisted Q-switched Nd:YAG laser treatment with two different sets of pulse width parameters offers a useful treatment modality for severe inflammatory acne: a case report. Photomed Laser Surg. 2011;29:131-5.
8. Kim S, Cho KH. Treatment of facial postinflammatory hyperpigmentation with facial acne in Asian patients using a Q-switched neodymium-doped yttrium aluminum garnet laser. Dermatol Surg. 2010;36:1374-80.
9. Lee MC, Chang CS, Huang YL. Treatment of melasma with mixed parameters of 1,064-nm Q-switched Nd:YAG laser toning and an enhanced effect of ultrasonic application of Vit C: a split-face study. Lasers Med Sci. 2014;30:159-63.
10. Polder KD, Bruce S. Treatment of melasma using a novel 1,927-nm fractional thulium fiber laser: a pilot study. Dermatol Surg. 2012;38:199-206.
11. Polder KD, Harrison A, Eubanks LE, Bruce S. 1,927-nm fractional thulium fiber laser for the treatment of nonfacial photodamage: a pilot study. Dermatol Surg. 2011;37:342-8.
12. Saedi N, Metelitsa A, Petrell K, Arndt KA, Dover JS. Treatment of tattoos with a picosecond Alexandrite laser: a prospective trial. Arch Dermatol. 2102;148:1360-3.
13. Kossida T, Rigopoulos D, Katsambas A, Anderson RR. Optimal tattoo removal in a single laser session based on the method of repeated exposures. J Am Acad Dermatol. 2012;66:271-7.
14. Marini L. Combining fractional Er:YAG and Q-switched lasers for tattoo removal. Journal of Laser and Health Academy. 2013;1:S15.
15. Alster TS, Tanzi EL. Combined 595 nm and 1064 nm laser irradiation of recalcitrant and hypertrophic port-wine stains in children and adults. Dermatol Surg. 2009;35:914-9.
16. Huang YC, Tran N, Shumaker PR, Kelly K, Ross EV, Nelson JS, et al. Blood flow dynamics after laser therapy of port wine stain birthmarks. Lasers Surg Med. 2009;41:563-71.
17. Jia W, Sun V, Tran N, Choi B, Liu SW, Mihm MC, et al. Long-term blood vessel removal with combined laser and topical rapamycin antiangiogenic therapy: implications for effective port wine stain treatment. Lasers Surg Med. 2010;42:105-12.
18. Reddy KK, Brauer JA, Idriss MH, Anolik R, Bernstein L, Brightman L, et al. Treatment of Port-wine stains with a short pulse width 532-nm Nd:YAG Laser. J Drugs Dermatol. 2013;12:66-71.
19. Majid I, Imran S. Fractional CO2 laser resurfacing as monotherapy in the treatment of atrophic facial acne scars. J Cutan Aesthet Surg. 2014;7(2):87-92.
20. Preissig J, Hamilton K, Markus R. Current Laser Resurfacing Technologies: A Review that Delves Beneath the Surface. Semin Plast Surg. 2012;26:109-16.
21. DeHoratius DM, Dover JS. Nonablative tissue remodeling and photorejuvination. Clin Dermatol. 2007;25:474-79.
22. Bogle MA. Fractionated mid-infrared resurfacing. Semin Cutan Med Surg. 2008;27:252-8.
23. Kim ST, Lee KH, Sim HJ, Suh KS, Jang MS. Treatment of acne vulgaris with fractional radiofrequency microneedling. J Dermatol. 2014;41:586-91.
24. Dover J, Burns J, Coleman S, Fitzpatrick R, Garden J, Goldberg D, et al. A prospective clinical study of noninvasive cryolipolysis™ for subcutaneous fat layer reduction. Lasers Surg Med. 2009;45:S 21.
25. Di Bernardo BE. Cellulite treatment using the Nd:YAG 1440 nm wavelength laser with side-firing fiber: 3-year follow-up. Plastic surgery Pulse News. 2013;5:1.
26. Pak CS, Lee YK, Jeong JH, Kim JH, Seo JD, Heo CY. Safety and efficacy of Ulthera in the rejuvenation of ageing lower eyelids: a pivotal clinical trial. Aesthetic Plastic Surg. 2014;38:861-8.
27. Lanzafame RJ, Blanche RR, Bodian AB, Chiacchierini RP, Fernandez OA, Kazmirek ER. The growth of human scalp hair mediated by visible red light laser and LED sources in males. Lasers Surg Med. 2013;45:487-95.

Appendices

Appendix 1

Consent Forms and Patient Record Sheets

Asad Ansari, Projna Biswas

Pre- and Post-treatment Instructions for Laser Patients

A. Pretreatment Instructions for Laser Patients

Your results with laser therapy are highly dependent on your cooperation. There are many things you can inadvertently do to decrease the safety or effectiveness of the treatment. Please follow these directions carefully regarding tanning, shaving, and topical agents, or we may have to cancel your appointment and reschedule.

1. Avoid direct sun exposure, tanning, tanning product, use broad spectrum sunscreen SPF 30 or more daily for 4 weeks before and after the treatment
2. Avoid deep facial peeling procedure for 4 weeks prior (aggressive chemical peeling, dermabrasion etc.)
3. Depending upon your skin type, a bleaching regimen may be started 2–6 weeks before treatment
4. Avoid medication that causes photosensitivities (like doxycycline, minocycline) for 72 hours prior to treatment
5. Avoid medication which causes blood thinning and have anti-inflammatory action for 2 weeks prior to procedure to minimize risk of bruising (such as aspirin, vitamin E, ibuprofen, naproxen etc.)
6. Tell us if you have taken systemic retinoids within the past 6 months
7. Discontinue use of glycolic acid or retinoic acid containing products 1 week before treatment
8. If you have history of or recent break out of herpes (oral or genital cold sore) or shingles in the treatment area start your antiviral medications 2 days prior to treatment and continue for 3 days after treatment
9. Please notify us of any history of diabetes, herpes, blood coagulation disorders, keloid, or hypertrophic scarring
10. For hair removal treatment, avoid any depilatory creams, plucking or waxing 2 weeks prior to treatment
11. Shave the area to be treated at the night before or morning of the procedure
12. Do not wear makeup or use moisturizer on the area to be treated in the morning of the procedure
13. The area to be treated must be free of any open sore, wound, or infection
14. You may experience a slight vibration or heat on your teeth or dental work if being treated around the mouth area—this is normal
15. Bring sun protective items like wide-brimmed hat and sunglasses for postprocedure.

What to Expect

1. A mild sunburn sensation
2. Minor redness and swelling at the treatment site
3. Pigment areas will turn a dark gray and flake off in 1–2 weeks
4. Healing on the face can take 1–2 weeks or longer
5. Healing on the body can take 2–4 weeks or longer
6. A temporary lightening or darkening of the treated skin can occur.

B. Post-treatment Instructions

1. After treatment, the area will be red and there may be temporary localized swelling. Sleep and rest with your head and shoulder elevated to reduce the swelling for 3–4 days postoperatively
2. If redness or swelling occurs, ice packs, cold packs, aloe vera, or any other cooling preparation may be used for temporary discomfort
3. Oral analgesics, nonsteroidal anti-inflammatory agents, or other medications may be used at the discretion of your physician for discomfort
4. Keep applying layers of moisturizer to the treated area for protection and to promote the healing process. Reapply and keep face moist as needed until peeling has stopped, about 3–5 days
5. Avoid heat and hot water on the treated areas for 24 hours, exposure to fumes while cooking, sweating, and exercise should be avoided for a period of 1 week
6. Avoid direct sun exposure and use broad spectrum sunscreen of SPF 30, with UVB and UVA ray coverage, should be worn daily [2–3 hourly] regardless of sun exposure for 4 weeks. It is important that you commit to staying out of the sun
7. Use mild soap that do not contains ingredient that may irritate the treated area
8. After showering, do not rub the area only pat dry the skin
9. Avoid aggressive facial treatment or any topical product that can cause facial irritation minimum 4 weeks following treatment
10. If any scabbing, blistering, or crusting appears, do not pick or scratch it, apply an antibiotic ointment and notify your treating doctor
11. Avoid activities that can cause flushing for 2 weeks after treatment
12. Anywhere from 20 days after the treatment, shedding of the surface hair may occur and this appears as new hair growth. This is not new hair growth
13. Do not use Retin-A or glycolic acid to the treated area for 5 days post-treatment
14. If you feel any discomfort (typically this does not last more than 6 hours), use acetaminophen
15. Avoid swimming and contact sports while the skin is healing
16. You can start wearing light makeup after 5th day
17. No creams or lotions should be applied to the skin except prescribed by the doctor.

Fractional Laser Resurfacing for Treatment of Scars

A. Informed Consent Form

Name:____________________________________

Registration No.:___________________________ Age:________ Sex:_______

Phone No.:________________

Address:____

My lesion(s) being treated are called______________________________________

The laser to be used on me is ____

I have been explained about my condition and the treatment in my regional language.

I, the undersigned, authorize Dr __________________________ or his/her assistant ____________________ to perform laser therapy on me.

I have been informed that the numbers of sessions required for complete clearing of my lesion are variable. I have also understood that it may not be possible to clear my lesion completely and no guarantees can be given for the results. I understand that I may need to undergo many sessions for optimum resolution of my lesion.

I also give consent to the use of any form of anesthesia if my doctor feels it fit to use the same. I also understand that a cooling device in the form of a cryogen spray or ice pack may be used during the procedure to reduce any discomfort and to protect my skin.

I have been informed that laser light can damage my eyes. Therefore, during the session I will have my eyes covered with laser protective glasses to protect my eyes from the intense laser light.

I have been informed that this laser is not the only treatment for my condition and other treatment options have also been discussed with me in detail. I acknowledge that I have understood all treatment options and their possible complications and benefits. I have also understood the health consequences that may arise if I do not take this laser treatment. Considering all the information that I have been provided with by my doctor, I consent to undergo laser therapy for my scars.

All the contraindications to laser treatment have been fully explained to me.

I understand that, side effects and complications of ablative fractional carbon dioxide laser resurfacing include, but are not limited to:

1. Pain: the stinging or burning sensation from the laser can produce a moderate amount of discomfort. An anesthetic cream, oral and injectable pain relievers, and antianxiety medications will typically be used to minimize discomfort
2. Redness: redness resembling sunburn can occur in treated area. The redness will typically subside in 1–6 weeks, but could last longer
3. Swelling: treatment may cause swelling which subsides in 1–2 weeks and can be minimized with application of cool water compresses
4. Allergic reactions: in rare cases, local allergies to tape, preservatives used in cosmetics, or topical preparations have been reported. Systemic reactions which are more serious may result from drugs used during medical procedures and prescription medicines. Allergic reactions may require additional treatment
5. Skin color alteration: darkening of the skin or loss of pigmentation rarely occurs in the treated areas and will usually fades or repigment within 1–6 months. This reaction is more common when treated areas are exposed to the sun. It is extremely important to protect the treated area from sun exposure with a hat and sunscreen for 6 weeks after treatment and carefully adhere to all post-treatment instructions

Continued

Continued

6. Blisters or scabs: blistering is uncommon but can develop with treatment. Blisters will go away within 2–5 days and may be followed by a scab. The scab will disappear during the natural wound healing process of the skin. During this time, the area should not be manipulated or picked, which can lead to scarring
7. Infection: swelling, crusting, pain, or fever could indicate an infection or reactivation of cold sores or fever blisters. This may require use of topical or oral antibiotics and/or antiviral agents
8. Acneiform eruptions or milia: breakouts from acne or milia have been reported to occur after treatment with laser resurfacing. If this occurs, topical or oral antibiotics may be required
9. Scarring: there is a risk of skin scarring, including abnormal raised and/or depressed scars with any resurfacing procedure. Careful adherence to all advised postoperative instructions will help reduce the possibility of this occurrence
10. Lesion persistence or failure to respond: some skin conditions may not improve or go away completely despite the best efforts made by the doctor. No guarantees can be made regarding any individual's response to treatment with laser resurfacing
11. Delayed healing: it may take longer than anticipated for healing to occur after laser treatments. Skin healing may result in thin, easily injured skin. This is different from the normal redness in skin after a laser treatment
12. Surgical anesthesia: both local and general anesthesia involve risk. There is the possibility of complications, injury, and even death from all forms of surgical anesthesia and sedation.

For young women of child-bearing age: I give my consent for laser treatment with the absolute knowledge that I am not pregnant. I have been advised to avoid pregnancy during the course of my treatment. I have also been advised to inform immediately if I become pregnant during the course of my treatment.

I give my consent for taking photographs before and after each laser session. I understand that taking photographs is necessary for maintaining records and optimizing my treatment. These photographs can also be used for teaching purposes.

I understand that I have to start using a sunscreen (SPF 30) 2 weeks before the procedure and continue using it during the course of treatment and even after it. I understand that failure to do so would result in suboptimal results and lead to complications.

I understand that additional treatment may be necessary—there are many variable conditions which influence the long-term result of laser skin treatments. Even though risks and complications occur infrequently, the risks cited are the ones that are particularly associated with these procedures. The practice of medicine and surgery is not an exact science. Although good results are expected, there is no guarantee or warranty expressed or implied on the results that may be obtained.

I understand that for optimal results and minimal side effects, I need time to time follow-up visits as prescribed by the doctor/clinic and also I need to strictly follow the postoperative care instructed to me.

Financial Responsibilities:

I have been explained about the cost of each laser session.

I am going to pay per session/package basis. Package, if opted for, includes minimum number of sessions and I have to pay accordingly if any additional sessions or treatments are required. I understand that no guarantees have been made and all payments are nonrefundable.

I consent to the treatment or procedure and I certify that I have read, and fully understand the above paragraphs and that i have had sufficient opportunity for discussion to have any questions answered.

Patient signature:______________________ Date:_____________________________

Signature of parent/guardian:______________________________

(In case of minors)

Witness:_________________________________ Time:__________

B. Patient Record Sheet (Fractional Laser Resurfacing for Treatment of Scars)

Name:______________________________ Age:________ Sex:_______

Address:______________________________ Mobile No.:_______________

Registration No.:_____________ Diagnosis:____________________________

General Information

1. Any photosensitive disorder: SLE/rosacea/blooms, etc.
2. Photosensitive medication: captopril/NSAID/tetracyclines, retinoids, etc.
3. Bleeding disorders: yes/no
4. Any implants/prosthesis: yes/no
5. Keloidal tendencies: yes/no
6. Any infections at the site: herpes labialis, genitalis, zoster, etc.
7. Pregnancy: yes/no
8. History of convulsions: yes/no
9. Isotretinoin within the last 6 months: yes/no.

Fitzpatrick's skin type: I, II, III, IV, V, VI

Information of scar:

1. Site of scar:________
2. Onset: acute/insidious
3. Duration: ________
4. Dimension: ________
5. Hypertrophic/atrophic: acne scar
6. Cause of scar: acne/varicella/trauma/burn/others
7. Grade of acne scar: I/II/III/IV
8. Any superficial skin changes: ________
9. Color of the scar: dark/red/whitish
10. Keloidal tendency: yes/no
11. Symptoms on the scar: pruritus/pain
12. Any contracture/deformity:________.

C. Treatment Record Sheet (Fractional Laser Resurfacing for Treatment of Scars)

Name:________________________ Age:________ Sex:_______

Registration No.:____________________ Mobile No.:______________

Skin type:_______________________ Diagnosis:___________________________

Treating doctor:____________________ Treatment area:_____________________

No. of session	1	2	3	4	5	6
Date						
Anesthesia used (yes/no)						
Consent taken (yes/no)						
Name of laser						
Wavelength						
Fluence/energy						
Pulse duration						
Pulse delay						
Density						
Mode (superficial/deep)						
Scanner type used						
No. of pass						
Subcision						
Spot size						
Frequency (Hz)						
No. of pulses						
Any complications						
Signature of patients						
Signature of doctor						

Laser Hair Reduction

A. Informed Consent Form

Name:_______________________________

Registration No.:_______________________ Age:________ Sex:_______

Phone No.:______________

Address:____

Indication of laser hair reduction:____

The laser to be used on me is ____

I have been explained about my condition and the treatment in my regional language.

I, the undersigned, authorize Dr _______________________ or his/her assistant __________________ to perform hair reduction laser therapy on me.

The laser is a device that produces an intense but gentle burst of laser light. This light gets absorbed by the melanin pigment in hair. This causes heating and destruction of the hair follicles without harming the surrounding tissue.

The purpose of laser hair reduction is to diminish or remove unwanted hair. I have also understood that it may not be possible to remove my hair completely and no guarantees can be given for the results.

I have also been informed that rarely there are patients who do not respond to laser hair reduction. I have been informed that laser works only on active (anagen) hairs and not on dormant hairs. Therefore, I will need to undergo an average of 6–8 sessions for optimum, long-term hair reduction.

I understand that the number of sessions required varies between individuals. I have also been informed of the need for repeated maintenance sessions at regular intervals for obtaining optimum results.

I understand that my hair will become finer with successive sessions and their growth rate will decrease. However, even with many laser sessions, there will be very fine hair over the treated area.

I understand that laser is most effective on coarse, black hair, and that white or grey hair will not respond to laser treatment.

I understand that hair growth is dependent on hormones. Therefore, in case of hormonal imbalance (polycystic ovarian syndrome), results will be suboptimal and I will require greater number of sessions.

I have been informed that topical anesthesia is usually not required for the procedure. However, I give my consent to the use of any form of anesthesia if my doctor feels it fit to use the same. I also understand that a cooling device in the form of a cryogen spray or ice pack may be used during the procedure to reduce any discomfort and to protect my skin.

I have been informed that this laser is not the only treatment for my unwanted hair and other treatment options do exist. These include electrolysis, threading, shaving, plucking, and waxing. These treatment options have also been discussed with me in detail. I acknowledge that I have understood all treatment options and their possible complications and benefits. Considering all the information that I have been provided with by my doctor, I consent to undergo laser therapy for my unwanted hair.

During laser treatment, slight pinching sensation will be felt. The hairs in the follicles are usually extruded in 1–3 weeks after the treatment.

All the contraindications to laser treatment have been fully explained to me.

I have been informed that laser light can damage the retina of my eyes. Therefore, during the session, I will have my eyes covered with laser protective glasses to protect my eyes from the intense laser light.

Continued

Continued

I have been informed of the following complications that may occur while undergoing laser treatment:

1. Discomfort in the form of mild pain or tingling sensation during laser session
2. Redness, swelling, purpura (red-blue discoloration), or bruising: it usually lasts a few hours
3. Itching (hives): it may last for a few hours
4. Wounds in the form of burns, blisters or pin-point bleeding: It usually heals with crusting and scab formation
5. Skin color changes in the form of hyperpigmentation (darker skin) or hypopigmentation (lighter skin color): these color changes are usually temporary and resolve over 2–4 weeks. However, it may be permanent at times
6. Infection: either bacterial infection or reactivation of herpes viral infection can occur. It is important to follow the postprocedure instructions carefully to prevent any infections and to report them immediately if they occur
7. Scarring: it is a rare complication and can be avoided by following the postprocedure instructions carefully. It can be permanent.
8. Paradoxical hair growth: this can rarely occur with laser hair reduction. However, these hairs can also be treated with laser.

I give my consent for taking photographs before and after each laser session. I understand that taking photographs is necessary for maintaining records and optimizing my treatment. These photographs can also be used for teaching purposes.

I understand that I have to start using a sunscreen (SPF 30) 2 weeks before the procedure and continue using it during the course of treatment and even after it. I understand that failure to follow the postprocedure instructions would result in suboptimal results and lead to complications.

For young women of child-bearing age: I give my consent for laser treatment with the absolute knowledge that I am not pregnant. I have been advised to avoid pregnancy during the course of my treatment. I have also been advised to inform immediately if I become pregnant during the course of my treatment.

I have read and understood all information presented to me before signing this consent.

Patient signature:____________________ Date:__________________________

Signature of parent/guardian:____________________________

(In case of minors)

Witness:______________________________ Time:____________

Pretreatment instructions:

1. Start using sunscreen daily 1 month before the laser treatment to avoid tanning
2. Avoid waxing, threading, or plucking your hair 1 month before treatment as these procedures remove the hair by its root. Shaving can be done in this period
3. Avoid using irritant products, such as tretinoin or glycolic acid creams, 5–7 days before the procedure
4. Avoid using bleach or hair removal creams 2 weeks before the session as they can cause skin irritation
5. Inform about any history of herpes recently. Antiviral medication needs to be started before 1 day before laser session
6. Avoid shaving the area for the last 48 hours before laser session for better appreciation of hair growth.

Post-treatment instructions:

1. Use sunscreen for the entire duration of the treatment
2. Some swelling and redness may be visible after the laser session. Apply ice packs to reduce this swelling and redness
3. Avoid using irritant products, such as tretinoin or glycolic acid creams, 5–7 days after the treatment
4. If any crusting or scabbing occurs, do not scratch it. Apply antibiotic cream to the area for 5–7 days and aloe vera cream. Contact the clinic/doctor without delay
5. Some remaining hairs in the follicles will extrude in 1–3 weeks.

B. Patient Record Sheet (Laser Hair Reduction)

Name:______________________________ Age:________ Sex:_______

Address:______________________________ Mobile No.:________________

Registration No.:______________ Diagnosis:____________________________

General information:

1. Any photosensitive disorder: SLE/rosacea/blooms, etc.
2. Photosensitive medication: captopril/NSAIDs/tetracyclines, retinoids, etc.
3. Bleeding disorders: yes/no
4. Any implants/prosthesis: yes/no
5. Keloidal tendencies: yes/no
6. Any infections at the site: herpes labialis, genitalis, zoster, etc.
7. Pregnancy: yes/no
8. History of convulsions: yes/no
9. Isotretinoin within the last 6 months: yes/no.

Fitzpatrick's skin type: I, II, III, IV, V, VI

Other history:

1. Clinical signs of hormonal disturbances: obesity, menstrual irregularities, acanthosis, FPHL, acne
2. Any documented hormonal disturbances: PCOS, hypothyroidism, etc.
3. Specific investigations:
   - Serum testosterone level
   - LH/FSH ratio
   - Fasting and postprandial insulin level
   - Ultrasound of abdomen and pelvis
   - Serum TSH, free T4, free T3.
4. History of ingestion of drugs like phenytoin, cyclosporine, OCPs, etc.

Areas to be treated:

1.
2.
3.
4.

Hair types:

1. Thick, dense
2. Thick, less dense
3. Thinner, less dense
4. Very fine hair (vellus), very low hair density.

C. Treatment Record Sheet (Laser Hair Reduction)

Name:________________________ Age:________ Sex:_______

Registration No.:____________________ Mobile No.:______________

Skin type:________________________ Diagnosis:____________________________

Treating doctor:____________________ Treatment area:________________________

Modified Ferriman-Gallwey score for hirsutism :

Site	Upper lip	Chin	Chest	Upper back	Lower back	Upper abdomen	Lower abdomen	Upper arms	Thighs
Score (0–4)									
Total score									

No. of session	1	2	3	4	5	6
Date						
Anesthesia used (yes/no)						
Consent taken (yes/no)						
Name of laser						
Wavelength						
Fluence/energy						
Pulse duration						
Pulse delay						
Spot size						
Frequency (Hz)						
No. of pulses						
Any complications						
Signature of client						
Signature of doctor						

Laser Treatment for Pigmentation Removal

A. Informed Consent Form

Name:__________________________________

Registration No.:__________________________ Age:________ Sex:_______

Phone No.:________________

Address:____

Laser and machine used:

My lesions(s) being treated are called____

The laser to be used on me is ____

I have been explained about my condition and the treatment in my regional language.

I, the undersigned, authorize Dr _________________________ or his/her assistant ___________________ to perform laser therapy on me.

The laser is a device that produces an intense but gentle burst of laser light. This light gets selectively absorbed by the melanin pigment without harming the surrounding tissue. This causes heating and dispersion of the melanin pigment into smaller particles which are eventually eliminated by the body over a period of time.

I have been informed that the number of sessions required for complete clearing of my lesion are variable. I have also understood that it may not be possible to clear my lesion completely and no guarantees can be given for the results. I understand that I may need to undergo 4–6 sessions for optimum resolution of my lesion. However, I have also been informed of the need for repeated follow-up sessions for obtaining optimum benefits.

I have been informed that topical anesthesia is usually not required for the procedure. However, I give consent to the use of any form of anesthesia if my doctor feels it fit to use the same. I also understand that a cooling device in the form of a cryogen spray or ice pack may be used during the procedure to reduce any discomfort and to protect my skin.

I have been informed that laser light can damage the retina of my eyes. Therefore, during the session, I will have my eyes covered with laser protective glasses to protect my eyes from the intense laser light.

I have been informed that this laser treatment is not the only treatment for my condition and other treatment options have also been discussed with me in detail. I acknowledge that I have understood all treatment options and their possible complications and benefits. I have also understood any possible health consequences that may arise if I do not take this laser treatment. Considering all the information that I have been provided with by my doctor, I consent to undergo laser therapy for my pigmented lesion(s).

All the contraindications to laser treatment have been fully explained to me.

I have been informed of the following complications that may occur while undergoing laser treatment:

1. Discomfort in the form of mild pain or tingling sensation during laser session
2. Redness, swelling, purpura (red-blue discoloration), or bruising: it usually lasts a few hours
3. Itching (hives): it may last for a few hours
4. Wounds in the form of burns, blisters, or pin-point bleeding: it usually heals with crusting and scab formation
5. Skin color changes in the form of hyperpigmentation (darker skin) or hypopigmentation (lighter skin color): these color changes are usually temporary and resolve over 2–4 weeks. However, it may be permanent at times
6. Infection: either bacterial infection or reactivation of herpes viral infection can occur. It is important to follow the postprocedure instructions carefully to prevent any infections and to report them immediately if they occur
7. Scarring: it is a rare complication and can be avoided by following the postprocedure instructions carefully. It can be permanent.

Continued

Continued

I give my consent for taking photographs before and after each laser session. I understand that taking photographs is necessary for maintaining records and optimizing my treatment. These photographs can also be used for teaching purposes.

I understand that I have to start using a sunscreen (SPF 30) 2 weeks before the procedure and continue using it during the course of treatment and even after it. I understand that failure to do so would result in suboptimal results. I also understand that some of these lesions can recur if strict sun protection is not done.

For young women of child-bearing age: I give my consent for laser treatment with the absolute knowledge that I am not pregnant. I have been advised to avoid pregnancy during the course of my treatment. I have also been advised to inform immediately if I become pregnant during the course of my treatment.

I have read and understood all information presented to me before signing this consent.

Patient signature:____________________ Date:__________________________

Signature of parent/guardian:____________________________

(In case of minors)

Witness:______________________________ Time:____________

B. Patient Record Sheet (Laser Treatment for Pigmentation Removal)

Name:________________________________ Age:________ Sex:_______

Address:______________________________ Mobile No.:_______________

Registration No.:_____________ Diagnosis:___________________________

General information:

1. Any photosensitive disorder: SLE/rosacea/blooms, etc.
2. Photosensitive medication: captopril/NSAIDs/tetracyclines, retinoids, etc.
3. Bleeding disorders: yes/no
4. Any implants/prosthesis: yes/no
5. Keloidal tendencies: yes/no
6. Any infections at the site: herpes labialis, genitalis, zoster, etc.
7. Pregnancy: yes/no
8. History of convulsions: yes/no
9. Isotretinoin within the last 6 months: yes/no.

Fitzpatrick's skin type: I, II, III, IV, V, VI

Information of pigmented lesion:

1. Lesion present since: ________
2. Onset: acute/insidious/pregnancy/drug intake
3. Site: _______
4. Unilateral/bilateral
5. Size: _______
6. Number of lesions: single/multiple
7. Previous treatment: yes/no
8. History of similar lesion in family: yes/no
9. Any other dermatologic/systemic association: _______.

C. Treatment Record Sheet (Laser Treatment for Pigmentation Removal)

Name:________________________ Age:________ Sex:_______

Registration No.:____________________ Mobile No.:________________

Skin type:________________________ Diagnosis:________________________

Treating doctor:____________________ Treatment area:______________________

No. of session	1	2	3	4	5	6
Date						
Anesthesia used (yes/no)						
Consent taken (yes/no)						
Name of laser						
Wavelength						
Fluence/Energy						
Picosecond/nanosecond						
Standard/fractional						
Spot size						
Frequency (Hz)						
No. of pulses						
Any complications						
Signature of client						
Signature of doctor						

Laser Tattoo Removal

A. Informed Consent Form

Name:________________________________

Registration No.:________________________ Age:________ Sex:_______

Phone No.:______________

Address:____

The laser to be used on me is ____________________________________

I have been explained in detail about my condition and the treatment in my regional language.

I, the undersigned, authorize Dr __________________________ or his/her assistant __________________ to perform laser therapy on me.

The laser is a device that produces an intense but gentle burst of laser light. This light gets selectively absorbed by the ink particles of the tattoo without harming the surrounding tissue. This causes heating and dispersion of the ink particles into smaller particles which are eventually eliminated by the body over a period of time.

I have been informed that the number of sessions required for complete clearing of my tattoo are variable. I have also understood that it may not be possible to clear my tattoo completely and no guarantees can be given for the results. I understand that I may need to undergo 6–8 sessions for optimum resolution of my tattoo.

I have been informed that topical anesthesia is usually not required for the procedure. However, I give consent to the use of any form of anesthesia if my doctor feels it fit to use the same. I also understand that a cooling device in the form of a cryogen spray or ice pack may be used during the procedure to reduce any discomfort and protect my skin.

I have been informed that laser light can damage the retina of my eyes. Therefore, during the session, I will have my eyes covered with laser protective glasses to protect my eyes from the intense laser light.

I have been informed that this laser treatment is not the only treatment for my tattoo and other treatment options have also been discussed with me in detail. I acknowledge that I have understood all treatment options and their possible complications and benefits. I have also understood any possible health consequences that may arise if I do not take this laser treatment. Considering all the information that I have been provided with by my doctor, I consent to undergo laser therapy for my tattoo.

All the contraindications to laser treatment have been fully explained to me.

I have been informed of the following complications that may occur while undergoing laser treatment:

1. Discomfort in the form of mild pain or tingling sensation during laser session
2. Redness, swelling, purpura (red-blue discoloration), or bruising: it usually lasts a few hours
3. Itching (hives): it may last for a few hours
4. Wounds in the form of burns, blisters, or pin-point bleeding: it usually heals with crusting and scab formation
5. Skin color changes in the form of hyperpigmentation (darker skin) or hypopigmentation (lighter skin color): these color changes are usually temporary and resolve over 2–4 weeks. However, it may be permanent at times
6. Infection: either bacterial infection or reactivation of herpes viral infection can occur. It is important to follow the postprocedure instructions carefully to prevent any infections and to report them immediately if they occur
7. Scarring: it is a rare complication and can be avoided by following the postprocedure instructions carefully. It can be permanent.

I give my consent for taking photographs before and after each laser session. I understand that taking photographs is necessary for maintaining records and optimizing my treatment. These photographs can also be used for teaching purposes.

Continued

Continued

I understand that I have to start using a sunscreen (SPF 30) 2 weeks before the procedure and continue using it during the course of treatment and even after it. I understand that failure to do so would result in suboptimal results.

For young women of child-bearing age: I give my consent for laser treatment with the absolute knowledge that I am not pregnant. I have been advised to avoid pregnancy during the course of my treatment. I have also been advised to inform immediately if I become pregnant during the course of my treatment.

I have read and understood all information presented to me before signing this consent.

Patient signature:____________________ Date:___________________________

Signature of parent/guardian:____________________________

(In case of minors)

Witness:_______________________________ Time:_____________

B. Patient Record Sheet (Laser Tattoo Removal)

Name:_________________________________ Age:_______ Sex:_______

Address:________________________________ Mobile No.:_______________

Registration No.:____________ Diagnosis:___________________________

General information:

1. Any photosensitive disorder: SLE/rosacea/blooms, etc.
2. Photosensitive medication: captopril/NSAIDs/tetracyclines, retinoids, etc.
3. Bleeding disorders: yes/no
4. Any implants/prosthesis: yes/no
5. Keloidal tendencies: yes/no
6. Any infections at the site: herpes labialis, genitalis, zoster, etc.
7. Pregnancy: yes/no
8. History of convulsions: yes/no
9. Isotretinoin within the last 6 months: yes/no.

Fitzpatrick's skin type: I, II, III, IV, V, VI

Information of tattoo:

1. Tattoo was done in the year: _______
2. Tattoo done by: professional/amateur
3. Site: _______
4. Size: _______
5. Number of tattoos: single/multiple
6. Color of tattoo: black/blue/red/green
7. Previous treatment: no/yes.

Continued

Continued

Kirby-Desai score:

Feature	Score
Skin type	
Tattoo location	
Tattoo pigment color	
Amount of ink	
Scarring and tissue change amount	
Tattoo layering	
Total score	

C. Treatment Record Sheet (Laser Tattoo Removal)

Name:____________________________ Age:_______ Sex:______

Registration No.:____________________ Mobile No.:_____________

Skin type:________________________ Diagnosis:___________________________

Treating doctor:____________________ Treatment area:_______________________

No. of session	1	2	3	4	5	6
Date						
Anesthesia used (yes/no)						
Consent taken (yes/no)						
Name of laser						
Wavelength						
Fluence/energy						
Nanosecond/picosecond						
R20/R0						
Spot size						
Frequency (Hz)						
No. of passes						
Any complications						
Signature of client						
Signature of doctor						

Laser Treatment of Vascular Lesions

A. Informed Consent Form

Name:_______________________________

Registration No.:________________________ Age:________ Sex:_______

Phone No.:______________

Address:____

My lesions(s) being treated is/are called__________________________________

The laser to be used on me is ______________________________________

I have been explained about my condition and the treatment in my regional language.

I, the undersigned, authorize Dr _______________ or his/her assistant ____________ to perform vascular laser therapy on me.

The laser is a device that produces an intense but gentle burst of laser light. This light gets absorbed by the abnormal blood vessels seen in spider veins or other cutaneous vascular lesions. This causes heating and destruction of the unwanted vessels without harming the surrounding tissue. These lesions fade slowly due to destruction by laser and eventual elimination by the body over a period of time.

I have been informed that the number of sessions required for complete clearing of my lesion are variable. I have also understood that it may not be possible to clear my lesion completely and no guarantees can be given for the results. I understand that I may need to undergo many sessions for optimum resolution of my lesion.

I have been informed that topical anesthesia is usually not required for the procedure. However, I give consent to the use of any form of anesthesia if my doctor feels it fit to use the same. I also understand that a cooling device in the form of a cryogen spray or ice pack may be used during the procedure to reduce any discomfort and to protect my skin.

I have been informed that laser light can damage the retina of my eyes. Therefore, during the session, I will have my eyes covered with laser protective glasses to protect my eyes from the intense laser light.

I have been informed that this laser is not the only treatment for my condition and other treatment options have also been discussed with me in detail. I acknowledge that I have understood all treatment options and their possible complications and benefits. I have also understood the health consequences that may arise if I do not take this laser treatment. Considering all the information that I have been provided with by my doctor, I consent to undergo laser therapy for my vascular lesion(s).

All the contraindications to laser treatment have been fully explained to me.

I have been informed of the following complications that may occur while undergoing laser treatment:

1. Discomfort in the form of mild pain or tingling sensation during laser session
2. Redness, swelling, purpura (red-blue discoloration), or bruising: it usually lasts a few hours
3. Itching (hives): it may last for a few hours
4. Wounds in the form of burns, blisters, or pin-point bleeding: it usually heals with crusting and scab formation
5. Skin color changes in the form of hyperpigmentation (darker skin) or hypopigmentation (lighter skin color): these color changes are usually temporary and resolve over 2–4 weeks. However, it may be permanent at times
6. Infection: either bacterial infection or reactivation of herpes viral infection can occur. It is important to follow the postprocedure instructions carefully to prevent any infections and to report them immediately if they occur
7. Scarring: it is a rare complication and can be avoided by following the postprocedure instructions carefully. It can be permanent.

I give my consent for taking photographs before and after each laser session. I understand that taking photographs is necessary for maintaining records and optimizing my treatment. These photographs can also be used for teaching purposes.

I understand that I have to start using a sunscreen (SPF 30) 2 weeks before the procedure and continue using it during the course of treatment and even after it. I understand that failure to do so would result in suboptimal results and lead to complications.

Continued

Continued

For young women of child-bearing age: I give my consent for laser treatment with the absolute knowledge that I am not pregnant. I have been advised to avoid pregnancy during the course of my treatment. I have also been advised to inform immediately if I become pregnant during the course of my treatment.

I have read and understood all information presented to me before signing this consent.

Patient signature:______________________ Date:_____________________________

Signature of parent/guardian:______________________________

(In case of minors)

Witness:_________________________________ Time:_____________

B. Patient Record Sheet (Laser Treatment of Vascular Lesions)

Name:___________________________________ Age:________ Sex:_______

Address:__________________________________ Mobile No.:________________

Registration No.:_____________ Diagnosis:____________________________

General information:

1. Any photosensitive disorder: SLE/rosacea/blooms, etc.
2. Photosensitive medication: captopril/NSAIDs/tetracyclines, retinoids, etc.
3. Bleeding disorders: yes/no
4. Any implants/prosthesis: yes/no
5. Keloidal tendencies: yes/no
6. Any infections at the site: herpes labialis, genitalis, zoster, etc.
7. Pregnancy: yes/no
8. History of convulsions: yes/no
9. Isotretinoin within the last 6 months: yes/no.

Fitzpatrick's skin type: I, II, III, IV, V, VI

Information of vascular lesion:

1. Age of onset: at birth/later (years)
2. Site: _______
3. Symptoms: no/pain/pruritus
4. Size: constant/increasing/decreasing
5. Family history: negative/1st degree/2nd degree
6. Palpable pulsation: present/absent
7. Number of lesions: _______
8. Color of lesions: pink/blue
9. Surface: raised/flat/verrucous
10. Previous treatment: yes/no
11. Past Rx: steroids/propranolol/laser
12. Improvement with past Rx: yes/no.

Continued

Continued

Association of vascular lesion:

1. Arteriovenous fistula: yes/no
2. Syndromes:
   - With vascular tumor: PHACE syndrome
   - With low-flow malformations: Sturge-Weber/Klippel-Trennauny/proteus/blue rubber bleb nevus/Maffuci/Gorham-Stout syndromes
   - With high-flow malformations: Rendu-Osler-Weber, Cobb, Wyburn-Mason, and Parkes-Weber syndromes
3. Bone changes: _______
4. CNS changes: _______
5. Others: _______.

Lab investigations:

1. Blood count: _______
2. Hemoglobin: _______
3. Total count: _______
4. Platelets: _______
5. Doppler study: _______
6. CT scan: _______
7. Histopathology:
   - Pretreatment
   - Post-treatment.

C. Treatment Record Sheet (Laser Treatment of Vascular Lesions)

Name:________________________________ Age:________ Sex:_______

Registration No.:________________________ Mobile No.:________________

Skin type:_______________________________ Diagnosis:________________________________

Treating doctor:__________________________ Treatment area:_____________________________

No. of session	1	2	3	4	5	6
Date						
Anesthesia used (yes/no)						
Consent taken (yes/no)						
Name of laser						
Wavelength						
Fluence/energy						
Pulse duration						
Pulse delay						
Spot size						
Frequency (Hz)						
No. of pulses						
Any complications						
Signature of client						
Signature of doctor						

Appendix 2

Glossary of Terminologies in Laser

Samujjala Deb

A

Ablation: the procedure of removing the target tissue using a laser beam leading to melting, evaporation, or vaporization.

Absorption: the process of transformation of radiant energy into another type of energy with a resultant rise in temperature and heating up of the tissue, dependent on the wavelength of laser and the properties of the tissue.

Absorption coefficient factor: it is the ability of light to be absorbed per unit of the path length it travels.

Accessible emission: this is the amount of accessible laser radiation having a particular wavelength or duration of emission at a particular point and measured by specific devices. This is also a measure of maximum possible radiation exposure to humans.

Accessible radiation: laser radiation that may be exposed to human eye or skin during use.

Active medium: it is the collection of atoms or molecules that can be made to be stimulated to a state of population inversion and produce stimulated emission of radiation.

Afocal: an optical system where the object and system is at infinity.

Aiming beam: a laser beam or light source that is used as a guiding light.

Alignment: it is the deviation of laser beam with respect to the mechanical axis of the device.

Amplification: this is the process of increasing the stimulated emission on each pass through the lasing medium.

Amplitude: the maximum value of the electromagnetic wave, measured from the mean to the extreme; or simply the height of the wave.

Aperture: the small opening through which the electromagnetic radiation passes.

AR coatings: antireflection coatings used on optical instruments to minimize reflection.

Argon laser: a laser medium using argon ions. It emits blue/green light of wavelengths 448 and 515 nm.

Articulated arm: a carbon dioxide laser beam delivery device that has a series of hollow tubes and mirrors interconnected in such a manner as to maintain alignment of the laser beam along the path of the arm.

Attenuation: the decrease in radiation energy (power) as the laser beam passes through an absorbing or scattering medium.

Average power: the total energy output during exposure divided by the exposure duration.

Aversion response: this is a protective reflex where there is an involuntary movement of the eyelid or head to prevent exposure to a harmful light source, occurs within 0.25 seconds.

Axicon lens: the alignment of a conical lens with a conventional lens that can focus the beam of the laser light into a ring shape.

B

Beam bender: an optical device that can modify the direction of a laser beam to reorient the beam in compact or folded laser systems.

Beam diameter: the distance between diametrically opposed points in the cross section of a circular beam, and thus, the intensity is reduced by a factor of 1/e (0.368) of the peak level (for safety standards). The value is normally chosen at 1/e2 (0.135) of the peak level.

Beam divergence: angle of beam spread measured in radians or milliradians (1 milliradian = 3.4 minutes-of-arc or approximately 1 mil).

Beam expander: an optical device to increase beam diameter while decreasing beam divergence.

Beam splitter: an optical device used to divide the light from a laser into two separate beams—the reference beam and the object beam.

Beam: a collection of rays that may be parallel, convergent, or divergent.

Blink reflex: (see aversion response).

Brewster windows: these are the windows of the gas laser tube to achieve zero loss of reflection.

Brightness: the apparent sensation of luminosity of a light source, closely associated with radiance.

C

Calorimeter: an instrument to measure the heat generated due to the absorption of a laser beam.

Carbon dioxide laser: a gas laser in which carbon dioxide molecules are the active medium and emission in the infrared spectrum, with the strongest emission line at 10.6 μm. It can be operated in either continuous wave or pulsed mode.

Cathode: the negative electrode of a gas laser used for electrical excitation of the gas.

Chromophore: endogenous light absorbing chemicals, which absorb light of specific wavelength.

Closed installation: a location housing the laser apparatus and closed to persons without adequate protection against the laser beam.

Coaxial gas: an inert gas shield over the target material.

Coherence: the alignment between light wave wavelength and the position of that wave in its oscillation cycle. When the crests and troughs of several light waves are in alignment.

Collimated light: parallel rays of light.

Collimation: ability of the laser beam to not spread significantly (low divergence) with distance.

Collimator: optical device consisting of two lenses separated by the sum of their focal lengths. It is used to provide desired beam diameter to meet specific beam delivery requirements.

Combiner mirror: the mirror in a laser which combines two or more wavelengths into a coaxial beam.

Continuous mode: the duration of laser exposure is controlled by the user (by foot or hand switch).

Continuous wave: steady-state delivery of laser power: a laser which with a continuous output that is greater than or equal to 0.25 seconds.

Controlled area: a locale where the activities of those within are subject to control and supervision for the purpose of laser radiation hazard protection.

Convergence: the bending of light rays toward each other, as by a positive (convex) lens.

Corrected lens: a compound lens that is made measurably free of aberrations through the careful selection of its dimensions and materials.

Crystal: a solid with a regular array of atoms. Sapphire (ruby laser) and yttrium-aluminium-garnet (neodymium doped yttrium-aluminium-garnet laser) are two crystalline materials used as laser sources.

Current regulation: laser system regulation in which discharge current is kept constant.

Current saturation: the maximum flow of electrical current in a conductor; in a laser, the point at which further electrical input will not increase laser output.

D

Depth of field: the working range of the beam in or near the focal plane of a lens; a function of wavelength, diameter of the unfocused beam, and focal length of the lens.

Depth of focus: the distance over which the focused laser spot has a constant diameter and thus, constant irradiance.

Diachronic filter: filter that allows selective transmission of colors desired wavelengths.

Diffraction: a wave property which creates deviation from a straight line when the beam passes near an edge of an opaque object.

Diffraction limited: electromagnetic waves diffract around the edges of opaque objects, or on passing through or reflecting off a finite aperture, like a dish, lens, or mirror.

Diffuse reflection: takes place when different parts of a beam incident on a surface are reflected over a wide range of angles in accordance with Lambert's law. The intensity will fall off as the inverse of the square of the distance away from the surface, and also obey a cosine law of reflection.

Diffuser: an optical device or material that homogenizes the output of light causing a very smooth, scattered, even distribution over the area affected.

Diode laser: a laser that emits coherent light through the injection of electric current into a semiconductor diode.

Diode: an electronic device that conducts a current in only one direction.

Divergence: the angular measurement of laser beam spread with distance. The projected dot of a laser will increase in size the farther it is projected. Laser divergence is measured in milliradians (mrad).

Dosimetry: measurement of the power, energy, irradiance, or radiant exposure of light delivered to tissue.

Drift (angular): any unintended change in direction of the beam before, during, and after warm-up; measured in milliradians (mrad).

Drift: all undesirable variations in output (either amplitude or frequency).

Duty: cycle ratio of total "on" duration to total exposure duration for a repetitively pulsed laser.

E

Electromagnetic radiation (spectrum): a wave which propagates in vacuum with the speed of light, and composed of simultaneous oscillations of electric field and magnetic field perpendicular to each other, and perpendicular to the direction of propagation of the beam. It is created by accelerating electric charge, and includes X-rays, visible spectrum, infrared spectrum, microwave, etc.

Electromagnetic spectrum: the range of frequencies and wavelengths emitted by atomic systems. The total spectrum includes radio waves as well as short cosmic rays. Frequencies cover a range from 1 Hz to perhaps as high as 1,020 Hz.

Electromagnetic wave: a disturbance which propagates outward from an electric charge that oscillates or is accelerated. It includes radio waves, X-rays, γ-rays; and infrared, ultraviolet, and visible light.

Electron volt (eV): a unit of energy; the amount of energy that the electron acquires while accelerating through a potential difference of 1 volt. 1 eV = 1.6×10^{-19} joules.

Electron: negatively charged particle of an atom.

Embedded laser: a laser with an assigned class number higher than the inherent capability of the laser system in which it is incorporated, where the system's lower classification is appropriate to the engineering features limiting accessible emission.

Emergent beam diameter: diameter of the laser beam at the exit aperture of the system in centimeters defined at 1/e or 1/e2 irradiance points.

Emission: act of giving off radiant energy by an atom or molecule.

Emissivity: the ratio of the radiant energy emitted by any source to that emitted by a black body at the same temperature.

Emittance: the rate at which emission occurs.

Enclosed laser device: any laser or laser system located within an enclosure which does not permit hazardous optical radiation emission from the enclosure. The laser inside is termed an "embedded laser".

Energy: the capacity for doing work. Energy is commonly used to express the output from pulsed lasers and it is generally measured in joules. It is the product of power (watts) and duration (seconds); 1 watt-second = 1 joule.

Energy source: high voltage electricity, radio waves, flashes of light, or another laser used to excite the laser medium.

Enhanced pulsing: electronic modulation of a laser beam to produce high peak power at the initial stage of the pulse. This allows rapid vaporization of the material without heating the surrounding area. Such pulses are many times the peak power of the continuous wave mode (also called "superpulse").

Excimer laser: a gas laser which emits in the ultraviolet spectrum. The active medium is an "excited dimer" which does not have a stable ground state.

Excitation: energizing the active medium to a state of population inversion.

Excited state: atom with an electron in a higher energy level than it normally occupies.

Extinction length: the thickness of material necessary to absorb 98% of incident energy.

F

Failsafe interlock: an interlock where the failure of a single mechanical or electrical component of the interlock will cause the system to go into, or remain in a safe mode.

Fan angle: the measure of angular spread of a line generating laser.

Femtoseconds (fs): 10–15 seconds; 1 fs = 0.000,000,000,000,001 seconds.

Fiber optics: a system of flexible quartz or glass fibers that use total internal reflection to pass light through thousands of glancing (total internal) reflections.

Flash lamp: a tube typically filled with krypton or xenon. It produces a high intensity white light in short duration pulses.

Fluence: fluence measures the laser energy absorbed per unit of area treated. It is affected by beam energy/power density, laser pulse duration, wavelength, and absorption of the tissue. Fluence is measured by joules/cm^2 and this equals laser pulse energy (joules) divided by focal spot area (cm^2).

Fluorescence: emission of light of particular wavelength, as a result of absorption of light at shorter wavelength. It is a property of some materials; each material has a specific wavelength of absorption and emission.

Flux: the radiant, or luminous, power of a light beam; the time rate of the flow of radiant energy across a given surface.

Focal length: distance between the center of a lens and the point on the optical axis to which parallel rays of light are converged by the laser.

Focal point: that distance from the focusing lens where the laser beam has the smallest diameter.

Fractional photothermolysis: here, pinpoint laser pulses create thousands of microthermal zones, which are microscopic epidermal and dermal thermal wounds interspersed within untreated tissue. The small wound size and short migratory distance for keratinocytes facilitate rapid epidermal repair resulting in effective skin rejuvenation and quick recovery.

Frequency: the number of times that the wave oscillates per second (the number of periods of oscillations per second). Also, the number of light waves passing a fixed point in a given unit of time, or the number of complete vibrations in that period of time.

G

Gas discharge laser: a laser containing a gaseous lasing medium in a glass tube in which a constant flow of gas replenishes the molecules depleted by the electricity or chemicals used for excitation.

Gas laser: a laser in which the active medium is a gas. The gas can be composed of molecules (like carbon dioxide), atoms (like helium-neon), or ions [like argon (Ar^+)].

Gated pulse: a discontinuous burst of laser light, made by timing (gating) a continuous wave output, usually in fractions of a second.

Gaussian curve: statistical curve showing a peak with normal even distribution on either side.

Ground state: lowest energy level of an atom or molecule.

H

Half-power point: the value on either the leading or trailing edge of a laser pulse at which the power is one-half of its maximum value.

Heat sink: a substance or device used to dissipate or absorb unwanted heat energy.

Helium-neon laser: a gas laser in which helium and neon atoms are the active medium. This laser emits primarily in the visible spectrum, primarily at 633 nm, but also have some lines in the near infrared. Used widely for alignment, recording, printing, and measuring.

Hertz: unit of frequency in the International System of Units, abbreviated as Hz; replaces cps for cycles per second.

I

Infrared radiation: invisible electromagnetic radiation with wavelengths which lie within the range of wavelength from 700 nm to 1 mm. This region is often broken up into infrared-A, infrared-B, and infrared-C.

Infrared spectrum: invisible electromagnetic radiation between 0.7 and 1,000 μm.

Injection laser: (also see diode laser), a type of laser which produces its output from semiconductor materials such as gallium arsenide.

Intensity: the magnitude of radiant energy.

Ion laser: a laser in which the active medium is composed of ions of a noble gas (gas such as argon or krypton). The gas is usually excited by high discharge voltage at the ends of a small bore tube.

Ionizing radiation: radiation commonly associated with X-ray or other high energy electromagnetic radiation which will cause deoxyribonucleic acid damage with no direct, immediate thermal effect, contrasts with nonionizing radiation of lasers.

Irradiance: radiant flux (radiant power) per unit area incident upon a given surface. Units: watts/cm^2. Sometimes, it is referred to as power density.

Irradiation: exposure to radiant energy such as heat, X-rays, or light.

J

Joule: a unit of energy (1 watt-second) used to describe the rate of energy delivery. It is equal to 1 watt-second or 0.239 calorie. It is a basic unit of energy. A 1 watt transmitter radiates 1 joule of energy every second. Joule/cm^2 is a unit of radiant exposure used in measuring the amount of energy incident upon a unit area.

K

KTP (potassium titanyl phosphate): a crystal used to change the wavelength of a neodymium doped yttrium-aluminium-garnet laser from 1,060 nm (infrared) to 532 nm (green).

L

Laser: an acronym for light amplification by stimulated emission of radiation. A laser device is an optical cavity, with mirrors at the ends, filled with material such as crystal, glass, liquid, gas, or dye. A device which produces an intense beam of light with the unique properties of coherence, collimation, and monochromaticity. Lasers can operate in the infrared, visible, and ultraviolet regions of the optical spectrum. Some, called continuous wave lasers, produce a continuous beam of light. Others, called pulsed lasers, emit more light in brief pulses.

Laser accessories: the hardware and options available for lasers, such as secondary gases, Brewster windows, Q-switches, electronic shutters, and optical components used to control laser radiation.

Laser class: in order to regulate laser safety, the Center for Devices and Radiological Health classifies lasers into different categories based on wavelength and output power.

Laser diode module: a complete laser assembly including all circuits, a laser diode, and optics packaged in a protective housing. All that is required for operation is an appropriate external power supply.

Laser medium (active medium): material used to emit the laser light and for which the laser is named.

Laser oscillation: the buildup of the coherent wave between laser cavity end mirrors producing standing waves.

Laser pulse: a discontinuous burst of laser radiation, as opposed to a continuous beam. A true laser pulse achieves higher peak powers than that attainable in a continuous wave output.

Laser rod: a solid-state, rod-shaped lasing medium in which ion excitation is caused by a source of intense light (optical pumping) such as a flashlamp. Various materials are used for the rod, the earliest of which was synthetic ruby crystal.

Laser safety officer: one who has authority to monitor and enforce measures to the control of laser hazards, and effect the knowledgeable evaluation and control of laser hazards.

Laser system: an assembly of electrical, mechanical, and optical components which includes a laser; under the United States Federal Standard, a laser in combination with its power supply (energy source).

Leading edge spike: the initial pulse in a series of pulsed laser emissions, often useful in starting a reaction at the target surface. The trailing edge of the laser power is used to maintain the reaction after the initial burst of energy.

Lens: a curved piece of optically transparent material, which depending on its shape, is used to either converge or diverge light.

Light: usually refers to the visible spectrum; the range of electromagnetic radiation frequencies detected by the eye, or the wavelength range from about 400 to 700 nm. The term is sometimes used loosely to include radiation beyond visible spectrum limits.

Limiting aperture: the maximum circular area over which radiance and radiant exposure can be averaged when determining safety hazards.

Limiting exposure duration: an exposure duration which is specifically limited by the design or intended use(s).

Longitudinal (axial) modes: specific wavelengths in the laser output, determined by standing waves within the laser cavity. Only longitudinal modes under the laser gain curve, above the laser threshold, are found in the laser output. Individual longitudinal modes are produced by standing waves within a laser cavity.

Lossy medium: a medium which absorbs or scatters radiation passing through it.

M

Maximum permissible exposure: the level of laser radiation to which person may be exposed without hazardous effect or adverse biological changes in the eye or skin.

Metastable state: the state of an atom, just below a higher excited state, which an electron occupies momentarily before destabilizing and emitting light; the upper of the two lasing levels.

Micron: an abbreviated expression for micrometer which is the unit of length equal to one millionth of a meter (10^{-6} m).

Microprocessor: a digital chip (computer) that operates, controls, and monitors some lasers.

Milliamperes: a unit of electrical current equal to one thousandth of an ampere.

Milliradian: a unit of angular measure equal to one thousandth of a radian (1 radian = 57.295 degrees); 1 milliradian = 0.057 degrees.

Milliwatt: a unit of power equal to one thousandth of a watt.

Mode locked: a method of controlling the length of the output laser pulse. It produces very short (10–12 seconds) bursts of pulses.

Mode: a term used to describe how the power of a laser beam is geometrically distributed across the cross section of the beam; also used to describe the operating mode of a laser such as continuous or pulsed.

Modulation: the ability to superimpose an external signal on the output beam of the laser as a control.

Monochromatic light: theoretically, light at one specific wavelength; practically, light with very narrow bandwidth. The light out of a laser is the most monochromatic source known. No light is absolutely single frequency since it will have some bandwidth. Lasers provide the narrowest of bandwidths that can be currently achieved.

Multimode: laser emission at several closely spaced frequencies.

N

Nanometer: a unit of length in the International System of Units equal to one billionth of a meter. It is the usual measure of light wavelengths. Visible light ranges from about 400 nm in the purple to about 700 nm in the deep red.

Nanosecond: one billionth of a second; longer than a picosecond or femtosecond, but shorter than a microsecond; associated with Q-switched lasers.

Neodymium glass laser: a solid-state laser of neodymium glass offering high power in short pulses in which a neodymium doped glass rod is used as a laser active medium, to produce 1,064 nm wavelength.

Neodymium doped yttrium-aluminium-garnet laser: a solid-state laser in which neodymium doped yttrium-aluminium-garnet is used as a laser active medium, to produce 1,064 nm wavelength. Yttrium-aluminium-garnet is a synthetic crystal.

Near field imaging: a solid-state laser imaging technique offering control of spot size and hole geometry, adjustable working distance, uniform energy distribution, and a wide range of spot sizes.

Neodymium: the rare earth element that is the active element in neodymium doped yttrium-aluminium-garnet lasers and neodymium glass lasers.

Noise: unwanted minor currents or voltages in an electrical system.

Nominal hazard zone: the nominal hazard zone (NHZ) describes the space within which the level of the direct, reflected, or scattered radiation during normal operation exceeds the applicable maximum permissible exposure (MPE). Exposure levels beyond the boundary of the NHZ are below the appropriate MPE level.

Nominal ocular hazard distance: the axial beam distance from the laser where the exposure or irradiance falls below the applicable exposure limit.

O

Object: the subject matter or figure imaged by, or seen through, an optical system.

Object beam: the light from a laser beam that illuminated the object and is reflected to the holographic film.

Opacity: the condition of being nontransparent.

Open installation: any location where lasers are used which will be open to operating personnel during laser operation and may or may not specifically restrict entry to observers.

Operating voltage: the range of specified input voltage required to operate a laser. Laser operating voltage is measured in volts.

Operation: the performance of the laser or laser system over the full range of its intended functions (normal operation).

Optic disk: the portion of the optic nerve within the eye which is formed by the meeting of all the retinal nerve fibers at the level of the retina.

Optical: that part of the electromagnetic spectrum covering the spectral range from the far infrared to the ultraviolet. It is a superset of the visible and infrared spectral regimes.

Optical cavity (resonator): space between the laser mirrors where lasing action occurs.

Optical density: a logarithmic expression for the attenuation produced by an attenuating medium such as an eye protection filter.

Optical fiber: a filament of quartz or other optical material, capable of transmitting light along its length by multiple internal reflections and emitting it at the end.

Optical pumping: the excitation of the active medium in a laser by the application of light, rather than electrical discharge. Light can be from a conventional source like xenon or krypton lamp, or from another laser.

Optical resonator: the mirrors (or reflectors) making up the laser cavity including the laser rod or tube. The mirrors reflect light back and forth to build up amplification.

Optically pumped lasers: a type of laser that derives energy from another light source such as a xenon or krypton flashlamp or other laser source.

Output coupler: the part of the laser which enable light to come out of the laser. Usually, it is a partially reflecting mirror at the end of the laser optical cavity.

Output power: the energy per second (measured in watts) emitted from the laser in the form of coherent light.

P

Phase: the position of a wave in space, measured at a particular point in time. Waves are in phase with each other when all the troughs and peaks coincide and are "locked" together. The result is a reinforced wave in increased amplitude (brightness).

Photocoagulation: use of the laser beam to heat tissue below vaporization temperatures with the principal objective being to stop bleeding and coagulate tissue.

Photometer: an instrument which measures luminous intensity.

Photon: in quantum theory, the elemental unit of light, having both wave and particle behavior. It has motion, but no mass or charge.

Photosensitizers: chemical substances or medications which increase the sensitivity of the skin or eye to irradiation by optical radiation, usually to ultraviolet.

Photoacoustic effect: the ability of Q-switched laser light to generate a rapidly moving wave within living tissue that destroys melanin pigment and tattoo ink particles.

Picosecond: a period of time equal to 10–12 seconds.

Pigment epithelium: a layer of cells at the back of the retina containing pigment granules, i.e., a cloud of charged particles surrounding a laser impact.

Plasma shield: the ability of plasma to stop transmission of laser light.

Pockel's cell: an electro-optical crystal used as a Q-switch.

Point source: ideally, a source with infinitesimal dimensions. Practically, a source of radiation whose dimensions are small compared with the viewing distance.

Pointing errors: beam movement and divergence, due to instability within the laser or other optical distortion.

Polarized light: they are nonstandard on industrial lasers, but some polarizing element must be used if a polarized output is desired.

Population inversion: a state in which a substance has been energized, or excited, so that more atoms or molecules are in a higher excited state than in a lower resting state. This is a necessary prerequisite for laser action.

Power: the rate of energy delivery in a unit of time, expressed in watts (joules per second). Thus, 1 watt = 1 joule/1 s.

Power density: laser output per unit area, such as watts/cm^2.

Power meter: an accessory used to measure laser beam power.

Protective housing: a protective housing is a device designed to prevent access to radiant power or energy.

Pulse duration: the "on" time of a pulsed laser. It may be measured in terms of millisecond, microsecond, or nanosecond as defined by half peak power points on the leading and trailing edges of the pulse.

Pulse frequency: the rate at which pulses are generated. Pulse frequency is expressed in pulses per second (Hz).

Pulse length: time, expressed in fractions of seconds, in which energy is delivered.

Pulse mode: operation of a laser when the beam is intermittently on in fractions of a second.

Pulse modulation: a method akin to digital modulation where the intensity of a carrier is modulated between two states, either maximum or zero. If the pulse width is small and the repetition rate slow, the peak power in the pulse can be vastly above that of the mean power.

Pulse repetition frequency or rate: the number of pulses produced per second by a laser.

Pulse: a discontinuous burst of laser, light or energy, as opposed to a continuous beam. A true pulse achieves higher peak powers than that attainable in a continuous wave output.

Pulsed laser: a laser which delivers energy in the form of a single pulse, or train, of laser pulses.

Pulsing: electrical modulation of a laser power supply to produce discreet pulses of energy at a given pulse length and pulse period (pulse repetition rate).

Pump: to excite the lasing medium; pumping addition of energy (thermal, electrical, or optical) into the atomic population of the laser medium, necessary to produce a state of population inversion.

Q

Q-switch: a device that has the effect of a shutter to control the laser resonator's ability to oscillate. Control allows one to spoil the resonator's "Q-factor", keeping it low to prevent lasing action. When a high level of energy is stored, the laser can emit a very high peak power pulse.

Q-switched laser: a laser which store energy in the active medium, to produce short pulse with high energy. It is done by blocking the resonator ability to oscillate, keeping the "Q-factor" of the optical cavity low.

Quality factor: it is defined as the ratio of the energy stored in the optical resonant cavity to the energy loss per cycle. The higher the quality factor, the lower the losses. In the technique of Q-switching, energy is stored in the amplifying medium by optical pumping while the cavity Q is lowered to prevent the onset of laser emission. When a high cavity Q is restored, the stored energy is suddenly released in the form of a very short pulse of light. Q-switched lasers are often used in applications which demand high laser intensities in nanosecond pulses

R

Radiant energy: energy in the form of electromagnetic waves usually expressed in units of joules (watt-seconds).

Radiant exposure: the total energy per unit area incident upon a given surface. It is used to express exposure to pulsed laser radiation in units of J/cm^2.

Rayleigh scattering: scattering of radiation in the course of its passage through a medium containing particles, the sizes of which are small compared with the wavelength of the radiation.

Repetitively pulsed laser: a laser with multiple pulses of radiant energy occurring in sequence with a pulse repetition frequency more than 1 Hz.

Resonator: the mirrors (or reflectors) making up the laser cavity, including the laser rod or tube. The mirrors reflect light back and forth to build up amplification.

Rotating lens: a beam delivery lens designed to move in a circle and thus, rotate the laser beam around a circle.

Ruby laser: the first laser type; a crystal of sapphire (aluminium oxide) containing trace amounts of chromium oxide as an active medium.

S

Semiconductor laser: (also see diode laser); a type of laser which produces its output from semiconductor materials such as gallium arsenide.

Selective photothermolysis: a concept used to localize thermal injury to a specific target based on its absorption characteristics, the wavelength of light used, the duration of the pulse, and the amount of energy delivered. Extended theory of selective thermolysis distinguishes between an "absorber" chromophore (e.g., melanin in hair shaft) in which heat is generated and a distant target (e.g., stem cells of isthmus), to which heat is transmitted and which is damaged as a result.

Solid state laser: a laser in which the active medium is in solid state (usually not including semiconductor lasers).

Source: the term "source" means either laser or laser-illuminated reflecting surface, i.e., source of light.

Spot size: the mathematical measurement of the radius of the laser beam.

Stability: the ability of a laser system to resist changes in its operating characteristics. Temperature, electrical, dimensional, and power stability are included.

Stimulated emission: coherent emission of radiation, stimulated by a photon absorbed by an atom (or molecule) in its excited state.

Superpulse: electronic pulsing of the laser driving circuit to produce a pulsed output (250–1,000 times per second), with peak powers per pulse higher than the maximum attainable in the continuous wave mode. Average powers of superpulsed lasers are always lower than the maximum in continuous wave. Process often used on carbon dioxide surgical lasers.

T

TEA laser: an acronym for transversely excited atmospheric laser. This carbon dioxide gas laser uses a transverse flow of gas and operates at higher pressures than other gas lasers, generally near atmospheric pressure. The result is a higher energy beam.

Thermal relaxation time: the time to dissipate the heat absorbed during a laser pulse.

Thermal damage time: it is the time required, for the entire target, including the primary chromophore (e.g., melanin) and the surrounding target (e.g., hair follicle), to cool by about 63%. It includes cooling of the primary chromophore as well as the entire target.

Thermomodulation: the ability of low energy light to upregulate certain cellular biologic activities without producing an injury.

Threshold: the input level at which lasing begins during excitation of the laser medium.

Transmission: passage of electromagnetic radiation through a medium.

Transverse electromagnetic mode: used to designate the shape of a cross section of a laser beam.

Transverse mode: the geometry of the power distribution in a cross section of a laser beam.

Tunable dye laser: a laser whose active medium is a liquid dye, pumped by another laser or flashlamps, to produce various colors of light. The color of light may be tuned by adjusting optical tuning elements and/or changing the dye used.

Tunable laser: a laser system that can be "tuned" to emit laser light over a continuous range of wavelengths or frequencies.

U

Ultraviolet radiation: electromagnetic radiation with wavelengths between soft X-rays and visible violet light, often broken down into ultraviolet-A (315–400 nm), ultraviolet-B (280–315 nm) and ultraviolet-C (100–280 nm).

V

Vaporization: conversion of a solid or liquid into a vapor.

Vignetting: the loss of light through an optical element when the entire bundle of light rays does not pass through; an image or picture that shades off gradually into the background.

Visible radiation (light): electromagnetic radiation which can be detected by the human eye. It is commonly used to describe wavelengths which lie in the range between 400 and 700 nm. The peak of the human spectral response is about 555 nm.

W

Wall plug efficiency: the ratio of the transmitter output power, be it microwave or optical, to the (electrical) power consumed by the transmitter.

Watt/cm^2: a unit of irradiance used in measuring the amount of power per area of absorbing surface, or per area of continuous wave laser beam.

Watt: a unit of power (equivalent to one joule per second) used to express laser power.

Wave: a sinusoidal undulation or vibration; a form of movement by which all radiant electromagnetic energy travels.

Wavelength: the length of the light wave, usually measured from crest to crest, which determines its color. Common units of measurement are the micrometer (micron), the nanometer, and the angstrom unit.

White light: light that contains most of the wavelengths in the visible spectrum such as light from the sun or from a spotlight. White light is incoherent, while laser light is coherent.

Window: a piece of glass (or other material) with plane parallel sides which admits light into or through an optical system and excludes dirt and moisture.

X

X-ray laser: a device that uses stimulated emission to produce coherent X-rays.

Y

Yttrium-aluminium-garnet: a widely used solid-state crystal which is composed of yttrium and aluminum oxides which is doped with a small amount of the rare earth neodymium.

Z

Z-cavity: a term referring to the shape of the optical layout of the tubes and resonator inside a laser.

SUGGESTED READINGS

1. Berlien H, Müller G. Applied laser medicine. Berlin: Springer-Verlag Berlin Heidelberg; 2003.
2. Carruth J. The principles of laser surgery. Scott Brown's Otolaryngology. 5th ed. London: Butterworths; 1987.
3. Chii WL. Laser surgery and therapy. Biophotonics. 2000.
4. Clayman L, Kuo P. Lasers in maxillofacial Surgery and Dentistry. New York: Thieme; 1997.
5. Baxter GD. Therapeutic Laser, Theory and Practice. London: Churchill Livingstone; 1994.
6. Muller GJ, Berlien P, Scholz C. Medical laser. Medí LASER Appl. 2006;21:99-108.
7. Neimz MH. Laser tissue interaction. Heidelberg: Springer-Verlag Berlin Heidelberg; 1996.
8. Karu TI. Low-power laser therapy. Biomedical Photonics Handbook. 2003.
9. Vij DR, Mahesh K. Medical Applications of Lasers. Norwell: Kluwer Academic Publishers; 2002.
10. Waynant R. Lasers in Medicine. Boca Raton: CRC Press; 2002.
11. Wolbarsht M. Laser Applications in Medicine and Biology. Plenum Press: New York; 1991.
12. Yadav RK. Definitions in Laser Technology. J Cutan Aesthet Surg. 2009;2(1):45-6.
13. Glossary of laser terminology. Saleh J Jany.

Index

Page numbers followed by *f* refer to figure, *t* refer to table, and *b* refer to box.

I

K

L

M

N

T

U

V

W

X

Z